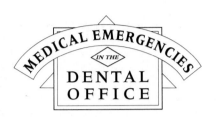

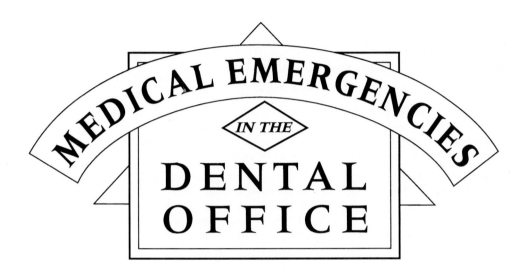

MEDICAL EMERGENCIES
IN THE
DENTAL OFFICE

Stanley F. Malamed, D.D.S.
Professor and Chair
Section of Anesthesia and Medicine
University of Southern California School of Dentistry
Los Angeles, California

Chapter 4, Medicolegal Considerations, by

Kenneth S. Robbins, B.A., J.D.
Attorney in private practice;
Law offices of Kenneth S. Robbins
Honolulu, Hawaii

FOURTH EDITION
with 192 *illustrations*

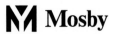 **Mosby**

St. Louis Baltimore Boston Chicago London Philadelphia Sydney Toronto

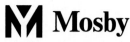
Mosby

Dedicated to Publishing Excellence

Publisher: George Stamathis
Editor: Robert W. Reinhardt
Assistant Editor: Melba Steube
Project Supervisor: Barbara Bowes Merritt
Editing and Production: The Wheetley Company
Designer: David Zielinski

FOURTH EDITION

Printed in the United States of America

Mosby–Year Book, Inc.
11830 Westline Industrial Drive
St. Louis, Missouri 63146

Library of Congress Cataloging in Publication Data

Malamed, Stanley F.
    Medical emergencies in the dental office / Stanley F. Malamed ; chapter 4, Medicolegal considerations, by Kenneth S. Robbins.—4th ed.
        p.   cm.
    Rev. ed. of: Handbook of medical emergencies in the dental office. 3rd ed. 1987.
    Includes bibliographical references and index.
    ISBN 0-8016-6386-5
    1. Medical emergencies—Handbooks, manuals, etc. 2. Dental emergencies—Handbooks, manuals, etc. I. Robbins, Kenneth S. II. Malamed, Stanley F. Handbook of medical emergencies in the dental office.   III. Title.
    [DNLM: 1. Dentistry. 2. Emergencies. WB 105 M236m]
RC86.8.M34   1993
616'.025'0246176—dc20
DNLM/DLC
for Library of Congress   92-49542
                                                              CIP

92 93 94 95 96 GW/MB 9 8 7 6 5 4 3 2 1

To my
mother and **father,**
who made it all possible, and
to my wife **Beverly** and children,
Heather, Jennifer, and **Jeremy,**
who make it all so worthwhile,
I dedicate this book

Foreword

In the past 25 years, dental physicians have truly joined the ranks of health professionals by developing competence in internal medicine, psychosedation, physical evaluation, and emergency medicine. Although technical excellence must never be sacrificed, the role of dentistry is broadening to include adequate pain and anxiety control, significant health screening, and emergency preparedness.

Is there anything more noble than the saving of a life? It is just as noble to avoid mortality or serious morbidity by proper pretreatment physical evaluation and by appropriate modification of dental therapy. It is equally as noble to discover undiagnosed disease and to refer the patient for proper care, thus adding significantly to longevity.

In a time when the credibility and motives of health professionals are under constant scrutiny, dentistry has added immeasurably to its public and professional image by extending its treatment scope in the public interest. This book on medical emergencies will be a valued addition to the library of the dental physician who has extended his or her horizons to include the broad health picture and has made the transition from the oral cavity to the complete patient. It is an excellent contribution to our literature.

Frank M. McCarthy, M.D., D.D.S.

Note

The treatment modalities and the indications and dosages of all drugs in *Medical Emergencies in the Dental Office* have been recommended in the medical literature. Unless specifically indicated, drug dosages are those recommended for adult patients.

The package insert for each drug should be consulted for use and dosages as approved by the FDA. Because standards of usage change, it is advisable to keep abreast of revised recommendations, particularly those concerning new drugs.

Preface

In December of 1975 I began writing the manuscript for *Medical Emergencies in the Dental Office.* The book was completed and published in April of 1978. As was mentioned in the preface to that first edition, my primary aim in writing the book was to stimulate the members of the dental profession—the doctor, dental hygienist, dental assistant, and all other office personnel—to improve and to maintain their skills in the prevention of medical emergencies and in the management of emergencies that inevitably occur. This aim is ever more focused in my mind as this, the fourth edition of *Emergencies,* is written in 1992.

It is acknowledged that with proper patient management most medical emergency situations within the dental office can be prevented. What then is the need for a textbook on the management of medical emergencies? This thought has recurred to me on several occasions over the years. Do life-threatening situations really happen? The answer, unfortunately, is yes, they definitely do. I have received numerous letters and telephone calls and have met with many doctors and other dental personnel who have had real-life experiences with life-threatening medical problems. Virtually all of these situations have occurred within the dental office, but a significant number happened outside: on family outings, driving in a car, or at home.

There is a need for an ever-increasing awareness by the dental profession in the area of emergency medicine. Although many states and provinces currently mandate continued certification in basic life support (cardiopulmonary resuscitation—CPR) for dental relicensure, all too many states and provinces have not yet addressed this important issue. As a person with a long-term commitment in the teaching of basic life support and advanced cardiac life support, I see the immense value in training all adults in the simple procedures collectively known as basic life support. Local and state dental societies, as well as specialty groups should continue to present courses in basic life support or should initiate them posthaste.

Some progress has been made. The awareness of our profession has been elevated and laudable achievements continue. Yet because of the very nature of the problem, what we require in dentistry is a continued maintenance of our high level of skill in the prevention, recognition, and management of medical emergencies. To do so we must all participate in ongoing programs designed by individual doctors to meet the needs of their offices. These programs should include attendance at continuing education seminars in emergency medicine, constant access to up-to-date information on this subject (through journals and texts), semiannual or annual recertification in basic life support or advanced cardiac life support, and in-office practice sessions in emergency procedures for the entire office staff. Such a program is discussed more completely in Chapter 3. The ultimate goal in preparation of a dental office for emergencies should be for you, the reader, to be able to put yourself into the position of a victim of a serious medical emergency in your dental office, and for you to be confident that your office staff would be able to react promptly and effectively in the recognition and management of your problem.

Emergency medicine is a constantly evolving medical specialty, and because of this many changes have occurred since publication of the first three editions of this text. My goal now, as it was then, is to enable you to manage a given emergency situation in an effective yet uncomplicated manner. Alternative treatments and alternative drugs, which are also effective, are advocated by some authors. Our goal, as well as theirs, is simply to preserve the life of the victim.

Continual revision and updating of essential materials is evident in this fourth edition. Significant changes have occurred in the design of the emergency drug and equipment kit in Chapter 3 (Preparation), as well as Airway Obstruction (Chapter 11), Asthma (Chapter 13), Cerebrovascular Accident (Chapter 19), Seizure Disorders (Chapter 21), Drug-Related Emergencies (Chapter 22), Chest Pain (Chapter 26), and Cardiopulmonary Resuscitation (Chapter 30). The American Heart Association met in Dallas, Texas in February, 1992 to review its guidelines for basic and advanced life support. Many of these findings have been incorporated into this text.

The basic format of the text—based upon clinical signs and symptoms rather than on a systems-oriented approach—remains quite well received and is continued in this fourth edition.

As with the previous editions of this text, I have been quite fortunate to have been associated with a number of persons who helped to make the task of revision somewhat more tolerable and, to whatever degree possible, enjoyable. As I have discovered with each previous edition it is impossible to mention everyone involved in the production of this book. However I must mention several persons without whose help and guidance this volume would not have been completed: Jerry Drucker, Dr. Andrew Chen, Dr. Nicholas Gadler, Dr. Mitzi Goldstein, Dr. Susan DeGruccio, Dr. John Rokhsarzadeh, and Adam Kleiger all of whom participated as photographic models and tolerated all sorts of injustices in the name of science and education. I would also like to acknowledge Dr. Susan Sprau and Mr. Jerry Drucker for their assistance in reviewing the section on cardiopulmonary resuscitation and last, but by no means least, Mr. Kenneth Robbins for his well-written material on Medico-

legal Considerations (Chapter 4). The staff of the library at the U.S.C. School of Dentistry deserve acknowledgement for having worked with me locating many of the (obscure) references cited in this book. In this regard I wish to thank especially Mr. John Glueckert. And, as always, I wish to thank my friends at Mosby–YearBook, especially Ms. Melba Steube for her ever ready telephone calls to the AWOL author, and to my editor, Robert W. (Sandy) Reinhardt, for whom it has been a pleasure to work.

Reader input concerning the previous editions of this text and their suggestions of new items for inclusion in future editions have proven to be of inestimable value. I greatly appreciate, and indeed wish to solicit, comment from my readers.

Stanley F. Malamed

Contents

1 *Introduction*

Life-threatening emergencies can and do occur in the practice of dentistry. They may happen to anyone: the dental patient, the doctor, members of the dental office staff, even a person who is simply waiting to accompany a patient home from the dental office. Although life-threatening emergency situations do not occur frequently within the typical dental practice, a number of factors may increase the rate at which these incidents arise. These include (1) the increasing number of older persons seeking dental care, (2) therapeutic advances by the medical profession, (3) the growing trend toward longer dental appointments, and (4) the increasing utilization and administration of drugs in the practice of dentistry. On the other hand, there are factors that the dental profession has at its disposal that will minimize the risk of life-threatening situations occurring. Included are (1) the pretreatment physical evaluation of the dental patient, consisting of the patient-completed medical history questionnaire, physical examination of the patient, and the dialogue history; and (2) possible modification in dental care to decrease medical risk to the patient. It has been estimated by McCarthy[1] that through the effective use of stress-reduction procedures, all but about 10% of life-threatening situations can be prevented (10% of all nonaccidental deaths are classified as sudden, unexpected deaths).

MORBIDITY IN DENTAL PRACTICE

In spite of the most meticulous protocols designed to prevent life-threatening situations from arising, some will still occur. Just consider, for example, articles in local newspapers describing the sudden and unexpected death of a young, well-conditioned athlete (Fig. 1-1).[2,3] Such deaths may occur at any time and in any place. That such situations may occasionally develop within the confines of the dental office is therefore to be expected.

What is the nature of the emergency situations that develop in dental practice? It must be stated at the outset that there is no medical emergency situation that is entirely unique to the practice of dentistry (even local anesthetic overdose is seen outside of dentistry with abuse of cocaine). Any acute medical situation may arise. Table 1-1 presents the findings of a 1985 survey of dentists in the states of Kentucky and Florida. A total of 1605 respondents (out of 6505 dentists—a 24.6% return rate) reported 16,826 emergencies developing within their practices during the preceding 10 years.[4] The overwhelming majority of these situations (11,247) were of a relatively benign nature (syncope), but a very significant number were related to the cardiovascular (2284), central nervous (951), and/or respiratory systems (1007)—all were potentially life-threatening. In a recently completed survey of 2704 dentists throughout North

Schoolgirl Dies During Basketball Drill

DANBURY, Conn., Nov. 20 (AP)— A female high school basketball player who became ill during a practice session collapsed and died as she was being led out of a gymnasium Monday night.

Fig. 1-1. Sudden death of athlete.

Table 1-1. Occurrence of medical emergencies: results from 1605 practicing dentists

Emergency	Number reported	Notes
Syncope	11,247	98% in office
Cardiovascular	2,284	
Angina pectoris	1,908	Most in office
Cardiopulmonary arrest	183	Most out of office
Myocardial infarction	102	Most in office
Heart failure	37	Most in office
Acute asthmatic attacks	1,007	
Epileptic seizures	951	
Epinephrine "reversal" reactions	913	
Insulin shock	181	
Anaphylactic shock	135	
Diabetic coma	109	

Adapted from Fast TB, Martin MD, Ellis TM: *J Am Dent Assoc* 112:499-501, 1986.

Table 1-2. Occurrence of medical emergencies: results from 2704 practicing dentists

Emergency	Number reported	
Fainting		4160
Mild allergic reaction		2583
Postural hypotension		2475
Hyperventilation		1326
Hypoglycemia		709
Grand mal epilepsy		644
Angina pectoris		584
Asthmatic attack		385
Local anesthetic overdose		204
Acute myocardial infarction		187
Anaphylaxis		169
Cardiac arrest		148
Acute heart failure		104
Stroke		68
Acute adrenal insufficiency		25
Thyroid storm		4
Cardiovascular		**1091**
Angina pectoris	584	
Myocardial infarction	187	
Cardiac arrest	148	
Heart failure	104	
Stroke	68	
Allergy		**2752**
Mild	2583	
Anaphylaxis	169	
Total number of emergencies = 13,775		

From Malamed SF: The incidence of medical emergencies in dentistry, submitted for publication, *J Am Dent Assoc*, 1992.

America, Malamed[5] reported 13,775 emergencies within the past 10 years. A description of the nature of the emergencies and their incidence is found in Table 1-2.

On a somewhat smaller scale, Table 1-3 presents a summary of those life-threatening situations that occurred at the clinics of the School of Dentistry of the University of Southern California, from 1973 through mid-1992. Although most of these situations arose during dental treatment with the patient seated in the dental chair, others developed elsewhere in the dental school: patients experienced episodes of orthostatic (postural) hypotension in the restroom, several patients suffered convulsive seizures while in the patient waiting room, and another patient suffered a seizure just outside the entrance to the clinic. Patients were not the only victims of these emergencies: an adult accompanying a patient developed an allergic skin reaction following ingestion of aspirin for a headache,[6] and a dental student seated in a lecture hall suffered episodes of vasodepressor syncope (while viewing pictures of acute maxillofacial injuries), as did a dentist during the treatment of a patient. As is vividly demonstrated by the headline in Figure 1-2, it is not just the dental patient who is at risk during dental treatment!

Although all medical emergencies may develop in the dental office, some will be seen with a greater frequency than others. These are situations produced entirely by stress or those that are exacerbated when the patient is placed in a stressful environment. Stress-induced situations include vasodepressor syncope and hyperventilation,

Table 1-3. Summary of medical emergency situations occurring at the USC School of Dentistry (1973-1992)

Nature of situation	
Convulsive seizures	41
Hyperventilation	36
Vasodepressor syncope	24
Hypoglycemia	21
Angina pectoris	13
Postural hypotension	13
Allergic reactions	12
Acute asthmatic attacks	8
Acute myocardial infarction	1
Site of occurrence	
Patient (during treatment)	108
Patient (before or after treatment)	35
Dental personnel	19
Other persons in dental office	7

Part II/Sunday, February 7, 1988.★

Patient Has Heart Attack, Dies; Dentist Also Stricken

Fig. 1-2. Patient and dentist stricken with heart attacks.

whereas preexisting medical problems that are exacerbated by stress include acute cardiovascular emergencies, bronchospasm (asthma), and convulsions. The effective management of stress in the dental environment therefore becomes an essential element in our effort to minimize the occurrence of these potentially catastrophic situations.

Other life-threatening situations that occur with a greater than expected frequency in dentistry are those reactions associated with the administration of drugs. The most frequently observed adverse reactions are those associated with the administration of local anesthetics, the most used drugs in dentistry. Drug administration may bring with it a variety of adverse responses, most frequently psychogenic reactions, but also drug overdose and drug allergy. The overwhelming majority of these adverse reactions are stress related (psychogenic); however, other reactions (overdose, allergy) are produced in response to the drug itself. Although not all adverse drug responses are preventable, most are. Thorough knowledge of drug pharmacology and of proper drug administration technique are critical in minimizing adverse drug reactions.

DEATH IN DENTAL PRACTICE

Most of the emergency situations that arise in dental practice are life threatening. Fortunately however, it is only on rare occasions that a patient actually dies in the dental office. Although accurate statistics on dental morbidity and mortality are extremely difficult to obtain, surveys of dental practices have been undertaken by various investigators and organizations, including the Southern California Society of Oral Surgeons[7,8] and the American Dental Association.[9] In the 1962 American Dental Association survey, which included almost 4000 dentists, 45 deaths in dental offices were reported. Seven of these deaths occurred in the waiting room before the patients had been treated. In a survey

of dentists in the state of Texas, Bell[10] reported eight deaths occurring in dental offices. Six occurred in the offices of general practitioners and two in oral surgery practices. One death occurred in the waiting room prior to treatment. Only two deaths were associated with the administration of general anesthetics. More recently, Lytle[8] reported eight deaths associated with the administration of general anesthesia in a 20-year period (one death in every 673,000 general anesthetic administrations); Robinson[11] reported eight deaths related to the use of anesthetics; and Adelman[12] reviewed three deaths resulting from aspiration of dental appliances.

In actual fact any life-threatening situation has the potential to become a fatality. Failure to properly recognize and treat clinical signs and symptoms may change a relatively "innocuous" situation into an office tragedy.

Adequate physical evaluation of the patient prior to treatment, combined with the proper use of the many techniques of pain and anxiety control available in dentistry will go far to prevent much of the morbidity and many of the mortalities. Unfortunately however, people will still die in dental offices, just as people will die while asleep in bed or while watching a football game.

It is my firm conviction that the prevention of all life-threatening situations is the goal we must pursue. Chapter 2 is devoted to this goal, as are three excellent textbooks. *Dental management of the medically compromised patient*, ed 3, by Little and Falace (St Louis, 1988, Mosby–Year Book), and *Essentials of safe treatment for the medically compromised patient* by Frank M. McCarthy (Philadelphia, 1989, WB Saunders) are concise texts that are applicable for chairside use, whereas *Internal medicine for dentistry*, ed 2, by Rose and Kaye (St Louis, 1988, Mosby–Year Book) is a much more comprehensive review of medicine in dentistry.

However, as effective as certain steps may be in preventing most life-threatening situations, it is a fact that not all are preventable. Ten percent of all nonaccidental deaths that occur each year in the United States are of a sudden, unexpected nature, occurring in persons supposedly in good health and who are relatively young. The usual cause of death in these cases is cardiac arrest, most frequently ventricular fibrillation. Because preventive measures cannot yet entirely eliminate this occurrence, preparation becomes extremely important. All members of a dental office team must be well versed in the recognition and management of life-threatening situations. The survey by the Southern California Society of Oral and Maxillofacial Surgeons (SCSOMS) reported two dental patients who suffered cardiac arrest and were successfully resuscitated.[7] In both cases the necessary resuscitative equipment was available, and proper resuscitative measures were promptly and effectively carried out by the dental office team.

Not all dentistry related deaths occur within the confines of the dental office. The stress of dental treatment may trigger events that result in the death of the patient within a few days after the appointment. In the SCSOMS survey, 10 such incidents were reported.[7] Of particular interest are three deaths caused by myocardial infarction and one caused by cerebral vascular accident. Another death was reported to have been related to an allergic reaction to propoxyphene hydrochloride prescribed for postoperative pain relief.

McCarthy[1] estimates that one or two treatment-related deaths will occur over the practice lifetime of the typical dental practitioner. He further estimates that the number of office-related deaths would increase to five if dental patients were observed for seven days following treatment.

FACTORS INCREASING THE INCIDENCE OF LIFE-THREATENING EMERGENCIES
Increased Number of Older Patients

The life expectancy of persons born in the United States has increased steadily during this century (Table 1-4). In fact the most rapidly growing segment of the U.S. population is persons above the age of 60 years (Table 1-5). Greater numbers of older persons are therefore seeking dental care. Although many of these persons appear to be in good health, it is important to remember that significant disease of a subclinical nature may be present. Although all major organ systems (cardiovascular, hepatic, renal, pulmonary, and central nervous) are of importance, of primary concern will be the cardiovascular system. In the normal aging

Table 1-4. Years of life expected at birth in the United States

Year	Total	White male	White female	Black male	Black female
1981	74.2	71.1	78.5	64.4	73.0
1980	73.7	70.7	78.1	63.7	72.3
1979	73.8	69.9	77.8	—	—
1978	73.3	69.5	77.2	—	—
1975	72.5	68.7	76.5	—	—
1970	70.8	67.1	74.6	60.0	68.3
1960	69.7	66.6	73.1	—	—
1950	68.2	66.6	71.1	—	—
1940	62.9	60.8	65.2	—	—
1930	59.7	58.1	61.6	—	—
1920	54.1	53.6	54.6	—	—
1910	47.3	46.3	48.2	—	—

Data from Division of Vital Statistics, National Center for Health Statistics, 1985.

process, cardiovascular function decreases in efficiency. In some instances, this decreased efficiency may become clinically evident as heart failure or angina pectoris; however, in many other persons no overt clinical manifestations will appear. Yet when subjected to stress, demands on the cardiovascular system for increased supplies of oxygen and other nutrients may not be met; a condition that can lead to the development of acute cardiovascular complications. Disease of the cardiovascular system represents the leading cause of death in the United States today in persons over 45 years of age (Table 1-6). It is evident, then, that the older patient becomes more stress intolerant. Situations that might have proved innocuous to a person at a younger age may well prove to be harmful 20 years later. This relative inability of older persons to tolerate undue stress was demonstrated in a sur-

Table 1-5. Percent of U.S. population 65 years and over

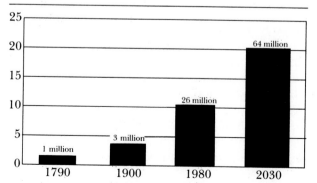

Table 1-6. Causes of death by age (in years)

1–9 years	10–20 years	21–40 years	41–60 years	61–80 years	81–89 years
1. Congenital anomalies	Accident/injury	Accident/injury	Neoplasms	Disorder of circulatory system	Disorder of circulatory system
2. Accident/injury	Neoplasms	Neoplasms	Disorder of circulatory system	Neoplasms	Neoplasms
3. Disorder of nervous system	Disorder of circulatory system	Infections	Accident/injury	Disorder of respiratory system	Disorder of respiratory system
4. Disorder of respiratory system	Disorder of nervous system	Disorder of circulatory system	Disorder of digestive system	Disorder of digestive system	Disorder of digestive system
5. Disorder of circulatory system	Congenital anomalies	Disorder of digestive system	Disorder of respiratory system	Endocrine	Disorder of genitourinary system

Data from Vital Statistics of the United States, 1988. U.S. Department of Health and Human Services, Hyattsville, MD, 1991.

vey on the effects of age in fatally injured automobile drivers. Baker and Spitz[13] found the proportion of drivers aged 60 years or older to be five times as high among those killed as among drivers who survived multivehicle crashes.

Many of the fatally injured drivers aged 60 and over died following crashes that did not prove fatal to younger drivers. The association between age and length of survival suggests that whereas younger drivers recover from injuries, many older ones succumb to complications.

The aging process involves both physiologic and pathologic changes that may alter the patient's ability to respond to stress. Table 1-7 lists the many changes frequently encountered in the geriatric patient. Decrease in tissue elasticity is a major physiologic change that has a significant effect on organs throughout the body. For example, at 75 years of age, cerebral blood flow is but 80% of what it was at the age of 30, cardiac output has declined to 65%, and renal blood flow has decreased to 45% of its earlier volume. This decrease in renal perfusion has a potentially significant bearing on the actions of certain drugs, primarily those in which

Table 1-7. Physiologic and pathologic changes in geriatric patients

Central nervous system
Decreased number of brain cells
Cerebral arteriosclerosis
 CVA
 Decreased memory
 Emotional changes
Parkinsonism

Cardiovascular system
Coronary artery disease
 Angina pectoris
 Myocardial infarction
 Arrythmias
 Decreased contractility
High blood pressure
 Renovascular disease
 Cerebrovascular disease
 Cardiac disease

Respiratory system
Senile emphysema
Arthritic changes in thorax
Pulmonary problems related to pollutants
Interstitial fibrosis

Genitourinary system
Decreased renal blood flow
Decreased number of functioning glomeruli
Decreased tubular reabsorption
Benign prostatic hypertrophy

Endocrine system
Decreased response to stress
Maturity—type one adult-onset diabetes mellitus

Modified from Lichtiger M, Moya F: *Curr Rev Nurse Anesth* 1(1):1, 1978.

urinary excretion is a principal means of removing the drug and its metabolites from the body. Drugs such as penicillin, tetracycline, and digoxin exhibit greatly increased beta half-lives in geriatric patients.

Decreased tissue elasticity also affects the lungs. Pulmonary compliance decreases with age and in fact may progress to senile emphysema. Other pulmonary factors that tend to decrease respiratory function include the chronic exposure of the geriatric patient to smoke, dust, and pollutants, which may produce respiratory disorders such as asthma and chronic bronchitis. Pulmonary function in the geriatric patient is considerably diminished when compared to that in the younger patient (Table 1-8).

A major change in dental care has also occurred within the past two decades. It is commonplace today to see older patients (>60 years) who possess most of their natural dentition, seeking dental care. These patients require a full range of dental care: periodontics, endodontics, crown and bridge and restorative work, and oral surgery, yet due to their age, and the possible presence of other physical disabilities, they are much less able to tolerate the stresses normally involved in planned treatment.

Because of these factors, the older patient is less able to tolerate stress than a younger patient and should therefore be considered a greater medical risk during the dental therapy even in the absence of clinically evident disease (see box). In addition, steps must be taken to minimize this risk as much as possible (see the section entitled, Stress Reduction Protocols[11] in Chapter 2).

Advances Made by the Medical Profession

With increasing age, the incidence of many diseases rises greatly. Diabetic patients and patients with cardiovascular disease (heart failure, arteriosclerosis) faced significantly shorter life expectancies a decade or two ago than they do today. This was also true for many other medical disorders, all of which commonly proved fatal at a relatively early

---

FACTORS INCREASING RISK DURING DENTAL CARE

1. Increased number of older patients
   a. Conservation of teeth by dentistry
2. Advances made by the medical profession
   a. Pharmaceutical
   b. Surgical
3. Longer dental appointments
4. Increased use of drugs
   a. Local anesthetics
   b. Sedatives
   c. Analgesics
   d. Antibiotics

---

age. At best, many of these patients lived lives confined to home or to a wheelchair, unable to work for a living, and unlikely to seek dental care. Today, however, because of unprecedented advances in drug therapy and surgical technique, many of these patients live apparently normal lives. Radiation and chemotherapy enable many cancer victims to live longer; surgical procedures such as the coronary artery bypass and graft operation (CABG) and heart valve replacement have become commonplace and enable previously incapacitated patients to become virtually asymptomatic. Single and multiple organ transplants have higher success rates and are performed with greater frequency. Newer and more effective drug therapies have been introduced for the management of many disorders, such as high blood pressure and diabetes, that were previously untreatable and were associated with a high mortality rate at a young age.

These medical advances are truly significant. Yet they also mean that the dentist will be called on to manage the oral health needs of these patients who are at a greater potential risk. It is necessary to keep in mind that most of these patients have not been cured of their illnesses; these chronic disorders are merely being kept under control or managed, with the underlying disease still present. McCarthy[1] has termed these persons "the walking wounded, accidents looking for a place to happen."

Longer Dental Appointments

In recent years a significant number of doctors have increased the length of their typical dental appointment. Although appointments of less than 60 minutes are still commonplace, many doctors now schedule 1- to 3-hour treatment sessions. Dental therapy is stressful to the patient (and to the doctor and the staff) and longer appointments are naturally more stressful than shorter ones. Medi-

---

Table 1-8. Pulmonary changes in geriatric patients (age 65 and older)

Function	Percentage compared to capacity at age 30
Total lung capacity	100
Vital capacity	58
O_2 uptake during exercise	50
Maximum breathing capacity	55

From data in Lichtiger M, Moya F: *Curr Rev Nurse Anesth* 1(1):1, 1978.

cally compromised patients are more likely to react adversely under these conditions than are healthy individuals, yet even the so-called normal, healthy patient becomes stressed during longer procedures and is more likely to exhibit unwanted reactions. Stress reduction has become an important part of many dental procedures.

Increased Use of Drugs

Drugs are an integral part of the practice of dentistry. Drugs for the prevention of pain, the reduction of anxiety, and the treatment of infection are an important component of every doctor's armamentarium. Yet drug use carries with it an inherent risk. All drugs exert multiple actions, and no drug is absolutely free of risk. Knowledge of the pharmacologic actions of a drug and of the proper administration technique will greatly decrease the occurrence of drug-related emergencies.

Drugs not prescribed by the doctor are yet another source of increased risk. Halpern[14] found that 18% of his patient population was taking medication of one form or another. This incidence rose with age, with 41% of patients over the age of 60 years taking medication regularly. Many patients take multiple drugs in order to manage a variety of disorders. Situations may arise in dentistry that are related either to the pharmacologic actions of these drugs or to complex drug interactions between commonly used dental drugs and other medications. An example of a pharmacologic action is orthostatic hypotension, which is associated with many drugs used to manage high blood pressure. Potentially fatal interactions between the monoamine oxidase (MAO) inhibitors and narcotics (such as meperidine) or between epinephrine and β-adrenergic blockers exemplify drug interactions between dental drugs and other medications.

One of the aims of this textbook is to increase the awareness of the dental team to possible high-risk patients so that appropriate modifications may be incorporated into dental therapy to minimize the risk to these patients. A second aim relates to the prompt recognition and effective management of those situations that occur in spite of our efforts at prevention. Goldberger[15] wrote in the preface to his textbook, *Treatment of cardiac emergencies,* "When you prepare for an emergency, the emergency ceases to exist." Adequate preparation of the staff and the office *before* an emergency arises will greatly increase the probability of a successful outcome. The ultimate aim in the management of any emergency is the preservation of life. This primary goal is the thread that runs through all sections of this textbook.

CLASSIFICATION OF LIFE-THREATENING SITUATIONS

Several methods are available for the classification of medical emergencies. The approach traditionally employed has been the systems-oriented classification. In such a classification, major organ systems are listed, and life-threatening situations associated with those systems are discussed. The following is an example of a systems-oriented classification:

Systems-Oriented Classification

Infectious diseases
Immune system
  Allergies
    Angioneurotic edema
    Contact dermatitis
    Anaphylaxis
Skin and appendages
Eye
Ear, nose, and throat
Respiratory tract
  Asthma
Cardiovascular system
  Arteriosclerotic heart disease
    Angina pectoris
    Myocardial infarction
  Heart failure
Blood
Gastrointestinal tract and liver
Obstetrics and gynecology
Nervous system
  Unconsciousness
    Syncope
    Hyperventilation
    Vasodepressor syncope
    Orthostatic hypotension
  Convulsive disorders
    Epilepsy
Drug overdose reactions
Cerebrovascular accident
Endocrine disorders
  Diabetes mellitus
    Hyperglycemia
    Hypoglycemia
  Thyroid gland
    Hyperthyroidism
    Hypothyroidism
  Adrenal gland
    Acute adrenal insufficiency

Although this may be considered the approach of choice for educational purposes, from a clinical viewpoint it is insufficient.

A second method of classifying emergency situations is to divide them into two broad categories: cardiovascular and noncardiovascular emergencies, which can both be broken down further into stress-related and non–stress-related emergencies. This system offers a very general breakdown of life-threatening emergencies that may be of use in dentistry. Combining the two systems, we have four categories with which to work:

Cardiovascular Versus Non-Cardiovascular Emergencies, Stress-Related Versus Non-Stress Related

Noncardiovascular emergencies
  Stress related
  Non-stress related
Cardiovascular emergencies
  Stress related
  Non-stress related

This system can assist the doctor in preparing a workable treatment protocol for the prevention of such situations. The risk of developing a stress-related emergency may be reduced through the employment of several stress-reducing modifications in dental therapy. Such factors will include psychosedative techniques, effective pain control, and limitations on the length of the dental appointment. A complete description of these factors may be found in Chapter 2. Classification by this system follows:

Noncardiovascular emergencies

Stress related
  Vasodepressor syncope
  Hyperventilation
  Hypoglycemic reactions
  Seizures
  Acute adrenal insufficiency
  Thyroid crisis
  Asthma (bronchospasm)
Non-stress related
  Orthostatic hypotension
  Overdose reaction
  Hyperglycemia
  Allergy

Cardiovascular emergencies

Stress related
  Angina pectoris
  Acute myocardial infarction
  Heart failure
  Cerebral ischemia and infarction
Non-stress related
  Acute myocardial infarction

As effective as this system will be in the prevention of emergencies, we also need a system that will be effective in the clinical recognition and management of these situations. For this to be effective we must abandon classification based on organ systems, because in most real-life clinical situations the underlying pathologic conditions that produce the symptoms are not immediately known to those who must manage them.

The doctor (the term *doctor* will be applied generically throughout this book; it relates to the person who is charged with directing the management of the emergency situation) is forced to recognize and to initiate management of a potentially life-threatening situation with only the most obvious clinical signs and symptoms as a guide. For this reason, a classification of emergency situations based on clinically apparent signs and symptoms appears to be useful and indeed has proven to be so over the years. Initial management of emergency situations will, of necessity, be based on these clinical clues until a more definitive diagnosis can be obtained. Commonly seen signs and symptoms include unconsciousness, respiratory difficulty, altered consciousness, seizures, drug-related emergencies, and chest pain. In all of these situations a definite treatment protocol must be adhered to if a successful outcome is to be achieved. Once these basic management steps have been successfully employed, additional (secondary) steps that lead to a more definitive diagnosis and to management of the situation may be instituted.

This textbook has been designed to be used in this manner. Each major section of this textbook is devoted to one of the commonly seen presenting symptoms. Within each section will be a list of the most common emergencies that initially exhibit that particular symptom. The basic management of that particular problem will be discussed, followed by a detailed review of the most common emergencies falling in that category. At the close of each section a differential diagnosis is presented. The following outline will be adhered to throughout the remainder of this text.

Clinical Signs and Symptoms

Unconsciousness
  Vasodepressor syncope
  Orthostatic hypotension
  Acute adrenal insufficiency
Respiratory difficulty
  Airway obstruction
  Hyperventilation
  Asthma (bronchospasm)

Heart failure and acute pulmonary edema
Altered consciousness
    Hyperglycemia and hypoglycemia
    Hyperthyroidism and hypothyroidism
    Cerebrovascular accident
Seizure disorders
Drug-related emergency situations
    Drug overdose reactions
    Allergy
Chest pain
    Angina pectoris
    Acute myocardial infarction
Cardiac arrest

In designing these classifications, the aim was to place each life-threatening situation in the category that most closely represents the usual clinical manifestation of the problem. Several life-threatening situations might also be included in classifications other than the ones in which they have been placed. For example, acute myocardial infarction and cerebrovascular accident are possible causes of unconsciousness, yet full discussion of these emergencies is found elsewhere in the text because the most commonly encountered clinical manifestations of these emergencies are chest pain for myocardial infarction and altered consciousness for cerebrovascular accident.

OUTLINE OF SPECIFIC EMERGENCY SITUATIONS

In the discussion of each emergency situation, various factors will be presented. Included are the following headings and the aim of each:

1. *Introduction.* An introductory section presents relevant general information. Definitions and synonyms are included when necessary.
2. *Predisposing factors.* Discussions of the incidence and cause of the disorder and of those factors that might predispose a patient to develop an acute life-threatening situation in the dental office are presented.
3. *Prevention.* Employing information obtained from the previous sections, this section is devoted to preventing the acute exacerbation of the disorder. The medical history questionnaire, vital signs, and dialogue history are used to determine a degree of risk for each patient. This discussion closes with suggestions for specific modification in dental management to minimize patient risk.
4. *Clinical manifestations.* Those clinically evident signs and symptoms that lead to recognition of the acute disorder are presented.
5. *Pathophysiology.* A discussion of the pathology underlying clinical signs and symptoms is presented in the hope that a fuller understanding of the cause of a problem will better enable the doctor to manage the situation in a more rational and efficient manner.
6. *Management.* The management of the clinical signs and symptoms of the emergency situation is presented in step-by-step fashion.
7. *Disposition.* New to this fourth edition, this section is designed to provide information to the doctor on the ultimate disposition of the "victim"; recovery in the office and dismissal to home, immediate referral to a primary care physician, or hospitalization.

REFERENCES

1. McCarthy EM: Sudden, unexpected death in the dental office, *J Am Dent Assoc* 83:1091, 1971.
2. Drooz A: Gathers collapses, then dies. *Los Angeles Times*, March 5, 1990, p C-1.
3. Schoolgirl dies during basketball drill. *New York Times*, November 20, 1988.
4. Fast TB, Martin MD, Ellis TM: Emergency preparedness: a survey of dental practitioners, *J Amer Dent Assoc* 112:499-501, 1986.
5. Malamed SF: The incidence of medical emergencies in dentistry, submitted for publication, *J Am Dent Assoc*, 1992.
6. Gill CJ, Michaelides PL: Dental drugs and anaphylactic reactions: report of a case, *Oral Surg* 50:30, 1980.
7. Lytle JJ: Anesthesia morbidity and mortality survey of the Southern California Society of Oral Surgeons, *J Oral Surg* 32:739, 1974.
8. Lytle JJ, Stamper EP: The 1988 anesthesia survey of the Southern California Society of Oral and Maxillofacial Surgeons, *Oral Surg* 47(8):834-842, Aug 1989.
9. Moen BD, Ogawa GY: *The 1962 survey of dental practice*, Chicago, 1963, American Dental Association.
10. Bell WH: Emergencies in and out of the dental office: a pilot study of the State of Texas, *J Am Dent Assoc* 74:778, 1967.
11. Robinson EM: Death in the dental chair, *J Forensic Sci* 34(2):377-380, March 1989.
12. Adelman GC: Asphyxial deaths as a result of aspiration of dental appliances: a report of three deaths, *J Forensic Sci* 23(2):389-395, March 1985.
13. Baker SP, Spitz WU: Age effects and autopsy evidence of disease in fatally injured drivers, *JAMA* 214:1079, 1970.
14. Halpern IL: Patient's medical status: a factor in dental treatment, *Oral surg* 39:216, 1975.
15. Goldberger E: *Treatment of cardiac emergencies*, ed 5, St Louis, 1990, Mosby—Year Book.

2 *Prevention*

Through the use of a complete system of physical evaluation of all prospective patients, approximately 90% of life-threatening situations can be prevented.[1] The remaining 10% (the so-called "sudden unexpected death") will occur in spite of all preventive efforts. "When you prepare for an emergency, the emergency ceases to exist,"[2] is an accurate statement to the degree that preparation for an emergency will diminish the danger or possibility of death and morbidity. Prior knowledge of a patient's physical status will enable the doctor to incorporate modifications into the planned dental treatment. Prior knowledge is important. "To be forewarned is to be forearmed," or, stated another way, "Never treat a stranger."

This chapter* provides a detailed discussion of the most important components of physical evaluation, which, when properly employed, can lead to a significant reduction in the occurrence of acute medical emergencies. Continual reference to this chapter will be made throughout the text as the prevention of specific emergencies is discussed.

GOALS OF PHYSICAL AND PSYCHOLOGIC EVALUATION

In the following discussion a comprehensive but easy to employ program of physical evaluation is described. Its recommended use will enable a doctor to accurately assess the potential risk presented by a patient before the start of treatment.† The following are goals that are sought in the use of this system:

1. To determine the patient's ability to physically tolerate the stress involved in the planned treatment.

2. To determine the patient's ability to psychologically tolerate the stress involved in the planned treatment.
3. To determine whether or not treatment modification will be required to enable the patient to better tolerate the stress involved in the planned treatment.
4. To determine whether or not the use of psychosedation is indicated.
5. To determine which sedation technique is most appropriate for the patient.
6. To determine whether or not contraindications exist to any of the medications employed.

The first two goals involve the patient's ability to tolerate the stress involved in planned dental treatment. Stress may be of either a physiologic or a psychologic nature. Patients with underlying medical problems will usually be less able to tolerate the levels of stress commonly associated with various forms of dental care. These patients will be more likely to undergo an acute exacerbation of their medical problems during these periods of stress. Examples of such disease processes include angina pectoris, epilepsy, asthma, and sickle-cell disease. Although most of these patients will be able to safely tolerate dental care, it is the obligation of the doctor and staff to determine, prior to the start of treatment, (1) whether or not a potential problem exists, and (2) the degree of severity of the problem.

Excessive stress can also be detrimental to the patient who is not medically compromised; fear and anxiety produce acute changes in the normal homeostasis of the body. Many dental patients experience fear-related emergencies, including hyperventilation and vasodepressor syncope (fainting).

The third goal is to determine whether or not the usual treatment regimen for a patient requires modification to better enable the patient to tolerate the stress involved in the planned treatment. In many instances a healthy patient will be unable to

---

*Portions of this chapter have appeared in a slightly different form in *Sedation: a guide to patient management* (Malamed, St. Louis, ed 2, 1989, Mosby-Year Book).
†I am often asked, "What is this risk?" It is the risk that an adverse situation will develop that is related to dental care.

GOALS OF PHYSICAL EVALUATION

1. To determine the patient's ability to physically tolerate the stress involved in the planned treatment.
2. To determine the patient's ability to psychologically tolerate the stress involved in the planned treatment.
3. To determine whether or not treatment modification will enable the patient to better tolerate the stress involved in the planned treatment.
4. To determine whether or not the use of psychosedation is indicated.
5. To determine which sedation technique is most appropriate.
6. To determine whether or not contraindications exist to any of the medications employed.

psychologically tolerate the planned treatment. Treatment may be modified to minimize this stress. The medically compromised patient will also benefit from treatment modifications aimed at minimizing stress. Always remember that medically compromised patients may also be fearful of dental care. The stress reduction protocols will be introduced later in this chapter; they are designed to aid the doctor in minimizing treatment-related stress in both the healthy and the medically compromised patient.

In those instances in which the patient requires some assistance in coping with dental care, the use of psychosedation will be considered. The last three goals involve the determination of the need for use of these techniques (goal #4), selection of the most appropriate technique (goal #5), and selection of the most appropriate medication(s) for the patient (goal #6). The accompanying box summarizes the goals of physical evaluation in the dental environment.

PHYSICAL EVALUATION

The term *physical evaluation* will be employed to discuss the steps involved in fulfilling the aforementioned goals. Physical evaluation in dentistry consists of the following three components: (1) medical history questionnaire; (2) physical examination, and (3) dialogue history.

With the information collected from these three sources, the doctor will be better able to (1) determine the physical and psychologic status of the patient (and thus establish a risk factor classification for the patient); (2) seek medical consultation, if it

appears to be indicated; and (3) institute appropriate modifications in dental treatment, if indicated. Each of the three steps in this information-gathering process will now be discussed.

Medical History Questionnaire

The use of a written, patient-completed medical history questionnaire is a moral and legal necessity in the practice of both medicine and dentistry. In addition, a questionnaire provides the doctor with valuable information about the physical, and in some cases, the psychologic condition of the prospective patient.

Many forms of medical history questionnaires are available. However, most are simply modifications of two basic types: the American Dental Association's (ADA) short form and the ADA long form. The short form medical history questionnaire, usually one page in length, provides basic information concerning a patient's medical history and is ideally suited for the doctor who has obtained considerable clinical experience in physical evaluation. When employing the short form, the doctor must have a firm grasp of the appropriate dialogue history required to aid in determination of the relative risk presented. He or she must also be experienced in the use and interpretation of physical evaluation techniques. Unfortunately, most doctors will employ the short form or a modification of it primarily as a convenience to the patient. The long form medical history questionnaire, usually two or more pages in length, provides a more detailed data base concerning the past physical condition of the prospective patient. It is used most often in teaching situations and represents an ideal instrument for teaching physical evaluation techniques.

With the increasing use of computers in dentistry, several computer-generated history questionnaires are now available. By entering a "yes" response to a question, the computer then proceeds to ask a patient the appropriate questions of dialogue history in order to better determine the degree of risk associated with an indicated problem.

Any form of medical history questionnaire may be used to accurately determine the physical status of a patient. Any form of medical history questionnaire can also prove to be entirely worthless. The ultimate value of the questionnaire will rest on the ability of the doctor to interpret its meaning and to then elicit additional information through the physical examination and dialogue history. The adult and pediatric medical history questionnaires used at the University of Southern California (USC) School of Dentistry (Figs. 2-1 and 2-2, re-

MEDICAL HISTORY

CIRCLE

1. Are you having pain or discomfort at this time? .... YES NO
2. Do you feel very nervous about having dentistry treatment? .... YES NO
3. Have you ever had a bad experience in the dentistry office? .... YES NO
4. Have you been a patient in the hospital during the past two years? .... YES NO
5. Have you been under the care of a medical doctor during the past two years? .... YES NO
6. Have you taken any medicine or drugs during the past two years? .... YES NO
7. Are you allergic to (i.e., itching, rash, swelling of hands, feet or eyes) or made sick by
   penicillin, aspirin, codeine, or any drugs or medications? .... YES NO
8. Have you ever had any excessive bleeding requiring special treatment? .... YES NO
9. Circle any of the following which you have had or have at present:

Heart Failure	Emphysema	AIDS
Heart Disease or Attack	Cough	Hepatitis A (infectious)
Angina Pectoris	Tuberculosis (TB)	Hepatitis B (serum)
High Blood Pressure	Asthma	Liver Disease
Heart Murmur	Hay Fever	Yellow Jaundice
Rheumatic Fever	Sinus Trouble	Blood Transfusion
Congenital Heart Lesions	Allergies or Hives	Drug Addiction
Scarlet Fever	Diabetes	Hemophilia
Artificial Heart Valve	Thyroid Disease	Venereal Disease (Syphilis, Gonorrhea)
Heart Pacemaker	X-ray or Cobalt Treatment	Cold Sores
Heart Surgery	Chemotherapy (Cancer, Leukemia)	Genital Herpes
Artificial Joint	Arthritis	Epilepsy or Seizures
Anemia	Rheumatism	Fainting or Dizzy Spells
Stroke	Cortisone Medicine	Nervousness
Kidney Trouble	Glaucoma	Psychiatric Treatment
Ulcers	Pain in Jaw Joints	Sickle Cell Disease
		Bruise Easily

10. When you walk up stairs or take a walk, do you ever have to stop because of pain in your chest,
    or shortness of breath, or because you are very tired? .... YES NO
11. Do your ankles swell during the day? .... YES NO
12. Do you use more than 2 pillows to sleep? .... YES NO
13. Have you lost or gained more than 10 pounds in the past year? .... YES NO
14. Do you ever wake up from sleep short of breath? .... YES NO
15. Are you on a special diet? .... YES NO
16. Has your medical doctor ever said you have a cancer or tumor? .... YES NO
17. Do you have any disease, condition, or problem not listed? .... YES NO
18. WOMEN: Are you pregnant now? .... YES NO
             Are you practicing birth control? .... YES NO
             Do you anticipate becoming pregnant? .... YES NO

*To the best of my knowledge, all of the preceding answers are true and correct. If I ever have any change
in my health, or if my medicines change, I will inform the doctor of dentistry at the next appointment
without fail.*

_____   _____   _____
Date   *Faculty Signature*   *Signature of Patient, Parent or Guardian*

MEDICAL HISTORY / PHYSICAL EVALUATION UPDATE

Date   *Addition*   *Student/Faculty Signatures*

_____   _____   _____   _____

_____   _____   _____   _____

_____   _____   _____   _____

Fig. 2-1. Medical history questionnaire. Room is provided for periodic updates on USC
medical history questionnaire. (From Malamed SF: *Sedation*, St Louis, 1985, Mosby—Year
Book.)

Child's Name: _____ Date of Birth: _____ Age _____ Date: _____

Address: _____ Telephone: (___) _____

Physician's name (Medical Doctor): _____ Telephone: (___) _____

Please circle the appropriate answer

1. Does your child have a health problem? .... YES NO
2. Was your child a patient in a hospital? .... YES NO
3. Date of last physical exam: _____
4. Is your child now under medical care? .... YES NO
5. Is your child taking medication now? .... YES NO
   If so, for what? _____
6. Has your child ever had a serious illness or operation? ...... YES NO
7. If so, explain: _____
8. Does your child have (or ever had) any of the following diseases?
   a. Rheumatic fever or rheumatic heart disease .... YES NO
   b. Congenital heart disease .... YES NO
   c. Cardiovascular disease (heart trouble, heart attack, coronary insufficiency, coronary occlusion, high blood pressure, arteriosclerosis, stroke) .... YES NO
   d. Allergy? Food □, Medicine □, Other □ .... YES NO
   e. Asthma □ Hay Fever □ .... YES NO
   f. Hives or a skin rash .... YES NO
   g. Fainting spells or seizures .... YES NO
   h. Hepatitis, jaundice or liver disease .... YES NO
   i. Diabetes .... YES NO
   j. Inflammatory rheumatism (painful or swollen joints) .... YES NO
   k. Arthritis .... YES NO
   l. Stomach ulcers .... YES NO
   m. Kidney trouble .... YES NO
   n. Tuberculosis (TB) .... YES NO
   o. Persistent cough or cough up blood .... YES NO
   p. Veneral disease .... YES NO
   q. Epilepsy .... YES NO
   r. Sickle Cell disease .... YES NO
   s. Thyroid disease .... YES NO
   t. AIDS .... YES NO
   u. Emphysema .... YES NO
   v. Psychiatric treatment .... YES NO
   w. Cleft lip / palate .... YES NO
   x. Cerebral palsy .... YES NO
   y. Mental retardation .... YES NO
   z. Hearing disability .... YES NO
   aa. Developmental disability .... YES NO
   If yes, explain: _____
   bb. Was your child premature? .... YES NO
   If yes, how many weeks _____
   cc. Other: _____
9. Does your child have to urinate (pass water) more than six times a day? .... YES NO
10. Is your child thirsty much of the time? .... YES NO
11. Has your child had abnormal bleeding associated with previous surgery, extractions or accidents? .... YES NO

12. Does he/she bruise easily? .... YES NO
13. Has he/she ever required a blood transfusion? .... YES NO
14. Does he/she have any blood disorders such as anemia, etc? .... YES NO
15. Has he/she ever had surgery, x-ray or chemotherapy for a tumor, growth, or other condition? .... YES NO
16. Does your child have a disability that prevents treatment in a dental office? .... YES NO
17. Is he/she taking any of the following?
    a. Antibiotics or sulfa drugs .... YES NO
    b. Anticoagulants (blood thinners) .... YES NO
    c. Medicine for high blood pressure .... YES NO
    d. Cortisone or steroids .... YES NO
    e. Tranquilizers .... YES NO
    f. Aspirin .... YES NO
    g. Dilantin or other anticonvulsant .... YES NO
    h. Insulin, tolbutamide, Orinase, or similar drug .... YES NO
    i. Any other? _____
18. Is he/she allergic to, or has he/she ever reacted adversely to, any of the following?
    a. Local anesthetics .... YES NO
    b. Penicillin or other antibiotics .... YES NO
    c. Sulfa drugs .... YES NO
    d. Barbituates, sedatives, or sleeping pills .... YES NO
    e. Aspirin .... YES NO
    f. Any other? _____
19. Has he/she any serious trouble associated with any previous dental treatment? .... YES NO
    If so, please explain: _____
21. Has your child been in any situation which could expose him/her to x-rays or other ionizing radiators? .... YES NO
22. Last date of dental examination: _____
23. Has he/she ever had orthodontic treatment (worn braces)? .... YES NO
24. Has he/she ever been treated for any gum diseases (gingivitis, periodontitis, trenchmouth, pyorrhea)? .... YES NO
25. Does his/her gums bleed when brushing teeth? .... YES NO
26. Does he/she grind or clench teeth? .... YES NO
27. Has he/she often had toothaches? .... YES NO
28. Has he/she had frequent sores in his/her mouth? .... YES NO
29. Has he/she had any injuries to his/her mouth or jaws? ...... YES NO
    If yes, explain: _____
30. Does he/she have any sores or swellings of his/her mouth or jaws? .... YES NO
31. Have you been satisfied with your child's previous dental care? .... YES NO

ADOLESCENT WOMEN:

32. Are you pregnant now, or think you may be? .... YES NO
33. Do you anticipate becoming pregnant? .... YES NO
34. Are you taking the Pill? .... YES NO

To the best of my knowledge, all of the preceding answers are true and correct. If my child ever has a change in his/her health or his/her medicines change, I will inform the doctor at the next appointment without fail.

Parent's Signature: _____ Date _____

....

MEDICAL HISTORY / PHYSICAL EXAMINATION REVIEW

Date   Addition   Student/Faculty Signatures

_____ _____ _____ _____

_____ _____ _____ _____

_____ _____ _____ _____

Fig. 2-2. USC pediatric medical history questionnaire.

spectively) have combined the best of both short and long forms.[3]

Although both the long and short forms of medical history questionnaires are valuable in the determination of a patient's physical risk during treatment, a criticism of most available health history questionnaires is their lack of questions relating to the patient's attitudes toward dentistry. It is recommended therefore that one or more questions be added that relate to this all-important subject. The following questions are included in the USC School of Dentistry adult health history questionnaire:

Do you feel very nervous about having dentistry treatment?

Have you ever had a bad experience in the dental office?

It has been my experience that many adult patients are reluctant to verbally express their fears about the upcoming treatment to the doctor, hygienist, or assistant for fear of being labeled a "baby." This is especially true of young men, usually in their late teens and early twenties. Rather than admitting their fears, these persons will attempt to "take it like a man" or "grin and bear it." Unfortunately, all too often the outcome of such macho behavior is an episode of syncope. Whereas an open admission of their fears before the episode usually is nonexistent, experience has demonstrated that these same patients will volunteer this information in writing if questions are included in the medical history questionnaire. Other means of identifying anxiety will be discussed later in this chapter.

The USC adult medical history questionnaire will be reviewed, with a discussion of the basic significance of each of the questions.

QUESTION 1. Are you having pain or discomfort at this time?

COMMENT. The primary thrust of this question is related to dentistry. The question is asked to try to determine what it was that actually brought the patient to seek dental care at this time. Should pain or discomfort be present, it may be necessary for the doctor to institute treatment at this first visit, whereas in a more normal situation, treatment would not begin until future visits.

QUESTION 2. Do you feel very nervous about having dentistry treatment?

QUESTION 3. Have you ever had a bad experience in the dentistry office?

COMMENT. The inclusion of questions relating to a patient's attitudes toward dentistry is a significant addition to the medical history questionnaire. Un-

fortunately, most questionnaires ignore questioning along this important line. It has been my experience that many adult patients, who would never verbally admit to being fearful, will indicate their fears or prior negative experiences in these questions.

QUESTION 4. Have you been hospitalized during the past 2 years?

COMMENT. Knowledge of the reason(s) for hospitalizations will better enable the doctor to adequately evaluate the patient's ability to tolerate the stress involved in the planned dental care.

QUESTION 5. Have you been under the care of a medical doctor during the past 2 years?

COMMENT. As with question 4, knowledge of any problem(s) for which the patient required medical intervention can greatly increase the doctor's ability to fully evaluate the patient prior to the start of treatment.

QUESTION 6. Have you taken any medicine or drugs during the past 2 years?

COMMENT. An explanation about the wording of the question is necessary. Because many patients make a distinction between the terms *drugs* and *medications*, it becomes important to use both terms when determining what drugs (implying any pharmaceutically active substance) a patient has taken. Unfortunately, in today's world, the term *drug* has come to connote the illicit use of medications (e.g., narcotics). People "do" drugs; however, medications are used (in the minds of our patients) for the management of their ills—people "take" medicine.

Knowledge of those medications and drugs taken by a patient for the control or treatment of medical disorders is vitally important. Frequently, patients take medications but are unaware of the condition for which they are being taken; in addition, many patients do not even know the names of medications they are taking. For these two reasons it is essential that the doctor have available one or more means of identifying these medications (which patients may or may not carry with them) and of determining their indications, side effects, and potential drug interactions. Many sources are available, including the *Physicians' Desk Reference* (PDR)[4] and Mosby–Year Book's 1990 *Nursing Drug Reference.*[5] The PDR, though primarily a compilation of drug package inserts, is an invaluable reference that is highly recommended for inclusion in every doctor's office. It contains sections that permit the visual identification of a drug should the patient be unaware of its name, and also includes indices that list drugs by therapeutic category, proprietary name, and generic name. Because of the significant number of new drugs added to therapeutic armamentaria almost daily, a current PDR should be readily available.

Knowledge of the drugs and medications being taken by a patient is essential because (1) it permits identification of the medical disorder being treated; (2) there are potential side effects to most medications, some of which may be of significance in dentistry (such as postural hypotension); and (3) drug interactions can develop between a patient's medication and the drugs administered during dental treatment. The box on pp. 16–17 lists interactions of drugs that might occur in dentistry.

QUESTION 7. Are you allergic to (i.e., do you experience itching; rash; swelling of hands, feet, or eyes) or made sick by penicillin, aspirin, codeine, or any other drugs or medications?

COMMENT. Question 7 seeks to determine whether or not the patient has experienced any adverse drug reactions (ADRs). Adverse drug reactions are not uncommon; the most frequently reported reactions are commonly labeled as "allergic." However, in spite of the great frequency with which they are reported, true allergic drug reactions are relatively uncommon. The doctor must thoroughly evaluate all ADRs, especially in those situations in which closely related medications are to be administered to or prescribed for the patient during dental care. Evaluation of alleged allergic and other adverse drug reactions is discussed in considerable detail in Section VI.

QUESTION 8. Have you ever had any excessive bleeding that required special treatment?

COMMENT. Bleeding disorders such as hemophilia can lead to modification of certain forms of dental therapy (for example, surgery, local anesthetic administration) and must therefore be made known to the doctor prior to the start of treatment.

QUESTION 9. Circle any of the following ailments that you have had or have at present.

COMMENT. This question presents a list (which follows) of many of the more common ailments afflicting the adult population in the United States.

Heart Failure

COMMENT. The degree of heart failure must be assessed through the dialogue history. In the presence of more serious congestive heart failure (CHF), such as dyspnea at rest, the patient will require strict modification in therapy and possibly the administration of supplemental oxygen throughout treatment. While most CHF patients will be classified as an ASA II (mild CHF without disabil-

ity) or ASA III (disability developing with exertion or stress), dyspnea observed at rest implies an ASA IV risk.*

Heart Disease or Attack

COMMENT. Heart attack is the lay term for myocardial infarction (MI). Knowledge of its severity, residual damage, and time that has elapsed since its occurrence is essential because therapy modifications may be warranted for this patient. Dental treatment should be postponed for 6 months following the MI. Most status postmyocardial infarction patients represent an ASA III risk; however, when the MI occurred less than 6 months prior, an ASA IV risk is present. When little or no residual damage to the myocardium is present, an ASA II risk exists.

Angina Pectoris

COMMENT. A history of angina (defined as a chest pain brought on by exertion and alleviated by rest) usually indicates the presence of a significant degree of coronary artery atherosclerosis. The risk factor for the typical anginal patient is an ASA III. Stress reduction is strongly recommended in these patients. Patients with unstable angina or angina of recent onset represent ASA IV risks.

High Blood Pressure

COMMENT. Elevated blood pressure measurements are not uncommon in the dental environment primarily because of the added stress associated (in the minds of many dental patients) with dental treatment. Whenever patients report a history of high blood pressure, the doctor must seek to determine the names of those medications being taken to manage the problem, their potential side effects, and drug interactions. Guidelines for clinical evaluation of risk (ASA categories) based on adult blood pressure determinations are discussed on page 41 and summarized in Table 2-1.

Heart Murmur

COMMENT. Heart murmurs are not uncommon; however, not all murmurs are clinically significant. The doctor should determine if a murmur is functional (nonpathologic—ASA II) or if clinical signs and symptoms of either valvular stenosis or regurgitation are present (ASA III or IV) and if antibiotic prophylaxis is warranted. A major clinical symptom of a signifi-

---

*For a detailed discussion of the American Society of Anesthesiologists (ASA) physical evaluation system, refer to page 41.

DENTAL DRUG INTERACTIONS

Dental drug	Interacting agents	Resulting effect
Anesthetics, general	Antidepressants	Hypotension
	Antihypertensives	Hypotension
Antihistamines	Alcohol	CNS* depression
	Phenothiazine (Compazine, Thorazine)	Increased sedation
Anticholinergics (atropine)	Antihistamines	Increased anticholinergic effect
	Levodopa	Increased anticholinergic effect
	Phenothiazine	Increased anticholinergic effect
	Antidepressants, tricyclic (Vivactil, Surmontil, Tofranil)	Increased anticholinergic effect
Barbiturates	Alcohol	Enhanced sedation, increased
	Anticoagulants, oral	Decreased anticoagulant effect
	Antidepressants, tricyclic (Vivactil, Surmontil, Tofranil)	Decreased antidepressant effect
	β-adrenergic blockers (Lopressor, Inderal)	Decreased beta-blocker effect
	Corticosteroids	Decreased steroid effect
	Digitoxin (digitalis)	Decreased digitoxin effect
	Doxycycline	Decreased doxycycline effect
	Griseofulvin (Fulvicin, Grisactin, Grifulvin [II])	Decreased griseofulvin effect
	Phenothiazine	Decreased phenothiazine effect
	Quinidine	Decreased quinidine effect
	Rifampin	Decreased barbiturate effect
	Valproic acid	Increased phenobarbital effect
Benzodiazepines	Alcohol	Enhanced sedation
	Barbiturates	Enhanced sedation and increased respiratory depression
Carbamazepine	Anticoagulants, oral	Decreased anticoagulant effect
	Doxycycline	Decreased doxycycline effect
	Propoxyphene	Increased carbamazepine effect
Cephalosporin antibiotics	Aminoglycoside antibiotics	Increased nephrotoxicity
	Ethacrynic acid	Increased nephrotoxicity
	Furosemide	Increased nephrotoxicity
Clindamycin	Curariform drugs	Neuromuscular blockade
	Lomotil	Increased diarrhea, colitis
Corticosteroids	Barbiturates	Decreased corticosteroid effect
	Ephedrine	Decreased dexamethasone effect
	Phenytoin	Decreased corticosteroid effect
	Rifampin	Decreased corticosteroid effect
Erythromycin	Lincomycin	Decreased antimicrobial effect
Fluoride	Aluminum hydroxide	Decreased fluoride absorption
Lincomycin	Curariform drugs	Neuromuscular blockade
	Kaolin-pectin	Decreased lincomycin effect
	Diphenoxylate-atropine and similar products (Lomotil)	Increased diarrhea, colitis

Modified from Council on Dental Therapeutics; *J Am Dent Assoc* 107:885, 1983.

DENTAL DRUG INTERACTIONS—*cont'd*

Dental drug	Interacting agents	Resulting effect
Meperidine	Barbiturates	Increased CNS depression
	Curariform drugs	Increased respiratory depression
	MAO* inhibitors (Marplan, Nardil, Parnate)	Hypertension
Phenothiazine	Alcohol	Increased sedation (Promethazine)
	Guanethidine	Decreased phenothiazine effect
	Levodopa	Decreased levodopa effect
	Lithium	Decreased phenothiazine effect
Propoxyphene	Alcohol	Increased respiratory depression
	Carbamazepine	Increased carbamazepine effect
	Curariform drugs	Increased respiratory depression
Salicylates (aspirin)	Acetazolamide	Increased salicylate CNS toxicity
	Antacids	Decreased salicylate levels
	Anticoagulants, oral	Increased bleeding risk
	Dipyridamole	Increased effect on platelet function
	Hypoglycemics	Increased hypoglycemia
	Methotrexate	Increased methotrexate toxicity
	Probenecid	Decreased uricosuric effect
Sympathomimetic amines (epinephrine, phenylephrine, nordefrin)	Antidepressants, tricyclic (Vivactil, Surmontil, Tofranil)	Hypertension, hypertensive crisis
	Antihypertensive drugs	Decreased hypertensive effect
	β-adrenergic blockers (Lopressor, Inderal)	Hypertension with epinephrine
	Halogenated anesthetics	Cardiac dysrhythmias
	Digitalis drugs	Tendency for cardiac dysrhythmias
	Indomethacin	Severe hypertension
	MAO inhibitors (Marplan, Nardil, Parnate)	Hypertensive crisis
Tetracycline	Antacids	Decreased tetracycline effect
	Barbiturates	Decreased doxycycline effect
	Bismuth subsalicylate	Decreased tetracycline effect
	Carbamazepine	Decreased doxycycline effect
	Iron, oral	Decreased tetracycline effect
	Methoxyflurane	Increased nephrotoxicity
	Milk and dairy products	Decreased tetracycline effect
	Phenytoin	Decreased doxycycline effect
	Zinc sulfate	Decreased tetracycline effect

*CNS, central nervous system; MAO, monoamine oxidase.

Table 2-1. Recommended standard and alternate prophylactic regimens for dental, oral, or upper respiratory tract procedures[A]

For patients able to take amoxicillin/penicillin[A]

Amoxicillin 3.0 g orally one hour before procedure, then 1.5 g six hours after initial dose.

For patients allergic to amoxicillin/penicillin[B]

Erythromycin ethylsuccinate 800 mg or erythromycin stearate 1.0 g orally 2 hours before procedure, then one-half the dose 6 hours after initial dose.
Or:
Clindamycin 300 mg 1 hour before procedure, then 150 mg 6 hours after initial dose.

For standard risk patients unable to take oral medications

Ampicillin 2.0 g IV or IM 30 minutes before procedure, then 1.0 g ampicillin IV or IM (or 1.5 g amoxicillin orally)* 6 hours after initial dose.
For ampicillin/amoxicillin/penicillin-allergic patients unable to take oral medications:
Clindamycin 300 mg IV 30 minutes before a procedure and 150 mg IV (or orally)* 6 hours after initial dose.

For high-risk patients for whom the practitioner desires to use a parenteral regimen

Ampicillin 2.0 g IV or IM plus gentamicin 1.5 mg/kg IV or IM (not to exceed 80 mg) one-half hour before procedure, followed by 1.5 g oral amoxicillin 6 hours after the initial dose. Alternatively, the parenteral regimen may be repeated 8 hours after the initial dose.
For amoxicillin/ampicillin/penicillin-allergic patients considered to be at high risk:
Vancomycin 1.0 g IV administered over one hour, starting 1 hour before the procedure. No repeat dose is necessary.

From Committee on Rheumatic Fever, Endocarditis, and Kawasaki Disease of the Council on Cardiovascular Disease in the Young of the American Heart Association: Prevention of bacterial endocarditis—recommendations by the American Heart Association, *JAMA* 264:2919, 1990.
NOTE: Initial pediatric doses are listed below. Follow-up doses should be one-half the initial dose. Total pediatric dose should not exceed total adult dose.
Amoxicillin: 50 mg/kg[B]
Erythromycin ethylsuccinate or stearate: 20 mg/kg
Clindamycin: 30 mg/kg
[A]Includes those with prosthetic heart valves and other high risk patients.
[B]The following weight ranges may also be used for the initial pediatric dose of amoxicillin:
<15 kg (33 lbs), 750 mg amoxicillin
15-30 kg (33-66 lbs), 1500 mg amoxicillin
>30 kg (66 lbs), 3,000 mg amoxicillin (full adult dose)
NOTE: Initial pediatric dosages are listed below. Follow-up oral doses should be one-half the initial dose. Total pediatric dose should not exceed total adult dose.
Ampicillin: 50 mg/kg
Clindamycin: 10 mg/kg
Gentamicin: 2.0 mg/kg
Vancomycin: 20 mg/kg
Amoxicillin: No initial dose recommended in this table. 25 mg/kg is the follow-up dose.
*Some patients unable to take oral medications prior to a procedure may be able to take them after the procedure.

Table 2-2. Cardiac conditions[A]

Endocarditis prophylaxis recommended

*Prosthetic cardiac valves, including bioprosthetic and homograft valves

*Previous bacterial endocarditis, even in the absence of heart disease

*Surgically constructed systemic-pulmonary shunts

Most congenital cardiac malformations

Rheumatic and other acquired valvular dysfunction, even after valve surgery

Hypertrophic cardiomyopathy

Mitral valve prolapse with valvular regurgitation

Endocarditis prophylaxis not recommended

Isolated secundum atrial septal defect

Surgical repair without residua beyond six months of:
   Secundum atrial septal defect
   Ventricular septal defect
   Patent ductus arteriosus

Previous coronary artery bypass graft surgery

Mitral valve prolapse without valvular regurgitation[B]

Physiologic, functional, or innocent heart murmurs

Previous Kawasaki disease without valvular dysfunction

Previous rheumatic fever without valvular dysfunction

Cardiac pacemakers and implanted defibrillators

From Council on Dental Therapeutics and American Heart Association: Preventing bacterial endocarditis: a statement for the dental profession, *J Amer Dent Assoc* 122:87, 1991.

[A]This chart lists selected conditions but is not meant to be all-inclusive.

[B]Individuals with mitral valve prolapse associated with thickening and/or redundancy of the valve leaflets may be at increased risk for bacterial endocarditis, particularly men over the age of 45 years.

*These patients are at high risk for developing bacterial endocarditis.

Table 2-3. Dental or oral surgical procedures

Endocarditis prophylaxis recommended

Dental procedures likely to induce gingival or mucosal bleeding, including professional cleaning

Surgical operations involving respiratory mucosa (maxillary sinus)

Incision and drainage of infected tissue

Intraligamentary injections

Endocarditis prophylaxis not recommended

Dental procedures not likely to induce gingival or mucosal bleeding such as simple adjustment of orthodontic appliances or fillings above the gum line

Injection of local intraoral anesthetic (except intraligamentary injections)

Shedding of primary teeth

New denture insertion

From Council on Dental Therapeutics and American Heart Association: Preventing bacterial endocarditis: a statement for the dental profession, *J Amer Dent Assoc* 122:87, 1991.

This chart lists selected procedures but is not meant to be all-inclusive.

would indicate an ASA II, III, or IV risk, depending upon severity and the presence of disability.

Congenital Heart Lesions

COMMENT. An in-depth dialogue history is required to determine the nature of the lesion and, of greater significance, the degree of disability it produces. Patients will represent ASA II, III, or IV risks. Medical consultation may be required to help determine severity, especially for the pediatric patient. Prophylactic antibiotics may be required for most dental treatment.

Scarlet Fever

COMMENT. Produced by group A beta-hemolytic streptococci, scarlet fever rarely produces cardiovascular sequelae such as valvular damage. However, where such damage is present, antibiotic prophylaxis will be required. An adult patient may be considered an ASA I risk with a history of scarlet fever in childhood and with no negative permanent sequelae (all other history factors being negative).

Artificial Heart Valve

COMMENT. Patients with artificial heart valves are no longer uncommon. The primary concern of the doctor is to determine which antibiotic regimen is appropriate during dental treatment. The prophylactic guidelines list these requirements; however, medical consultation with the patients' physicians (e.g., cardiologist) before the start of treatment may be recommended in many of these patients. These patients usually represent an ASA II or III risk.

cant murmur is undue fatigue. Guidelines for antibiotic prophylaxis underwent revision in December 1990 and are presented in Table 2-1.[6,7] Table 2-2 lists those cardiac problems which do or do not necessitate antibiotic prophylaxis, while prophylactic requirements for dental procedures are listed in Table 2-3.

Rheumatic Fever

COMMENT. A history of rheumatic fever should lead the doctor to an in-depth dialogue history to seek the possible presence of rheumatic heart disease (RHD). If RHD is present, antibiotic prophylaxis is indicated to minimize the risk of developing subacute bacterial endocarditis (SBE). Additional therapy modification may be desirable to further minimize risk to the patient, depending on the degree of cardiac involvement. The presence of RHD

Heart Pacemaker

COMMENT. Pacemakers are implanted beneath the skin of the upper chest or the abdomen, with pacing wires extending into the myocardium. The most frequent indication for the use of a pacemaker is the presence of a clinically significant dysrhythmia. Fixed-rate pacemakers provide the heart with a regular, continuous rate of firing regardless of the inherent rhythm of the heart, whereas the much more commonly employed demand pacemakers remain inactive while the rhythm of the heart is normal but take over pacing of the heart when the inherent rhythm of the heart becomes abnormal. Although there is little indication for the administration of antibiotics in these patients, medical consultation is suggested prior to the start of treatment in order to obtain the specific recommendations of the patient's physician. The patient with a pacemaker usually represents an ASA II or III risk during dental treatment.

In recent years patients who represent a significant risk of sudden unexpected death (e.g., cardiac arrest) due to electrical instability of the myocardium (e.g., ventricular fibrillation) have had implantable defibrillators placed below the skin of their abdomen. This question may provoke a "yes" response in these high-risk patients (ASA III or IV).

Heart Surgery

COMMENT. This is a very general term that may include any procedure, from the implantation of a pacemaker to a valve replacement to coronary artery bypass surgery to a heart transplant. A "yes" response must elicit a vigorous dialogue history from the doctor in order to more accurately determine the nature of the surgery and its dental implications. The degree of risk in these patients will vary from ASA II to V.

Artificial Joint

COMMENT. The replacement of hip, knee, and elbow joints with prosthetic devices is becoming more common. However, it is unknown at this time whether bacteremia produced in many dental procedures significantly increases the risk of joint infection. For this reason it is recommended that consultation with the patient's surgeon be obtained before the start of any dental procedure. When antibiotic prophylaxis is required, the regimens described in Table 2-1 are employed.

Anemia

COMMENT. Anemia is relatively common in the adult population, especially among younger women (iron deficiency anemia). It is important to determine the type of anemia present. One major concern with anemic patients is the decreased ability of their blood to carry oxygen or to give up oxygen molecules to cells requiring it. This may be of special significance during procedures in which hypoxia is more likely to develop. Although hypoxia should never occur during dental treatment, the use of deeper levels of intramuscular (IM) or intravenous (IV) sedation without supplemental oxygen administration is more likely to produce hypoxia, which will be of considerably greater significance in these patients. ASA risk factors will vary from ASA II to IV, depending upon the severity of the oxygen deficit.

Sickle cell anemia will be seen in some black patients. A differentiation between sickle cell disease and sickle cell trait must be made.

The presence of congenital or idiopathic methemoglobinemia represents a relative contraindication to the administration of the amide local anesthetics articaine and prilocaine.

Stroke

COMMENT. Stroke or cerebrovascular accident (CVA) must be evaluated carefully, because patients with a history of CVA are also at greater risk of another CVA or a seizure when exposed to hypoxic levels of oxygen. If sedation is considered necessary for proper patient management, only lighter levels, such as those provided by inhalation sedation, are recommended. Transient cerebral ischemia (TCI) is a prodromal syndrome to CVA and must be evaluated carefully. This patient represents an ASA III risk. The status post-CVA patient represents an ASA IV risk within 6 months of the CVA and an ASA III risk more than 6 months after the initial incident (if recovery is uneventful). In rare cases the status post-CVA patient may represent an ASA II risk.

Kidney Trouble

COMMENT. The nature of the renal disorder should be evaluated. Treatment modifications, including antibiotic prophylaxis, may be appropriate for several chronic forms of kidney disease. Functionally anephric patients are categorized as ASA IV risks, whereas patients with most other forms of renal dysfunction represent either ASA II or III risks.

Ulcers

COMMENT. The presence of stomach or intestinal ulcers may indicate acute or chronic anxiety and the possible use of medications such as tranquilizers, H_1-inhibitors, and antacids. Knowledge of which drugs are being taken is important before

---

DENTAL REFERRAL LETTER

Dear Doctor:

The patient who bears this note is on long-term chronic hemodialysis treatment because of chronic kidney disease. In providing dental care to these patients, there are certain precautions to observe:

1. Dental manipulations are most safely done one day after their last dialysis treatment, or at least 8 hours thereafter. Residual heparin may make hemostasis difficult. (Some patients are on long-term anticoagulant therapy.)

2. We are concerned about bacteremic seeding of the arteriovenous shunt devices and heart valves. We recommend prophylactic antibiotics pre- and postdental manipulation. Antibiotic selection and dosage can be tricky in renal failure.

We recommend 3 g of amoxicillin 1 hour before procedure and 1.5 g 6 hours later. For patients with penicillin allergy, 1 g of erythromycin 1 hour before procedure and 500 mg 6 hours later is recommended.

Sincerely,
Courtesy Kaiser Permanente Medical Center, Los Angeles, California. Reprinted by permission.

---

additional drugs are administered in the dental office. The presence of ulcers does not in and of itself represent an increased risk during treatment. In the absence of additional medical problems, this patient may represent an ASA I or ASA II risk.

Emphysema

COMMENT. Emphysema is a form of chronic obstructive pulmonary disease (COPD). The patient with emphysema has a decreased respiratory reserve from which to draw upon in the event that his or her cells require additional oxygen, as may develop during stress. Supplemental oxygen therapy during dental treatment is strongly recommended in more severe cases of emphysema; however, the more severely afflicted emphysematous patient (ASA III to IV) should not receive oxygen in excess of 3 L per minute.[8] This minimizes the risk of eliminating the patients hypoxic drive, which is their stimulus for breathing. The emphysematous patient will be categorized as an ASA II, III, or IV risk dependent upon the degree of disability present.

Cough

COMMENT. The presence of a chronic cough may indicate active tuberculosis or other chronic respiratory disorders such as chronic bronchitis. Cough associated with an upper respiratory infection (URI) provides an ASA II classification, whereas chronic bronchitis observed in a patient who has smoked more than one pack of cigarettes daily for many years may be indicative of chronic lung disease and provides an ASA III classification. The risk versus the benefits of administration of central nervous system (CNS) depressants, especially those with greater respiratory depressant properties such as narcotics and barbiturates, must be carefully evaluated in those patients with signs of diminished respiratory reserve (ASA III and IV).

Tuberculosis

COMMENT. The status of the disease (active, arrested) should be determined before the start of dental care. Medical consultation is recommended if doubt persists, as is the consideration for possible modifications of dental care. Inhalation sedation with nitrous oxide and oxygen is not recommended for patients with active tuberculosis (ASA III or IV) because of the likelihood of contamination of the rubber goods (reservoir bag and conducting tubing) and the difficulty in sterilizing them. If the doctor treats many patients with tuberculosis or other infectious diseases, disposable rubber goods for inhalation sedation units are available. Arrested tuberculosis represents an ASA II risk.

Asthma

COMMENT. Asthma (bronchospasm) represents a partial obstruction of the lower airway. The doctor must seek to determine the nature of the asthma (intrinsic versus extrinsic), the frequency of episodes, any causative factors in its onset, the patient's method of management of the acute episode, and any drugs that the patient may be taking on a regular basis to minimize the risk of an acute episode developing. Stress is a very common cause of acute asthmatic episodes. The well-controlled asthmatic patient represents an ASA II risk, well-controlled but stress-induced asthma is an ASA III risk, whereas patients in whom the acute asthmatic episode is uncontrolled or difficult to terminate (requiring hospitalization) represent ASA III or IV risks.

Hay Fever

COMMENT. Hay fever indicates the presence of allergy to a foreign protein (for example, pollen, cat dander, dust, dirt) and represents an ASA II risk. Dental care should be avoided, if possible, during periods in which acute exacerbations of a patient's allergy are more frequent.

Sinus Trouble

COMMENT. Sinus trouble may indicate the presence of allergy (ASA II), to be pursued in the dialogue history, or of an upper respiratory infection (ASA II), such as a cold. The patient may experience some respiratory distress when placed in a supine position or if a rubber dam is used. Specific treatment modifications, such as postponement of treatment until the patient is better able to breathe comfortably, limiting the degree of recline of the dental chair, or foregoing the use of a rubber dam, may be warranted.

Allergies or Hives

COMMENT. Any allergy must be thoroughly evaluated before the start of dental treatment and possible administration of drugs. The importance of this question and of its full evaluation cannot be overstated. A complete dialogue history must be completed prior to the start of any dental care, especially where a presumed or a documented history of drug allergy is present. Allergy itself represents an ASA II risk. In the context of the emergency situations to be discussed in this text, there is none that is as frightening to health professionals as the acute, systemic allergic reaction—anaphylaxis. Prevention of this life-threatening situation is ever so much more gratifying than treatment once it develops.

Diabetes

COMMENT. A "yes" response requires further inquiry to determine the type, severity, and degree of control of the diabetic condition. The patient with type I diabetes mellitus (insulin-dependent diabetes mellitus or IDDM) or type II (non–insulin-dependent diabetes mellitus or NIDDM) does not usually represent a great risk during dental care or during the administration of drugs for the management of pain or anxiety. The NIDDM patient usually represents an ASA II risk, the well-controlled IDDM patient represents an ASA III risk, whereas the IDDM patient who is poorly controlled is either an ASA III or IV risk. The greatest concerns during dental management of this type of patient relate to the possible effect of dental care on subsequent eating and to the development of hypoglycemia (low blood sugar). Patients leaving a dental office with residual soft tissue anesthesia, especially in the mandible, will defer eating until

sensation returns, a period of possibly many hours. Modification of insulin dosage will be required in situations in which the patient does not maintain normal food intake.

Thyroid Disease

COMMENT. The clinical presence of thyroid dysfunction, either hyper- or hypothyroidism, should lead the doctor to be more cautious in the administration of certain drug groups (epinephrine to hyperthyroid patients and CNS depressants to hypothyroid patients). In most instances, however, by the time the patient is seen in the dental office, he or she will already have seen a physician and probably will have undergone treatment for hyper- or hypothyroidism. The patient will be in a euthyroid state (normal blood levels of thyroid hormone) because of either surgical intervention, irradiation, or drug therapy. The euthyroid state represents an ASA II risk, whereas clinical evidence of hypo- or hyperthyroidism represents an ASA III or (rarely) an ASA IV risk.

X-ray or Cobalt Treatment
Chemotherapy (Cancer, Leukemia)

COMMENT. The presence or prior existence of cancer of the head or neck may require specific modification of dental therapy. Irradiated tissues usually have a decreased resistance to infection and a diminished vascularity with reduced healing capacity. There is no specific contraindication to the administration of any medication for pain or anxiety control in these patients. Many patients with cancer may also be receiving long-term therapy with central nervous system (CNS) depressants such as antianxiety drugs, hypnotics, or narcotics. Consultation with the patient's physician may be in order before dental treatment is begun. A past or current history of cancer does not necessarily increase the ASA risk status. However, patients who are cachectic, hospitalized, and in poor physical condition may be considered to be either ASA IV or V risks.

Arthritis
Rheumatism
Cortisone Medicine

COMMENT. A history of arthritis may be associated with chronic use of salicylates (aspirin) or other nonsteroidal antiinflammatory drugs (NSAIDs), some of which may alter blood clotting (indeed, low-dose aspirin has been demonstrated to be quite effective in minimizing the risk of another myocardial infarction in patients who are recovering from MI[9]). Arthritic patients may also be receiving long-term corticosteroid therapy that will possibly increase the risk of acute adrenal insufficiency, especially when the patient has recently ceased taking the steroid. Such patients may require reinstitution of steroid therapy or modification (increase) in the dosage of corticosteroids during the period of dental care to enable them to respond more appropriately to any additional stress that is associated with the planned dental care. An additional concern for the arthritic patient is the possible difficulty that may be encountered in positioning the patient comfortably for dental treatment. Modification in patient positioning may be necessary to accommodate the patient's physical disability. Most patients receiving corticosteroids will be categorized as ASA II or III risks, depending upon the reason for use of the drugs and the degree of disability present. Patients with arthritis that is significantly disabling will be categorized as ASA III risks.

Glaucoma

COMMENT. For patients with glaucoma, administration of an agent to diminish salivary gland secretions will be of concern. Use of the anticholinergics atropine, scopolamine, and glycopyrrolate are contraindicated in these patients as they produce an increase in intraocular pressure. Glaucoma usually represents an ASA II risk.

Pain in the Jaw Joints

COMMENT. Chronic temporomandibular joint (TMJ) pain is seen with increasing frequency today. Evaluation of the cause(s) should be sought. In and of itself, pain in the jaw does not serve to increase the risk categorization of a patient. Bruxism may be an indication of unusual stress that may be managed via oral antianxiety drugs or other psychotropics. The doctor should determine the names of those drugs employed, their potential side effects, and any drug interactions.

Acquired Immunodeficiency Syndrome (AIDS)

COMMENT. The presence of human immunodeficiency virus (HIV)-positive antibodies in dental patients has become increasingly more common in many areas of the United States and in other countries, both industrialized and rural. Employment of usual barrier techniques should serve to minimize the risk of cross infection to both the patient and the dental staff. The HIV-positive patient may be categorized as an ASA II, III, IV, or V risk depending upon the progress of the infection.

Hepatitis A (infectious)
Hepatitis B (serum)
Liver Disease
Yellow Jaundice
Blood Transfusion
Drug Addiction

COMMENT. The preceding diseases or problems are either transmissible (such as AIDS and hepatitis A and B) or are possible indicators of a degree of hepatic dysfunction. A history of blood transfusion or past or present history of drug addiction should serve to alert the doctor to a probable increase in the risk of hepatic dysfunction and/or AIDS (this is especially important in the parenteral drug abuser). When any of these disorders are uncovered, the doctor must seek to determine the present status of the disease process and of the patient's condition through consultation with the patient's physician. Risk factors for these problems may range from ASA II through V.

Most drugs used in dentistry undergo primary biotransformation in the liver. The presence of significant (ASA III or greater) liver dysfunction will lead to a decreased rate of drug inactivation (increased half-life) and to an increased risk of overdosage and/or prolonged clinical duration of action.

In addition, parenteral drug abusers also have a significantly greater risk of valvular damage in the heart and may therefore require antibiotic prophylaxis. The regimens outlined in Table 2-1 adequately cover these patients.

Hemophilia

COMMENT. Hemophilia and other bleeding disorders must be fully evaluated before the start of any procedure, especially those in which bleeding may occur. It is prudent to avoid (wherever possible) the administration of regional nerve blocks in which the risk of positive aspiration of blood is great. These include the inferior alveolar nerve block and the posterior superior alveolar nerve block. In most instances, alternative techniques of pain control are available. Hemophiliacs may be categorized as ASA II, III, or IV risks.

Venereal Disease (syphilis, gonorrhea)
Cold Sores
Genital Herpes

COMMENT. The possibility of infection of the dentist or other members of the dental staff is increased when treating these patients. When oral lesions are present, dental care should be postponed if at all possible. Standard barrier techniques, protective gloves, eyeglasses, and a mask provide the operator with a degree of protection but not absolute protection. The patients described in this question usually represent ASA II and III risks, but in extreme situations may be either ASA IV or V risks.

Epilepsy or Seizures

COMMENT. Seizures are a commonly observed emergency situations in the dental office. Even otherwise well-controlled epileptics may have seizures in a stressful environment, such as the dental office. The type of seizure, frequency of occurrence, and the drug(s) used to control the seizures must be determined before the start of dental treatment. Treatment modifications, including the use of the stress reduction protocol, are frequently in order during the management of patients with known seizure disorders. Epileptics who are well controlled represent ASA II risks, with less well-controlled patients posing either an ASA III or IV risk.

Fainting or Dizzy Spells

COMMENT. The presence of chronic postural (orthostatic) hypotension or of symptomatic hypotension or anemia may be detected with this question. Transient ischemic attacks (TIA), a form of "prestroke," may also be detected by this question. Additionally, patients with certain types of seizures, such as the "drop attack," may circle "yes" in this question. Further evaluation, including possible consultation with the patient's physician, may be desirable. Transient ischemic attacks represents an ASA III risk, whereas chronic postural hypotension, in most instances, is an ASA II or III risk.

Nervousness
Psychiatric Treatment

COMMENT. The presence of undue nervousness (in general or specifically related to dentistry) and a history of psychiatric care should place the doctor on guard before the start of dental therapy. These patients may be receiving any number of medications for the management of their disorders—drugs that in some instances may interact with other drugs used in dentistry for the control of pain and anxiety (see box on pp. 16–17). Medical consultation should be considered in many of these cases. Patients with extreme levels of dental fear represent an ASA II risk, whereas patients receiving psychiatric care and drugs represent ASA II or III risks.

Sickle Cell Disease

COMMENT. Sickle cell disease is seen exclusively in the black patient. A sickle cell crisis can be precipitated during periods of unusual stress or when the patient does not receive an adequate oxygen supply (becomes hypoxic). When sickle cell disease is present, the use of supplemental oxygenation during treatment is strongly recommended. Patients with sickle cell trait represent an ASA II risk, whereas those with sickle cell disease are ASA II or III risks.

Bruise Easily

COMMENT. A positive response to this statement may indicate the presence of a bleeding disorder, which should be evaluated before the start of dental treatment. Any ASA category may be represented by this question.

> **Question 10. When you walk upstairs or take a walk, do you ever have to stop because of pain in your chest, shortness of breath, or because you are very tired?**
> **Question 11. Do your ankles swell during the day?**
> **Question 12. Do you use more than two pillows to sleep?**
> **Question 13. Have you lost or gained more than 10 pounds in the past year?**
> **Question 14. Do you ever wake up from sleep short of breath?**

Questions 10 through 14 have been included in the history because of the fact that a patient must have prior knowledge of a disease being present in order to answer "yes" to anything in question 9. Unfortunately, many persons do not have an accurate gauge of their current health status. Many persons do not receive annual or at least regular physical examinations simply because they are "in good health." However, many diseases begin insidiously, producing a gradual onset of clinical signs and symptoms over a period of many months to years. Patients who are diagnosed as diabetic are almost universally amazed to hear that they have probably been diabetic for many years prior to their diagnosis. When told of the presenting signs and symptoms, many state that they have had them for years.

Knowing that some patients will answer "no" to the aforementioned questions because they have never been told that they have the problem, a series of questions was designed that list possible signs and symptoms associated with many medical disorders. A positive response to any of these questions requires a detailed dialogue history in order to determine the dental implications, if any.

QUESTION 10. When you walk up stairs or take a walk, do you ever have to stop because of pain in your chest, shortness of breath, or because you are very tired?

COMMENT. Although the patient may have indicated in question 9 that he or she does not have angina, heart failure, or pulmonary emphysema, clinical signs and symptoms of heart or lung disease may be present. Though there are many significant reasons for a positive response to this question, there may also be any number of noncritical reasons, too. Further evaluation of the patient to more accurately determine his or her status prior to the start of dental care is suggested.

QUESTION 11. Do your ankles swell during the day?

COMMENT. Congestive heart failure immediately comes to mind when one thinks of swelling ankles (pitting edema or dependent edema); however, there are several other conditions in which ankle edema may be observed. These include varicose veins, pregnancy, and renal dysfunction. In addition, healthy persons who spend a great deal of time standing on their feet (for example, mail carriers or even dental personnel) may also exhibit edematous ankles.

QUESTION 12. Do you use more than two pillows to sleep?

COMMENT. Persons with more severe CHF exhibit orthopnea, which is the inability to breath comfortably when lying down. These patients usually require additional pillows under their back, in effect propping them up in bed, so that they may breathe more comfortably during sleep. This is referred to as four-pillow orthopnea and will represent an increase in risk during dental care, one that requires modification of treatment. A note placed on the chart stating that the patient should not be positioned at a greater than 45° recline (or the appropriate degree for that patient) will greatly increase his or her comfort during dental care. The use of a rubber dam may be contraindicated in patients who demonstrate difficulty in breathing at rest. Placement of a rubber dam may significantly impair their breathing.

QUESTION 13. Have you lost or gained more than 10 pounds in the past year?

COMMENT. The question refers primarily to an unexpected gain or loss of weight (as opposed to intentional dieting). Such unexpected weight changes may be observed in patients with heart failure or hypothyroidism (increased weight) or with widespread carcinoma, hyperthyroidism, or uncontrolled diabetes mellitus (weight loss), among other disorders.

QUESTION 14. Do you ever wake up from sleep short of breath?

COMMENT. Paroxysmal nocturnal dyspnea (PND), the sudden onset of shortness of breath while sleeping, is usually a clinical manifestation of more severe left ventricular failure or severe pulmonary disease. Patients exhibiting PND will require modifications in dental care, including changes in position. For these persons, ASA values range from III to V. There are other more benign reasons for this symptom to develop, such as the occurrence of nightmares.

QUESTION 15. Are you on a special diet?

COMMENT. This question will elicit dietary alterations resulting from certain medical disorders (diabetes, high blood pressure, heart failure, elevated cholesterol) and also diets that the patient may be on (either through a physician's consultation or a personal dieting plan) in an attempt to lose weight. Severe dieting (as in fasting or fad diets) may upset the biochemical homeostasis of the body and increase the risk of development of medical problems.

QUESTION 16. Has your medical doctor ever said you have a cancer or tumor?

COMMENT. This question refers to the comments made previously concerning x-ray or cobalt treatment, as well as chemotherapy (see the question 9 comment for such treatment on p. 22)

QUESTION 17. Do you have any disease, condition, or problem not listed here?

COMMENT. The patient is permitted to comment on specific matters not previously discussed. Examples of several possibly significant disorders that might be mentioned at this time include (acute intermittent) porphyria, atypical plasma cholinesterase, and malignant hyperthermia.

QUESTION 18. Women: are you pregnant now? Are you practicing birth control? Do you anticipate becoming pregnant?

COMMENT. Pregnancy is a relative contraindication to extensive elective dental care, particularly during the first trimester. Consultation with the patient's physician is usually recommended. Although the use of local anesthetics is indicated during pregnancy, the use of most sedative techniques should undergo scrutiny; their risks versus the benefits to be gained from their use should be weighed carefully. Of the available sedation techniques, inhalation sedation with N_2O-O_2 is the most highly recommended. Use of oral, intramuscular, or intravenous routes are not contraindicated, but should be reserved for those patients for whom other techniques are unavailable.

To the best of my knowledge, all of the preceding answers are true and correct. If I ever have any change in my health, I will inform the doctor of dentistry at the next appointment without fail.

This final statement is important from a medicolegal standpoint because even though instances of purposeful lying on health histories are apparently rare, they do occur. This statement must be accompanied by the date on which the history is completed and by signatures of the patient (or the patient's parent or guardian if the patient is a minor or is not legally competent) and of the doctor who reviews the history. In effect, this becomes a contract obliging the patient (or parent/guardian) to report any changes in the patient's health or medications. Brady and Martinoff[10] demonstrated that a patient's analysis of his or her own personal health is frequently overly optimistic and that pertinent health matters are sometimes not immediately reported. For these reasons the questionnaire must be updated regularly—approximately every 6 months—or following any prolonged lapse in treatment. In most instances the entire medical history questionnaire need not be redone, only the following questions need to be asked:

1. Has there been any change in your general health since your last dental visit?
2. Are you now under the care of a medical doctor? If so, what is the condition being treated?
3. Are you currently taking any drugs or medicine?

If a positive response is elicited to any of these questions, a detailed dialogue history must follow. The following are possible positive responses to these questions:

Response 1: no change

Response 2: minor change (i.e., pregnant 6 months ago, today no longer pregnant; or diagnosed as having asthma or non–insulin-dependent diabetes mellitus)

In either of these situations a written record of having updated the medical history should be entered into the patient's progress notes or on the health history form (if an area for periodic updates is available).

In a situation in which there has been a seemingly significant change in the patient's health status since the prior history was completed, it is recommended that the entire history be redone. This might be necessary in the situation in which a patient has recently been diagnosed with cardiovascular disease that is currently being managed by a multitude of drugs.

In reality most patients do not undergo major changes in their health with any regularity. Therefore, it is likely that one health history questionnaire may be kept for many years. The ability to demonstrate that a patient's medical history was updated regularly becomes all the more important in these circumstances.

Several other items to note concerning the medical history questionnaire are discussed here.

The questionnaire should be completed *in ink.* Any correction or deletion in the history that is subsequently made by the doctor should be done by drawing a single line through the original entry, not obliterating it. The change is then added, with the doctor initialing and dating the change.

It is strongly suggested that all positive responses on the medical history questionnaire be addressed by the doctor during the dialogue history and that a written notation be entered on the chart. As an example, when a patient answers "yes" to "heart attack," the notation on the chart might read "1986" (the year the myocardial infarction occurred).

Physical Examination

The medical history questionnaire, though an extremely important component in the overall assessment of a patient's physical and psychologic status, does have some limitations. For a health history to be a valuable part of our evaluation, the patient must (1) be aware of his or her state of health and of the presence of any medical condition, and (2) be willing to share this information with the dentist.

Most patients will not knowingly deceive the dentist by omitting important information from their medical history questionnaires, although cases in which such deception has been attempted are on record. For example, a patient seeking treatment for an acutely inflamed tooth decided to withhold from the doctor the fact that he had had a myocardial infarction $2\frac{1}{2}$ months earlier because he knew that to inform the doctor of this would mean that he would probably not receive the treatment he desired. Examples such as this, though quite rare, have occurred.[11]

The other factor, a patient's lack of knowledge of his or her physical status, is a much more likely cause of unintentional misinformation on the questionnaire. Most healthy persons do not visit their physicians for regular checkups. In fact, recent information has suggested that annual medical vistis be discontinued in the healthy patient under 40 years of age because the annual physical examination has not proved to be as valuable an aid in preventive medicine as was once thought.[12] Be that as it may, most patients simply do not visit their physicians on a regular basis, doing so instead only when they become ill. It therefore stands to reason that a patient's physical condition may be an unknown. Feeling well, although usually a reliable indicator of good health, does not guarantee good health. Many disease entities may be present for a considerable length of time in a subclinical state without exhibiting any overt signs or symptoms that might warn the patient of their presence. When such signs and symptoms, such as shortness of breath or undue fatigue, are present they are often mistaken for other, more benign problems. Although answering the questions in the medical history to the best of their ability, patients cannot give a positive response to a question unless they are aware that they do, in fact, have the problem.

The first few questions on most history forms establish the length of time since the patient's last physical examination. The value of answers to questions dealing with specific diseases (i.e., question 9) can be gauged from the patient's responses to these initial questions.

Because of these problems, which are inherent in the use of a patient-completed medical history questionnaire, the doctor must seek additional sources of information concerning the physical status of the prospective patient. Physical examination will provide much of the information. Physical examination in dentistry consists of these steps:

1. Monitoring of vital signs
2. Visual inspection of the patient
3. Function tests, as indicated
4. Auscultation of heart and lungs, monitoring (i.e., electrocardiogram), and laboratory tests, as indicated

A minimal physical evaluation of all prospective patients should consist of measurement of the vital signs and a visual inspection of the patient.

The primary value of the physical examination is that it provides the doctor with important information concerning the physical status of the patient immediately before the start of treatment, as contrasted with the questionnaire, which provides historical, anecdotal information. The physical examination should be completed at an initial visit prior to the start of any dental care. The vital signs obtained at this preliminary appointment (termed baseline vital signs) will serve two functions. First, as a means of screening our patient, vital signs help to determine a patient's ability to tolerate the stress involved in the planned treatment. Second, baseline vital signs are used as a standard during the management of emergency situations, to be compared with readings obtained during an incident.

Vital Signs

There are six vital signs:

1. Blood pressure
2. Heart rate (pulse) and rhythm
3. Respiratory rate
4. Temperature
5. Height
6. Weight

Baseline vital signs should be obtained prior to the start of any dental care in all patients in whom they are possible to record. This might be somewhat difficult to do with the screaming three-year-old patient or with the difficult to manage adult disabled patient. But in all other cases vital signs should be included as a regular part of patient evaluation.

Blood pressure and heart rate and rhythm should always be recorded unless it is physically impossible to do so. Respiratory rate should also be evaluated whenever possible, but must usually be done surreptitiously. Temperature recording may be a part of the routine evaluation, but is more commonly recorded in situations in which it is deemed necessary, as when infection is present or the patient appears feverish. Height and weight measurements may be obtained in most instances by asking the patient, but should be measured when the response appears inconsistent with visual appearance. Weighing of a patient is of considerable importance whenever parenteral (i.e., intramuscular) sedation is to be employed.

The technique of recording vital signs, as well as guidelines for the interpretation of the measurements obtained, follow.

Blood pressure

Technique. The following technique is recommended for the accurate determination of blood pressure (from the American Heart Association: *Recommendations for human blood pressure determination by sphygmomanometry,* Dallas, 1967, The American Heart Association). A stethoscope (Fig. 2-3) and sphygmomanometer, or blood pressure cuff (Figs. 2-4 and 2-5) are the required equipment. The most accurate and reliable of these devices is the mercury gravity manometer (Fig. 2-5). The aneroid manometer (Fig. 2-4), probably the most frequently employed, is calibrated to be read in millimeters of mercury (mm Hg, or torr) and is also quite accurate if well maintained. Rough han-

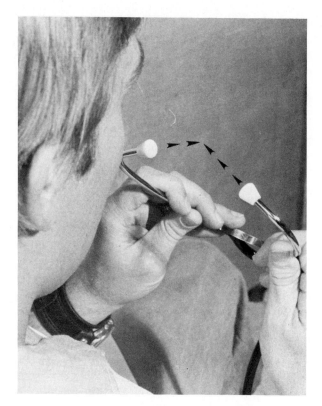

Fig. 2-3. Stethoscope ear pieces are inserted facing in an anterior direction.

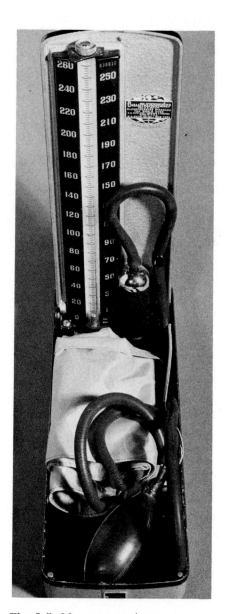

Fig. 2-5. Mercury gravity manometer.

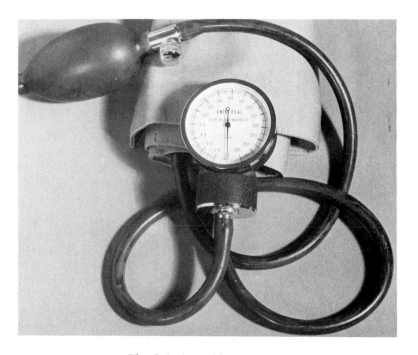

Fig. 2-4. Aneroid manometer.

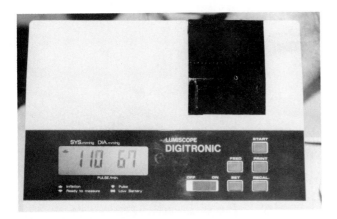

Fig. 2-6. Automatic blood pressure device.

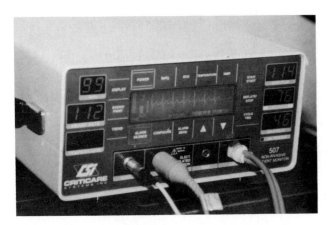

Fig. 2-7. Pulse oximeter.

dling of the aneroid manometer may lead to erroneous readings. The aneroid manometer should be recalibrated at least annually by checking it against a mercury manometer. In recent years many automatic blood pressure monitoring devices have been introduced on the market. The earliest of these devices left much to be desired in accuracy, sensitivity, and reliability; however, many of the more recent automatic blood pressure devices have proven to be quite acceptable. Their costs range from well under $100 (U.S.) (Fig. 2-6) to several thousands of dollars (Fig. 2-7).

For the routine preoperative recording of blood pressure, the patient should be seated in an upright position. The patient's arm should be at the level of the heart—relaxed, slightly flexed, and supported on a firm surface. The patient should be permitted to sit for at least 5 minutes before the blood pressure is recorded. This will permit the patient to relax somewhat so that the blood pressure recorded will be closer to the patient's usual baseline reading. During this time other nonthreatening procedures may be carried out, such as a review of the medical history questionnaire.

The blood pressure cuff should be deflated before it is placed on the arm. The cuff should be wrapped evenly and firmly around the arm, with the center of the inflatable portion over the brachial artery and the rubber tubing placed along the medial aspect of the arm. The lower margin of the cuff should be placed approximately 1 inch (2 to 3 cm) above the antecubital fossa. A cuff is too tight if two fingers cannot be placed under the lower edge of the cuff. Too tight a cuff will decrease venous return from the arm, leading to erroneous measurements. A cuff is too loose (a much more common problem) if it can be pulled off the arm with gentle tugging. A slight resistance should be present when a cuff is properly applied (Fig. 2-8).

The radial pulse must be palpated and then the pressure in the cuff increased rapidly to a point approximately 30 torr above the point at which the radial pulse disappears. The cuff should then be slowly deflated at a rate of 2 to 3 torr per second until the radial pulse reappears. This is termed the palpatory systolic pressure. Pressure in the cuff should then be released.

Determination of blood pressure by the more accurate auscultatory method requires palpation of the brachial artery, which is located on the medial aspect of the antecubital fossa (Fig. 2-9). The earpieces of the stethoscope should be placed facing forward (see Fig. 2-3), firmly in the recorder's ears. The diaphragm of the stethoscope must be placed firmly on the medial aspect of the antecubital fossa, over the brachial artery. To reduce extraneous noise, the stethoscope should not touch the blood pressure cuff or rubber tubing.

The blood pressure cuff should be rapidly inflated to a level 30 torr above the previously determined palpatory systolic pressure. Pressure in the cuff should be gradually released (2 to 3 torr per second) until the first sound is heard through the stethoscope. This is referred to as the systolic blood pressure.

As the cuff deflates further, the sounds undergo changes in quality and intensity (Fig. 2-10). As the cuff pressure approaches the diastolic pressure, sounds become dull and muffled and then cease. The diastolic blood pressure is best indicated at the point of complete cessation of sounds. In some instances, however, complete cessation of sound does not occur. In these instances, the point at which the sounds became muffled will be the diastolic pressure. The cuff should be slowly deflated to a point 10 torr beyond the point of disappearance and then totally deflated.

Should additional recordings be necessary, a wait of at least 15 seconds is required before reinflating

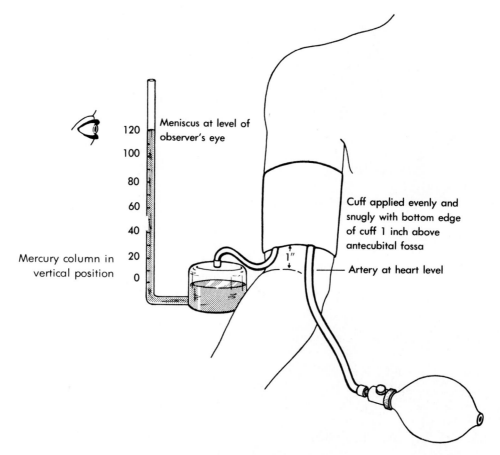

Fig. 2-8. Proper placement of blood pressure cuff (sphygmomanometer). (From Burch GE, DePasquale NP: *Primer of clinical measurement of blood pressure,* St Louis, 1962, Mosby—Year Book.)

the blood pressure cuff. This permits blood trapped in the arm to leave, providing more accurate readings.

Blood pressure is recorded on the patient's chart or sedation/anesthesia record as a fraction: 130/90 R (right) or L (left), depending on the arm used to obtain the blood pressure reading.

Common errors in technique. There are some relatively common errors associated with recording blood pressure. Lack of awareness of these errors may lead to unnecessary medical consultation, adding financial burden to the patient and a loss of faith in the doctor.

1. Applying the blood pressure cuff too loosely will give false elevated readings. This probably represents the most common error in recording blood pressure.
2. Use of the wrong cuff size can result in erroneous readings. A normal adult blood pressure cuff placed on an obese patient's arm will produce falsely elevated readings. This same cuff applied to the very thin arm of a child or adult will produce false-low readings. Sphygmomanometers are available in a variety of sizes. The width of the compression cuff should be approximately 20% greater than the diameter of the extremity on which the blood pressure is being recorded (Fig. 2-11). In many offices a pediatric cuff and perhaps a thigh cuff should be present along with the adult-sized cuff.
3. An auscultatory gap may be present (Fig. 2-12). This gap represents a loss of sound between systolic and diastolic pressures, with the sound reappearing at a lower level. For example, systolic sounds are noticed at 230 torr; however, the sound then disappears at 198 torr, reappearing at approximately 160 torr. All sound is lost at 90 torr. In this situation, if the person taking the blood pressure has not palpated (estimated) the systolic blood pressure before auscultation, the cuff might

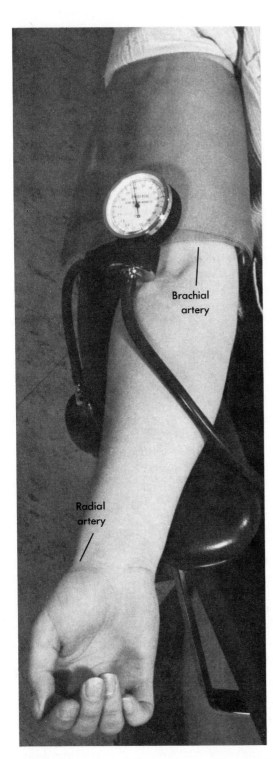

Fig. 2-9. Location of brachial artery and radial artery. Brachial artery is located on the medial half of the antecubital fossa; radial artery is located on the lateral volar aspect of the wrist.

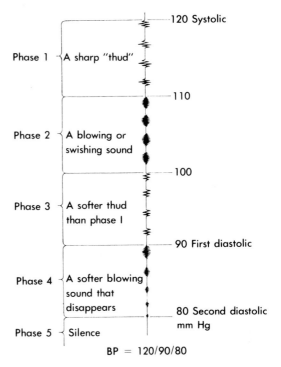

Fig. 2-10. Korotkoff sounds. Systolic blood pressure is recorded at the first phase, and diastolic blood pressure is recorded at the point of disappearance of sound (fifth phase). (From Burch GE, DePasquale NP: *Primer of clinical measurement of blood pressure,* St Louis, 1962, Mosby–Year Book.)

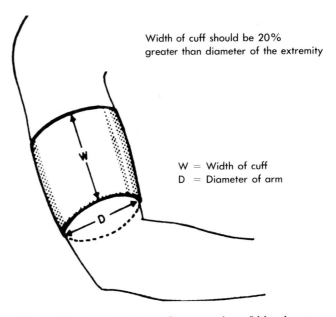

Fig. 2-11. Determination of proper size of blood pressure cuff. (From Burch GE, DePasquale NP: *Primer of clinical measurement of blood pressure,* St Louis, 1962, Mosby–Year Book.)

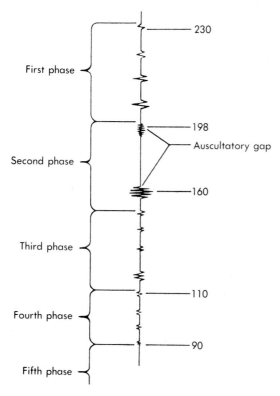

First phase

Second phase

— 230

— 198

— Auscultatory gap

Third phase

— 160

Fourth phase

— 110

Fifth phase

— 90

Blood pressure 230/110/90

Fig. 2-12. Korotkoff sounds, illustrating auscultatory gap. Sound is heard at 230 torr, disappears at 198 torr, and reappears at 160 torr. Sound disappears (fifth phase) at 90 torr. (From Burch GE, DePasquale NP: *Primer of clinical measurement of blood pressure,* St Louis, 1962, Mosby–Year Book.)

be inflated to some arbitrary pressure, such as 165 torr. At this level no sound would be heard because this lies within the auscultatory gap. Sounds would first be noticed at 160 torr, with disappearance at 90 torr, levels well within treatment limits for adults (see guidelines, Table 2-4). In reality, however, this patient has a blood pressure of 230/90, a significantly elevated pressure that represents a greater risk to the patient during dental care. Although the auscultatory gap occurs only infrequently, the possibility of error may be eliminated by first using the palpatory technique. A pulse will be palpable in the gap although the sound will disappear. Although there is no pathologic significance to its presence, the auscultatory gap is found most often in patients with high blood pressure.

4. The patient may be anxious. Sitting in the dental chair and having one's blood pressure monitored may produce anxiety, causing transient elevations in blood pressure, primarily the systolic pressure. This is even more likely to be noted in the patient who is to receive sedation to manage dental fears. For this reason it is recommended that baseline measurements of vital signs be taken at a visit prior to the start of any dental care, perhaps at the first office visit, when the patient will only be completing various forms. Measurements are more likely to be closer to the norm for the particular patient at this time.

5. Blood pressure is based on the Korotkoff sounds (see Fig. 2-10) produced by the passage of blood through obstructed, partially obstructed, or unobstructed arteries. Watching a mercury column or needle on an aneroid manometer for pulsations will lead to the recording of falsely elevated systolic pressures. These pulsations are observed approximately 10 to 15 torr before the first Korotkoff sounds are heard.

6. Use of the left or right arm will produce differences in recorded blood pressure. A difference of 5 to 10 torr exists between arms, with the left arm producing slightly higher measurements.

Guidelines for clinical evaluation. The University of Southern California (USC) physical evaluation system is based on the American Society of Anesthesiologists (ASA) Physical Status Classification System (see p. 41). It provides five risk categories based on a patient's medical history and physical evaluation. These categories for blood pressure recordings are presented in Table 2-4.

For the adult patient with a blood pressure in the ASA I range (<140/<90 torr) it is suggested that the blood pressure be recorded every 6 months, unless specific dental procedures demand more frequent monitoring. The administration of local anesthesia and the use of any parenteral or inhalation route of drug administration demand a more frequent recording of vital signs.

Patients falling into ASA, II, III, or IV categories for blood pressure should be monitored more frequently (as outlined in the guidelines). Patients with known high blood pressure should also have their blood pressure monitored at each visit to determine if it is adequately controlled. The routine monitoring of blood pressure in all patients according to the treatment guideline recommendations will minimize the occurrence of acute complications of high blood pressure (e.g., cerebrovascular accident, myocardial infarction).

When parenteral or inhalation sedation techniques or general anesthesia are employed, there is a greater need for recording baseline and preoperative vital signs. One of the factors employed to determine a patient's recovery from the effects

Table 2-4. Guidelines for blood pressure (adult)

Blood pressure (mm Hg, or torr)	ASA classification	Dental therapy considerations
<140 and <90	I	1. Routine dental management 2. Recheck in 6 months
140 to 159 and/or 90 to 94	II	1. Recheck blood pressure prior to dental treatment for three consecutive appointments; if all exceed these guidelines, medical consultation is indicated 2. Routine dental management 3. Stress reduction protocol as indicated
160 to 199 and/or 95 to 114	III	1. Recheck blood pressure in 5 minutes 2. If still elevated, medical consultation before dental therapy 3. Routine dental therapy 4. Stress reduction protocol
>200 and/or >115	IV	1. Recheck blood pressure in 5 minutes 2. Immediate medical consultation if still elevated 3. No dental therapy, routine or emergency,* until elevated blood pressure is corrected 4. Emergency dental therapy with drugs (analgesics, antibiotics) 5. Refer to hospital if immediate dental therapy indicated

*When the blood pressure of the patient is slightly above the cutoff for category IV, and when anxiety is present, the use of inhalation sedation may be employed in an effort to diminish the blood pressure (via the elimination of stress) below the 200/115 level. The patient should be advised that if the N_2O-O_2 succeeds in decreasing the blood pressure below this level, the planned treatment will proceed. However, should the blood pressure remain elevated, the planned procedure will be postponed until such time as the elevated blood pressure has been lowered to a more acceptable range.

of sedation and his or her readiness to be discharged from the office will be a comparison of the postoperative vital signs and baseline values.

Yet another reason for emphasizing the routine monitoring of blood pressure relates to the management of emergencies. After basic steps of assessment and management in each emergency are completed, certain specific steps are necessary for definitive treatment. Primary among these is the monitoring of vital signs, particularly blood pressure. Blood pressure recorded during an emergency situation is an important indicator of the status of the cardiovascular system. However, unless a baseline or nonemergency blood pressure had been recorded earlier, the measurement obtained during the emergency is of less significance. A recording of 80/50 torr is less ominous in a patient with a preoperative reading of 110/70 than if the preoperative recording were 190/110. In all situations the absence of blood pressure is an indication for cardiopulmonary resuscitation.

Normal blood pressures in younger patients will be somewhat lower than those already presented. Table 2-5 presents a normal range of blood pressure measurements in infants and children.

Heart rate and rhythm

Techniques of measurement. Heart rate or pulse may be measured using any readily accessible artery. Most commonly employed for routine (nonemergency) measurement are the brachial artery located the medial aspect of the antecubital fossa and the radial artery located on the radial and volar aspects of the wrist. Other arteries such as the carotid and femoral may be used; however, these are rarely used in routine situations because of their inaccessibility. In emergency situations it is recommended that the carotid artery be palpated in lieu of others, because the goal in managing life-threatening situations is the maintenance of life, and the carotid artery is the artery that carries oxygenated blood to the brain. Prompt and accurate location of this artery is essential in emergency situations. The technique of locating the carotid artery (in the neck) is reviewed in Chapter 5.

When palpating for a pulse, use the fleshy portions of the first two fingers, pressing gently enough to feel the pulsation but not so firmly that the artery is occluded and no pulsation is felt. The thumb should not be used to monitor any pulse, because the thumb contains a fair-sized artery that pulsates. Situations have arisen in which the measured heart rate has been the rescuer's, not the victim's.

In the infant the precordium is no longer recommended as the site to determine the presence of an effective heartbeat.[13] The brachial artery in the upper arm is recommended (Fig. 2-13).

Guidelines for clinical evaluation. Three factors should be evaluated while the pulse is monitored. These factors are as follows:

1. The heart rate (recorded as beats per minute)
2. The rhythm of the heart (regular or irregular)
3. The quality of the pulse (for example, thready, bounding, or weak)

The heart rate should be evaluated for a minimum of 30 seconds, and ideally for 1 minute. The normal resting heart rate for an adult ranges from 60 to 110 beats per minute. It is frequently lower in a well-conditioned athlete and elevated in the apprehensive individual. However, clinically significant pathology may also produce slow heart

Table 2-5. Normal blood pressure measurements for various ages*

Ages (yr)	Mean systolic ±2 SD	Mean diastolic ±2 SD
Newborn	80 ± 16	46 ± 16
6 mo-1	89 ± 29	60 ± 10†
1	96 ± 30	66 ± 25†
2	99 ± 25	64 ± 25†
3	100 ± 25	67 ± 23†
4	99 ± 20	65 ± 20†
5-6	94 ± 14	55 ± 9
6-7	100 ± 15	56 ± 8
7-8	102 ± 15	56 ± 8
8-9	105 ± 16	57 ± 9
9-10	107 ± 16	57 ± 9
10-11	111 ± 17	58 ± 10
11-12	113 ± 18	59 ± 10
12-13	115 ± 19	59 ± 10
13-14	118 ± 19	60 ± 10

From Nadas AS, Fyler DC: *Pediatric cardiology,* ed 3, Philadelphia, 1972, WB Saunders.
*Adapted from data in the literature; figures have been rounded off to nearest decimal place.
†In this study the point of muffling was taken as the diastolic pressure.

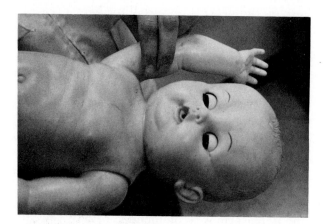

Fig. 2-13. Pulse determination in the infant is best accomplished in the brachial artery located on the medial side of the upper arm.

rates (bradycardia) or rapid heart rates (tachycardia). It is suggested that any adult heart rate under 60 or above 110 beats per minute be evaluated. When no obvious cause is determined (e.g., endurance sports, anxiety), medical consultation should be considered.

The normal pulse maintains a relatively regular rhythm. Occasional premature ventricular contractions (PVCs) are so common that they are not necessarily considered abnormal. These contractions may be produced by smoking, fatigue, stress, various medications (such as epinephrine), and alcohol. If, however, PVCs are present at a rate of five or more per minute in a patient with other risk factors of coronary artery disease, medical consultation should be considered. Clinically, PVCs are detected as breaks in a generally regular heart rate in which a longer than normal pause (skipped beat) is noted, followed by resumption of normal rhythm. Unusually frequent PVCs (more than five per minute in the presence of other cardiovascular disease risk factors) indicate myocardial irritability and may presage severe dysrhythmias such as ventricular fibrillation (Fig. 2-14).

A second important disturbance in pulse is termed pulsus alternans. It is not truly a dysrhythmia but is a regular heart rate characterized by a pulse in which strong and weak beats alternate. It is produced by the alternating contractile force of a diseased left ventricle. Pulsus alternans is observed frequently in left ventricular failure, severe arterial high blood pressure, and coronary artery disease. Medical consultation is indicated.

It is quite difficult, if not impossible, to accurately diagnose a cardiac dysrhythmia via palpation of an artery alone. However, consultation with a physician with possible testing such as electrocardiography will help to determine the nature of the dysrhythmia and its significance, if any, to the planned treatment of the patient.

The quality of the pulse is commonly described as bounding, thready, or weak. These adjectives relate to the feel of the pulse and are used to describe situations such as a full bounding pulse (as noted in severe arterial high blood pressure) or a weak thready pulse often noted in patients with hypotension and signs of shock. As may be noted in Table 2-6, normal heart rates in pediatric patients are more rapid than those seen in adults.

Respiratory rate

Technique. Determination of the respiratory rate must be made surreptitiously. Patients aware that their breathing is being observed will usually not breathe normally. Therefore it is recommended that respiration be monitored immediately after obtaining the heart rate. The observer's fingers are

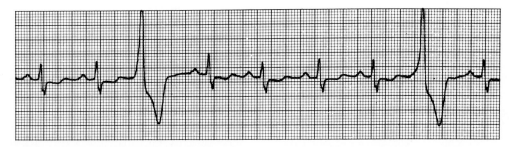

Fig. 2-14. The third and eighth complexes show unifocal premature ventricular contractions (PVC's) (From Zalis, EG, and Conover, MH: Understanding electrocardiography; physiological and interpretive concepts, St. Louis, 1972, The C.V. Mosby Co.)

Table 2-6. Average pulse rates at different ages

Age (yr)	Lower limits of normal	Average	Upper limits of normal
Newborn	70	120	170
1-11 mo	80	120	160
2	80	110	130
4	80	100	120
6	75	100	115
8	70	90	110
10	70	90	110

From Behrman RE, Vaughn VC, III: *Nelson textbook of pediatrics,* ed 12, Philadelphia, 1983, WB Saunders. Reprinted by permission.

Table 2-7. Respiratory rates by age

Age (yr)	Rate/minute
Neonate	40
1 wk	30
1	24
3	22
5	20
8	18
12	16
21	12

left on the patient's radial or brachial pulse after the pulse rate has been determined; however, the doctor counts respirations instead (by observing the rise and fall of the chest) for a minimum of 30 seconds, ideally for 1 minute.

Guidelines for clinical evaluation. The normal respiratory rate for an adult is 16 to 18 breaths per minute. Bradypnea (abnormally slow breathing rate) may be produced by opioid administration, and tachypnea (abnormally rapid breathing rate) is seen with fever and alkalosis. The most commonly observed change in breathing in dental practice will be hyperventilation, an abnormal increase in the rate and depth of respiration, which is usually a manifestation of anxiety. Hyperventilation is also seen in patients with diabetic acidosis. The most common cause of hyperventilation in dental settings is extreme psychologic stress.

Any significant variation in respiratory rate or depth should be fully evaluated before dental treatment commences. The absence of spontaneous ventilation is always an indication for artificial ventilation. Table 2-7 presents the normal range of respiratory rates at different ages.

Blood pressure, heart rate and rhythm, and respiratory rate are the vital signs that provide infor-

mation about the functioning of the patient's cardiopulmonary system. It is recommended that they be recorded as a part of the routine physical evaluation of all prospective patients. Recording of the remaining vital signs—temperature, height, and weight—is desirable but may be considered optional. However, in cases in which parenteral medications are to be administered, especially in lighter weight, younger patients, recording of a patient's weight becomes considerably more important.

Temperature

Technique. Temperature should be monitored orally, if possible. The thermometer, sterilized and shaken down, is placed under the tongue of the patient, who has not eaten, smoked, or had anything to drink in the previous 10 minutes. The thermometer remains in the closed mouth for 2 minutes before removal. Disposable thermometers (Fig. 2-15), digital thermometers (Fig. 2-16), as well as forehead thermometers (Fig. 2-17), are gaining acceptance today.

Guidelines for clinical evaluation. The normal oral temperature of 98.2°F (37°C) is only an average. The true range of normal is considered to be from 97°F to 99.6°F (36.1°C to 37.5°C). Temperatures vary (from 0.5°F to 2.0°F) throughout the day,

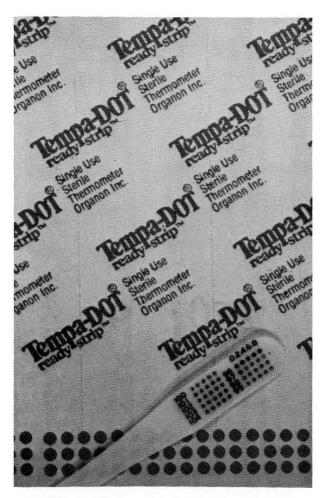

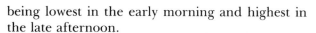

Fig. 2-15. Disposable thermometer. (From Malamed, S.F., Sedation, St. Louis, 1985, the C.V. Mosby Co.)

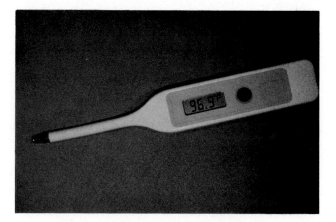

Fig. 2-16. Digital thermometer.

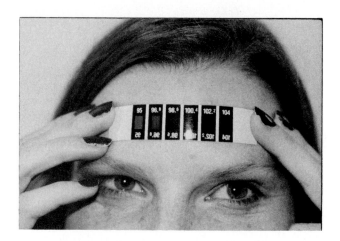

Fig. 2-17. Forehead thermometer.

being lowest in the early morning and highest in the late afternoon.

Fever represents an increase in temperature beyond 99.6°F (37.5°C). Temperatures in excess of 101°F (38.3°C) usually indicate the presence of an active disease process. Evaluation to determine the cause is necessary before treatment begins. When infection of dental origin is considered a probable cause of the elevated temperature, immediate treatment and antibiotic and antipyretic therapy are indicated. If the patient's temperature is 104°F (40°C) or higher, medical consultation is suggested. With elevated temperature, elective dental care is contraindicated and treatment should be limited to drug administration (antibiotics and antipyretics) because this patient is less able than usual to withstand stress.

Height and weight

Technique. Patients should be asked to state their height and weight. The ranges of normal height and weight are quite variable and are indicated on charts developed by various insurance companies.

Guidelines for clinical evaluation. Patients at either end of the normal distribution curve for height and/or weight should be carefully screened. Gross obesity or extreme underweight may be indicative of an active disease process. Obesity will be noted in various endocrine disorders such as Cushing's syndrome, whereas extreme underweight may be noted in pulmonary tuberculosis, malignancy, latter stages of AIDS, and hyperthyroidism. In all instances of gross obesity or extreme underweight, medical consultation prior to the start of treatment is recommended. Excessively tall persons are referred to as giants, whereas persons who are decidedly shorter than normal are called dwarfs. In both instances endocrine gland dysfunction may be present. Medical consultation relative to the planned dental care is usually not necessary for these patients.

Visual Inspection of the Patient

Visual observation of a patient may provide the doctor with valuable information concerning his or her medical status and the patient's level of apprehension toward dentistry. Observation of the patient's posture, body movements, speech, and skin can assist in a diagnosis of possibly significant disorders that may have gone previously undetected.

Patients with CHF and other chronic pulmonary disorders may find it necessary to sit in a more upright position in the dental chair because of the presence of more severe orthopnea (e.g., three- or four-pillow), whereas the arthritic patient with a rigid neck may need to rotate his or her entire trunk when turning toward the doctor or when viewing an object from the side. Recognition of these factors will better enable the doctor to determine necessary treatment modifications.

Involuntary body movements occurring in conscious patients may indicate significant disorders. Tremor is noted in disorders such as fatigue, multiple sclerosis, parkinsonism, hyperthyroidism, and, of great importance to dentistry, hysteria and nervous tension.

The character of a patient's speech may also be significant. Cerebrovascular accident may cause muscle paralysis leading to speech difficulties, whereas the speech of epileptic patients on long-term anticonvulsant therapy with barbiturates (and other anticonvulsants) may seen quite sluggish. Anxiety about the impending dental treatment may also be detected by listening to the patient. Rapid response to questions or a nervous quiver to the voice may indicate the presence of increased anxiety and the possible need for sedation during dental treatment.

Other possible disorders may be uncovered by the detection of specific, nondental odors on the patient's breath. A sweet, fruity odor of acetone is present in patients with diabetic acidosis and ketosis. The smell of ammonia is noted in patients with uremia. Probably the likeliest odor to be on the breath of a patient is that of alcohol. Detection of alcohol on a patient's breath should lead the doctor to consider the possibility of heightened anxiety.

The skin is an important source of information about the patient. It is my belief that the doctor should routinely greet patients by shaking hands. Much information can be gathered from the feel of a patient's skin. For example, the skin of a very apprehensive person will feel cold and wet, that of a patient with a hyperthyroid condition will be warm and wet, and that of a patient with diabetic acidosis will be warm but dry.

Looking at skin is also valuable. The color of a patient's skin is significant. Pallor may indicate anemia or heightened anxiety (i.e., presyncope). Cyanosis may indicate the presence of heart failure, chronic pulmonary disease, or polycythemia, and

will be most notable in the nail beds and mucous membranes (lips). Flushed skin may suggest apprehension, hyperthyroidism, or elevated temperature, and jaundice may indicate past or present hepatic disease. Remember too that each of these may also be benign, insignificant findings.

Additional factors revealed through a visual examination of the patient include the presence of prominent jugular veins in a patient seated upright; an indication of possible right ventricular failure (or of an overly tight collar!); clubbing of the fingers (cardiopulmonary disease); swelling of the ankles (seen in right ventricular failure, varicose veins, renal disease, and occasionally in near-term pregnancy); and exophthalomos (hyperthyroidism). Each of these findings will be discussed more completely in the section on prevention within each specific chapter.

For a more complete discussion of the art of observation and its importance in medical diagnosis, the reader is referred to *A Guide to Physical Evaluation*[14] (Bates, B) and to *Mosby's Guide to Physical Examination*, ed 2, (Seidel HM and others).[15]

Additional Evaluation Procedures

After the completion of the written medical history questionnaire, the recording of vital signs, and physical examination, a more in-depth evaluation of specific medical disorders uncovered is in order. This examination may include auscultation of the heart and lungs, testing for blood glucose levels, retinal examination, function tests for cardiorespiratory status (such as the breath-holding test), electrocardiographic examination, and blood chemistries. At present, many of these tests are used in dental offices but do not represent the standard of care in dentistry. Explanation and evaluation of many of the tests are beyond the scope of this text. Specific tests that may be used by the doctor in an effective and efficient manner will be referred to throughout this textbook. Examples are blood glucose testing and cardiopulmonary function tests.

Dialogue History

Once the medical history, vital signs, and physical examination of the patient have been completed, the doctor must next determine the significance, if any, of any disorder(s) that have been uncovered and the potential risk that these present to the planned dental treatment (the risk being discussed is that of the patient's medical problem becoming acutely exacerbated during or immediately following the dental appointment). The process of discussion with the patient is termed the dialogue history, and it forms an integral part of the process of patient evaluation. In the dialogue history the doctor must use all available knowledge of the disease to accurately assess the degree of risk it represents. Dialogue history will be emphasized in each chapter in the discussion on the prevention of specific emergency situations.

Two examples of dialogue history are presented. In response to a positive reply in question 9 to "Diabetes," the following questions might be included in the dialogue history:

QUESTION. At what age did you develop diabetes (adult or juvenile onset)?

COMMENT. Juvenile-onset diabetes is usually type I or insulin-dependent diabetes mellitus, whereas adult-onset diabetes is more likely to be the less severe non–insulin-dependent diabetes mellitus (type II).

QUESTION. How do you control your diabetes (insulin [IDDM] or non–insulin-dependent [NIDDM])?

COMMENT. IDDM is more likely to develop acute complications associated with diabetes, including hypoglycemia, than is NIDDM.

QUESTION. How often do you monitor your blood sugar and what are the recordings? (monitoring the degree of control the patient maintains over the disease)

QUESTION. Have you ever required hospitalization for your diabetic condition? Why?

COMMENT. A history of hospitalization for low blood sugar would prejudice a doctor toward seeking outside assistance more rapidly should a problem develop with the diabetic patient during treatment. Additionally, hospitalization due to the chronic complications of diabetes should alert the doctor to seek out signs and symptoms of arteriosclerosis.

The following dialogue history might be initiated if a patient answered yes to "angina pectoris" in question 9:

What precipitates your angina?
How frequently do you suffer anginal episodes?
How long do your anginal episodes last?
Describe a typical anginal episode.
How does nitroglycerin affect the anginal episode?
Has there been any change in the frequency, intensity, or radiation of pain of your angina in the past several weeks?

These questions and the responses will be discussed more completely in Chapter 27.

RECOGNITION OF ANXIETY

Thus far the primary aim of our evaluation of the prospective patient has been to determine his or her physical ability to handle the stress involved in the planned treatment. Few if any questions have been directed at the patient's psychological outlook

toward dentistry in general and the planned treatment in particular. The traditional (long-form) medical history questionnaire has questions that ask, "Do you have fainting spells or seizures?" and "Have you had any serious trouble associated with any previous dental treatment?" Most short-form medical histories contain no questions that relate to this important area.

Heightened anxiety and fear of dentistry are stresses that can lead to the acute worsening of medical problems such as angina, seizures, or asthma, or to other stress-related problems such as hyperventilation or vasodepressor syncope. One of the goals of patient evaluation is to determine whether or not the patient is psychologically able to tolerate the stress associated with the planned dental therapy.

Three methods are available to recognize the presence of anxiety. First is the medical history questionnaire, second is the anxiety questionnaire, and third is the art of observation.

PSYCHOLOGICAL EXAMINATION
Medical History Questionnaire

Earlier in this chapter it was recommended that one or more questions relating to a patient's attitudes toward dentistry be included in the medical history questionnaire. It has been our experience at the University of Southern California (USC) School of Dentistry that patients who will not verbally admit their fears to the doctor will in fact indicate on the questionnaire that they are apprehensive. An affirmative response to either question 2 or 3 should alert the doctor to begin a more in-depth dialogue history with the patient to determine the cause of the individual's fear of dentistry.

Anxiety Questionnaire

An additional aid in the recognition of anxiety is the anxiety questionnaire (see box on p. 39) devised by Corah.[16] Used since 1973 at the USC School of Dentistry, this questionnaire has proved to be a reliable aid in the recognition of anxiety. Answers to individual questions are scored 1 through 5 (a = 1, e = 5). The maximum score is 20. Scores of 8 or above indicate higher than usual levels of dental anxiety that should be addressed by the doctor prior to the start of treatment.

Observation

In the absence of such questions or in the absence of an affirmative response to such questions, careful observation of the patient will enable the doctor and staff members to recognize the presence of unusual degrees of anxiety. Some patients may admit to the doctor and staff that they are quite ap-

ANXIETY QUESTIONNAIRE

1. If you had to go to the dentist tomorrow, how would you feel about it?
   a. I would look forward to it as a reasonably enjoyable experience.
   b. I would not care one way or the other.
   c. I would be very uneasy about it.
   d. I would be afraid that it would be unpleasant and painful.
   e. I would be very frightened of what the dentist might do.
2. When you are waiting in the dentist's office for your turn in the chair, how do you feel?
   a. Relaxed
   b. A little uneasy
   c. Tense
   d. Anxious
   e. So anxious that I almost break out in a sweat or almost feel physically sick
3. When you are in the dentist's chair waiting for him or her to get the drill ready and begin working on your teeth, how do you feel?
   a. Relaxed
   b. A little uneasy
   c. Tense
   d. Anxious
   e. So anxious that I almost break out in a sweat or almost feel physically sick
4. You are in the dentist's chair to have your teeth cleaned. While you are waiting and the dentist is getting out the instruments with which to scrape your teeth around the gums, how do you feel?
   a. Relaxed
   b. A little uneasy
   c. Tense
   d. Anxious
   e. So anxious that I almost break out in a sweat or almost feel physically sick
5. In general, do you feel uncomfortable or nervous about receiving dental treatment?
   a. Yes
   b. No

From Corah NL: Development of a dental anxiety scale, *J Dent Res* 48:596, 1969.

prehensive; however, the vast majority of apprehensive adult patients will do everything within their power to conceal their anxiety. The usual feeling of these patients is that their fear of dentistry is irrational and probably even a bit childish. They do not wish to tell the doctor of their fears because they are afraid of being labeled "a baby." Because of this pervasive attitude, members of the dental staff must be trained to recognize clinical signs and symptoms of heightened anxiety in their patients.

Whereas there are a number of levels into which anxiety may be subdivided, for the purposes of this discussion two will be discussed: moderate anxiety and severe (neurotic) anxiety.

Patients with severe anxiety will usually not attempt to hide this fact from the doctor. In fact, these patients will usually do anything within their power to avoid having to be dental patients. It is estimated that between 6% and 14% (14,000,000 to 34,000,000) of the American population avoid dental visits completely because of fear and that another 20% to 30% dislike dental visits enough to make only occasional visits.[17] These persons constitute the severe anxiety group. When in the dental office, they may be recognized by the following:

1. Increased blood pressure and heart rate
2. Trembling
3. Excessive sweating
4. Dilated pupils

Severely anxious patients will most commonly appear in the dental office when they have a serious toothache or infection. On questioning, they state that they have had this problem for quite some time, not just a few days, and have attempted every available means of home remedy (for example, toothache drops), which have apparently worked for some time. The reason that they are finally in the dental office is that over the past few nights they have been unable to sleep because of intense pain that none of their home remedies has been able to alleviate. Therefore, these patients are driven by extreme discomfort to the dental office, where they usually expect to have the tooth removed. These patients represent quite a management problem. Although they desire to have their problem treated, when it comes time for treatment to begin (the moment of truth!), their underlying fear of dentistry comes to the forefront and often makes it impossible for them to tolerate the procedure. In addition, the doctor is often faced with the unpleasant prospect of having either to extract an acutely inflamed tooth or to extirpate the pulp of an acutely sensitive tooth—two situations in which achieving clinically adequate pain control can be difficult with even a nonfearful patient.

Because of these factors, severely anxious patients will very often be candidates for the use of either IV sedation or general anesthesia. Other techniques, such as oral, IM, or inhalation sedation, used as suggested, will have little likelihood of success primarily because of their limited effectiveness or the constraints that are properly placed on their use. Children with severe anxiety are frequently candidates for either IM or IV sedation or for general anesthesia.

Patients with more moderate degrees of anxiety will be much more frequently seen. Many of these patients will try to hide their fears from the doctor because they believe that, being adults, they should not admit to being afraid of the dentist. Children, on the other hand, being less inhibited than the typical adult, will immediately make their feelings toward dental treament known to the entire dental staff. Assuming then that adult patients may attempt to hide their dental fears, the doctor and staff should remain observant both before and during the dental treatment.

The front-office people, such as the receptionist, will be able to overhear patients in the waiting room talking among themselves. Patients might ask important questions of the receptionist, such as, "Is the doctor gentle?" or "Does the doctor use gas?" The receptionist should be trained to immediately inform the doctor whenever a patient makes statements that might indicate an increased level of concern about the upcoming treatment. This is also true for all chairside personnel. Touching the patient, as in shaking their hands when greeting them, may lead to a presumption of anxiety if the patient's palms are cold and sweaty, especially if the office is not especially cool.

Discussing a patient's prior dental experiences may give an indication of his or her dental anxiety status. A patient with a history of emergency treatment only (for example, extractions or incision and drainage), but who cancels or does not appear for subsequent appointments may be a fearful individual. A patient with a history of multiple canceled appointments may also be a fearful patient. This history should be discussed with the patient in an attempt to determine the reasons behind this pattern of treatment (or nontreatment).

Once the patient is seated in the chair, he or she should be watched and listened to. Apprehensive patients remain alert and on guard at all times. They sit at the edge of the chair; their eyes roam all around the room, taking everything in. They are afraid of being "snuck up on." Their posture appears unnaturally stiff, and their arms and legs are tense. They may nervously fiddle with a hand-

---

> ### *CLINICAL SIGNS OF MODERATE ANXIETY*
>
> #### *Reception area*
> 1. Questions to receptionist regarding injections or use of sedation
> 2. Overhearing patients talking in waiting room
> 3. History of emergency dental care only
> 4. History of canceled appointments for non-emergency treatment
> 5. Shaking hands with patient: cold, sweaty palms
>
> #### *In dental chair*
> 1. Unnaturally stiff posture
> 2. Nervous play with tissue or handkerchief
> 3. White-knuckle syndrome
> 4. Perspiration noted on forehead and hands
> 5. Overly willing to cooperate with doctor
> 6. Answers questions too quickly

kerchief or tissue, occasionally being unaware that they are doing so. The white-knuckle syndrome may be observed, in which the patient clutches the armrest of the dental chair tightly enough that their knuckles turn white. Profuse diaphoresis (sweating) of the palms or forehead may be noted, explained by the patient as, "Gee, it's hot in here!"

The moderately apprehensive patient will be overly willing to aid the dentist. Actions are carried out quickly, usually without thinking. Questions to this patient are answered very quickly, usually too quickly. The clinical signs of moderate anxiety are summarized in the accompanying box.

Once anxiety has been recognized, be it through the questionnaire or via observation, the patient must be confronted with it. The straightforward approach is surprisingly successful. The dentist might say, "Mr. Smith, I see from your medical history that you have had several unpleasant experiences in a dental office. Would you kindly describe these to me?" Or, when the anxiety is determined visually, "Mrs. Smith, you appear to be somewhat nervous today. Is something bothering you?" I have been truly astonished at how rapidly patients will drop all pretense at being calm once it is known to them that the doctor is aware of their fears. They will usually say, "Doctor, I didn't think you could tell." Once in the open, determination of the exact source of the patient's fears, such as injections or the drill, should be attempted. Once the source(s) of a patient's fears are known, steps may be instituted to minimize their occurrence.

The patient with moderate anxiety will usually prove to be treatable. In most cases, psychosedation will prove effective in the management of this patient. Psychosedation may involve the administration of a drug (pharmacosedation) or may be a nondrug form of sedation (iatrosedation). General anesthesia will only rarely be needed for the effective management of the moderately fearful patient.

• • •

With the information that has been gathered concerning the patient's past and present medical and dental histories, vital signs, and physical examination, the basic goals of physical evaluation can now be completed.

DETERMINATION OF MEDICAL RISK

Having completed all of the components of the physical evaluation in addition to a thorough dental examination and deciding on a tentative treatment plan, the doctor must then gather all of this information and answer the following questions:

1. Is the patient capable, physiologically and psychologically, of tolerating in relative safety the stress involved in the proposed dental treatment plan?
2. Does the patient represent a greater risk (of morbidity or mortality) than normal during the planned dental care?
3. If the patient does represent an increased risk, what treatment modifications, if any, should be employed during the planned dental treatment to minimize this risk?
4. Is this risk too great for the patient to be managed safely in the dental office?

In an attempt to answer these questions, the USC School of Dentistry has developed a physical evaluation system that attempts to assist the doctor in categorizing patients from the standpoint of risk factor orientation. The function of this evaluation system is to place each patient in an appropriate risk category so that dental care can be provided in greater comfort and safety. This system is based on the ASA Physical Status Classification System, which will now be described.

ASA PHYSICAL STATUS CLASSIFICATION SYSTEM

In 1962 the American Society of Anesthesiologists adopted what is now commonly referred to as the ASA Physical Status Classification System.[18] It represents a method of estimating the medical risk presented by a patient who is scheduled to receive anesthesia for a surgical procedure. The system was designed primarily for patients who were to receive a general anesthetic, but since its introduction the classification system has been used for all surgical patients regardless of anesthetic technique (for example, general anesthesia, regional anesthesia, or sedation). The system has been in continuous use since 1962 essentially without change and has proved to be a valuable method for determining surgical and anesthetic risk prior to the actual procedure. The classification system follows:

ASA I: A patient without systemic disease; a normal, healthy patient
ASA II: A patient with mild systemic disease
ASA III: A patient with severe systemic disease that limits activity but is not incapacitating
ASA IV: A patient with an incapacitating systemic disease that is a constant threat to life
ASA V: A moribund patient not expected to survive 24 hours with or without operation
ASA E: Emergency operation of any variety; E precedes the number, indicating the patient's physical status (for example, ASA E-III)

When this system was adopted for use in a typical outpatient dental setting, the ASA V classification was eliminated. An effort has been made to correlate the remaining four classifications with possible treatment modifications for dental therapy. Figure 2-18 illustrates the USC physical evaluation record on which a summary of the patient's physical and psychologic status can be presented. Each of the classifications will be reviewed, with specific examples of each listed.

ASA I

ASA I patients are considered to be normal and healthy. Review of their medical histories, physical evaluations, and any other parameters that have been evaluated indicate no abnormalities. The heart, lungs, liver, kidneys, and central nervous system in these patients are in apparent good health. Physiologically, these patients should be capable of tolerating the stress involved in a proposed dental treatment with no added risk of serious complications. Psychologically, these patients should present little or no difficulty in handling the proposed treatment. Healthy patients with little or no anxiety are classified ASA I. Treatment modifications are usually not necessary for patients in this group.

ASA I patients are able to walk up one flight of stairs or two level city blocks without distress.* An ASA I classification represents a "green flag" for treatment.

---

*Distress is considered to be shortness of breath, undue fatigue, or chest pain.

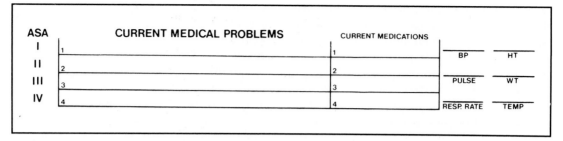

Fig. 2-18. The physical evaluation section on the health history form provides room for summary of medical problems, vital signs, and ASA classification. (From Malamed SF: *Sedation*, St Louis, 1985, Mosby–Year Book.)

ASA II

ASA II patients have a mild systemic disease or are healthy (ASA I) patients who demonstrate a more extreme anxiety and fear toward dentistry. These patients are generally somewhat less stress tolerant than ASA I patients; however, they still represent a minimal risk during dental treatment. Routine treatment is in order with consideration given toward possible treatment modifications or special considerations as warranted by the particular condition. Examples of such modifications include the use of prophylactic antibiotics or sedative techniques, limiting the duration of treatment, and possible medical consultation.

ASA II patients are able to walk up one flight of stairs or two level city blocks, but will have to stop after completion of the exercise because of distress. An ASA II classification represents a "yellow flag" (proceed with caution). Elective dental care is warranted with little increase in risk to the patient during therapy. Consideration should be given to possible treatment modifications.

Examples of ASA II patients include those with:
1. Well-controlled, non–insulin-dependent diabetes mellitus (NIDDM)
2. Well-controlled epilepsy
3. Well-controlled asthma
4. Well-controlled hyperthyroid or hypothyroid disorders who are under care and presently have normal thyroid function (euthyroid)
5. ASA I patients with upper respiratory infection (URI)
6. Healthy, pregnant women (during their pregnancy)
7. Otherwise healthy patients with allergies (especially to drugs)
8. Otherwise healthy patients with extreme dental fears
9. The healthy patient over the age of 60 years
10. Adult blood pressure between 140 to 159 torr and/or 90 to 94 torr

In general, the ASA II patient will be able to perform normal activities without experiencing distress such as undue fatigue, dyspnea, or precordial pain.

ASA III

ASA III patients have severe systemic disease that limits activity but is not incapacitating. At rest ASA III patients will not exhibit signs and symptoms of distress, but will do so when stressed either physiologically or psychologically. An example of this would be the anginal patient who, while in the waiting room is normal, but develops chest pain when seated in the dental chair.

ASA III patients are able to walk up one flight of stairs or two level city blocks, but will have to stop en route because of distress.

Like the ASA II classification, the ASA III classification represents a "yellow flag" (proceed with caution). Elective dental care is not contraindicated, though this patient does represent a greater risk during treatment. Serious consideration should be given to possible implementation of treatment modifications.

Examples of ASA patients include those with:
1. Stable angina pectoris
2. Status postmyocardial infarction >6 months with no residual signs and symptoms
3. Status postcerebrovascular accident >6 months with no residual signs and symptoms
4. Well-controlled insulin-dependent diabetes (IDDM)
5. Congestive heart failure (CHF) with orthopnea and ankle edema
6. Chronic obstructive pulmonary disease (COPD)—emphysema or chronic bronchitis
7. Exercise-induced asthma
8. Less well-controlled epilepsy
9. Hyperthyroid or hypothyroid disorders who are symptomatic
10. Adult blood pressure between 160 to 199 torr and/or 95 to 114 torr

ASA III patients are usually able to perform normal activities without experiencing distress such as undue fatigue, dyspnea, or precordial pain; however, they may need to stop and rest during an activity should they become distressed.

ASA IV

ASA IV patients have an incapacitating disease that is a constant threat to life. Patients in this category have a severe medical problem of greater importance to the patient than the planned dental treatment. Whenever possible, elective dental care should be postponed until such time as the patient's medical condition has improved to at least an ASA III classification.

ASA IV patients are unable to walk up one flight of stairs or two level city blocks. Distress is present even at rest. This patient will present in the dental office showing clinical signs and symptoms of disease.

An ASA IV classification represents a "red flag"—a warning flag indicating that the risk involved in treating the patient is too great to allow elective care to proceed.

The management of dental emergencies, such as infection or pain, should be treated as conservatively as possible until the patient's condition improves. When possible, treatment should be noninvasive, consisting of the prescription of medications such as analgesics for pain and antibiotics for infection. In situations in which it is felt that immediate intervention is required (I & D, extraction, pulpal extirpation), it is suggested that the patient receive such care within the confines of an acute care facility (i.e., a hospital). Although a hospitalized patient can still be at risk, his or her chance of survival will perhaps be increased should an acute medical emergency arise.

Examples of ASA IV patients include those with:
1. Unstable angina pectoris (preinfarction angina)
2. Myocardial infarction within the past 6 months
3. CVA within the past 6 months
4. Adult blood pressure greater than 200 torr and/or 115 torr
5. Severe CHF or COPD (requiring oxygen supplementation and/or confined to wheelchair)
6. Uncontrolled epilepsy (with history of hospitalization)
7. Uncontrolled insulin-dependent diabetes (with history of hospitalization)

ASA V

ASA V patients are moribund and are not expected to survive more than 24 hours with or without the planned surgery.

ASA V patients are almost always hospitalized, terminally ill patients. They might be considered in many institutions to be "DNAR" (do not attempt resuscitation) patients. Elective dental treatment is definitely contraindicated; however, emergency care, in the realm of palliative treatment (i.e., relief of pain), may be necessary. An ASA V classification represents a "red flag" for dental care.

Examples of ASA V patients include those with:
1. End-stage renal disease
2. End-stage hepatic disease
3. Terminal cancer
4. End-stage infectious disease

The ASA classification system is quite easy to employ in dentistry. This is especially the case when a patient has but one isolated medical problem (see examples provided with each ASA category). However, many patients will have a history of multiple diseases, in which case determination of the appropriate ASA classification might be clouded. In these situations the doctor must weigh the significance of each disease and then choose the appropriate ASA category.

The ASA physical status classification system is not meant to be inflexible; rather, it is meant to function as a relative value system based on a doctor's clinical judgment and assessment of the relevant clinical data that are available.

When the doctor is unable to determine the clinical significance of one or more disease entities, consultation with the patient's physician or other medical or dental colleagues is recommended. In all cases, however, the ultimate decision either to treat or to postpone treatment must be made by the treating doctor. The ultimate responsibility rests solely in the hands of the doctor who treats or does not treat the patient.

To summarize the ASA physical status classification system, ASA I, II, and III patients are candidates for both elective and emergency dental care. The degree of risk represented by these patients increases with the category (I<II<III) as do the indications for treatment modification.

MEDICAL CONSULTATION

The accompanying box lists the steps involved in a typical medical consultation. It is strongly suggested that a medical consultation not be sought until the patient's dental and physical evaluations have been completed. The dentist should be fully prepared to discuss with the patient's physician the proposed dental treatment plan and any anticipated problems. One of the most important considerations in medical consultation is to determine the ability of the patient to tolerate in relative safety the stress involved in the planned dental treatment.

MEDICAL CONSULTATION

1. Obtain the patient's dental and medical histories.
2. Complete the physical examination, including both oral and general examination.
3. Provide a tentative treatment plan based on the patient's oral needs.
4. Make a general systemic assessment (choose a physical status category).
5. Consult the patient's physician, when appropriate, via telephone:
   a. Physician's receptionist:
      - Introduce yourself and give the patient's name.
      - Ask to speak with the physician.
   b. Physician:
      - Introduce yourself.
      - Give the patient's name and the reason for his or her visit to you.
      - Relate briefly your summary of the patient's general condition.
      - Ask for additional information about the patient.
      - Present your treatment plan briefly, including medications to be used and the degree of stress anticipated.
      - Discuss any problems if necessary.
   c. Following consultation:
      Write a complete report of the conversation for records and if possible obtain a written report from the physician.

Modified with permission from WH Davis, DDS, Bellflower, California.

The physician's advice should be carefully considered. Whenever doubt remains following consultation, a second opinion, perhaps from a specialist in the specific area of difficulty, is recommended. Following a satisfactory consultation the dentist must next consider implementing steps to minimize the perceived risk to the patient. The final responsibility for the dental treatment plan and the risks of treatment rests solely with the treating dentist. Risk cannot be shared with the patient's physician.

In most cases medical consultation will lead to little or no alteration in planned dental care. Specific treatment modifications, such as those listed in the following section on stress reduction protocol, represent potentially important steps in decreasing the risk to a patient during dental treatment.

STRESS REDUCTION PROTOCOL

At this point in our pretreatment evaluation we have reviewed all of the history and physical evaluation data and have assigned a physical status classification. Most patients will be assigned an ASA I or II status, with fewer categorized as ASA III and only a very small percentage as ASA IV.

As discussed earlier, virtually every dental procedure is potentially stress-inducing in certain patients. Stress may be of either a physiologic nature (pain, strenuous exercise) or of a psychologic nature (anxiety, fear). In either case, however, one of the body's responses to stress involves an increase in the release of catecholamines (epinephrine and norepinephrine) from the adrenal medulla into the cardiovascular system, resulting in an increase in cardiovascular workload (increased heart rate, increased strength of myocardial contraction, increased myocardial oxygen requirement). Although ASA I patients may be quite able to tolerate such changes in cardiovascular activity, ASA II, III, and IV patients will be increasingly less able to safely tolerate these changes. For example, patients with angina may respond to increased stress with episodes of chest pain, and various dysrhythmias may develop. Patients with CHF may develop pulmonary edema. Patients with noncardiovascular disorders may also respond adversely when faced with increased levels of stress. For example, patients with asthma may develop acute episodes of breathing difficulty, whereas epileptics may have seizures.

Unusual degrees of stress in ASA I patients may be responsible for several psychogenically induced emergency situations, such as hyperventilation or vasodepressor syncope.

Interviews with apprehensive dental patients have demonstrated that many persons will begin to worry one or two days before their upcoming dental appointments. These persons may be unable to sleep well the night prior to an appointment, thus arriving fatigued and even more stress-intolerant. The risk presented by these patients during dental treatment is increased even further.

The stress reduction protocol[19] includes two series of procedures that, when used either individually or collectively, act to minimize stress to the patient during treatment and thereby decrease the degree of risk presented by the patient. This protocol is predicated on the belief that the prevention of or reduction of stress ought to begin before the start of an appointment, continue throughout treatment, and, if indicated, into the postoperative period.

Stress Reduction Protocol: Normal, Healthy, Anxious Patient (ASA I)

1. Recognize the patient's level of anxiety.
2. Premedicate the evening before the dental appointment, as needed.
3. Premedicate immediately before the dental appointment, as needed.
4. Schedule the appointment in the morning.
5. Minimize the patient's waiting time.
6. Use psychosedation during therapy.
7. Use adequate pain control during therapy.
8. Length of appointment variable.
9. Follow up with postoperative pain/anxiety control.
10. Telephone the highly anxious or fearful moderate-to-high-risk patient later on the same day that treatment was given.

Stress Reduction Protocol: Medical Risk Patient (ASA II, III, IV)

1. Recognize the patient's degree of medical risk.
2. Complete medical consultation before dental therapy, as needed.
3. Schedule the patient's appointment in the morning.
4. Monitor and record preoperative and postoperative vital signs.
5. Use psychosedation during therapy, as needed.
6. Use adequate pain control during therapy.
7. Length of appointment—variable; do not exceed the patient's limits of tolerance.
8. Follow up with postoperative pain/anxiety control.
9. Telephone the higher medical risk patient later on the same day that treatment was given.
10. Arrange the appointment for the highly anxious or fearful moderate-to-high-risk patient during the first few days of the week when the office will be open for emergency care and when the treating doctor is available.

Recognition of Medical Risk and Anxiety

Recognition of these factors represents the starting point for the management of stress in the dental or surgical patient. Medical risk assessment will be accurately determined by strict adherence to the measures previously described in this chapter, which include completing the medical history questionnaire, performing the physical examination, and obtaining the dialogue history. The recognition of anxiety is often a more difficult task. As has been described previously, visual observation, as well as verbal communication with the patient, can provide the doctor with important clues to the presence of dental anxiety.

Medical Consultation

Medical consultation with a patient's physician should be considered in those situations in which the doctor is uncertain about the degree of risk represented by the patient. Medical consultation is neither required nor recommended for all patients with medical problems. A consultation should be sought when the treating doctor is uncertain about the nature of the patient's disorder(s) or of possible interaction of the disorder(s) with the planned dental care. In all cases it must be remembered that a consultation is but a request for additional information concerning a specific patient or disease process. The doctor is seeking information that will aid in determining the degree of risk present and therapy modification that may be needed. The final responsibility for the care and safety of a patient rests with the person who ultimately treats them.

Premedication

Many apprehensive patients state that their fear of dental treatment is so great that they are unable to sleep well the night before scheduled treatment. Fatigued the next day, these patients are even less able to tolerate the additional stress placed on them by the actual dental treatment performed. Should a patient be medically compromised, the risk of an acute exacerbation of the patient's medical problem is greatly increased. In an ASA I patient, such additional stress may provoke a psychogenically induced reponse. Clinical manifestations of increased fatigue include a lowered pain reaction threshold. Such a patient is more likely to interpret what is usually perceived as a nonpainful stimulus as being painful than is the well-rested patient.

Restful sleep the night before a scheduled appointment is desirable. Therefore, whenever it has been determined that heightened anxiety exists, it should also be determined if this anxiety interferes with sleep. Oral sedation is one method of achieving restful sleep. An antianxiety or sedative-hypnotic drug such as triazolam or flurazepam may be prescribed to be taken one hour before sleep.*

As the scheduled appointment time approaches, the patient's anxiety level will heighten. In many

---

*Doses of these and other medications may be found in *Sedation: a guide to patient management*, ed 2, St Louis, 1989, Mosby–Year Book.

instances, the administration of an antianxiety or sedative-hypnotic agent approximately one hour prior to the scheduled appointment will decrease the patient's anxiety level to such a degree that the thought of dental treatment is no longer frightening. Oral medications should be administered approximately one hour before the scheduled start of treatment to permit a therapeutic blood level of the agent to develop. Oral agents may be taken by the patient while at home or at the dental office. Whenever an oral antianxiety drug has been prescribed to be taken by the patient at home, the doctor must advise the patient (and document in the chart) against driving a car or operating other potentially hazardous machinery.

The appropriate use of oral antianxiety or sedative-hypnotic agents is an excellent method of diminishing preoperative stress. Agents such as diazepam, oxazepam, hydroxyzine, promethazine, and chloral hydrate have proven effective. Use of barbiturates, such as secobarbital, pentobarbital, or even hexobarbital, is not recommended.

Appointment Scheduling

Apprehensive or medically compromised patients are best able to tolerate stress when they are well rested. In most cases, therefore, the most appropriate time to schedule these patients will be early in the day. This is also the case for the management of apprehensive or medically compromised children.

When the appointment is scheduled for the afternoon, the apprehensive patient must contend with the ominous specter of the dental appointment, which casts a pall over everything the patient does before it, allowing him or her more time to think and to worry about it. The patient becomes more anxious, thereby increasing the likelihood of adverse psychogenic reactions. A morning appointment permits this patient to get it over with and to then continue with his or her usual activities, unburdened by dental anxiety.

For the medically compromised patient the situation is somewhat similar. As fatigue sets in during the day the patient becomes less able to manage additional increases in stress. A dental appointment scheduled for later in the day may result in a medically compromised patient who has spent many hours at work, has driven through traffic, and possesses little or no ability to adequately handle any additional stress. An earlier appointment provides the doctor and patient with a degree of flexibility in patient management.

The doctor should also try to schedule the moderately to highly anxious medical-risk patient for treatment early in the week so that if postoperative complications should arise, the patient will be able to contact and be seen promptly by the original treating doctor. In addition, the doctor should routinely contact the moderately to highly anxious, medically compromised patient later on the same day of dental treatment to see how he or she is doing. Such personal contact is greatly appreciated by the patient and serves as a means of preventing or at least minimizing posttreatment complications.

Minimized Waiting Time

Once in the dental office setting, the apprehensive patient should not be required to sit in the waiting room or dental chair for extended periods of time before treatment starts. It is well known that anticipation of a procedure can induce more fear that the actual procedure itself.[20] Sitting and waiting allows the patient to smell dental office "smells," to hear dental office sounds, and to fantasize about the "horrible things" that are going to happen to them. Cases of serious morbidity and of death have occurred in dental office waiting rooms prior to a patient ever being treated.[21] Minimized waiting time is of even greater significance for the apprehensive patient.

Vital Signs (Preoperative and Postoperative)

Before the start of dental treatment on the medically compromised patient, the doctor should routinely measure and record the patient's vital signs. (Vital signs can be recorded by a trained member of the auxiliary staff.) Those signs recorded should include blood pressure, heart rate and rhythm, and respiratory rate. Comparison of these signs to the baseline values recorded at an earlier visit can serve as indicators of the patient's physical status on any given day. Although vital sign recordings are particularly relevant for patients with cardiovascular disease, it is strongly suggested that they be taken and recorded on all medically compromised (all ASA III and appropriate ASA II) patients. Postoperative vital signs should also be measured and recorded in these same patients on a routine basis.

Psychosedation During Therapy

Should additional stress reduction be considered necessary during dental treatment, any of the techniques of sedation or general anesthesia may be considered. Nondrug techniques include iatrosedation and hypnosis, whereas the more commonly used pharmacosedation procedures include oral, inhalation, intramusuclar (IM), and intravenous (IV) sedation. The primary goal of all these techniques is the same: to decrease or eliminate stress in a conscious patient. When appropriate techniques are properly employed, this goal may usually be achieved without the addition of any risk to the patient. The use of these techniques in various medical problems will be discussed in subsequent chapters.

Adequate Pain Control During Therapy

For stress reduction to be successful, it is absolutely essential that adequate pain control be achieved. The successful management of pain is probably of greater importance in the medically compromised patient than in the ASA I individual. The potentially significant actions of endogenously released catecholamines on cardiovascular functioning in the patient with clinically significant heart or blood vessel disease almost always warrants the inclusion of a vasoconstrictor in the local anesthetic solution. Judicious use of these agents along with proper injection technique must, of course, be effected. Without adequate control of pain, sedation and stress reduction are impossible to achieve.

Duration of Dental Treatment

The length of the treatment period is significant to both the medically compromised and the apprehensive patient. In the absence of any medical factors dictating the need for shorter appointments, the length of the appointment should be decided by the doctor after consideration of the patient's desires. In many cases the apprehensive patient (ASA I or II) may prefer to have as few dental appointments as possible regardless of their length. Appointments three hours or longer may constitute preferred management for this otherwise healthy patient. However, attempting to satisfy the patient's desire for a longer appointment is inadvisable when the doctor believes that there is appropriate justification for a shorter appointment. Cases of serious morbidity and of death have occurred when the doctor complied with parents' wishes to complete treatment of their child in one long appointment as opposed to multiple shorter visits.[22]

Unlike the anxious ASA I patient, the medically compromised patient should not be permitted to undergo longer appointments. For many persons, being seated in a dental chair for one hour is quite stressful. Even a "good" ASA I patient may have some difficulty tolerating two or three-hour dental procedures. To allow a higher risk patient to undergo such extended treatment will unnecessarily increase risk. Dental appointments in the medically compromised patient should therefore be of shorter duration, never exceeding the limit of the patient's tolerance. Signs that this limit of tolerance has been reached include evidence of fatigue, rest-lessness, sweating, and evident discomfort. The most prudent way of managing the patient at this time is to terminate the procedure as expeditiously as possible and reschedule the treatment for a later date.

Postoperative Control of Pain and Anxiety

Of equal importance to preoperative and intraoperative pain and anxiety control is the management of pain and anxiety in the posttreatment period.[23] This is especially relevant for the patient who has undergone a potentially traumatic procedure such as endodontics, periodontal or oral surgery, extensive oral reconstruction, or restorative procedures. The doctor must carefully consider the possible complications that might arise during the 24 hours immediately following dental care, discuss these with the patient, and then take steps to assist the patient in managing them. These steps include any or all of the following when indicated:

1. Be available by telephone 24 hours a day.
2. Monitor pain control and prescribe analgesic medication as needed.
3. Prescribe antibiotics if a possibility of infection exists.
4. Prescribe antianxiety agents, if in the doctor's opinion they may be required by the patient.
5. Prescribe muscle relaxant agents after prolonged therapy or following multiple injections into one area (such as inferior alveolar nerve block).

Availability of the doctor by telephone 24 hours a day has become a standard of care in dentistry. With answering services, telephone answering machines, and portable pagers readily available, the patient should be able to contact their doctor whenever necessary.

Several studies have demonstrated that unexpected pain is rated as being more uncomfortable than expected pain.[24] Should the possibility of discomfort exist following a procedure, the patient should be forewarned and an analgesic medication made available. Where the possibility of posttreatment pain has not been discussed and it does develop, the patient will immediately think that something has gone wrong. Such pain is recorded as being more intense and anxiety provoking than pain that is expected. Should posttreatment discomfort, which has been discussed, fail to materialize, the patient will be all the more relaxed and confident in the doctor's abilities.

In addition to the general modifications in patient management discussed in the stress reduction protocol, there are specific therapy modifications that will benefit certain groups of medically compromised patients. Both the general and specific

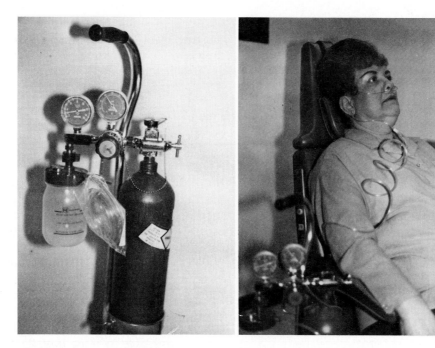

Fig. 2-19. Supplemental oxygen may be administered through a nasal cannula and humidifier.

therapy modifications indicated for a given patient should be entered on a patient's permanent record for future reference (See Fig. 2-18). Examples of specific therapy modification include:

1. The intraoperative administration of oxygen through a nasal cannula at a flow of 3 to 4 L per minute; the oxygen should be humidified (Fig. 2-19). This might be necessary for patients with degrees of CHF or COPD.
2. Modification of patient positioning during treatment; the patient may be unable to tolerate the recommended supine or semisupine position and will require placement in a more upright position. Patients with significant degrees of orthopnea (three to four pillow) may be unable to breathe comfortably while supine.
3. The use of a rubber dam—highly recommended for all dental procedures when its placement is possible—may be contraindicated in patients with certain cardiovascular or respiratory disorders, or allergy; if a rubber dam cannot be used, the patient should be warned about the danger of swallowing or aspirating a foreign body (i.e., dental instrument), and a note to this effect should be entered on the patient's chart.

Through the use of the stress reduction protocols and specific treatment modifications, patient management has been increased to include the preoperative and postoperative periods as well as the intraoperative period. These protocols have made it possible to manage the dental health needs of a broad spectrum of both anxious and medically compromised patients with a minimal complication rate.

REFERENCES

1. McCarthy EM: Sudden, unexpected death in the dental office, *J Am Dent Assoc* 83:1091, 1971.
2. Goldberger E: *Treatment of cardiac emergencies*, ed 5, St Louis, 1990, Mosby–Year Book.
3. McCarthy, FM: A new, patient-administered medical history developed for dentistry, *J Am Dent Assoc* 111:595, 1985.
4. *Physicians' Desk Reference*, ed 45, Oradell, NJ, 1991, Medical Economics.
5. Skidmore-Roth L: *Mosby's 1990 nursing drug reference*, St Louis, 1990, Mosby–Year Book.
6. Committee on Rheumatic Fever, Endocarditis, and Kawasaki Disease of the Council on Cardiovascular Disease in the Young of the American Heart Association: Prevention of bacterial endocarditis—recommendations by the American Heart Association, *JAMA* 264:2919, 1990.
7. Council on Dental Therapeutics and American Heart Association: Preventing bacterial endocarditis: a statement for the dental profession, *J Amer Dent Assoc* 122:87, 1991.
8. McCarthy, FM: *Essentials of safe treatment for the medically compromised patient*, Philadelphia, 1989, WB Saunders.
9. Ridker PM, Manson JE, Goldhaber SZ, Hennekens CH: Clinical characteristics of nonfatal myocardial infarction among individuals on prophylactic low-dose aspirin therapy, *Circulation* 84(2):708-711, 1991.
10. Brady WF, Martinoff JT: Validity of health history data

collected from dental patients and patient perception of health status, *J Am Dent Assoc* 101:642, 1980.

11. Prior AJ, Drake-Lee AB: Auditing the reliability of recall of patients of minor surgical procedures, *Clin Otolaryngol* 16(4):373-375, 1991.

12. Dorman JM: The annual physical comes of age (editorial), *J Amer Coll Health* 38(5):205-206, 1990.

13. Cavallaro D, Melker R: Comparison of two techniques for determining cardiac activity in infants, *Crit Care Med* 11:189, 1983.

14. Bates B: *A guide to physical examination*, Philadelphia, 1900, JB Lippincott.

15. Seidel HM, Ball JW, Dains JE, Benedict GW: *Mosby's guide to physical examination,* ed 2, St Louis, Mosby Yearbook.

16. Corah NL, Gale EN, Illig SJ: Assessment of a dental anxiety scale, *J Am Dent Assoc* 97:816, 1981.

17. Milgrom P, Weinstein P, Kleinknecht R, Getz T: *Treating fearful dental patients*, Reston, Va., 1985, Reston Publishing.

18. American Society of Anesthesiologists: New classification of physical status, *Anesthesiology* 24:1, 1963.

19. McCarthy, FM: Stress reduction and therapy modifications, *CDAJ* 9:41, 1981.

20. Gale EN: Fears of the dental situation, *J Dent Res* 51:964, 1972.

21. Bell WH: Emergencies in and out of the dental office: a pilot study in the state of Texas, *J Am Dent Assoc* 74:778, 1967.

22. deJulien LE: Causes of severe morbidity/mortality cases, *J Cal Dent Assoc* 11:45, 1983.

23. Goodsen JM, Moore PA: Life-threatening reactions after pedodontic sedation: an assessment of narcotic, local anesthetic, and antiemetic drug interaction, *J Am Dent Assoc* 107:239, 1983.

24. Corah N: Development of a dental anxiety scale. *J Res Dent* 48:596, 1969.

3 *Preparation*

In spite of our efforts, described in the preceding chapter, at preventing life-threatening emergencies, these situations will occur on occasion. Prevention, as successful as it may be, will not be enough. The entire dental office staff must also be fully prepared to assist in the recognition and management of any emergency situation that may develop. Unless all office personnel are capable of effectively managing those few serious emergencies that might develop during the practice lifetime of the doctor, such situations might well become office catastrophes.

What constitutes adequate preparation of the dental office and staff for the rapid and effective management of life-threatening situations? Surprisingly, there are few guidelines that have been developed to assist the dentist in this important area. Most have been developed by a state's Board of Dental Examiners in relation to the certification of doctors who wish to employ parenteral sedation techniques, such as intramuscular or intravenous sedation, or general anesthesia in their offices.[1] Specialty groups such as the American Association of Oral & Maxillofacial Surgeons[2], and the Academy of Pediatric Dentistry[3], and the American Association of Periodontists have developed similar guidelines for their membership. The American Association of Dental Schools has developed curricular guidelines for teaching anesthesia and pain control, which include recommendations for emergency preparation.[4] The groups of dentists affected by these guidelines are, as a whole, persons who have received a significant degree of advanced education and training in various techniques of drug administration. Development of such guidelines for these groups is quite appropriate. These guidelines list the requirements for available personnel, equipment, and emergency drugs for the safe and effective management of emergency situations, as well as providing suggested protocol for the management of specific problems.

Unfortunately (or fortunately perhaps), no such guidelines exist for the overwhelming majority of dentists who have not received such advanced training in drug administration or who are not members of these specialty societies. In addition, the level of training in emergency medicine among dentists varies considerably, as it does among all health professionals, including physicians. There are but a few who possess an expertise in emergency medicine, whereas the vast majority have only a basic knowledge of emergency care.

Regardless of the level of prior training in emergency medicine possessed by a doctor, the preparation of the dental staff and of the office will be remarkably similar. Indeed, in all situations it will be expected that the doctor will initiate emergency management and be capable of sustaining a victim's life through application of basic life support. Subsequent management steps, including the administration of drugs, will depend upon the level of training of the doctor managing the situation.

There are some doctors who will find themselves in special situations that require them to become significantly better trained than the level described here. There are still a good number of areas in the United States, many more areas in Canada, and in all other countries, where population is sparse and medical services (routine and emergency) are not readily available. In my travels over the years I have met many dentists, assistants, and hygienists from very small towns in Montana, North Dakota, eastern Nevada, Alaska, and throughout Canada, who are the only medical professionals in a large geographical area. Many state that they are their area's primary source for emergency medical care, the nearest ambulance company being over one hour away. It behooves these persons to seek additional training in emergency medicine. Many of these persons have received advanced cardiac life support (ACLS) training, emergency medical technician (EMT) training at varying levels, and in some situations even advanced trauma life support (ATLS) certification. Morrow[5] describes in detail the added training requirements for these doctors and suggests appropriate levels of emergency training as well as providing recommendations for emergency kits based upon the distance between a dental office and nearest emergency medical services.

The following steps are involved in the preparation of the dental staff and of the office for medical emergencies regardless of the level of training available:

1. Staff training should include:
   • Basic Life Support training for all members of the dental office staff
   • Training in the recognition and management of specific emergency situations
   • Emergency "fire drills"
2. Office preparation should include:
   • Posting emergency assistance numbers
   • Stocking emergency drugs and equipment

These steps of preparation will be described in depth in the remainder of this chapter.

GENERAL INFORMATION
Office Personnel
Training

Emergency courses. Without any doubt the most important step in the preparation of a dental office for medical emergencies will be the training of all office personnel, including nonchairside personnel (i.e., receptionist and laboratory personnel), in the recognition and management of these situations. This training should include an annual refresher course in emergency medicine that provides a general review of all aspects of the subject, such as seizures, chest pain, and respiratory difficulty, rather than just a review of basic life support (BLS). Such continuing education courses are presented at most major dental meetings and through most local dental societies. Lists of scheduled courses are available from the American Dental Association.

Basic life support. The aforementioned training must include an understanding of and the ability to perform the steps of basic life support (cardiopulmonary resuscitation or CPR). *All* office personnel should be required as a part of their employment process to receive certification at the BLS-provider level–C course (American Heart Association) at least once a year. Include BLS training as a part of the job description for every member of the dental office staff. The ability of a fellow worker to administer BLS could be a life assurance policy for you!

The ability of all staff members to perform basic life support effectively represents the single most important step in preparation of the dental office staff for medical emergencies. In all emergency situations, without exception, initial management will always entail the application, as needed, of the steps of basic life support. The technique of basic life support will be described in Chapters 5 and 30. Most emergency situations that occur in dental practice will be readily manageable through the use of these steps. Drug therapy is always relegated to a secondary role.

Advanced cardiac life support. Interestingly, and soberingly, statistics from the American Heart Association and other sources[6,7] have demonstrated that the application of basic life support alone does not provide the victim of an out-of-hospital cardiac arrest with a great chance of survival. Survival rates of only 16% are found when BLS is initiated promptly and efficiently, but implementation of further, more advanced steps of advanced cardiac life support (ACLS) is delayed for more than 16 minutes. Though 16% may appear a dismal rate of survival, it contrasts dramatically with the 0% survival rate when BLS is not employed. In Seattle, King County Washington,[7] on the other hand, survival rates for out-of-hospital cardiac arrest victims reached 43% because of the combination of rapid implementation of BLS and the more ready availability (<8 minutes) of ACLS.

These figures have been used by some in medicine and dentistry to argue against the requirement that dentists and physicians be CPR-certified for licensure. This argument is faulty for two reasons: first and foremost because CPR (BLS) is not only used in situations of cardiac arrest.* In fact it is likely that most health professionals working outside of a hospital may never find themselves in a situation where all three steps of BLS are necessary (i.e., as with cardiac arrest). However, it is a virtual certainty that *all* health professionals, especially dentists, will be required on multiple occasions during their careers to employ airway management and on fewer occasions to maintain breathing in the management of medical emergencies other than cardiac arrest.

The second reason that CPR should be a requirement for dental licensure is that dentists are one of the four groups of health professionals who

---

*The author prefers to call this technique basic life support (BLS) instead of cardiopulmonary resuscitation (CPR) for this same reason. The term *CPR* conjures up the picture of a cardiac arrest victim on whom chest compression is being performed. In reality it is airway and breathing that are, without doubt, the most often used steps of basic life support, thus the author's preference for BLS.

are permitted to learn and administer ACLS. Though the author does not advocate mandatory ACLS for dentists or for physicians (though there are some groups for whom such training should be required, as described shortly), it is a plain and simple fact that ACLS is not effective in the absence of adequate BLS.

Training in advanced cardiac life support should be considered, especially by dentists who practice in more remote areas of the country where emergency medical assistance is less readily available. Advanced cardiac life support training involves the following:

- Adjuncts for airway control and ventilation (including intubation)
- Patient monitoring and dysrhythmia recognition
- Defibrillation and synchronized cardioversion
- Cardiovascular pharmacology
- Acid-base balance maintenance
- Venipuncture
- Resuscitation of infants, including the newborn

Although not essential for all dentists, the knowledge of and ability to use these techniques in emergency situations is invaluable. Advanced cardiac life support programs are usually given by hospitals under the sponsorship of the American Heart Association. Such training is especially valuable for doctors employing parenteral sedation or general anesthetic techniques in their offices. For information concerning ACLS training, contact your local American Heart Association affiliate or the in-service training department of a nearby hospital.

Team Management

With all office personnel trained in the recognition and management of life-threatening situations, it is possible for each person to maintain the life of a victim alone or as a member of a trained emergency team. Although management of most emergencies is possible with a single rescuer, the combined efforts of several trained persons are usually more efficient. Because most dental offices will have more than one staff person present during working hours (when most emergencies would logically occur), a team approach to management is possible.

The emergency team consists of a minimum of two or three members, each having a predefined role in the management of the emergency. The doctor will usually lead the team and will be responsible for directing the actions of all other team members.

Team member 1 is the person, usually the doctor, who is with the victim when the emergency situation is noticed or who first reaches the victim. The primary task assigned to member 1 is the initiation of the steps of basic life support (**A**irway **B**reathing **C**irculation), as indicated by physical assessment of the victim. The other task assigned to member 1 is to activate the office emergency system by calling for help to alert other office personnel to the need for assistance (in the hospital this signal might be "code blue"). Member 1 should remain with the victim throughout the emergency unless relieved by another team member. If the initial person at the scene of the incident is not the doctor, the doctor will assume the role of team member 1 on arrival at the scene.

Duties of team member 1:
Provide basic life support as indicated
Stay with victim
Alert office staff

Team member 2 is responsible for gathering up the emergency kit and portable oxygen system. This equipment must be kept in a convenient, readily accessible place during usual office hours. This person is also assigned to regularly check the supply of emergency drugs and oxygen to be certain they will be readily available and current when needed (see discussion of emergency drugs and equipment in this chapter). When an emergency does occur, team member 2 will immediately bring this material to the site of the emergency. In the absence of a third team member, member 2 will assume the duties listed for member 3.

Duties of team member 2:
Bring emergency kit and oxygen to site of emergency
Check oxygen daily
Check emergency kit weekly

Team member 3 will act as a circulating nurse or assistant. For example, a chairside assistant working alongside the doctor will serve in this capacity if the patient is the victim. In another situation, member 3 may be the next person to come to the aid of member 1. Primary assignments for member 3 are to assist member 1 with basic life support as required; monitor the vital signs of the victim (blood pressure, heart rate and rhythm, respirations); and otherwise assist as needed, such as preparing emergency drugs for administration (and in certain situations even administering them), positioning the victim, loosening a collar or belt, or activating the EMS (emergency medical services) system by dialing 9-1-1 or the appropriate telephone number. In the absence of other tasks to perform, member 3 will keep a written chronological record of all events, such as vital signs, drug administration, and patient response to this treatment. In a large medical office building, member 3 may be sent to the building's main entrance to meet the rescuers and hold an elevator (if necessary) for their use.

Duties of team member 3:

Assist with basic life support
Monitor vital signs
Prepare emergency drugs for administration
Activate EMS system
Assist as needed
Keep records
Meet rescue team at building entrance

It is important that all office personnel be capable of joining the team. In addition, all team members should be able to carry out any of the functions of the entire team. Practice thus becomes a vitally important factor.

Emergency Practice Drills

If life-threatening situations occurred with any regularity in dentistry, there would be little need for emergency practice sessions. Team members would receive their training under actual emergency conditions. Fortunately, life-threatening situations do not occur with any frequency. Because of this, members of the dental office emergency team quickly become "rusty" from the lack of opportunity to use their newly gained knowledge and skills. For this reason, annual refresher courses are invaluable in maintaining the overall knowledge of the team. Of even greater importance, however, is the ability of the team to perform well in the office setting. In-office emergency drills are a means of maintaining an efficient emergency team in the absence of true emergency situations. On an irregular basis, the doctor may stage a simulated life-threatening situation. All members of the team should be able to respond exactly as they must under emergency conditions. Many doctors have even purchased mannequins for practicing cardiopulmonary resuscitation and hold frequent practice sessions for all staff members.

A recent addition as a teaching aid in this area are videotapes that provide the entire office staff with visual examples of emergency situations and their management in the dental environment.[8,9] In addition, these tapes demonstrate the manner in which emergency drugs are prepared and administered.

An example of an emergency situation and the team approach to its management follows: The doctor is preparing to administer a local anesthetic to a patient. As the syringe is inserted in the patient's mouth, the patient loses consciousness. The doctor (member 1) calls the other members of the team (with a code word or communication device, such as a light or buzzer). Member 2, an assistant working in the back room, gets the portable oxygen supply and the emergency drug kit and brings them to the site of the emergency, while member 3, the chairside assistant working with the doctor, remains with the doctor and victim, ready to assist as needed. Member 1, in this case the doctor in charge of the situation, initiates basic life support by positioning the victim and establishing a patent airway. Member 3 monitors the victim's vital signs, first recording the heart rate (carotid, brachial, or radial pulse). Under the doctor's supervision, member 2 prepares the oxygen for possible use and locates the aromatic ammonia vaporoles. If possible, member 3 will record in chronological fashion the management of this situation. Should the victim not regain consciousness in a reasonable period of time, member 2 or 3 will be sent to activate the emergency medical services system, meet the emergency personnel (extremely important in a large facility or office building), and escort them to the site of the emergency. Should emergency drug administration be considered necessary, it is the doctor who should, if at all possible, administer the drugs. Should this not be possible (e.g., when airway management is difficult), the author has absolutely no difficulty in assigning a member of the auxiliary staff to administer the drug under supervision.

The remaining sections of this book will provide the dental staff with the proper knowledge of how to prevent, recognize, and manage these situations. It is only through repeated practice, however, that efficiency can be expected in these difficult circumstances.

Office Preparation
Medical Assistance

There are two items to consider in this area: first, whom to call when help is needed, and second, when to call them.

Whom to call? Although most office emergencies are readily manageable by the office emergency team, there may be occasion to seek additional assistance. It is important that this matter be given consideration by the doctor *before* a situation actually develops in which assistance is needed. These emergency telephone numbers must be readily available and conspicuously displayed by all telephones in the dental office. Persons and their telephone numbers to be considered for inclusion are: local emergency medical services (EMS), a well-trained (in emergency care) dental or medical professional in close proximity to the office, an emergency ambulance service, and a nearby hospital emergency room.

Most communities in the United States, and increasingly in other countries throughout the world, have instituted the use of a universal emergency number, 9-1-1*, to expedite activation of the EMS. Though present in varying degrees of sophistication, this number connects the caller to an emergency operator who screens the call (fire, police, medical) and activates the appropriate response. When emergency medical care is required in the dental office, the community EMS is the preferred source for immediate assistance. However, since not all areas have as yet instituted the 9-1-1 system, proper emergency telephone numbers must be posted.

When contacting the EMS operator, it is important for the caller to try to remain calm and to clearly give the operator any and all requested information. This may include the nature of the emergency in general terms (e.g., consciousness, unconsciousness, chest pain, or seizures) and the location of the emergency (office address). For this reason, the address of the dental office should also be posted by every telephone in the office. Should the doctor's office be located in a large professional building, a member of the staff should be sent to the main entrance to the building to (1) hold an elevator for immediate use by emergency personnel and (2) escort them directly to the appropriate office.

A well-trained dental or medical professional can also serve as a source of assistance in an emergency. It is important, however, to discuss this arrangement before its actual need. Be absolutely certain that the person called in for assistance is, in fact, well-trained in emergency medicine and likely to be available during office hours. It has been my experience that the best-trained individuals in emergency medicine are emergency medicine physicians, anesthesiologists (both MD and DDS), surgeons (MD), and oral and maxillofacial surgeons (DDS). Unfortunately, the first two groups of physicians are hospital-based and are not readily available for assistance outside of the hospital. However, most surgeons (MD), oral and maxillofacial surgeons (DDS), and dentist anesthesiologists maintain private practices in the community and may

---

*It is important to note that the telephone number for emergency medical services is 9-1-1 (nine-one-one) and not 911 (nine-eleven). In moments of panic persons may not think clearly and will be unable to locate the 11 (eleven) on the telephone pad. There have been a number of recorded incidents in which this precise problem has led to the delayed arrival (or nonarrival) of EMS personnel and the death of the victim.

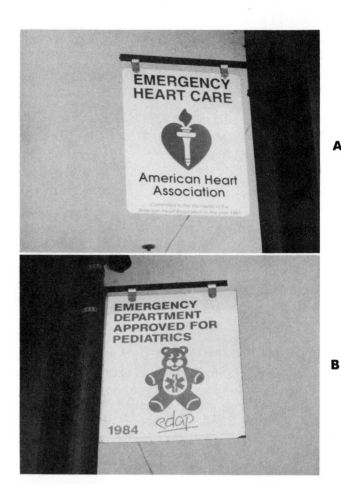

Fig. 3-1. A, Emergency heart care seal from American Heart Association. **B,** Pediatric emergency care seal.

be available. Prior arrangement with these persons will avoid potential misunderstandings and increase their potential usefulness in emergency situations in your office.

Many emergency ambulance services require that their personnel be trained as emergency medical technicians (EMTs). This can be an alternate source of assistance should the other sources be unavailable. The degree of assistance available in this case will vary, ranging from basic life support only, to advanced cardiac life support.

The location of the hospital closest to the dental office should be determined; it should have a 24-hour emergency department staffed with fully trained emergency personnel. It is also recommended that all staff members determine the nearest fully equipped hospital emergency room to their place of residence. The American Heart Association (AHA) evaluates hospital emergency departments and provides a list of AHA-approved sites (Fig. 3-1).

Emergency medical services (9-1-1)

Nearby MD or DDS well-trained in emergency medicine

Ambulance service

Nearby hospital with AHA-approved emergency department

When to call? When should assistance be sought to aid in the management of an emergency situation? Quite simply put, it is prudent to seek outside assistance when you (as team member 1) feel that the situation has gotten the upper hand—when, despite your efforts, the condition of the victim has not improved. Seeking assistance is more than justified in this situation; it is the appropriate action to take. If, conversely, the victim appears to improve, that is, the skin or mucous membranes become more pink, blood pressure increases, wheezing or seizures cease, chest pain stops, or consciousness returns, then you may elect to continue with your emergency management without seeking outside assistance. The question of when to seek outside assistance is a very personal one. The doctor's prior training, experience, and personality will dictate the need to summon assistance. Always remember that it is better to err on the side of caution—to seek help a little too soon rather than a little too late.

As soon as team member 1 feels it is necessary

Sooner is always better than later

Emergency Drugs and Equipment

Emergency drugs and equipment must be available in every dental office. In a recent survey of 2704 dentists in the United States and Canada, 84% had emergency drugs and kits available.[10]

Although most emergency situations do not demand the administration of drugs, in other situations drug utilization may prove to be life-saving. In the acute systemic allergic response (anaphylaxis), the administration of epinephrine is essential. In most other situations, however, drug administration will play a secondary role to the steps of basic life support in overall management.

Commercial versus homemade emergency kits. A number of emergency kits are produced commercially for sale to the dental and medical professions. Though some of these kits are rather well designed, others are not and contain drugs and equipment of little practical value in a typical medical or dental office. These kits are produced after discussion between the manufacturer and persons who are considered experts in this field. The drugs and equipment found in these kits all too often reflect the personal expertise of these individuals, but not the level of training of the doctor for whom it is designed.

The Council on Dental Therapeutics[11] of the American Dental Association issued a report on the subject of drug emergency kits in October, 1973. The following statement, equally true in 1992, is excerpted from this report:

"None of these kits is compatible with the needs of all practitioners, and their promotion is sometimes misleading. All dentists must be prepared to diagnose and treat expeditiously life-threatening emergencies that may arise in their practices. The best way to accomplish this objective is by taking continuing education courses on the subject of emergencies to remain informed on current practices recommended for handling emergencies in the office. A false sense of security may be engendered by the purchase of a kit if the purchaser presumes that it will fulfill all the needs of an emergency situation. The most important factors in the effective treatment of emergencies are the knowledge, judgment, and preparedness of the dentist . . . Since emergency kits should be individualized to meet the special needs and capabilities of each clinician, no stereotyped kit can be approved by the Council on Dental Therapeutics. Practitioners are encouraged to assemble their own individual kit that will be safe and effective in their hands or to purchase a kit that contains drugs that they are fully trained to administer."

Figs. 3-2 through 3-7 illustrate a variety of commercially available and self-made emergency kits.

The most desirable approach to emergency drug kits for the dental office is for the doctor to prepare a kit that is individualized to meet his or her special requirements and capabilities. In the author's experience, commercially prepared emergency kits are quickly placed in a cabinet where they will not be touched until they are needed. The doctor and staff do not spend any time familiarizing themselves with the contents of the kit or the indications for the use of these agents, and the emergency kit quickly becomes a security blanket. It is there, ready for use, but in many instances it will prove useless when needed because the doctor and staff are unfamiliar with the kit. Worse yet, the doctor might be tempted to use it when he or she is not familiar with the drug or the nature of a patient's problem. This is the primary reason the author advocates homemade kits. By preparing an individualized kit, the doctor will of necessity become familiar with all of the drugs and equipment included in it. This intimate knowledge will prove to be of immense benefit when the doctor is called on to use the kit during an emergency situation.

Items included in the emergency kit will be selected based upon the doctor's training in emer-

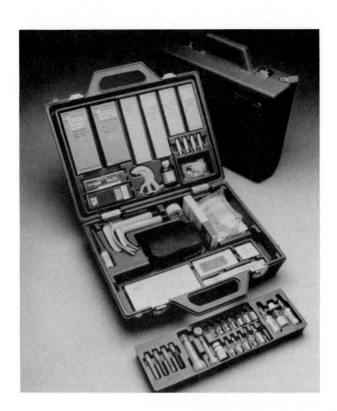

Fig. 3-2. Banyan STAT KIT 600 (Courtesy Banyan International Corporation, Abilene, Texas 79601).

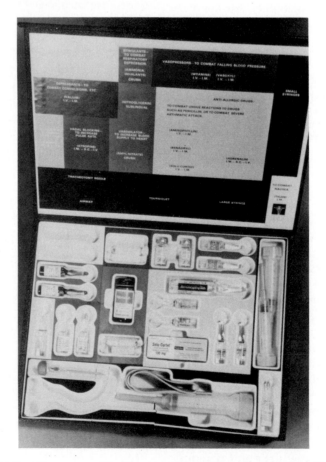

Fig. 3-3. Healthfirst Emergency Kit (Courtesy Healthfirst Corporation, Edmonds, WA).

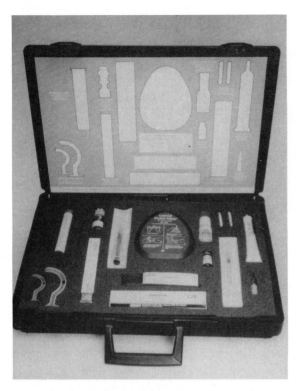

Fig. 3-4. Vital response crisis management system (Courtesy Block Drug Company, Jersey City, NJ).

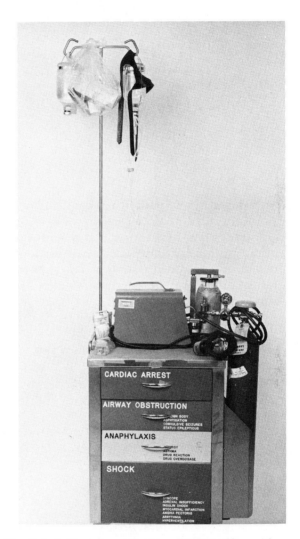

Fig. 3-6. Self-made emergency kit for office with personnel who are well trained in emergency medicine.

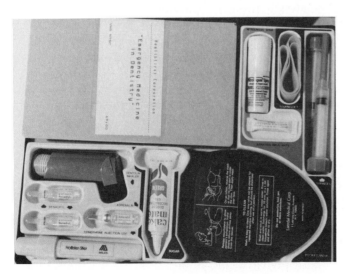

Fig. 3-5. SM-1 emergency drug kit (Courtesy Healthfirst Corporation, Edmonds, WA).

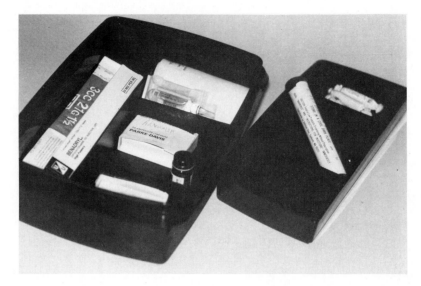

Fig. 3-7. Basic, self-made drug emergency kit.

gency medicine, the importance of the drug in the successful outcome of the situation, and in some cases by regulations that provide a list of mandatory drugs and equipment. The latter is usually found in specialty practice, such as anesthesiology or parenteral sedation,[1] oral surgery,[2] pedodontics,[3] and periodontology.

EMERGENCY DRUG KITS

The dental office emergency kit need not, and indeed should not, be complicated. It ought to remain as simple to use as possible. Pallasch's statement[12] that "complexity in a time of adversity breeds chaos" is all too true.

Remember:

1. Drugs are *not* necessary for the immediate management of most emergencies.
2. Primary management of all emergency situations is basic life support (BLS).
3. When in doubt, *never* medicate.

The emergency kit described in the following sections is a simple organized collection of drugs and equipment that has been found to be highly effective in managing those life-threatening situations requiring the administration of drugs. However, it cannot be emphasized too much that in most emergency situations drugs are not necessary for the proper management of a patient. First and foremost in the management of these situations will be the steps of basic life support. It is only after these steps have been employed that the doctor should consider the administration of drugs. Even in the acute anaphylactic reaction in which there is immediate respiratory embarrassment or circulatory collapse or both, basic life support constitutes

the immediate response followed almost as rapidly by the administration of epinephrine.

Management of emergency situations will then follow the A-B-C-D protocol: **A**irway, **B**reathing, **C**irculation, **D**rugs.

What should be included in the emergency kit? The following guidelines will be useful in the development of a useful and effective dental office emergency kit. Specific categories of drugs will be listed, with suggestions for specific agents within each grouping offered, along with an explanation of the selection criteria for each drug mentioned.

All of the categories of drugs presented here should be considered for inclusion in the emergency kit; however, the doctor should select only those drugs with which he or she is familiar and that they are able to employ. Suggested drugs are listed with alternatives presented in many instances. The doctor must carefully evaluate everything that goes into the office emergency kit. If doubt remains concerning any of the categories or specific agents, consult first with a physician (preferably a specialist in emergency medicine) or a hospital pharmacist, but above all determine their reasons for suggesting a certain drug over another one.

All drugs come with a package insert. Save this insert from each drug included in your kit, read it, and make note of important information concerning the drug, such as indications, usual dose (both pediatric and adult), adverse reactions, and expiration date. Many doctors transfer this information to a 3-by-5- card for quick reference.

The emergency drugs and equipment described in the following sections will be presented in four levels or modules. These modules are based upon the level of training and experience in emergency medicine possessed by the doctor.

- Module one—basic emergency kit (critical drugs and equipment)
- Module two—noncritical drugs and equipment
- Module three—advanced cardiac life support
- Module four—antidotal drugs

For each of the four modules, two categories of drug will be described: (1) injectable drugs and (2) noninjectable drugs, as well as emergency equipment. In reading the following material, always remember that the types of drugs and equipment included in the emergency kit must be appropriate for the level of training of the office personnel who will be using it. Simple but effective is the goal to work toward in preparing an emergency kit. The KISS principle (keep it simple, stupid) is quite applicable in this situation. A complete description of when and how each item is to be employed will be presented in the sections on management of specific emergencies.

The drugs and equipment included in the emergency kit to be described are intended for use with either the adult or pediatric patient. The primary distinction between their use in these patients will be the therapeutic dose of the drug to be administered, pediatric doses being somewhat smaller than adult doses. Specific dosages of drugs will not be emphasized in this chapter, rather, they will be presented in the section on the management of each emergency situation.

Most injectable emergency drugs are prepared in a 1-mL ampule or vial. The number of milligrams of drug present in 1 mL of solution will vary from drug to drug. For example, diazepam is 5 mg/mL, whereas diphenhydramine is 50 mg/mL, and ephedrine 10 mg/mL. This 1-mL form of the drug is called the *therapeutic dose* or the *unit dose.* Thus, 1 mL of solution will be the usual dose of the drug administered to the adult patient in an emergency situation. For pediatric patients aged 1 year through 8 years, the dose of injectable drug is 0.5 mL or one half of the adult dose, whereas for infants under the age of 1 year, the equivalent dose is 0.25 mL, one quarter of the adult dose (Table 3-1).

One major exception to this basic dosing statement is epinephrine. Although the 1-mL form of 1:1000 epinephrine is considered the adult therapeutic dose, a smaller dose—0.3 to 0.5 mL—is initially recommended, with subsequent doses based on the patient's response. Pediatric and infant doses of epinephrine are reduced accordingly.

Noninjectable drugs are usually prepared in a

Table 3-1. Injectable drug dosages

	Age range (years)	mL (cc) of solution	Epinephrine (1:1000) (mL)
Adult	>8	1.0	0.3-0.5
Child	1-8	0.5	0.15-0.25
Infant	<1	0.25	0.075-0.125

manner such that one tablet or one spray is the adult therapeutic dose. Many noninjectables are prepared in pediatric dosage forms for simplicity of administration. In the dental office in which both adults and children are treated, both forms of the agents should be considered for inclusion in the emergency kit.

Items of emergency equipment should also be available in both adult and pediatric sizes. These items include the face mask, and the oropharyngeal and nasopharyngeal airways (if included). Indeed, the pediatric dentist must have a wider range of equipment available, in both pediatric (for the patient-victim) and adult (for the doctor- or staff-victim) sizes, than the doctor who does not treat younger patients.

Administration of Injectable Drugs

How and where are these injectable drugs to be administered to the victim? For a drug to exert a therapeutic action a minimum therapeutic blood level must be achieved in the target organ (such as the brain or heart) or target system. In other words, enough of the drug has to get into the bloodstream and then be transported to the part of the body in which it is needed. With this in mind, then, the ideal technique of emergency drug administration will be the intravenous (IV) technique. Onset of action is quite rapid (approximately 20 seconds), and the drug effect is the most reliable using this route of administration. Unfortunately, unless an IV line has been established in this patient before the onset of the emergency, it often becomes quite difficult if not impossible to secure an IV line during an emergency. Unless the doctor is quite adept at venipuncture, this route, although the most nearly ideal, ought not be considered. Emergency medications may be administered intramuscularly (IM) into various sites, most often the anterolateral aspect of the thigh (vastus lateralis), the mid-deltoid region of the upper arm, and the upper-outer quadrant of the gluteal region. Onset of drug action may be expected in about 10 minutes (given normal tissue perfusion, somewhat slower with decreased blood pressure). Of these three traditional IM injection sites, the mid-deltoid region provides the most rapid uptake of most medications (a result

Fig. 3-8. A, Intralingual injection—intraoral approach. **B,** Intralingual injection—extraoral approach.

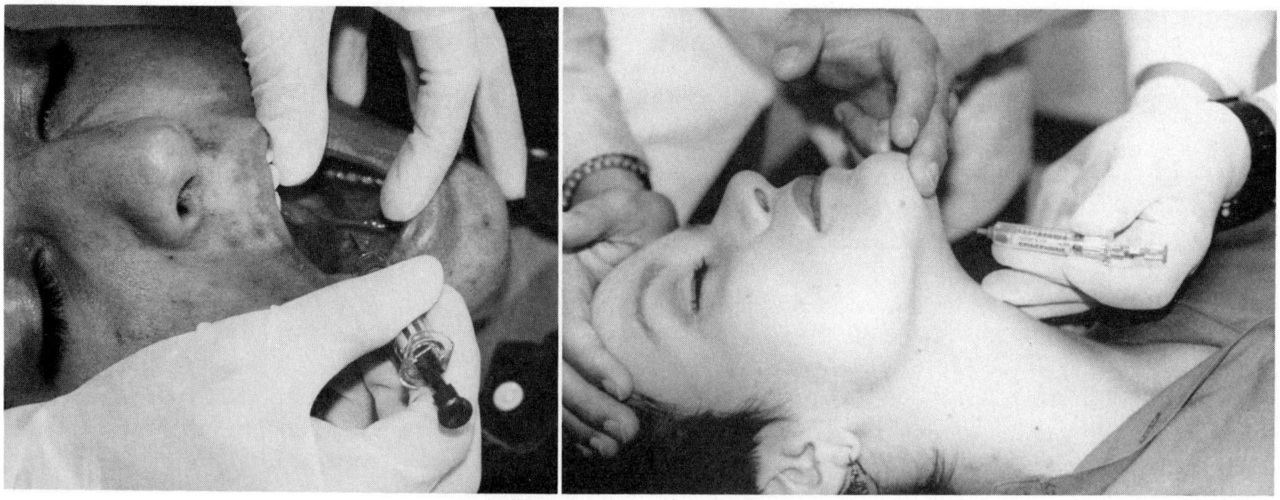

of greater tissue perfusion) and is therefore the site of choice, with the vastus lateralis a very close second because of its accessibility and anatomical safety. Indeed, in the younger pediatric patient the vastus lateralis represents the preferred IM injection site. The gluteal region, because of its relative lack of vascularity and its anatomical considerations (especially in the pediatric patient) should not be employed for emergency drug administration.

One additional site provides a somewhat more effective and more rapid uptake than even the mid-deltoid region: the tongue. Emergency medications can be injected into the body of the tongue or into the sublingual region with every expectation of a somewhat more rapid uptake and onset of clinical action. The drug may be administered into the body of the tongue or into the floor of the mouth, either intraorally (Fig. 3-8*A*) or extraorally (Fig. 3-8*B*). Onset of action is approximately 5 to 10 minutes if there is effective circulation, somewhat slower with hypotension.

The steps of basic life support must always be continued as needed while the emergency team awaits the onset of the drug's action. Remember that in the absence of effective circulation, neither intravenously nor intramuscularly administered drugs will be effective. In this situation (as in all emergency situations), drugs ought not be the first consideration in treatment—the implementation of the ABCs of basic life support should take precedence.

When possible, there is another route of drug administration that provides an onset of action somewhat faster than even the intravenous route.

In situations in which a patient has been successfully intubated, the administration of certain drugs into the endotracheal tube will provide an extremely rapid response as the drug is absorbed from the highly perfused pulmonary vascular bed. Drugs that may be administered via the endotracheal tube are epinephrine, lidocaine, atropine, and naloxone.

Parenteral Drug Administration

The different routes of drug administration are outlined in the accompanying box.

Virtually all injectable emergency drugs can be purchased preloaded in syringes. The author feels strongly that these drugs *not* be available in this preloaded form in the typical dental office because they become too easy to administer.* In most emergencies, there is absolutely no urgent need to administer any drug other than oxygen to the victim. The only critical drug the author recommends having available in a preloaded form is epinephrine, because in the acute allergic reaction this drug needs to be administered as promptly as possible. With only this one drug available in a preloaded form in the emergency kit, there will be less confusion over drug selection in a time of possibly near panic. Advance cardiac life support drugs are nor-

---

*In dental offices in which the doctor is thoroughly conversant with emergency drugs and their administration and has a well-trained emergency team, well-labeled preloaded syringes of emergency drugs are more appropriate. This situation is most apt to be found when the doctor has been trained in the techniques of general anesthesia or, in certain instances, intravenous sedation.

ROUTE OF DRUG ADMINISTRATION
(BY RATE OF ONSET)

1. Endotracheal (when available): epinephrine, lidocaine, atropine, naloxone only
2. Intravenous
3. Sublingual or intralingual
4. Intramuscular
   a. Vastus lateralis
   b. Mid-deltoid
   c. Gluteal region

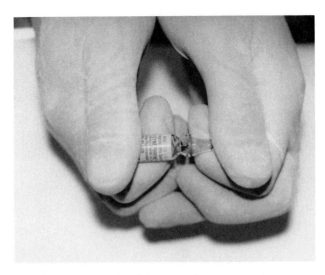

Fig. 3-9. Ampule, held between fingers, cracks at prescored neck.

mally available in preloaded form but should be kept separate from the other emergency drugs. It takes time to prepare a drug for administration in a syringe, time that might be better spent in basic management of the patient (i.e., by following ABC) and not in the administration of drugs that may be inappropriate to administer at that time.

Preparation of Drugs for Parenteral Administration

To prepare an injectable emergency drug for either intramuscular or intravenous administration, the rescuer breaks the unit dose ampule by covering the prescored neck with a gauze pad (Fig. 3-9), and then loads the syringe with the medication (Fig. 3-10). Always identify the name of the drug and its dosage prior to loading the syringe by checking its printed label. This is especially important with certain drugs, such as epinephrine, naloxone, and meperidine, which are available in more than one dosage form. When time permits (in nonurgent situations), a label should be applied to the loaded syringe that contains the name and concentration (in mg/mL) of the drug in the syringe. The technique of intramuscular drug administration and of venipuncture is summarized here, but is reviewed in depth in other texts.[13]

Intramuscular Administration

1. Cleanse the area of needle insertion.
2. Grab the muscle and pull it away from the bone (Fig. 3-11).
3. Holding the syringe like a dart, quickly insert the needle into the muscle mass to a depth of approximately 1 inch (one half the length of the needle, Fig. 3-12).
4. Aspirate to ensure nonvascular penetration.
5. Quickly administer the drug.
6. Remove the syringe, placing a dry gauze under pressure at the injection site for a minimum of 1 to 2 minutes.

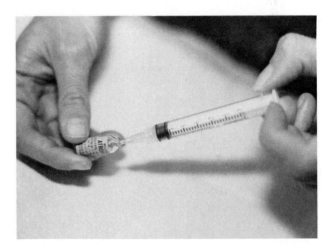

Fig. 3-10. Syringe is loaded with medication.

7. Rubbing the area may increase vascularity and somewhat speed the rate of drug absorption.

Intravenous Administration

1. Place a tourniquet above the antecubital fossa (Fig. 3-13).
2. If possible, have the patient open and close the fist to help distend the vein (Fig. 3-14).
   a. When the patient cannot open and close his or her fist (as with the unconscious or noncooperative patient) the arm should be placed below the level of the patient's heart to help distend the veins (Fig. 3-15).

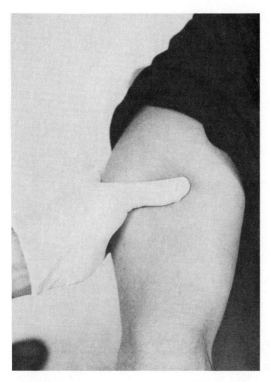

Fig. 3-11. Intramuscular injection—muscle pulled away from bone.

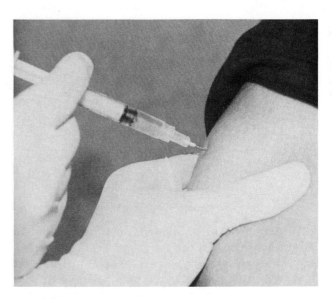

Fig. 3-12. Intramuscular injection—syringe held like dart, needle advanced 1 inch into tissue.

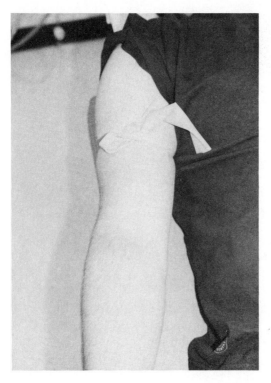

Fig. 3-13. Intravenous tourniquet placed above antecubital fossa.

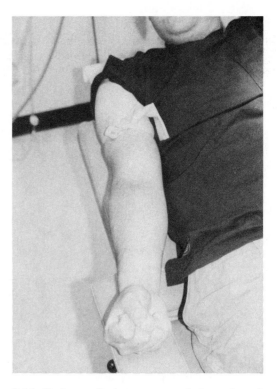

Fig. 3-14. Patient asked to open and then close fist to help distend veins.

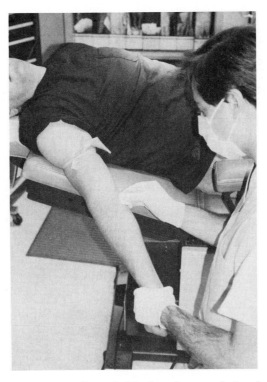

Fig. 3-15. Veins may be distended by keeping arm below level of heart.

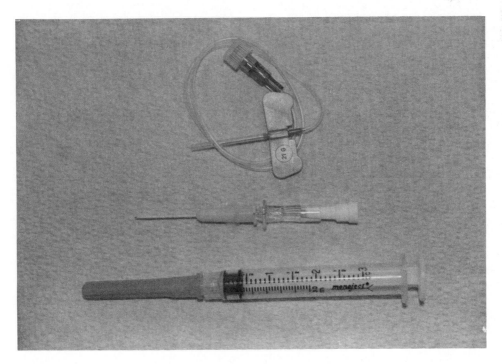

Fig. 3-16. Scalp vein needle, indwelling catheter, and syringe (top to bottom).

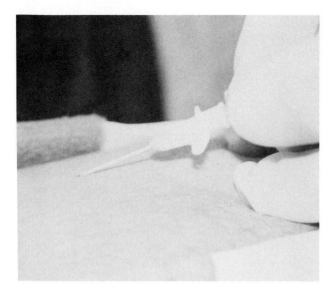

Fig. 3-17. Needle held at 30° angle for penetration of skin.

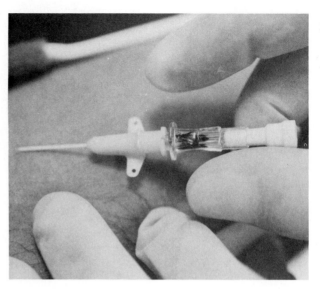

Fig. 3-18. Return of blood into needle is sign of successful venipuncture.

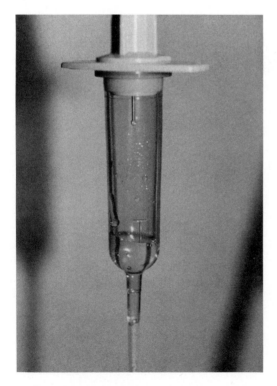

Fig. 3-19. Infusion set for continuous intravenous infusion.

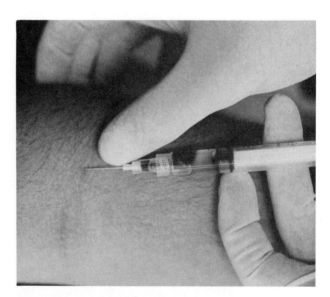

Fig. 3-20. Needle/syringe in vein. Drug injected directly into vein.

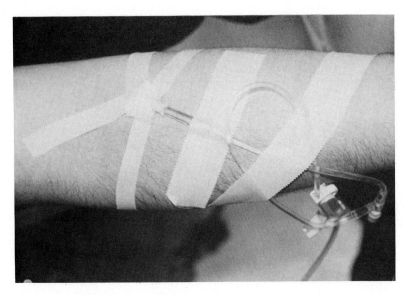

Fig. 3-21. Continuous infusion secured by tape.

3. Cleanse and then dry the area in which the venipuncture is to be placed.
4. Use an indwelling catheter, scalp vein needle, or syringe (Fig. 3-16), with the bevel of the needle facing up, held at about a 30° to 45° angle to the vein to be entered (Fig. 3-17).
5. Advance the needle into the vein until a return of blood is noted (Fig. 3-18).
   Note: the return of blood into the needle is the only consistent sign of a successful venipuncture.
6. Remove the tourniquet and either start the intravenous infusion (Fig. 3-19) or administer the desired drug (Fig. 3-20).
7. Secure the needle with tape to maintain venous access (Fig. 3-21).

Module One: Critical (Essential) Emergency Drugs and Equipment (Table 3-2)

What constitutes the minimum (absolutely basic) emergency kit for a dental or medical office? As always, basic life support training is the most significant asset and the first technique to be used in emergency management. However, there are a number of injectable and noninjectable drugs and items of equipment that must be considered as absolutely essential for inclusion in the emergency kit of the properly prepared dental office. These items will be listed followed by an in-depth discussion about each.

Injectable Drugs

There are two categories of injectable drugs that are considered to be critical in any emergency kit. Both of these drugs are employed for the man-agement of the same emergency—acute allergy—one of the most feared of all emergency situations faced by the health professional.
1. Epinephrine
2. Antihistamine
Noninjectable Drugs: There are two noninjectable drugs that are also considered to be critical:
1. Oxygen
2. Vasodilator
Emergency equipment: Critical items of emergency equipment include:
1. Oxygen delivery system
2. Suction and suction tips
3. Tourniquets
4. Syringes

Primary injectable: drug for acute allergic reaction

Drug of choice: Epinephrine
Drug class: Natural catecholamine
Alternative drug: None available

Epinephrine (Adrenalin) is the drug of choice for the management of the acute allergic reaction. Epinephrine will be of primary value in the management of the respiratory and cardiovascular manifestations of allergic reactions. Desirable properties of this agent include a rapid onset of action; potent action as a bronchial smooth muscle dilator (beta$_2$ properties); antihistaminic actions; vasopressor actions; and its actions on the heart, which include an increased heart rate (21%), increased systolic blood pressure (5%), decreased diastolic blood pressure (14%), increased cardiac output (51%), and increased coronary blood flow. Undesirable actions include its tendency to predispose

Table 3-2. Module one—critical (essential) drugs and equipment

Category	Primary drug		Alternative	Recommended for kit	
	Generic	Proprietary		Quantity	Availability
Injectables					
Antiallergy	Epinephrine	Adrenalin	None	1 preloaded syringe *and* 3-4 1-mL ampules	1:1000 (1 mg/mL)
Antihistamine	Chlorpheniramine	Chlor-Trimeton	Diphenhydramine	2-3 1-ml ampules	10 mg/mL
Noninjectables					
Oxygen	Oxygen	Oxygen	None	Minimum of 1 "E" cylinder	
Vasodilator	Nitroglycerin	Nitrolingual spray	Nitrostat tablets	1 spray bottle	0.4 mg/dose

Equipment	Description	Quantity for office
Emergency equipment		
Oxygen delivery system	Positive pressure/demand valve, *or* bag-valve-mask device and clear full face masks of various sizes	Minimum of one O$_2$ delivery system Minimum of 1 small (child) and 1 large (adult) mask
	Pocket mask is recommended for all office employees	1 pocket mask per employee
Suction and suction tips	High-volume suction system	Office suction system
	Large diameter, round-ended suction tips or tonsillar suction	Minimum of two
Syringes for drug administration	Disposable syringes	2-3 2-mL syringes with attached needle for parenteral drug administration
Tourniquets	Rubber or Velcro tourniquet, rubber tubing, or sphygmomanometer	Minimum of 1, up to 3
Magill intubation forceps	Magill intubation forceps	One forceps

the heart to dysrhythmias and its relatively short duration of action.

Therapeutic indications: Acute allergic reactions (see Chapter 24); acute asthmatic attacks (see also noninjectable drugs and Chapter 13); cardiac arrest (ACLS, see Chapter 30).

Side effects, contraindications, and precautions: Tachydysrhythmias, both supraventricular and ventricular, may develop. Epinephrine should be used with caution in pregnant women because it decreases placental blood flow and may induce premature labor. When used, all vital signs must be monitored frequently. In the setting of the dental practice, epinephrine will usually be considered for administration in situations that are considered to be life threatening (anaphylaxis, cardiac arrest). Under such situations the advantages of administering this agent clearly outweigh any risk. In effect there are no contraindications to the administration of epinephrine under these conditions.

Availability: Epinephrine for parenteral administration is supplied in either a 1:1000 concentration (1g [1000 mg]/L); thus each milliliter will contain 1 mg of the agent, or as a 1:10,000 concentration (for intravenous administration). Because the dosage of this drug is critical, it is advisable to have parenteral epinephrine available in a 1-mL dosage form rather than in a multidose vial. Another factor relevant to the available dosage forms of epinephrine is time. In the acute allergic reaction, it is desirable to administer this agent as soon as possible after the onset of symptoms. It is therefore recommended that epinephrine be available in a preloaded syringe as well as in 1-mL ampules. Because of the relatively short duration of action of epinephrine, multiple administrations may be necessary during the acute phase of treatment. Unit dose (1-mL) ampules are preferred over multidose vials because the unit dose form will prevent the rescuer from inadvertently over-administering epinephrine. A little epinephrine may be life-saving, but a lot can produce additional complications.

Dose: Although the 1-mL ampule of 1:1000 epinephrine is considered to be the adult therapeutic dose, it is usual to start administration of epinephrine with 0.3 to 0.5 mL of solution, IM or subcu-

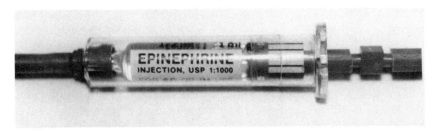

Fig. 3-22. 3-dose epinephrine syringe administers 0.3 mg per dose.

taneously (SC), with additional doses administered as needed. Unfortunately, in what may be a near-panic situation (for example, anaphylaxis or cardiac arrest) the doctor may administer an overly large dose of this agent to the victim. Preloaded syringes are available that make it impossible to administer in excess of the predetermined dose (Fig. 3-22).[14,15] The plunger on this syringe is rectangular, as is its guide channel. However, at the 0.3-mL mark the rectangle shifts 90°, making it impossible to administer more than 0.3 mL (0.3 mg) at a time. To administer an additional dose, the plunger must be rotated. Such a syringe is highly recommended for inclusion in the dental emergency drug kit. Pediatric dosage forms of these syringes are also available that deliver a pediatric dose of 0.15 mg.

Suggested for emergency kit: One preloaded syringe (1 mL of 1:1000 [1 mg epinephrine] and three to four ampules of 1:1000 epinephrine (anaphylaxis; IM, SC); also available in a preloaded syringe as 1 mg diluted in 10 mL fluid for intravenous administration 1:10,000 (cardiac arrest—ACLS; IV)

Primary injectable: antiallergy

Drug of choice: Chlorpheniramine
Drug class: Antihistamine
Alternative drug: Diphenhydramine

Antihistamines will be of value in the treatment of the delayed allergic response and in the definitive management of the acute allergic reaction (administered after epinephrine has terminated the acute life-threatening phase of the reaction). Antihistamines act as competitive antagonists of histamine. They do not prevent the release of histamine from cells in response to injury, drugs, or antigens, but do prevent access of histamine to its receptor site in the cell and thereby block the response of the effector cell to histamine. Thus, antihistamines are more potent in preventing the actions of histamine than in reversing these actions once they develop. An interesting action of many antihistamines is that they are also potent local anesthetics, diphenhydramine and tripelennamine being par-

ticularly potent in this regard.[16,17] The choice of an antihistamine for the emergency kit was made after considering that most patients seeking dental care are ambulatory and desire to leave the dental office unescorted (probably to drive a car). A potential side effect of most antihistamines is a degree of cortical depression (sedation) that will prevent the patient from leaving the dental office unescorted. Diphenhydramine HCl (Benadryl) causes sedation in nearly 50% of individuals. Chlorpheniramine (Chlor-Trimeton), on the other hand, produces less sedation (10%) than diphenhydramine for an equivalent antihistaminic action.

Therapeutic indications: Delayed allergy; definitive management of acute allergy; for local anesthesia, when history of alleged allergy to local anesthetics is present (Chapter 24)

Side effects, contraindications, and precautions: Side effects of antihistamines include central nervous system (CNS) depression, decreased blood pressure, and a thickening of bronchial secretions resulting from the drug's drying action. Antihistamines, because of this latter action, are contraindicated in the management of acute asthmatic episodes.

Availability: Chlorpheniramine, 10 mg/mL (1-mL ampule), 10 mg/mL (2-mL ampule), also in 1-mL preloaded syringe; diphenhydramine, 10 mg/mL (10- and 30-mL multidose vial), 50 mg/mL (1-mL ampule and 10-mL multidose vial); and in 1-mL preloaded syringe (50 mg/mL)

Suggested for emergency kit: Chlorpheniramine, 10 mg/mL (three to four 1-mL ampules), or diphenhydramine, 50 mg/mL (three to four 1-mL ampules); preloaded syringes of antihistamines are not recommended because there is no urgency in their administration

Critical Noninjectable Drugs

There are two noninjectable drugs that are also considered critical.
1. Oxygen
2. Vasodilator

Primary noninjectable: oxygen

Drug of choice: Oxygen
Drug class: None
Alternative drug: None

Unquestionably the most important drug in the entire emergency kit is oxygen. Oxygen is supplied in a variety of cylinder sizes but the recommended size is the E cylinder, which is quite portable. In emergency situations the E cylinder will provide oxygen for approximately 30 minutes. Larger cylinders (H cylinder) provide significantly more oxygen but are less portable; smaller cylinders (A through D) contain too little oxygen to be clinically effective for more than a short duration. Oxygen that is produced through a chemical reaction in small canisters is not adequate for an emeregncy kit and will not be considered. A portable E cylinder of oxygen should also be available in offices in which nitrous oxide-oxygen is available. Because emergencies may occur in other parts of the dental office than in the dental chair, oxygen delivery must be available anywhere within the office.

Therapeutic indications: The administration of oxygen is indicated in any emergency situation in which respiratory distress is evident.

Side effects, contraindications, and precautions: None with the emergency use of oxygen, although oxygen administration is not indicated in hyperventilation.

Availability: Compressed gas cylinders come in a variety of sizes. Portability of the oxygen cylinder is a desirable characteristic.

Suggested for emergency kit: A minimum requirement for the emergency kit is one E cylinder.

Primary noninjectable: vasodilator

Drug of choice: Nitroglycerin
Drug class: Vasodilator
Alternative drug: Amyl nitrite

Vasodilators are used in the immediate management of chest pain (such as may occur with angina pectoris or acute myocardial infarction). Two varieties of vasodilator are available: nitroglycerin (TNG) as a tablet and a spray, and an inhalant, amyl nitrite. A patient with a history of angina pectoris will usually carry a supply of nitroglycerin. Tablets remain the most popular form of TNG, although most patients prefer the translingual spray once they have used it. During dental care a patient's nitroglycerin source should be readily accessible. Placed sublingually or sprayed onto the lingual soft tissues, nitroglycerin acts in 1 to 2 minutes. A patient's drug should be used if at all possible, but if it is not available or is ineffective, the 0.4-mg dosage form should be available in the

emergency kit. The shelf life of TNG tablets once exposed to air is quite short (about 6 weeks). This is especially true when the container is not adequately sealed or the tablets are stored in a pill box. In these cases the active nitroglycerin vaporizes, leaving behind an inert filler. This is not normally a problem with patients most of whom will use a bottle of tablets in 4 to 6 weeks. Inactivation of the TNG is more likely to occur in the dental office supply where its use is extremely sporadic. Nitroglycerin tablets placed sublingually usually taste bitter and sting. Suspect that the drug has become ineffective if the bitter taste is absent.

A translingual nitroglycerin spray introduced in the United States in January 1986 (following its earlier introduction in Europe), has a significantly longer shelf life than sublingual tablets and is highly recommended for inclusion in the emergency drug kit.

Amyl nitrite, another vasodilator, is available for use as an inhalant. It is supplied in a yellow vaporole or a gray cardboard vaporole with yellow printing in a dose of 0.3 mL, which when crushed between one's fingers and held under the victim's nose will act in about 10 seconds to produce a profound vasodilation. The duration of action of amyl nitrite is shorter than that of TNG; however, the shelf life of the vaporole is considerably longer. Side effects occur with all vasodilators (see text that follows), but are more significant with amyl nitrite.

Therapeutic indications: With chest pain, as an aid in differential diagnosis; definitive management of angina pectoris (Chapter 27); in early management of acute myocardial infarction (Chapter 28); management of acute hypertensive episodes.

Side effects, contraindications, and precautions: Side effects of nitroglycerin include a transient pulsating headache, facial flushing, and a degree of hypotension (noted especially if the patient is in an upright position). Because of its mild hypotensive actions, nitroglycerin is contraindicated in patients who are hypotensive, but may be used with some degree of effectiveness in the management of acute hypertensive episodes. Because nitroglycerin as a tablet is an unstable drug (short shelf life once opened), it must be replaced, usually within 6 weeks of its initial use. Side effects of amyl nitrite are similar to but more intense than those of nitroglycerin. These include facial flushing, pounding pulse, dizziness, intense headache, and hypotension. Amyl nitrite should not be administered to patients who are in an upright position because significant postural changes develop.

Availability (Fig. 3-23): Nitroglycerin tablets, 0.1; 0.3, 0.6-mg sublingual tablets; translingual nitro-

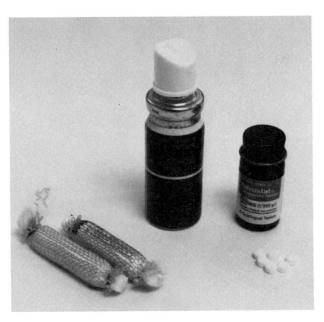

Fig. 3-23. Vasodilators.

glycerin spray (Nitrolingual, 0.4 mg/dose); amyl nitrite vaporoles (yellow), 0.3 mL

Suggested for emergency kit: One bottle of translingual nitroglycerin spray (0.4 mg) (Fig. 3-23)

Critical Emergency Equipment

Critical items of emergency equipment include:
1. Oxygen delivery system
2. Suction and suction tips
3. Tourniquets
4. Syringes

Merely having various items of emergency equipment available does not of itself make the dental office any better equipped or the staff any more prepared to manage emergency situations. Personnel expected to use this equipment must be well trained in their proper use as well as in patient selection. Unfortunately, many of the items of emergency equipment commonly found in dental and medical offices can prove to be useless or, more significantly, hazardous if employed improperly or in the wrong situation. Training in the proper use of such equipment as the laryngoscope and the oropharyngeal airway can best be obtained only by caring for patients under general anesthesia, a situation not readily available to most dental personnel. Many of the items listed in this section are therefore recommended for use only by properly trained individuals. All of the items of emergency equipment listed as secondary require special training, unfortunately, several items listed as primary also require training (such as the oxygen delivery system). Although all dentists and physicians should be trained in the use of oxygen delivery systems, courses in which these techniques are taught are particularly difficult to locate. (Readers interested in such hands-on programs should contact their local dental society, dental school, hospital, or American Heart Association affiliate—the most common providers of such training.)

It is important that dental personnel use only those pieces of emergency equipment with which they are intimately familiar and have been trained to use properly. The usefulness of the items described here will, of course, vary with the training of the office personnel. All dental personnel should become proficient in use of the primary items of equipment.

Syringes. Plastic disposable syringes equipped with an 18- or 21-gauge needle will be needed for parenteral drug administration. Although many sizes are available, the 2-mL syringe will be adequate (Fig. 3-24).

Suggested for emergency kit: Two to four 2-mL disposable syringes with an 18- or 21-gauge needle.

Tourniquets. A tourniquet will be required if intravenous drug administration is contemplated. In addition, three tourniquets will be needed for a bloodless phlebotomy in the management of acute pulmonary edema (Chapter 14). A sphygmomanometer (blood pressure cuff) may be employed as a tourniquet, as may a simple piece of latex tubing (Fig. 3-24).

Suggested for emergency kit: Three tourniquets and a sphygmomanometer

Suction and aspirating apparatus. An essential item of emergency equipment is a strong suction system and a variety of large diameter suction tips. The disposable saliva ejector is entirely inadequate in situations in which anything other than tiny objects must be evacuated from a patient's mouth. Aspiration tips should be rounded to ensure that there is little risk of bleeding should it become necessary to suction the hypopharynx. Plastic evacuators and tonsil suction tips are quite adequate for this purpose (Fig. 3-24).

Suggested for emergency kit: Two (minimum) plastic evacuators or tonsil suction tips

Magill intubation forceps. The Magill intubation forceps is designed to help place an endotracheal tube in the trachea during nasal intubation. The Magill intubation forceps is a blunt-ended scissors that has a right-angle bend in it (Fig. 3-25). This design permits the forceps to readily grasp objects that are found deep in the hypopharynx (such as the endotracheal tube).

In prior editions of this text, the Magill intubation forceps was considered a secondary item. Its

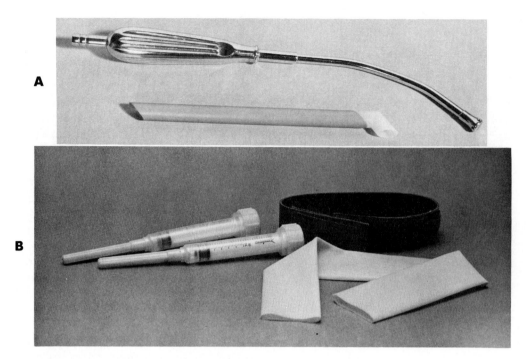

Fig. 3-24. A, and **B,** Primary emergency equipment: tourniquet, syringes, suction and suction tips.

Table 3-3. Comparison of methods of ventilation

Technique	% Oxygen
Mouth-to-mouth	16
Mouth-to-mask	16
Bag-valve-mask	21
Bag-valve-mask + O_2	>21-<100
Positive pressure mask	100

status has been upgraded to primary because of its importance and its simplicity of use. With the use of gloves now a standard for all areas of dental care, increasing numbers of reports have appeared of items of dental equipment, such as crowns and endodontic files, being dislodged and lying in the posterior region of the patient's oral cavity. There is usually nothing readily available on the instrument tray that adequately serves the purpose of retrieving such an object easily. The Magill intubation forceps is designed for just this function and is highly recommended for inclusion in the emergency kit.

Suggested for emergency kit: One Magill intubation forceps

Oxygen delivery system (Table 3-3)

Positive pressure oxygen. An oxygen delivery system adaptable to the E cylinder of oxygen allows for the delivery of positive pressure oxygen to the victim. Examples of this device include the positive pressure/demand valve (Fig. 3-26) and the reservoir bag on many inhalation sedation units. These devices should be fitted with a clear face mask, allowing for the efficient delivery of 100% O_2 to a patient while permitting the rescuer to visually inspect the mouth for the presence of foreign matter (e.g., vomitus, blood, saliva, water). Face masks should be available in several sizes (child, small adult, and large adult).

Bag-valve-mask device. A portable, self-inflating, bag-valve-mask device (Ambu-bag; PMR; Fig. 3-27) is a self-contained unit that may be easily transported to any site within the dental office. This is an important feature because not all emergences will occur within the dental operatory, and it may become necessary to resuscitate a patient in other areas, such as the waiting room or restroom. A source of positive pressure oxygen or ambient air must also be available in these areas. With either device the rescuer must be able to maintain both an airtight seal and a patent airway with one hand

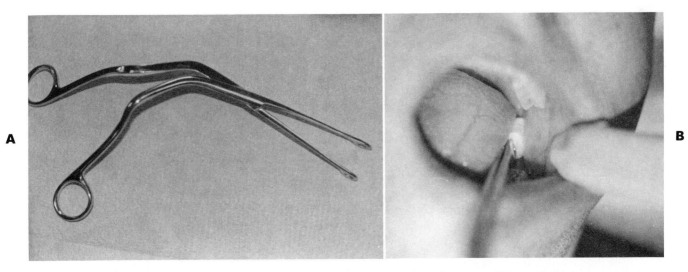

Fig. 3-25. A, Magill intubation forceps. **B,** Magill intubation forceps enable small objects to be readily removed from oral cavity.

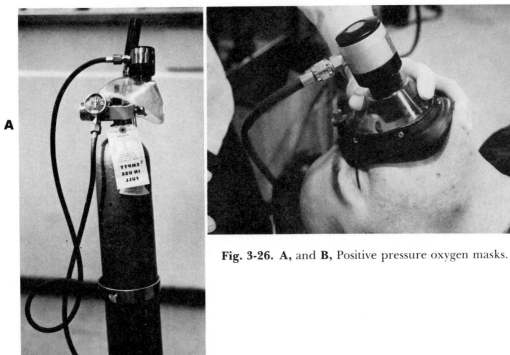

Fig. 3-26. A, and **B,** Positive pressure oxygen masks.

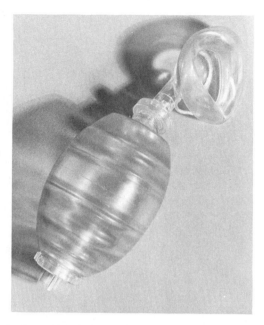

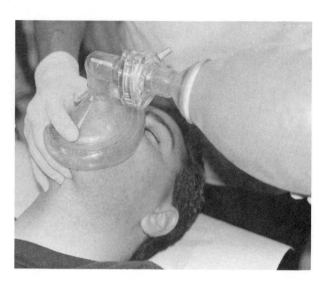

Fig. 3-28. Hand positions with bag-valve-mask device.

Fig. 3-27. Self-inflating resuscitation bag and mask. Permits delivery of atmospheric air (21% oxygen) or oxygen-enriched air. Clear face mask is preferred to opaque.

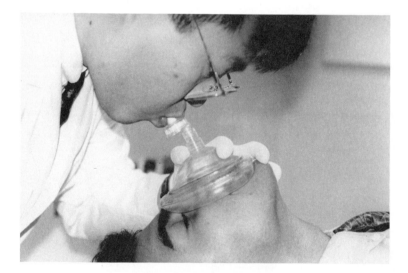

Fig. 3-29. Pocket mask.

while using the other hand to activate the device and ventilate the patient (Fig. 3-28). The bag-valve-mask device delivers either 21% O_2 or enriched O_2 (>21%, <100%), if it is attached to an oxygen delivery tube.

Pocket mask. A recent addition to the airway management armamentarium, the pocket mask (Fig. 3-29) has quickly become an integral component of emergency equipment. The pocket mask is a clear full-face mask, identical in shape and application to the positive pressure and bag-valve-mask devices. Unlike these devices however, the

rescuer applies exhaled air ventilation (16% O_2) into the inlet on the top of the mask to ventilate the victim. Exhalation occurs passively through a one-way valve located on the side of the mask. There is no rebreathing of the victim's exhaled air by the rescuer. The pocket mask is also available with a supplemental oxygen port, permitting the mask to be attached to an oxygen tube and deliver enriched oxygen ventilation.

Small enough to fit easily into a pocket or purse, the availability of a pocket mask enables a rescuer to provide mouth-to-mask ventilation to a non-

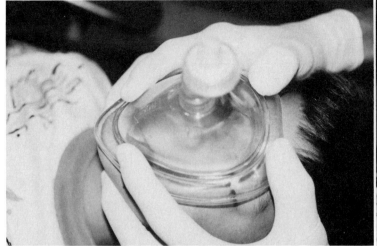
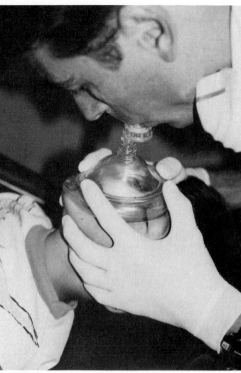

Fig. 3-30. A, B, Pocket mask for a child.

breathing victim in place of mouth-to-mouth ventilation in any rescue situation. The pocket mask may be used to ventilate the pediatric patient by simply inverting the mask (nose side held in cleft of chin; chin side in bridge of nose; Fig. 3-30). With increasing concern in the health professions over hepatitis and HIV infection from direct physical contact with bodily fluids, the pocket mask provides positive psychological support for the potential rescuer. The low cost of the mask (under $20 U.S. [10/92]) enables all dental office personnel to have their own individual pocket masks.

Suggested for emergency kit: One portable oxygen supply (E cylinder) with positive pressure mask, and/or one portable self-inflating bag-valve-mask device, and one pocket mask per staff member; several sizes of clear full-face masks must be available, such as child, small adult, large adult; other mask sizes should be available in specialty practices.

NOTE: Advanced training is required for the safe and effective use of masks used for ventilation.

Module Two: Non-critical (Secondary) Emergency Drugs and Equipment (Table 3-4)

Drugs and equipment included in this level, though important and valuable in the management of emergency situations, are not considered to be essential or critical elements of the office emergency kit. Doctors who have received training in the use of these drugs should consider their inclusion in the emergency kit. Doctors who administer parenteral sedation may be required by their state or specialty society to maintain many of these drugs in their emergency kits.

Secondary Injectable Drugs

Seven drug categories are included in this level:
1. Anticonvulsant
2. Analgesic
3. Vasopressor
4. Antihypoglycemic
5. Corticosteroid
6. Antihypertensive
7. Anticholinergic

Noninjectable drugs: There are three noninjectable drugs that are considered at this level:
1. Respiratory stimulant
2. Antihypoglycemic
3. Bronchodilator

Emergency equipment: Secondary emergency equipment should include:
1. Device for cricothyrotomy
2. Artificial airways
3. Laryngoscope and endotracheal tubes

Secondary injectable: anticonvulsant
Drug of choice: Midazolam
Drug class: Benzodiazephine
Alternative drug: Diazepam

Seizure disorders may occur in the dental office under several circumstances: overdose reactions to local anesthetics, epileptic seizures, and febrile convulsions. Only rarely will an anticonvulsant be re-

Table 3-4. Module two—secondary (noncritical) drugs and equipment

Category	Primary drug Generic	Primary drug Proprietary	Alternative	Recommended for kit Quantity	Recommended for kit Availability
Injectables					
Anticonvulsant	Midazolam	Versed	Diazepam	1 × 5-mL vial	5 mg/mL
Analgesic	Morphine	—	Meperidine	2 × 2-mL ampules	10 mg/mL
Vasopressor	Methoxamine	Vasoxyl	Phenylephrine	2-3 × 1-mL ampules	10 mg/mL
Antihypoglycemic	50% Dextrose solution	—	Glucagon	1 × 50-mL ampule (IV)	
Corticosteroid	Hydrocortisone sodium succinate	Solu-Cortef	Dexamethasone	1 × 2-mL vial	50 mg/mL
Antihypertensive	Labetalol HCl	Normodyne	—	1 × 20-mL vial	5 mg/mL
Anticholinergic	Atropine	—	—	3 × 1-mL ampules and/or 2 × 10-mL syringes	0.5 mg/mL 1.0 mg/10 mL
Noninjectables					
Respiratory stimulant	Aromatic ammonia	—	—	1-2 boxes	0.3 mL vaporole
Antihypoglycemic	Carbohydrate	Many	—	1-2 tubes or several bottles for oral use	
	Decorative icing	Many	—	1-2 tubes for transmucosal use	
Bronchodilator	Albuterol	Ventolin, Proventil	Metaproterenol	1 inhaler	
Antihypertensive	Nifedipine	Procardia	—	1 bottle	10-mg capsules

Equipment	Description	Quantity
Emergency equipment		
Cricothyrotomy equipment*	Scalpel or cricothyrotomy device	1 Scalpel or cricothyrotomy device
Artificial airways*	Oropharyngeal airways	Assorted adult and pediatric airways
	Nasopharyngeal airways	Assorted adult and pediatric airways
Equipment for endotracheal intubation:*	Laryngoscope and blades (curved or straight)	Minimum of one and spare batteries
	Endotracheal tubes	Assorted adult and pediatric sizes

*Use of these devices requires significant advanced training to ensure their safe and effective use.

quired to terminate seizure activity. However, an anticonvulsant drug should be considered for inclusion in the emergency kit so that it will be readily available when required. The choice of an anticonvulsant has become somewhat simpler since the introduction of the benzodiazepines into clinical use. Until about 30 years ago, barbiturates were the drugs of choice in the management of acute seizure disorders. With its introduction, diazepam became the preferred anticonvulsant. Because seizure disorders are characterized by a stimulation of the central nervous and cardiorespiratory and cardiovascular systems, followed by a period of depres-

sion of these same systems, drugs that depress these systems at therapeutic doses are more likely to produce postseizure complications. When barbiturates are administered to terminate seizure activity, the degree of postseizure depression is accentuated and its duration prolonged because of the pharmacologic actions of the barbiturate. When seizure activity itself has been significant, the ensuing postictal period of depression tends to be profound, leading to compromised respiration and a period of hypotension. When barbiturates are used to terminate seizures, the ensuing depression will likely be intensified, leading to respiratory arrest and a profound cardiovascular depression or collapse. If the doctor is not adept at recognizing and managing this situation, the patient may be in a more difficult situation after the seizure than during it. The benzodiazepines, unlike barbiturates, will usually terminate seizure activity without the pronounced depression of the respiratory and cardiovascular systems.

Diazepam was the anticonvulsant drug of choice because of its ability to terminate seizures and not produce profound postictal depression. Its lack of water solubility, however, limited the use of diazepam to the intravenous route of administration. It was highly unlikely that a physician or dentist who was not proficient in the technique of venipuncture would be able to readily start an IV line on a patient during a seizure. When possible, diazepam was the preferred drug. With the recent introduction of the water-soluble benzodiazepine, midazolam, an agent that is effective as an anticonvulsant via either the intravenous route or intramuscularly, became available. Though IV administration is preferred, the IM route is always available. Midazolam will provide clinical action after IM administration within 10 to 15 minutes (time of onset is dependent upon blood pressure and perfusion of tissue).[18]

Therapeutic indications: Termination of prolonged seizures (status epilepticus—Chapter 21; local anesthetic seizures (Chapter 23); hyperventilation (for sedation—Chapter 12); thyroid storm (for sedation—Chapter 18)

Side effects, contraindications, and precautions: The major side effect of benzodiazepines is respiratory depression or arrest; however, with careful titration during administration, this is unlikely to occur. Compared with barbiturates, benzodiazepine-induced respiratory depression is considerably more mild.

Availability: Midazolam (Versed [USA], Hypnovel and Dormicum [Europe, United Kingdom]): 5 mg/mL in 1-, 2-, 5-, and 10-mL vials, and 2-mL preloaded syringes; 1 mg/mL in 2-,5-, and 10-ml vials, Diazepam (Valium): 5 mg/mL in 2-mL ampules and 10-mL vials, and 2-mL preloaded syringes

Suggested for emergency kit: One 5-mL vial of midazolam, 5 mg/mL

Secondary injectable: analgesic
Drug of choice: Morphine sulfate
Drug class: Narcotic agonist
Alternative drug: Meperidine

Analgesic medications will be useful during emergency situations in which acute pain or anxiety is present. In most instances the presence of pain or anxiety will cause an increase in the workload of the heart (and an increased myocardial oxygen requirement) that may prove detrimental to the well-being of the patient. Two such circumstances are acute myocardial infarction and congestive heart failure. The choice of analgesic drugs includes the narcotic agonists morphine sulfate and meperidine (Demerol).

Therapeutic indications: Intense, prolonged pain and/or anxiety; acute myocardial infarction (Chapter 28); congestive heart failure (Chapter 14).

Side effects, contraindications, and precautions: Narcotic agonists are potent CNS and respiratory depressants. Vigilant monitoring of vital signs is mandatory whenever these agents are used. Use of narcotic agonists is contraindicated in victims of head injury and multiple trauma; they should be used with care in persons with compromised respiratory function.

The respiratory depressant actions of narcotic agonists, as well as other narcotic actions, may be reversed through administration of naloxone. Analgesic action is also reversed by naloxone (see Module Four: antidotal drugs)

Availability: Morphine sulfate, 8, 10, and 15 mg/mL (in 2-mL ampules and 20-mL vials); meperidine 50 and 100 mg/mL (in 1-mL ampules and 20 and 30-mL vials).

Suggested for emergency kit: Morphine sulfate, 10 mg/mL (two 2-mL ampules), *or* meperidine 50 mg/mL (2 mL ampules).

NOTE: In recent years emergency medical services in many countries have employed mixtures of nitrous oxide (N_2O) and oxygen (O_2) in place of narcotic analgesics in the management of pain associated with acute myocardial infarction. Concentrations of N_2O have varied between 35% and 50%. At these levels, a mixture of 35% to 50% N_2O and 50% to 65% O_2 decreases pain, relaxes the victim, and provides the victim with 2 ½ to 3 times the ambient level of oxygen. Clinical use of nitrous oxide and oxygen in this situation is discussed in Chapter 28. When the dental office has N_2O-O_2 available, it may be used in place of the narcotic analgesics. In its absence, however, a narcotic analgesic should be available.

Narcotic agonists are schedule II drugs, and as such should be maintained in a secure location in the dental office. This precludes their being left in the emergency drug kit, which should be readily accessible at all times.

Secondary injectable: vasopressor
Drug of choice: Methoxamine
Drug class: Vasopressor
Alternative drug: Phenylephrine

Although one potent vasopressor, epinephrine, has already been included in the emergency kit, it is important that a second one be considered for inclusion. In most emergency situations in which a vasopressor is indicated in the dental office (see discussion on therapeutic uses that follows), an agent such as epinephrine will not be the drug of choice. Epinephrine will be used primarily in the management of acute allergic reactions and is rarely employed in cases of clinically mild to moderate hypotension. One reason for this is that epinephrine elicits an extreme antihypotensive response. In addition to an increase in blood pressure, epinephrine causes an increase in the workload of the heart through its effect on heart rate and cardiac contraction; it also increases the irritability of the myocardium by sensitizing it to dysrhythmias. In most of the situations listed here, the systolic blood pressure of the victim has fallen to a level of about 60 to 80 mm Hg and has not returned to its baseline level in an appropriate period of time. An agent is called for that will elevate the blood pressure approximately 30 to 40 mmHg for a sustained period of time, allowing the body to return to its normal functioning state. Furthermore, in most instances the cardiovascular status of the patient will be unknown unless electrocardiographic monitoring is being carried out. For this reason, it seems desirable to utilize a vasporessor that will produce a moderate increase in blood pressure without unduly stimulating the myocardium. Vasopressors such as methoxamine (Vasoxyl) and phenylephrine (Neo-Synephrine) are drugs that produce moderate blood pressure elevations through peripheral vasoconstriction.

Methoxamine is a clinically useful vasopressor with sustained action and little effect on the myocardium or central nervous system. Its vasopressor action is associated with a marked increase in peripheral resistance and no increase in cardiac output. A compensatory bradycardia accompanies the rise in blood pressure produced by methoxamine. The onset of the pressor action is almost immediate following IV administration and may persist for up to 60 minutes. After IM injection the response occurs within 15 minutes and persists for 90 minutes.

Phenylephrine acts in a similar fashion, with a 5-mg IM dose causing a 30-mmHg elevation of systolic blood pressure and a 20-mmHg elevation of diastolic blood pressure, with the response persisting for 50 minutes. As with methoxamine, a pronounced and persistent bradycardia will be noted (average decline in heart rate from 70 to 44 beats per minute).

Therapeutic indications: The vasopressors will be useful in the management of hypotension, in which the status of the heart is unknown and the intent is to raise the blood pressure without cardiac stim-

ulation. Possible uses are in:
   Syncopal reactions (Section II)
   Drug overdose reactions (Chapter 23)
   Postseizure states (Chapter 21)
   Acute adrenal insufficiency (Chapter 8)
   Allergy (Chapter 24)

Side effects, contraindications, and precautions: Parenteral administration of most vasopressors is contraindicated in patients with high blood pressure or ventricular tachycardia, and such drugs are to be used with extreme caution in patients with hyperthyroidism, bradycardia, partial heart block, myocardial disease, or severe atherosclerosis.

Availability: Methoxamine (Vasoxyl), 10 mg/mL and 20 mg/mL (in 1-mL ampules and 10-mL vials); phenylephrine (Neo-Synephrine), 10 mg/mL (in 1-mL ampules)

Suggested for emergency kit: Methoxamine, 10mg/mL (two to three 1-mL ampules *or* phenylephrine, 10 mg/mL (two to three 1-mL ampules)

NOTE: Vasopressors are only infrequently used for the management of hypotensive states. Other nonpharmacologic means of elevating blood pressure are available, such as positioning the patient in the supine position with feet elevated and/or administration of intravenous fluids (D5&W, lactated Ringers) to increase the fluid compartment and elevate blood pressure. The author has been told by anesthesiologists (not entirely joking either) that the only vasopressor they will administer is epinephrine and then only when there is no blood pressure present.

Secondary injectable: antihypoglycemic
Drug of choice: 50% Dextrose
Drug class: Antihypoglycemic
Alternative drug: Glucagon

In the management of low blood sugar (hypoglycemia), the mode of therapy will depend in large part on the patient's level of consciousness. Oral carbohydrate is the preferred mode of therapy; however, if a patient is unconscious or is severely obtunded, the oral route should not be employed. In this situation 50 mL of a 50% dextrose solution may be administered intravenously. When the intravenous route is not available, glucagon may be administered intramuscularly. Glucagon is normally produced in the pancreas and acts to elevate the blood glucose level by mobilizing hepatic glycogen and converting it to glucose. Glucagon will therefore only be effective if hepatic glycogen is available. It will not be effective in starvation or chronic hypoglycemic states. Oral carbohydrate is then administered as soon as the patient begins to respond, that is, regains consciousness.

Therapeutic indications: Hypoglycemia (Chapter

17); diagnostic aid in unconsciousness or seizures of unknown origin (Chapter 9)

Side effects, contraindications, and precautions: 50% dextrose, which must be administered intravenously, may produce tissue necrosis should an extravascular infiltration occur. No specific contraindications exist to the use of 50% dextrose. If a bolus of 50% dextrose is given to an already hyperglycemic patient, the blood sugar level will not be elevated significantly.

Glucagon administered either IM or IV, is contraindicated in starvation states and in chronic hypoglycemia.

Availability: 50% Dextrose (50-mL vial); glucagon, 1 mg (1 unit) dry powder with 1 mL diluent; 10 mg dry powder with 10 mL diluent

Suggested for emergency kit: 50% Dextrose solution (1 vial) if IV route is available *or* glucagon, 1 mg/mL (two or three 1-mL vials) for IM or IV administration

Secondary injectable: corticosteroid

Drug of choice: Hydrocortisone sodium succinate
Drug class: Adrenal glucocorticosteroid
Alternative drug: Dexamethasone

Corticosteroids will be administered in the management of an acute allergic reaction, but only after the acute phase has been brought under control through the use of basic life support, epinephrine, and antihistamines. The primary value of the corticosteroids is in the prevention of recurrent episodes of anaphylaxis. Corticosteroids are also important in the management of acute adrenal insufficiency.

Studies have demonstrated that corticosteroids have a slow onset of action even when administered intravenously.[19] Because maximal effectiveness may not occur for up to 60 minutes after intravenous administration, many authorities question the effectiveness of these agents in the management of allergic reactions in patients with a normally functioning adrenal gland. It appears likely that the antiallergic effects of the corticosteroids are simply a manifestation of the nonspecific antiinflammatory action of the adrenal glucocorticoids (hydrocortisone and cortisone). Dexamethasone (Decadron) and methylprednisolone sodium succinate (Solu-Medrol) are both contraindicated for use in acute adrenal insufficiency. Therefore, hydrocortisone sodium succinate is considered the drug of choice for the dental emergency kit. Corticosteroids are considered second-line drugs primarily because of their slow onset of action.

Therapeutic indications: Definitive management of acute allergy (Chapter 24); acute adrenal insufficiency (Chapter 8)

Side effects, contraindications, and precautions: As used in the management of life-threatening medical emergencies, there are no contraindications to the corticosteroids. When administered for nonemergency treatment (i.e., prevention of edema during surgery, pruritis), there are many factors to be considered, such as the presence of preexisting infection, peptic ulcer, and hyperglycemia. (Consult a pharmacology textbook or the *PDR* for more detailed information.)

Availability: Hydrocortisone sodium succinate (Solu-Cortef), 50 mg/mL (2-mL vial); dexamethasone phosphate (Decadron) 4 mg/mL in various sizes of ampules and vials

Suggested for emergency kit: Hydrocortisone sodium succinate, 50 mg/mL (one 2-mL vial)

Secondary injectable: antihypertensive

Drug of choice: Labetalol
Drug class: β-Adrenergic blocker
Alternative drug: Propranolol

The need to administer drugs to decrease excessive elevations in blood pressure is extremely uncommon. First, the incidence of extreme acute blood pressure elevations is quite rare, and second, there are other means of decreasing blood pressure without resorting to parenteral antihypertensive drugs. Indeed, in interviews with hundreds of dentists who administer parenteral sedation and/or general anesthesia in their practices, this author has not discovered one who has had the occasion to administer a drug to decrease an excessively elevated blood pressure. Oral drugs, such as nifedipine or nitroglycerin, may be administered in most situations to provide a minor depression of blood pressure. The inclusion of a drug in this category is in response to state requirements for general anesthesia permits (and in a few states for parenteral sedation, too).

In the not too distant past, drugs such as diazoxide (Hyperstat) were employed for the management of acute hypertensive episodes or for controlled hypotensive anesthesia. Such a drug produces a decrease in blood pressure by relaxing vascular smooth muscle in peripheral arterioles. Cardiac output is increased as blood pressure is reduced and both coronary artery and renal blood flows are maintained. Its use in the dental office in emergency situations is no longer recommended because other more controllable agents are available.

Labetalol (Normodyne) is an adrenergic receptor blocking agent that has both selective α_1-adrenergic and nonselective β-adrenergic receptor blocking actions. Following IV administration, the ratio of alpha- to beta-blockade is 1:7. Labetalol produces a dose-related decrease in blood pressure without reflex tachycardia and without a significant reduction of heart rate (presumably through its mixture of both alpha- and beta-blockade). Because of its alpha-blockade, decreases in blood pressure are greater when the patient is standing than supine and signs of postural hypotension may develop in this situation. When administered to supine patients for management of severe hypertension, an initial IV dose of 0.25 mg/kg (17.5 mg for a 70-kg patient), decreased blood pressure by an average of 11/7 mmHg.

Therapeutic indications: Acute hypertensive episode

Side effects, contraindications, and precautions: Because of the likelihood of postural hypotension developing in an upright or semiupright patient receiving labetalol, it is recommended that the patient be in the supine position when the agent is administered. Labetalol is contraindicated for administration to patients with asthma, overt heart failure, greater than first degree heart block, cardiogenic shock, and severe bradycardia. Symptomatic postural hypotension (50% incidence) is likely to occur if a patient is tilted or assumes an upright position within 3 hours of receiving labetalol. It is therefore extremely important to ascertain the patient's ability to assume the upright position before permitting ambulation.

Availability: Labetalol HCI injection: 5 mg/mL in 20- and 40-mL multidose vials, and in 4-mL and 8-mL single-dose prefilled syringes

Suggested for emergency kit: Labetalol HCI 5 mg/mL, 20 ml vial or 2 × 4 mL or 1 × 8 mL preloaded syringe

Secondary injectable: parasympathetic blocking agent

Drug of choice: Atropine

Drug class: Anticholinergic

Alternative drug: None

Atropine, a parasympathetic blocking agent, is recommended for the management of symptomatic bradycardia (adult heart rate of <60 beats per minute). By enhancing discharge from the sinoatrial (SA) node, atropine may provoke tachycardia (adult heart rate > 100 beats per minute). Atropine will be of benefit in situations in which the patient has an overload of parasympathetic activity on the heart. Extremely fearful patients are likely candidates for this response. When stimulated, the vagus nerve acts to decrease SA node activity, thereby slowing the heart rate. When the heart rate becomes overly slow, cerebral blood flow is decreased and clinical signs and symptoms of cerebral ischemia are noted. By blocking this vagal effect, atro-

phine acts to maintain adequate cardiac output and cerebral circulation.

Atropine is also considered an essential drug in advanced cardiac life support (ACLS), in which it is employed in the management of bradydysrhythmias (hemodynamically significant heart block and asystole).

Therapeutic indications: Bradycardia and hemodynamically significant bradydysrhythmias (Chapter 30)

Side effects, contraindications, and precautions: Large doses of atropine (>2.0 mg) may produce clinical signs of overdosage, including: hot, dry skin; headache; blurred near vision; dryness of the mouth and throat; disorientation; and hallucinations. Administration of atropine is contraindicated in patients with glaucoma or prostatic hypertrophy. However, in life-threatening situations the benefits of atropine administration usually outweigh the possible risks. Atropine administration can increase the degree of partial urinary obstruction associated with prostatism; also, it should not be administered in the elderly with narrow-angle glaucoma.

Availability: 0.5 mg/mL in 1-mL vials and 1 mg in 10-mL syringe

Suggested for emergency kit: Two to three ampules of 0.5 mg/mL (for IM administration) and/or 2 × 10-mL syringes of 1 mg per syringe (for IV administration)

Secondary noninjectable drugs

There are three noninjectable drugs that are considered at this level:

1. Respiratory stimulant
2. Antihypolycemic
3. Bronchodilator

Secondary noninjectable: respiratory stimulant

Drug of choice: Aromatic ammonia

Drug class: Respiratory stimulant

Alternative drug: None

Aromatic ammonia is the agent of choice as a respiratory stimulant for inclusion in the emergency kit. It is available in a silver-gray vaporole, which is crushed and placed under the victim's nose until respiratory stimulation is effected. Aromatic ammonia has a noxious odor and acts by irritating the mucous membrane of the upper respiratory tract, thereby stimulating the respiratory and vasomotor centers of the medulla; this in turn increases respiration and blood pressure. Movement of the arms and legs often occurs in response to inhalation of ammonia. This too acts to increase the return of blood from the periphery and aids in raising blood pressure, especially if the patient has been positioned properly.

Therapeutic indications: Respiratory depression

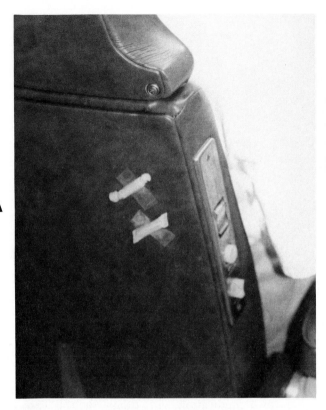

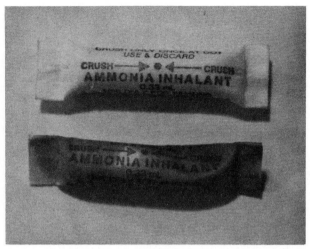

Fig. 3-31. A, Aromatic ammonia vaporoles on back of dental chair. **B,** Aromatic ammonia vaporole darkens (bottom) when used.

not induced by narcotic analgesics; vasodepressor syncope (Chapter 6)

Side effects, contraindications, and precautions: Ammonia should be employed with caution in persons with chronic obstructive pulmonary disease (COPD) or asthma because its irritating effects on the mucous membranes of the upper respiratory tract may precipitate bronchospasm.

Availability: Silver-gray vaporole (0.3 mL aromatic ammonia)

Suggested for emergency kit: One to two boxes of vaporoles

NOTE: After oxygen, aromatic ammonia will be the most commonly used drug in the emergency kit. The author has found it convenient to tape one or two vaporoles close to every dental unit (for example, behind the back of the headrest) so that when it is required, time need not be spent searching for it (Fig. 3-31). The vaporoles should be located so that the operator (dentist, hygienist, assistant) can reach them without having to leave the patient, assuming that there is no assistance close at hand. In addition, several vaporoles ought to be kept in the emergency kit for use in other areas of the dental office.

Secondary noninjectable: antihypoglycemic
Drug of choice: Sugar
Drug class: Antihypoglycemic
Alternative drug: None

Antihypoglycemic agents will be useful in the management of hypoglycemic reactions occurring in patients with diabetes mellitus or in the nondiabetic patient with hypoglycemia (low blood sugar). The diabetic patient will usually carry a ready source of carbohydrate such as a candy bar or hard candy. Such items should also be available in the dental office for use in the conscious patient with hypoglycemia. For management of the unconscious hypoglycemic patient, refer to the discussion of injectable drugs in this chapter. Thick, nonviscous forms of carbohydrate may be used in the management of unconscious hypoglycemic emergencies when no injectable form of the agent is available. This technique, transmucosal application of sugar, is presented in Chapter 17.

Therapeutic indications: Hypoglycemic states secondary to diabetes mellitus or fasting hypoglycemia in conscious patient (Chapter 17); emergency managment of unconscious hypoglycemic states in absence of parenteral medications (Chapter 17)

Side effects, contraindications, and precautions: Oral carbohydrates that are liquid or viscous should not be administered to patients who do not have an active gag reflex or who are unable to drink without assistance. Parenteral administration of antihypoglycemics is recommended in these situations. There are no side effects when oral carbohydrates are administered as directed.

Small tubes of decorative icing are useful in the management of unconscious hypoglycemic individuals. These tubes contain a thickened paste of concentrated sugar that can be applied in a thin ribbon

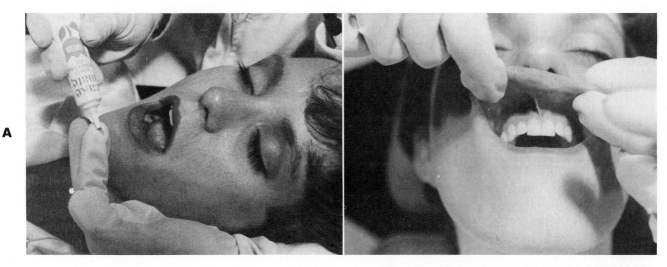

Fig. 3-32. A, Decorative icing applied transmucosally. **B,** Transmucosal sugar applied in thin layer on buccal mucosa.

to the buccal mucosa in the maxilla and mandible (Fig. 3-32). Because it is thick, this paste will not run and possibly obstruct the airway. Absorption into the cardiovascular system does not occur rapidly requiring a minimum of 20 to 30 minutes. Basic life support is continued during this continued period of unconsciousness.

Availability: Glucola®, Gluco-Stat®, Insta-Glucose®, cola beverages, fruit juices, granulated sugar, tubes of decorative icing

Suggested for emergency kit: Any of the aforementioned sources of carbohydrates listed

Secondary noninjectable: bronchodilator

Drug of choice: Albuterol

Drug class: Adrenergic agonist

Alternative drug: Metaproterenol

Asthmatic patients and patients with allergic reactions manifested primarily by respiratory difficulty will require the use of brochodilator drugs. Although epinephrine remains the drug of choice in the management of bronchospasm, its wide-ranging actions on systems other than the respiratory tract has resulted in the introduction of newer, more specific agents known as β_2-adrenergic agonists. These agents, of which albuterol is an example, have specific bronchial smooth muscle-relaxing properties (β_2) with little or no stimulatory effect on the cardiovascular and gastrointestinal systems (β_1). In the dental situation in which the patient's true cardiovascular status may be unknown, β_2 agonists appear more attractive for management of the acute asthmatic episode than agents

that have both β_1 and β_2 agonist properties, such as epinephrine and isoproterenol. As is also the case with anginal patients, most asthmatics will keep their own medication with them—in this case a bronchodilator. In most situations the bronchodilator will be in the form of an inhalator that dispenses a calibrated dosage of the bronchodilator. The patient inhales as the agent is dispensed, allowing the drug to reach the bronchial mucosa, where it acts directly on bronchial smooth muscle (Fig. 3-33).

Before dental treatment is started, the asthmatic patient who is at greater risk of bronchospasm (i.e., a dental phobic) should be asked to make his or her bronchodilator available. Bronchodilators must be administered precisely as directed. One to two inhalations every 4 to 6 hours is the recommended dosage for albuterol. Nebulized epinephrine (e.g., Primatene-Mist®) should be administered one to two inhalations per hour. In situations in which these nebulized agents fail to terminate the attack, other bronchodilators (e.g., epinephrine, aminophylline, isoproterenol) must be administered parenterally (intramuscularly or subcutaneously).

Therapeutic indications: Bronchospasm—asthma (Chapter 13); allergic reactions with bronchospasm (Chapter 24)

Side effects, contraindications, and precautions: Albuterol, like other β_2 agonists, may have a clinically significant cardiac effect in some patients. This response is less likely to develop with albuterol than with other bronchodilators, thus its selection for

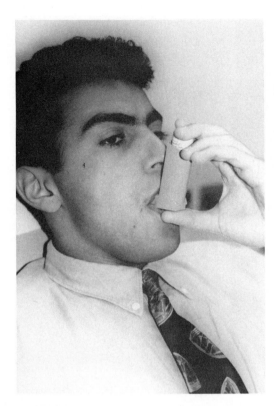

Fig. 3-33. Bronchodilator self-administered by asthmatic patient.

the emergency kit. Metaproterenol, epinephrine, and isoproterenol mistometers are more likely to produce cardiovascular side effects, including tachycardia and ventricular dysrhythmias. Administration of these latter drugs is contraindicated in patients with preexisting tachydysrhythmias from prior use of the drug (Chapter 13).

Availability: Albuterol inhaler (Ventolin, Proventil); metaproterenol inhaler (Alupent); epinephrine mistometer (Medihaler-epi); isoproterenol mistometer (Medihaler-iso)

Suggested for emergency kit: One inhaler of albuterol

Secondary noninjectable: antihypertensive

Drug of choice: Nifedipine

Drug class: Calcium channel blocker

Alternative drug: Nitroglycerin

Two drugs have been presented that are effective in the management of acute elevations of blood pressure: labetalol, for parenteral administration, and nitroglycerin, for sublingual administration. The need for yet another antihypertensive drug is minimal, especially in view of the fact that the need for antihypertensive drug administration in dental

situations is extremely slight. Nifedipine is primarily used for the management of angina, especially vasospastic or Prinzmetal's variant angina. As is also noted with nitroglycerin, a modest, and usually well-tolerated hypotension is a commonly observed side effect of nifedipine administration. The occasional patient may experience excessive and less well-tolerated hypotension, especially if standing or seated upright.

Therapeutic indications: Hypertension; acute anginal pain (Chapter 27)

Side effects, contraindications, and precautions: Excessive hypotension; this is noted especially when nifedipine has been administered to patients receiving beta blockers and are undergoing anesthesia with high doses of fentanyl.

Availability: 10-mg or 20-mg capsules

Suggested for emergency kit: One bottle of 10-mg capsules

Secondary Emergency Equipment

Items described in this section serve as adjuncts to the basic techniques of airway management presented in the primary equipment section in this chapter and in Chapter 5. Their use is recommended only for persons who have received the advanced training required to employ them safely and effectively.[20] They are not meant to serve as substitutes for the basic techniques of airway management.

Secondary emergency equipment includes the following:

1. Scalpel or cricothyrotomy needle
2. Artificial airways
3. Laryngoscope and endotracheal tubes

Scalpel or cricothyrotomy device. As a final step in airway maintenance, when all other noninvasive procedures have failed to maintain a patent airway, it may become necessary to perform a cricothyrotomy. The emergency kit should contain an instrument that can be used to make an opening into the trachea at a site below the obstruction. A scalpel or a specially designed cricothyrotomy device is recommended (Fig. 3-34). The use of these items and the technique of cricothyrotomy will be discussed in Chapter 11.

Suggested for emergency kit: One scalpel with disposable blade and/or one cricothyrotomy device

NOTE: Advanced training is required for safe and effective use of these devices.

Artificial airways. Plastic or rubber oropharyngeal or nasopharyngeal airways are used to assist in the maintenance of a patent airway in the unconscious patient (Fig. 3-35). They function by lift-

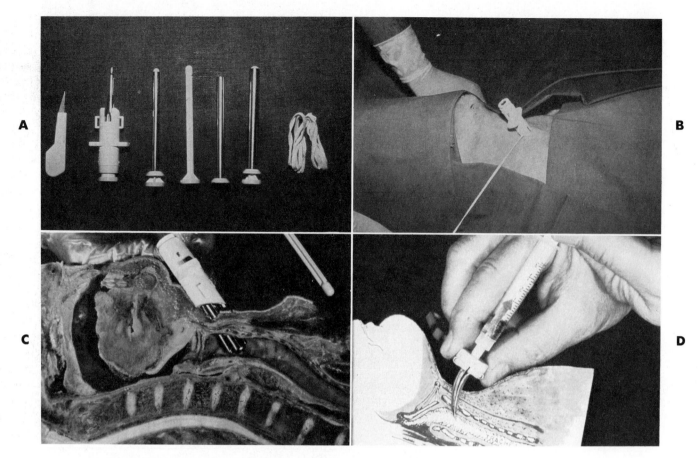

Fig. 3-34. A, (Left to right), stylet; needle and housing unit; airway; coturator; airways (2); tie. **B,** Airways secured in position. **C,** Anatomical view of positioned airway. **D,** Pediatric cricothyrotomy needle.

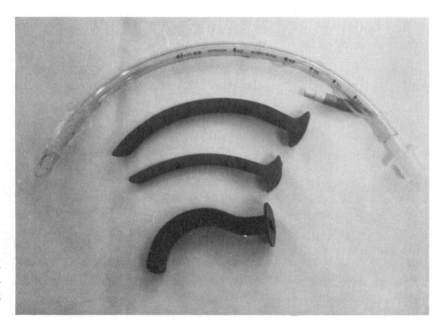

Fig. 3-35. Airway devices (top to bottom): endotracheal tube, nasopharyngeal airways (2), and oropharyngeal airway.

ing the base of the tongue off of the posterior pharyngeal wall. Their use is recommended by the American Heart Association[20] only in cases in which manual methods of maintaining an airway have proved ineffective. The nasopharyngeal airway is better tolerated by patients who are not deeply unconscious, whereas the oropharyngeal airway will produce gagging, regurgitation, or vomiting in patients who are not deeply unconscious. Therefore, the author's preference is for inclusion of the nasopharyngeal airway. Several sizes of airways should always be available (e.g., child, small adult, normal adult) when oropharyngeal or nasopharyngeal airways are included in the emergency kit.

Suggested for emergency kit: One set of adult and/or pediatric airways

NOTE: Advanced training is required for safe and effective use of these devices.

Laryngoscope and endotracheal tubes. Many devices are available to aid in the management of a patent airway in the unconscious or semiconscious patient. Among these are the S tube, esophageal obturator airway, laryngoscope, and endotracheal tube. As with the other devices listed in this section, advanced training in the use of each item is absolutely essential.

The S tube airway is a modification of the oropharyngeal airway that permits the rescuer to maintain a patent airway and deliver exhaled air ventilation without physically contacting the victim's mouth. Problems encountered with improper use include further obstruction of the airway, regurgitation, and/or laryngospasm. In order to ventilate the victim with the S tube, the rescuer must be positioned at the head of the victim, not astride, thus severely limiting the ability of the rescuer to perform one-rescuer CPR. Inclusion of the S-tube in the dental office emergency kit is *not* recommended.

The esophageal obturator airway or EOA is a large-bore tube, 37 cm in length, designed to occlude the esophagus (Fig. 3-36), thus permitting air forced into the airway to enter the victim's trachea and lungs, not the stomach.[21] Although it is usually easily inserted, even by untrained rescuers, problems can develop that will minimize the usefulness of this device. These include possible insertion of the tube into the trachea, thereby obstructing the airway, and the probability that the victim will vomit when the airway is removed. Because of these potential problems, the American Heart Association[22] lists the following considerations when EOAs are employed: they should be used only by trained individuals; they should not be used in victims younger than 16 years of age; they should not be used in conscious victims or

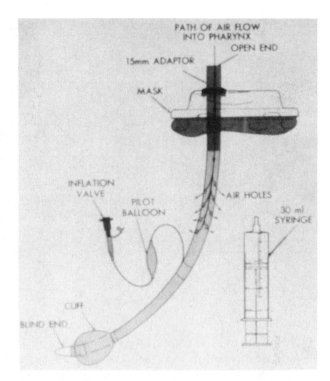

Fig. 3-36. Esophageal obturator airway (EOA).

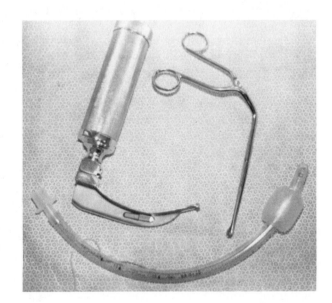

Fig. 3-37. Laryngoscope *(left)*, Magill intubation forceps *(right)*, and endotracheal tube *(bottom)*.

those who are breathing spontaneously; they should not be left in place for longer than 2 hours; force should not be used during insertion; and suction should be immediately available during insertion and removal. The EOA is not recommended for inclusion in the emergency kit unless the doctor and staff have received training in its proper insertion and removal.

Table 3-5. Module three—advanced cardiac life support—essential drugs

Category	Primary drug		Alternative	Recommended for kit	
	Generic	Proprietary		Quantity	Availability
Injectables					
Cardiac arrest	Epinephrine	Adrenalin	—	3 × 10-mL syringe	1 : 10,000 con-centration
Oxygen	Oxygen	—	—	1 E cylinder	
Antidysrhythmic	Lidocaine	Xylocaine	Procainamide	1 preloaded syringe	100 mg
				1 × 5-mL ampule	100 mg
Symptomatic bradycardia	Atropine	Atropine	Isoproterenol	2 × 10-mL syringe	1.0 mg/10 mL
Symptomatic hypotension	Dopamine	Intropin	Dobutamine	2 × 5-mL ampules	80 mg/mL
Analgesic	Morphine	Morphine	Meperidine	2 × 2-mL ampules	10 mg/mL
PSVT*	Verapamil	Isoptin	—	1 × 4-mL ampule	2.5 mg/mL

*PSVT, paroxysmal supraventricular tachycardia.

Endotracheal intubation using a laryngoscope (to visualize the trachea) and endotracheal tube (Fig. 3-37) is a technique of airway maintenance that must be strictly limited to persons extremely well-trained in its use. Realistically, this limits its usefulness to anesthesiologists, anesthetists, trained paramedical personnel, and those few dentists and physicians who have received extensive general anesthesia training.

Advantages of endotracheal intubation, which make it the preferred technique of airway control, include: isolation of the airway; preventing aspiration; facilitation of ventilation and oxygenation; and providing an avenue for administration of some drugs (epinephrine, lidocaine, atrophine, naloxone).[22] The most common mistakes in intubation are accidental intubation of the esophagus and taking too long to intubate (it should take no longer than 30 seconds to intubate a patient). In addition, improper intubation technique often results in fracture of the maxillary anterior teeth. When used by properly trained individuals, tracheal intubation is a preferred technique of airway management in the unconscious victim. Inclusion of the laryngoscope and an assortment of sizes of endotracheal tubes is suggested for the trained doctor only.

Module Three: Advanced Cardiac Life Support—Essential Drugs (Table 3-5)

A third category of injectable drugs to be included in the emergency kit are those classified as essential in the performance of advanced cardiac life support. It is recommended that these agents only be considered for inclusion by doctors who have received training in ACLS.

In recent years a number of ACLS drugs previously considered as essential have been deemphasized. These include sodium bicarbonate, calcium chloride, bretylium tosylate, and isoproterenol.

Essential ACLS drugs include the following:
1. Epinephrine
2. Oxygen
3. Lidocaine
4. Atropine
5. Dopamine
6. Morphine sulfate
7. Verapamil

ACLS essential: cardiac arrest
Drug of choice: Epinephrine
Drug class: Endogenous catecholamine
Alternative drug: None

Three items form the essentials of advanced cardiac life support treatment: epinephrine, oxygen, and defibrillation. Epinephrine has been previously discussed as an essential injectable drug for administration in anaphylaxis. Epinephrine is available as a 1-mg dose in preloaded syringes containing either 1 mL (1 : 1000 concentration) or 10 mL (1 : 10,000) of solution. The 1 : 10,000 concentration is for administration intravenously or instilled down the endotracheal tube of an intubated patient, whereas the 1 : 1000 solution is designed for subcutaneous or intramuscular administration.

Epinephrine is an important drug during cardiac arrest because no other drug is capable of maintaining coronary artery blood flow while CPR is in progress, which is essential for preserving the chances of survival from cardiac arrest. Epinephrine also preserves blood flow to the brain. In the absence of drug therapy, cerebral blood flow during CPR is minimal; most blood enters the common carotid artery and flows into the external carotid branch, not the internal carotid artery.[23] Following administration of a drug with α-adrenergic properties, such as epinephrine, cerebral blood flow is significantly increased.[24]

Therapeutic indications: Cardiac arrest (ventricular fibrillation, pulseless ventricular tachycardia, asystole, electromechanical dissociation [EMD] (Chapter 30)

Side effects, contraindications, and precautions: In the situations cited for administration of epinephrine, there are no contraindications to its use. However, one should be aware that when large doses are administered to patients who are not receiving CPR, hypertension is a common result. In addition, epinephrine may induce or exacerbate ventricular ectopy, especially in patients who are receiving digitalis.[25]

Availability: 1:10,000 concentration in preloaded 10-mL syringe

Suggested for emergency kit: Two to three preloaded syringes

ACLS essential: oxygen
Drug of choice: Oxygen
Drug class: None
Alternative drug: None

Oxygen has been included in the emergency kit as an essential noninjectable drug. It is essential to cardiac resuscitation and emergency cardiac care. Though exhaled air ventilation provides 16% to 17% oxygen and ambient air ventilation provides 21% oxygen, enriched oxygen ventilation or 100% oxygen ventilation precludes the possibility of hypoxia developing, if ventilation is adequate.

There are absolutely no contraindications to the administration of oxygen in emergency situations. Long-term administration of high concentrations of oxygen can produce oxygen toxicity, but the duration required far exceeds those encountered in virtually all emergency situations. Oxygen must never be withheld or diluted during resuscitation because of the mistaken belief that it will be harmful.[26]

The reader is referred to the previous discussion of oxygen, in Module one, under the section on critical noninjectable drugs, for a fuller description of oxygen's precautions, availability, and recommendations for the emergency kit.

ACLS essential: antidysrhythmic
Drug of choice: Lidocaine
Drug class: Local anesthetic
Alternative drug: Procainamide

Lidocaine has been used extensively in the management of cardiac dysrhythmias, especially those of ventricular origin that develop following acute myocardial infarction. It is considered to be the primary antidysrhythmic drug in advanced cardiac life support. Procainamide also effectively suppresses ventricular ectopy and is recommended for administration when lidocaine has not achieved suppression of life-threatening ventricular dysrhythmias.[27]

Therapeutic indications: Lidocaine is used in premature ventricular contractions (PVCs) occurring more than six times per minute, closely coupled PVCs, multifocal PVCs, and those occurring in bursts of two or more in succession. Lidocaine administration is also indicated in sustained ventricular tachycardia with a pulse and ventricular fibrillation that is refractory to defibrillation (Chapter 30).[28]

Side effects, contraindications, and precautions: Excessive doses of lidocaine produce myocardial, circulatory, and central nervous system depression. Clinical signs and symptoms of lidocaine overdose include drowsiness, paresthesias, and muscle twitching.[29] More severe overdose may produce tonic-clonic seizure activity.[30] Decreased hepatic function or hepatic blood flow slows the rate of lidocaine biotransformation, thus leading to prolonged elevated blood levels and a greater risk of lidocaine overdose. Impaired hepatic blood flow is frequently observed in the presence of acute reductions in cardiac output, as seen in myocardial infarction and congestive heart failure.[31]

Availability: Lidocaine is available for intravenous injection in 5-mL, 50-mg, and 100-mg prefilled syringes, and in 5 mL and 100-mg ampules.

Suggested for emergency kit: One preloaded syringe (100 mg) and one 5-mL ampule

ACLS essential: symptomatic bradycardia
Drug of choice: Atropine
Drug class: Parasympatholytic
Alternative drug: Isoproterenol

Atropine is the drug of choice for hemodynamically significant bradydysrhythmias and is also administered during asystole which is refractory to epinephrine. A bradydysrhythmia is considered hemodynamically unstable when the following are present: hypotension (defined by ACLS guidelines as a systolic blood pressure of <90 mmHg); premature ventricular contractions; altered mental status or symptoms (e.g., chest pain or dyspnea); ischemia; or infarction.[32]

Isoproterenol is a synthetic sympathomimetic amine with nearly pure β-adrenergic receptor activity. Despite producing a decrease in mean blood pressure, isoproterenol provides increased cardiac output. However, it also markedly increases myocardial oxygen consumption and may therefore induce or exacerbate myocardial ischemia. Though still considered for administration in the management of hemodynamically significant and atropine refractory bradycardias, isoproterenol has recently fallen from favor. Electronic pacing of the heart has proven more effective and it does not increase myocardial oxygen requirements.

Atropine is one of four drugs that may be administered endotracheally. It has been discussed previously in the section on secondary injectable drugs. Recommendations and other information concerning atropine are found there.

ACLS essential: symptomatic hypotension
Drug of choice: Dopamine
Drug class: Sympathomimetic amine
Alternative drug: Dobutamine

Dopamine is a chemical precursor of norepinephrine. In large doses it stimulates both α- and β-adrenergic receptors. At lower doses it dilates renal, mesenteric, and cerebral arteries.[33] Dopamine also stimulates the release of norepinephrine; it is indicated for administration in hemodynamically significant hypotension in the absence of hypovolemia. When administered, the dose of dopamine should be kept as low as possible in order to ensure adequate perfusion of vital organs.

Dobutamine is a synthetic sympathomimetic amine that exerts significant inotropic effects by stimulating β_1 and α-adrenergic receptors in the myocardium.[34] Its beta-stimulatory actions greatly outweigh its alpha actions, usually resulting in a mild vasodilation. In its usual dose, dobutamine is less likely than isoproterenol or dopamine to induce tachycardias. Dopamine is administered intravenously as a infusion. The infusion rate is altered according to the response of the patient.

Therapeutic indications: The primary therapeutic indication for dopamine is for hemodynamically significant hypotension in the absence of hypovolemia

Side effects, contraindications, and precautions: As dopamine produces an increase in heart rate, it may induce or exacerbate supraventricular or ventribular dysrhythmias. Additionally, dopamine may alter the imbalance between supply and demand of the myocardium for oxygen, thereby inducing or exacerbating myocardial ischemia.[35] Nausea and vomiting are frequently noted with dopamine administration. In patients receiving MOA-inhibitors (isocarboxazid, pargyline, tranylcypromine, or phenelzine), the activity of dopamine may be augmented. The dosage of dopamine administered to these patients should be no more than one tenth of the usual dose

Availability: Dopamine is available in 200 mg, 400 mg, and 800 mg in 5-mL ampules and syringes.

Suggested for emergency kit: One to two ampules of 400 mg dopamine (80 mg/mL)

ACLS essential: analgesia
Drug of choice: Morphine
Drug class: Narcotic agonist
Alternative drug: Meperidine

The management of pain and anxiety during ischemic chest pain is an essential part of overall patient care. Though a number of analgesics are available, morphine is the most recommended. Morphine has been reviewed in the prior section on secondary injectable drugs.

ACLS essential: paroxysmal supraventricular tachycardia (PSVT)
Drug of choice: Verapamil
Drug class: Calcium channel blocker
Alternative drug: None

Verapamil is the second calcium channel blocker discussed in this section. Nifedipine was presented as a secondary noninjectable drug for the management of hypertensive situations. Verapamil is included in the ACLS category because it has proven to be extremely effective in the management of patients who have supraventricular tachycardia.[36] Verapamil slows conduction through the atrioventricular node, thereby reducing ventricular response to atrial flutter and fibrillation. Though verapamil may be administered orally, in the context of ACLS, it should be administered intravenously.

Therapeutic indications: In emergency cardiac care, verapamil is employed primarily for the treatment of paroxysmal supraventricular tachycardia (PSVT) that does not require cardioversion. When verapamil proves ineffective in the management of PSVT, synchronized cardioversion is recommended.

Side effects, contraindications, and precautions: A transient decrease in arterial pressure may be noted because of peripheral vasodilation in response to verapamil.[37] Verapamil is not indicated for ventricular tachycardia; it may induce severe hypotension and predispose a patient to ventricular fibrillation.[38]

Availability: Verapamil is available for injection as 2.5 mg/mL in 2-mL and 4-mL ampules.

Suggested for emergency kit: One 4-mL ampule

• • •

For a complete discussion of all aspects of advanced cardiac life support, it is strongly suggested that the doctor consult one or both of the following references:

1. American Heart Association: *Textbook of advanced cardiac life support*, Dallas, 1987, American Heart Association.
2. Grauer K, Cavallaro D: *ACLS: certification, preparation, and a comprehensive review*, St Louis, 1987, Mosby–Year Book.

In addition, certification in advanced cardiac life

Table 3-6. Module four—antidotal drugs

	Primary drug			Recommended for kit	
Category	Generic	Proprietary	Alternative	Quantity	Availability
Injectables					
Narcotic antagonist	Naloxone	Narcan	Nalbuphine	2 × 1-mL ampules	0.4 mg/mL
Benzodiazepine antagonist	Flumazenil	Mazicon	—	1 × 10-mL vial	0.1 mg/mL
Antiemergence delirium	Physostigmine	Antilirium	—	2 × 2-mL ampules	1 mg/mL
Vasodilator	Procaine	Novocain	—	2 × 2-mL ampules	10 mg/mL

support at (minimally) the provider level is suggested in order to obtain a better understanding of the proper use of the drugs mentioned in this section.

Module Four: Antidotal Drugs (Table 3-6)

There are four categories of injectable drugs used for the management of emergency situations that arise in response to the administation of drugs used primarily for sedation via intramuscular and intravenous routes or general anesthesia. These drugs should be maintained in the emergency kit only as warranted by the nature of the dental practice. For example, a narcotic antagonist is not essential when narcotic agonists are not used for patient management.

Categories of antidotal drugs include:
1. Narcotic antagonist
2. Benzodiazepine antagonist
3. Antiemergence delirium drug
4. Vasodilator

Antidotal drug: narcotic antagonist

Drug of choice: Naloxone
Drug class: Thebaine derivative
Alternative drug: Nalbuphine

The most significant side effect of parenterally administered narcotic agonists is their ability to produce respiratory depression by diminishing the responsiveness of the respiratory centers of the brain to arterial carbon dioxide. The rate of breathing is thereby slowed. Narcotic antagonists have been available since 1951 (nalorphine, levallorphan). Though these agents had the ability to reverse narcotic-induced respiratory depression, when administered to patients with non–narcotic-induced respiratory depression, both nalorphine and levallorphan were capable of producing their own respiratory depression and of enhancing barbiturate-induced respiratory depression. Naloxone became available in the late 1960s and today re-

mains the only narcotic antagonist free of any agonistic properties. Naloxone will also reverse other properties of narcotics, namely analgesia, and sedation.[39] This action is not entirely innocuous because if narcotics have been employed for postsurgical analgesia naloxone administration will antagonize this effect and leave the patient with unmanaged postsurgical pain. Naloxone may be administered endotracheally in situations in which intravenous access is not available. Administered intravenously or endotracheally, improved respiratory functions will be noted within 2 minutes. Nalbuphine, a narcotic agonist-antagonist has been employed effectively to reverse respiratory depression induced by narcotic agonists.[40]

Therapeutic indications: Naloxone is indicated for use in narcotic-induced depression, including respiratory (Chapter 23).

Side effects, contraindications, and precautions: When administered intravenously or endotracheally, the duration of naloxone is but 30 minutes. A recurrence of respiratory depression may be observed if the narcotic employed is of longer duration (e.g., morphine). It is common for a second dose of naloxone to be administered intramuscularly following the intravenous dose. Though slower in onset, the duration of therapeutic action of IM naloxone is considerably longer than IV administration. This regimen will minimize the possibility of a recurrence of respiratory depression. It is important to remember that in the presence of narcotic-induced respiratory depression, naloxone is neither the most important drug nor the first step to be taken in patient management. Airway patency and ventilation are of significantly greater importance. Naloxone must be administered with extreme care to persons with known or suspected physical dependence on narcotics. The abrupt and complete reversal of narcotic agonist effects by naloxone may precipitate an acute withdrawal syndrome.

Availability: Adult availability: 0.4 mg/mL in 1-mL ampules and 10-mL vials; pediatric availability: 0.02 mg/mL in 2-mL ampules

Suggested for emergency kit: Two 1-mL ampules of 0.4 mg/mL naloxone

Antidotal drug: benzodiazepine antagonist

Drug of choice: Flumazenil

Drug class: Benzodiazepine antagonist

Alternative drug: None

Although the benzodiazepines have been described as the most nearly ideal agents for anxiety control and sedation, there are still a number of adverse reactions associated with their administration. Emergence delirium, excessive duration of sedation, and possible (though unlikely in most instances) respiratory depression are but a few side effects. The availability of a specific antagonistic agent for benzodiazepines adds another degree of safety to intravenous and, to a lesser extent, intramuscular sedation. Flumazenil has been demonstrated to produce a rapid reversal of sedation and improve a patient's ability to comprehend and obey commands.[41] The duration of anterograde amnesia produced with midazolam was reduced from 121 minutes (without flumazenil) to 91 mintues with flumazenil.[41,42] Flumazenil also decreased recovery time from midazolam sedation, increased alertness, and provided a decreased amnesic effect in a geriatric population (72 ± 9 years). Two patients, however, became anxious following flumazenil administration.[43]

Flumazenil is recommended whenever benzodiazepines such as diazepam, midazolam, or lorazepam are administered parenterally.

Therapeutic indications: Flumazenil is used to reverse clincial actions of parenterally administered benzodiazepines (Chapter 23).

Side effects, contraindications, and precautions: Flumazenil has been demonstrated to produce a rebound anxiety state is some patients.[43]

Availability: Flumazenil (Mazicon) 0.1 mg/ml in 1 0mL multidose vial.

Suggested for emergency kit: 1 × 10 mL multidose vial flumazenil

Antidotal drug: antiemergence delirium

Drug of choice: Physostigmine

Drug class: Reversible anticholinesterase

Alternative drug: None

Several drugs that are commonly employed parenterally to induce sedation have the ability to produce what is known as emergence delirium. Scopolamine and the benzodiazepines, diazepam and midazolam, are most likely to produce this phenomenon in which the patient appears to lose contact with reality. There may also be increased muscular movement, and the patient may seem to speak but the sounds are unintelligible. Physostigmine (Antilirium), a reversible cholinesterase with the ability to cross the blood-brain barrier, has become the drug of choice in the management of emergence delirium.

Physostigmine is recommended for inclusion in the emergency drug kit if scopolamine, benzodiazepines, or other drugs that may induce emergence delirium are administered parenterally.

Therapeutic indications: Physostigmine is used to reverse emergence delirium (Chapter 23).

Side effects, contraindications, and precautions: Side effects noted with physostigmine administration are increased salivation, possible emesis, and involuntary urination and defecation. The first two actions are most often noted. If administered too rapidly, physostigmine can produce the preceding effects as well as bradycardia and hypersalivation, leading to respiratory difficulty. Atropine should always be available whenever physotigmine is administered because it is an antagonist and antidote for physostigmine. Physostigmine should not be administered to patients with asthma, diabetes, cardiovascular disease, or mechanical obstruction of the gastrointestinal or genitourinary tracts.

Availability: Physostigmine is available as Antilirium in 1 mg/mL in 2-mL ampules.

Suggested for emergency kit: Two to three ampules

Antidotal drug: local anesthetic/vasodilator

Drug of choice: Procaine

Drug class: Ester local anesthetic

Alternative drug: None

A local anesthetic that also possesses significant vasodilating properties is recommended for inclusion in the emergency kit whenever IM or IV drugs are employed. Indications for the use of this drug are extravascular injection of an irritating chemical and accidental intraarterial administration of a drug. In both instances the problem is that of compromised circulation in either a localized area (extravascular administration) or a limb (intraarterial administration).

Procaine possesses excellent vasodilating properties along with its pain-relieving actions, both of which make this drug ideal for administration in the aforementioned situations.

Therapeutic indications: Management of vasospasm and compromised circulation following accidental intraarterial injection of a drug

Management of pain and vascular compromise following extravascular administration of irritating drugs

Side effects, contraindications, and precautions: Allergy to ester-type local anesthetics is not uncommon. Do not administer procaine to patients with histories (either documented or alleged) of allergy to Novocain.

Availability: Procaine is available as a 1% (10 mg/mL) solution in 2-mL and 6-mL ampules.

Suggested for emergency kit: Two 2-mL ampules

ORGANIZING THE EMERGENCY KIT

As stressed throughout this chapter, the emergency drug kit need not, and indeed should not, be complicated. Four levels or modules of drugs and equipment were presented: Module one—basic emergency kit (critical drugs and equipment): Module two—noncritical drugs and equipment; Module three—advanced cardiac life support; Module four—antidotal drugs. Doctors should review their educational background and experience with these different drugs before including them in the emergency kit. Only those drugs and items of equipment with which the doctor is thoroughly familiar should be considered for inclusion in the kit. Minimally, Module one (critical drugs and equipment) should be available in all offices.

A simple means of storing emergency drugs is in a fishing tackle box or plastic box with several compartments. Larger kits may be stored in mobile tool cabinets. Labels should be applied to compartments in which each drug is stored and should list both the drug's generic name (e.g., epinephrine) and proprietary name (e.g., Adrenalin) to avoid possible confusion during an emergency.

Written records should be kept of the expiration date of each of the drugs in the emergency kit, and each drug should be replaced prior to its expiration date. Expired drugs as well as empty oxygen cylinders are ineffective in the management of any emergency situation. Office personnel should be assigned the job of regularly checking the emergency kit at least once a week and checking daily all emergency equipment, especially oxygen cylinders, to ensure that all is in readiness. Records of emergency drug and equipment inspection should be entered in a bound, not a loose-leaf, notebook.

On occasion, difficulty may arise in the purchase of the small quantities of drugs required for this emergency kit. Most drug wholesalers usually sell these drugs in prepackaged boxes of 12 or 25 units, yet in most instances only two or three ampules are required for the emergency kit. This problem may be overcome by contacting a hospital pharmacy, which will be more likely to dispense these drugs in smaller quantities.

One potential advantage of commercially prepared emergency kits over self-made kits is a system whereby soon to be outdated drugs are automatically replaced (at a cost) by mail. In situations in which the doctor does not have ready access to a source for emergency drugs, this system may prove beneficial.

The emergency kit and equipment must be kept in a readily accessible area to all office personnel. The back of a storage closet is not the place for life-saving equipment.

To assess whether your office is adequately prepared to manage a life-threatening situation, ask yourself the following question: "If you were in need of emergency medical care, would you want it to be in your office and managed by your dental team?"

REFERENCES

1. American Dental Association House of Delegates. The use of conscious sedation, deep sedation, and general anesthesia in dentistry, November, 1985.
2. Office anesthesia evaluation manual, American Association of Oral & Maxillofacial Surgeons, ed 4, Chicago, 1992, The Association.
3. American Academy of Pediatric Dentistry: Guidelines for the elective use of conscious sedation, deep sedation, and general anesthesia in pediatric patients, *Ped Dent* 7:334-337, 1985.
4. Guidelines for teaching the comprehensive control of pain and anxiety in dental education, Chicago, 1989, American Dental Association.
5. Morrow, GT: Designing a drug kit, *Dent Clin North Amer* 26(1):21-33, 1982.
6. Weaver WD, Cobb LA, Hallstrom AP, and others: Factors influencing survival after out-of-hospital cardiac arrest, *J Am Coll Cardiol* 7:752, 1986.
7. Eisenber MS, Bergner L, Hallstrom A: Cardiac resuscitation in the community: importance of rapid provision and implications for program planning, *JAMA* 241:1905, 1979.
8. Block Drug Company - Vital Response Crisis Management System, Block Drug Company, Jersey City 1988.
9. Healthfirst Corporation: Emergency medicine videotape, Seattle, 1991.
10. Malamed SF: survey of EM, unpublished data 1992.
11. Council on Dental Therapeutics: Emergency kits, *J Am Dent Assoc* 87:909, 1973.
12. Pallasch TJ: This emergency kit belongs in your office, *Dent Management*, August 1976, pp 43-45.
13. Malamed SF: *Sedation: a guide to patient management*, ed 2, St Louis, 1991, Mosby–Year Book.
14. Hollister-Stier Laboratories, Spokane, Washington.
15. Epipen/Epipen Jr.; Center Laboratories, Division of EM Pharmaceuticals, Inc., 35 Channel Drive, Port Washington NY 11050
16. Malamed SF: The use of diphenhydramine HCl as a local anesthetic in dentistry, *Anesth Prog* 20:76, 1973.
17. Pollack CV Jr, Swindle GM: Use of diphenhydramine for local anesthesia in "caine"-sensitive patients, *J Emerg Med* 7(6):611-614, 1989.
18. Raines A, Henderson TR, Swinyard EA, Dretchen KL: Comparison of midazolam and diazepam by the intramuscular route for the control of seizures in a mouse model of status epilepticus, *Epilepsia* 31(3):313-317, 1990.
19. Streeten DHP: Corticosteroid therapy. I. Pharmacological properties and principles of corticosteroid use, *JAMA* 232:944, 1975.
20. American Heart Association and National Academy of Sciences: National Research Council: Standards for cardiopulmonary resuscitation (CPR) and emergency cardiac care (ECC), *JAMA* 255:2905, 1986.

21. Smith JP, Boadi BI, Seifkin A, and others: The esophageal obturator airway: a review, *JAMA* 250:1081, 1983.

22. American Heart Association: *Textbook of advanced cardiac life support*, Dallas, 1987, American Heart Association.

23. Parmley WW, Hatcher CR, Ewy GA, and others: Task force V: physical interventions and adjunctive therapy. Thirteenth Bethesda Conference on emergency cardiac care, *Am J Cardiol* 50:409, 1982.

24. Koehler RC, Michael JR, Guerci AD, and others: Beneficial effect of epinephrine infusion on cerebral and myocardial blood flows during CPR, *Ann Emerg Med* 14:744, 1985.

25. Packer M, Gottlieb SJ, Kessler PD: Hormone-electrolyte interactions in the pathogenesis of lethal cardiac arrhythmias in patients with control of arrhythmias, *Am J Med* 80(suppl 4A):23, 1986.

26. American Heart Association: *Textbook of advanced cardiac life support*, Dallas, 1987, American Heart Association, pg. 97.

27. Giardina EG, Heissenbuttel RH, Bigger JT Jr: Intermittent intravenous procainamide to treat ventricular arrhythmias, *Ann Intern Med* 78:183, 1973.

28. Olson DW, Thompson BM, Darin JL, and others: A randomized comparison study of bretylium tosylate and lidocaine in resuscitation of patients from out-of-hosptial ventricular fibrillation in a paramedic system, *Ann Emerg Med* 13:807, 1984.

29. Benowitz N, Forsyth RP, Melmon KL, and others: Lidocaine disposition kinetics in monkey and man. I. Prediction of a perfusion model, *Clin Pharmacol Ther* 16:87, 1974.

30. Collingsworth KA, Kalman SM, Harrison DC: The clinical pharmacology of lidocaine as an antiarrhythmic drug, *Circulation* 50:1217, 1974.

31. Thomson PD, Melmon KL, Richardson JA, and others: Lidocaine pharmacokinetics in advanced heart failure, liver disease, and renal failure in humans, *Ann Intern Med* 78:499, 1973.

32. American Heart Association: *Textbook of advanced cardiac life support*, Dallas, 1987, American Heart Association, p. 242.

33. Weiner N: Norepinephrine, epinephrine, and the sympathomimetic amines. In Gilman AG, Goodman LS, Rall TW, Murad F, editors: *The pharmacological basis of therapeutics*, New York, 1985, Macmillan.

34. Leier CV: Acute inotropic support. In Leier CV, editor: *Cardiotonic drugs: a clinical survey*, New York, 1986, Marcel Dekker.

35. Mueller HS, Evans R, Ayers S: Effect of dopamine on hemodynamics and myocardial metabolism in shock following acute myocardial infarction in man, *Circulation* 57:361, 1978.

36. McGoon MD, Vlietstra RE, Holmes DR, and others: The clinical use of verapamil, *Mayo Clin Proc* 57:495, 1982.

37. Singh BN, Collett JT, Chew CY: New perspectives in the pharmacologic therapy of cardiac arrhythmias, *Prog Cardiovasc Dis* 22:243, 1980.

38. Stewart RB, Bardy GH, Greene HL: Wide complex tachycardia: misdiagnosis and outcome after emergency therapy, *Ann Intern Med* 104:766, 1986.

39. Pallasch TJ, Gill CJ: Naloxone-associated morbidity and mortality, *Oral Surg* 52:602, 1981.

40. Magruder MR, Delaney RD, DiFazio CA: Reversal of narcotic-induced respiratory depression with nalbuphine hydrochloride, *Anesth Rev* 9(4):34, 1982.

41. Rodrigo MR, Rosenquist JB: The effect of Ro 15-788 (Anexate) in conscious sedation produced with midazolam, *Anaesth Intensive Care* 15:185, 1987.

42. Wolff J, Carl P, Clausen TG, and others: Ro 15-1788 for postoperative recovery: a randomized clinical trial in patients undergoing minor surgical procedures under midazolam anaesthesia, *Anaesthesia* 41:1001, 1986.

43. Ricou B, Forster A, Bruckner A, and others: Clinical evaluation of a specific benzodiazepine antagonist (Ro 15-1788): studies in elderly patients after regional anaesthesia under benzodiazepine sedation, *Br J Anaesth* 58:1005, 1986.

4 *Medicolegal Considerations*

KENNETH S. ROBBINS

Recently, much has been written about the legal implications of practicing dentistry. There is good reason for this because each year 7% to 8% of dentists are sued. These percentages represent well over 15,000 lawsuits against dentists per year; the growing tendency of patients to sue is disquieting. The magnitude of the problem comes into sharper focus when it is discovered that these lawsuits represent only a small fraction of all claims for malpractice made against dentists; most claims are settled by insurers before they become lawsuits. As the number of dentists and attorneys continues to increase, claims and lawsuits against dentists will also continue to increase.

Most claims and lawsuits are brought against dentists because of an allegedly undesired result arising from desired treatment. Complaints of physical damage to components of the mouth are frequent, particularly nerve damage resulting in temporary or permanent loss of sensation and/or loss of control of portions of the mouth. Although malpractice complaints because of medical emergencies in dental offices constitute a minority of the total number of lawsuits against dentists, the life-and-death nature of medical emergencies makes these cases among the most serious in terms of potential injury to the patient and of the dentist's liability. As Dr. Malamed demonstrates, medical emergencies for which the dentist and dentist's staff should be prepared have substantially more serious implications to both patient and dentist than the other, less severe circumstances that (as previously mentioned) give rise to most lawsuits. Lawsuits for damages because of temporary paresthesia, a broken needle, or permanent cosmetic injuries pale in comparison to lawsuits brought because of brain damage or death from improperly administered CPR during a cardiac arrest emergency. Lawsuits resulting from medical emergencies are based on injuries and medical consequences

to the patient that demand the highest jury verdicts and the highest defense costs; they are the multi-million-dollar cases. The high potential jury verdict and the high cost of defense create the maximum probability of an increase both in the individual practitioner's and the profession's dental malpractice insurance. Another potentially devastating risk to dentists in these cases is that the multimillion-dollar verdict may exceed the amount of insurance coverage available, thereby putting dentists' assets and their incomes at risk.

Therefore, it is appropriate and timely to consider how dentists can avoid being sued and, if they are sued, what it will take to win.

Several forms are provided in this section; they are commonly used and have been accepted nationally. They include the American Dental Association (ADA)-recommended medical history questionnaire (Fig. 4-1), as well as the University of Southern California (USC) medical history questionnaire (p. 12). These forms have been accepted throughout the profession and can be important evidence for the dentist in a lawsuit brought by a patient.

COMMONLY ASKED QUESTIONS

What is the standard of care expected when a patient or other person in the office presents the dentist with a medical emergency? Is the standard of care in a medical emergency lower than the standard of care in a nonemergency? In a genuine medical emergency, wouldn't the Good Samaritan statute exempt the dentist from civil liability? If an emergency is truly nothing more than an unforeseen combination of circumstances, how can a dentist be held liable for it?

I am a trial-oriented defense attorney, and these are some of the questions I have been asked. Ultimately, it is a judge sitting without a jury or, more frequently, a jury that furnishes the answer to each

**Copies of the Medical History are Available through the Order Department
of the American Dental Association**

MEDICAL HISTORY

Name ....   Sex ....   Date of Birth ....

Address ....

Telephone ....   Height ....   Weight ....

Date ....   Occupation ....   Marital Status ....

DIRECTIONS

If the answer is YES to the question, put a circle around "YES."
If the answer is NO to the question, put a circle around "NO."
Answer all questions by circling either YES or NO and fill in all blank spaces when indicated.

Answers to the following questions are for our records only and will be considered confidential.

1. Are you in good health ....   YES   NO
   a. Has there been any change in your general health within the past year ....   YES   NO

2. My last physical examination was on ....

3. Are you now under the care of a physician ....   YES   NO

   a. If so, what is the condition being treated ....

4. The name and address of my physician is ....
   ....
   ....

5. Have you had any serious illness or operation ....   YES   NO

   a. If so, what was the illness or operation ....

6. Have you been hospitalized or had a serious illness
   within the past five (5) years ....   YES   NO

   a. If so, what was the problem ....

7. Do you have or have you had any of the following diseases or problems.
   a. Rheumatic fever or rheumatic heart disease ....   YES   NO
   b. Congenital heart lesions ....   YES   NO
   c. Cardiovascular disease (heart trouble, heart attack, coronary insufficiency,
      coronary occlusion, high blood pressure, arteriosclerosis, stroke) ....   YES   NO
      1) Do you have pain in chest upon exertion ....   YES   NO
      2) Are you ever short of breath after mild exercise ....   YES   NO
      3) Do your ankles swell ....   YES   NO
      4) Do you get short of breath when you lie down, or do you require extra pillows
         when you sleep ....   YES   NO
   d. Allergy ....   YES   NO
   e. Asthma or hay fever ....   YES   NO
   f. Hives or a skin rash ....   YES   NO
   g. Fainting spells or seizures ....   YES   NO
   h. Diabetes ....   YES   NO
      1) Do you have to urinate (pass water) more than six times a day ....   YES   NO
      2) Are you thirsty much of the time ....   YES   NO
      3) Does your mouth frequently become dry ....   YES   NO
   i. Hepatitis, jaundice or liver disease ....   YES   NO
   j. Arthritis ....   YES   NO
   k. Inflammatory rheumatism (painful swollen joints) ....   YES   NO
   l. Stomach ulcers ....   YES   NO
   m. Kidney trouble ....   YES   NO
   n. Tuberculosis ....   YES   NO
   o. Do you have a persistent cough or cough up blood? ....   YES   NO
   p. Low blood pressure ....   YES   NO
   q. Venereal disease ....   YES   NO

   r. Other

Fig. 4-1. ADA long-form medical history questionnaire.

8. Have you had abnormal bleeding associated with previous extractions, surgery, or trauma .... YES NO
   a. Do you bruise easily .... YES NO
   b. Have you ever required a blood transfusion .... YES NO

   If so, explain the circumstances _____

   _____

9. Do you have any blood disorder such as anemia .... YES NO

10. Have you had surgery or x-ray treatment for a tumor, growth, or other condition of your head or neck .... YES NO

11. Are you taking any drug or medicine .... YES NO

   If so, what _____

12. Are you taking any of the following:
   a. Antibiotics or sulfa drugs .... YES NO
   b. Anticoagulants (blood thinners) .... YES NO
   c. Medicine for high blood pressure .... YES NO
   d. Cortisone (steroids) .... YES NO
   e. Tranquilizers .... YES NO
   f. Aspirin .... YES NO
   g. Insulin, tolbutamide (Orinase) or similar drug .... YES NO
   h. Digitalis or drugs for heart trouble .... YES NO
   i. Nitroglycerin .... YES NO
   j. Antihistamine .... YES NO
   k. Oral contraceptive or other hormonal therapy .... YES NO
   l. Other _____

13. Are you allergic or have you reacted adversely to:
   a. Local anesthetics .... YES NO
   b. Penicillin or other antibiotics .... YES NO
   c. Sulfa drugs .... YES NO
   d. Barbiturates, sedatives, or sleeping pills .... YES NO
   e. Aspirin .... YES NO
   f. Iodine .... YES NO
   g. Codeine or other narcotics .... YES NO

   h. Other_____

14. Have you had any serious trouble associated with any previous dental treatment .... YES NO

   If so, explain _____

   _____

15. Do you have any disease, condition, or problem not listed above that you think I should know about? .... YES NO

   If so, please explain _____

16. Are you employed in any situation which exposes you regularly to x-rays or other ionizing radiaton .... YES NO

17. Are you wearing contact lenses .... YES NO

WOMEN

18. Are you pregnant .... YES NO

19. Do you have any problems associated with your menstrual period? .... YES NO

Chief Dental Complaint:

_____
Signature of Patient

_____
Signature of Dentist

Fig. 4-1, cont'd. ADA long-form medical history questionnaire.

of these questions in any given lawsuit. Therefore it is appropriate first to examine the context within which a jury answers these difficult questions.

I believe a brief review of what is important at trial will provide a logical basis for understanding and applying the legal principles that pertain to medical emergencies in a dental office and legal expectations of dentists under those circumstances.

THE JURY SYSTEM—SOME IMPORTANT CONSIDERATIONS

Unless a dentist has agreed with a patient beforehand to resolve a dispute in any way other than the judicial system, such as through arbitration or mediation, the existing judicial system in each community and state is the mechanism through which a complaint of malpractice will be resolved. More particularly, if a medical emergency has arisen in a dental office and the patient claims to have been injured because of negligence during the medical emergency, and subsequently files a lawsuit, the case will be disposed of ultimately at trial by the jury.

Frequently, it appears unlikely that a jury will be able to make sense of the enormous volume of evidence presented in a trial and return to the proper verdict. They can, however, and they will. The result depends on the evidence, the law, and the quality of trial counsel.

Long ago, the manner in which well-heeled people resolved important disputes was by means of professionals who were adept at some form of one-on-one combat—for example, knights at a joust. Whoever hired the victorious combatant won the dispute. Those professionals of old have been replaced in the modern world by a different kind of combatant. Lawyers now oppose each other with legal, not lethal, results; the consequences, however, are just as important to those who hire them. The adversarial system between attorneys has evolved into a process that uncovers as many facts as possible to assist a nonpartisan third person (the judge) or group of third persons (the jury) in deciding who should win and lose. Ideally, if the plaintiff's attorney and the defendant's attorney excel equally at their craft, a judge and/or jury will be provided with sufficient enlightenment to reach a just conclusion. Sadly, advocates are not equal, and frequently, greater incentive to win cases is provided to patients' attorneys than to attorneys hired by insurance companies.

Plantiff's attorneys are usually hired on a contingency fee basis; that is, they will recover a percentage of whatever they obtain for their clients (generally 25% to 40%, but sometimes up to 75%).

Therefore, plantiffs' attorneys have a built-in incentive to win their clients' cases. Contingency fees have not been accepted as appropriate compensation in the defense of a party to a lawsuit. Therefore virtually all dentists are defended in a lawsuit by an attorney who is paid by the hour and is generally paid the same fee, win or lose. The professionalism among defense attorneys should be sufficiently high to negate the presumption that an attorney with a vested interest in a victory will do better for his client. The primary difference between the two types of attorneys is the fact that a plaintiff-oriented attorney who chooses his or her cases carefully will probably generate a substantially higher fee revenue than a defense attorney, who is often required to maintain highly competitive hourly rates. Thus, the insurance company, in a meritorious case, pays a fee to the plaintiff's lawyer that is usually higher than the fee paid to its own defense attorney. This is done to keep the carrier's expenses as low as can reasonably be expected and is particularly notable in a multimillion-dollar case, in which the patient's attorney will receive a substantial percentage of a gigantic award. Again, the professionalism and trial expertise of a community of defense attorneys should remain unaffected by the different fee arrangements, and the quality of services rendered should ideally be as high for defendants as for plaintiffs. This disparity in incentive, however, may create inequality of legal services.

A skilled attorney for the plantiff decides to take a case based on what the attorney believes the outcome of the potential lawsuit will be. If the facts of the potential lawsuit indicate that a jury may not decide favorably for the patient, the attorney will probably not take the case at all or will accept it with the understanding that the potential lawsuit has reduced settlement value. I believe that the unhappy practice of plaintiffs' attorneys taking weak cases and settling them for reduced but substantial amounts is encouraged everytime a dentist, his insurance company, and his defense attorney approve of such settlements.

An astute attorney for the plaintiff will request a copy of the patient's chart for the attorney's review and for the review of another dentist, as well—before agreeing to accept the patient's case. A well-documented chart demonstrating satisfactory care of the patient will discourage a decision to take the case. Therefore, good documentation by the dentist is not only important at trial but also extremely important in determining whether or not an attorney will take the case against the dentist.

Once a lawsuit is filed with the court, the dentist

is served by a sheriff with a complaint and a summons, either by mail or by notice in a newspaper. Within a prescribed time of service, usually 30 days or less, the dentist must file an answer or risk having a default judgment taken against him. Between the time of service and the time of answering the complaint, the dentist must secure the services of a defense attorney. Generally, the assignment of the case to a defense attorney is made by the dentist's insurance carrier. However, dentists are strongly urged to know whom they would wish to represent them before they are ever sued. Depending on the population, an insurance company usually employs one to three attorneys in any given community, to whom it gives all or most of its defense work on behalf of its insured. Sometimes the attorney selected is not the attorney whom the dentist may wish to have represent him or her. Therefore, it is urged that a dentist become familiar with those attorneys in the community who excel in dental malpractice defense. The dentist should make certain when he or she purchases malpractice insurance that he or she and the insurance carrier agree on the choice of an attorney in case the dentist is sued. The worst time to make a well-reasoned decision—one that could affect the rest of the dentist's life—is when the dentist is upset over having just been sued and has a month or less to agree on the selection of a defense attorney.

After the dentist's attorney has filed an answer to the complaint on the dentist's behalf, the process of discovery begins. There is no longer any excuse, in a case to be tried for a patient or dentist, for attorneys to be ignorant of any important facts. Liberal rules of discovery allow the use of many discovery tools. Among these are written interrogatories to be answered by each party; depositions, which are made up of testimony under oath during the discovery period; requests for production of records by the parties; and requests to admit certain facts. The period of discovery permits both parties and their attorneys to learn as much as possible about the merits of the patient's case and the dentist's defense. The dentist should expect to be kept abreast of all important developments in the lawsuit. A feeling of teamwork should develop between dentist and attorney; each has expertise the other needs.

A clear example of good teamwork is planning for the presence of the defendant dentist during the deposition of the patient's expert witness. It is more difficult for the expert to criticize the dentist if he is sitting across the table. Often, the dentist should be present during the patient's deposition, too. In addition, these depositions provide an excellent opportunity for the dentist to evaluate the quality of the attorney. Another example of teamwork is when the dentist offers assistance to his attorney on dental and medical issues. This also provides the defendant dentist with an excellent opportunity to evaluate for himself the most important evidence against him.

BURDEN OF PROOF AND RES IPSA LOQUITUR

With few exceptions, the plaintiff has what is called the burden of proof in any case, including a lawsuit against a dentist. This means that for a patient to win his or her case against a dentist, a jury must find that the plaintiff sustained the burden of providing the following:
1. That the dentist was at fault
2. That the dentist's fault was the cause of injuries to the patient
3. That those injuries must be compensated in dollars and cents (damages), which the dentist must pay to the patient and, in serious cases, to the patient's family

Therefore, in almost all cases in which a dentist has been sued, he or she may take comfort in the fact that the burden is *not* on the defendant to disprove any of the issues; rather, it is on the plaintiff. In practical terms, however, the best defense is often the offense for the dentist's attorney. He goes on the offense, by producing evidence to disprove his client's fault, that is, he proves the dentist did not injure the patient. A good defense attorney, like a good boxer, will be prepared at trial to take the lead or to counterpunch with appropriate evidence. This decision is made as late as possible.

The reader will note some qualification when I say that the patient has the burden of proof in all instances. The law has carved out an interesting and logical exception to a plaintiff's responsibility to prove fault. That exception is known as *res ipsa loquitur,* commonly shortened to *res ipsa.* Literally translated, this phrase means "the thing speaks for itself." Expressed simply, this concept applies to lawsuits in which the result itself indicates that there must have been some wrong committed by the dentist; otherwise, the harm would not have occurred. For instance, if the dentist or oral surgeon performed a surgical procedure that required the use of small sponges and a sponge was left in the gum and discovered later, the plaintiff would not have the burden of proving that the dentist was at fault. In this case, the dentist has the burden of proving that the sponge being left in the patient's tissue was not the dentist's fault. There are relatively few areas of dentistry in which the burden of proof is shifted to the dentist because of the doctrine of *res ipsa loquitur*. Few if any lawsuits arising out of medical emergencies fall into this category.

THE EXPERT WITNESS

Part of the plaintiff's burden of proving the three indispensable elements of a case against the dentist is the procurement of expert testimony. Except in cases of *res ipsa loquitur*, the plaintiff's burden of proving a case of malpractice against a dentist is accomplished through an expert witness. The expert witness, retained by the patient's lawyer, gives testimony that includes opinions on the appropriate standard of care and whether or not the dentist met it in treating the patient. Cases involving medical emergencies are included in those that require an expert witness. Because a lay jury is not considered competent to reach decisions without expert testimony in cases against dentists (except in *res ipsa loquitur* cases), an indispensable part of the plaintiff's case against the dentist is having an expert witness, qualified by the court as such, who will state under oath that the dentist fell below the standard of care and that the injuries complained about resulted from the dentist's breach of this standard of care. Except in cases of *res ipsa loquitur*, most courts in most states will dismiss a lawsuit against a dentist before trial if the plaintiff has not obtained expert testimony against the defendant dentist. On the other hand, the defendant dentist and his attorney may also retain an expert witness to counter the testimony of the plaintiff's expert witness. Because the plaintiff has the burden of proof, the dentist need not obtain an expert witness to testify at trial. But if a plaintiff has an expert witness, it is rare for an experienced defense trial attorney to fail to secure an expert witness on behalf of his or her own client; this witness is needed to counter the adverse testimony of the plaintiff's expert. In some cases, however, an expert need not be called on behalf of the dentist. An entire book could be written on the appropriate strategies and counter strategies of using or not using expert witnesses at trial. I have defended cases through trial that have proved the proposition that, in rare instances, the defendant dentist may well be his or her own best expert witness. However, the strategy must be used carefully. Of course, selection of the expert witness is extremely important. It is a rare person who can testify equally effectively at trial in many different professional and geographic areas. Selection and use of an expert witness is an example of the great care, thought, and psychology that

must be exercised in case preparation and trial.

A lawsuit tried solely on the basis of the strategy of the attorneys and the credibility of expert witnesses would be much like a football game without officials. From the beginning of the lawsuit to the conclusion of trial, a judge is always available to provide answers when the lawyers cannot agree and to interject into each case the principles of law by which all cases are governed, including those regarding standard of care, negligence, proximate cause of the injuries, and guidelines for awarding damages.

Although the precise wording of these legal concepts may vary somewhat from state to state, their interpretation is sufficiently broad to allow meaningful discussions about their application in virtually all states. Discussion of several of these important concepts provide the dentist with a better understanding of what the law expects of him or her in terms of anticipating, preventing, or successfully treating a medical emergency in the dental office. These concepts are the cornerstones of a successful defense for a lawsuit resulting from a medical emergency.

THE LAW OF EACH CASE—THE STANDARD OF CARE

A jury must find the dentist negligent before the patient can recover damages. The terms *negligence* and *malpractice* are used synonymously in lawsuits against health care providers. In defining *negligence* in a dental malpractice case, a judge will usually tell the jury that negligence is (1) doing something that an ordinarily prudent dentist would not do under the same or similar circumstances, or (2) not doing something that a reasonably prudent dentist would do under the same or similar circumstances. A judge will instruct the jury that negligence is the failure to use ordinary care. This seems easy enough to determine as it applies to an automobile driver or a shop owner who leaves a slippery substance on the floor of the shop. However, how does a jury apply the principle of negligence to a dentist?

This is where the testimony of the expert witness enters the picture. The judge's instructions will guide the jury with regard to the indispensable expert testimony in almost all cases against dentists; the judge will instruct the jury that in a case against the dentist, each side is permitted to call an expert witness to define the standard of care and testify about whether or not the defendant met the standard. The judge will inform the jury that people ordinarily are not permitted to come into the courtroom and offer opinions. Usually, witnesses may only testify to facts: what they saw or heard or what documents or other information they have that may assist the jury. However, the procedure differs in a lawsuit in which a jury must determine whether or not a dentist is at fault. In that case, expert witnesses—witnesses who have special training and experience and are acknowledged to possess the skill or education to qualify them to offer opinions to the jury—may so testify, and the jury may consider their opinions. The judge informs the jury that they need not consider any of the opinions given and may weigh the credibility of the expert witnesses by the same criteria they use for all other witnesses. The crux of the testimony of each expert witness in a dental malpractice lawsuit is whether or not the dentist was negligent. In most states, an expert witness is not permitted to testify whether he or she believes that the dentist was negligent or not. However, the expert witness may give opinion testimony about whether or not the dentist fell within or below the acceptable standard of care. In doing so, the expert may not use his or her own personal standards but must use what he or she believes to be the standards of the community. In recent years the community standard has been expanded to match the national community standard. Therefore, in almost all lawsuits in all courts across the country, each defendant dentist is held to a national standard of care, which the expert witnesses establish in their testimonies. However, experts frequently do not agree on what the national standard is. It should now be self-evident that expert witnesses are an indispensable part of the plaintiff's case and that without them the case must be dismissed. Without expert testimony on behalf of the plaintiff who, you will recall, has the burden of proof, there can be no evidence regarding the acceptable standard of care, which the jury must use to reach a conclusion about the dentist's treatment of the patient.

A multitude of people in different professions are qualified as experts in the proper response to medical emergencies in dental offices. They include cardiopulmonary resuscitation (CPR) instructors, paramedics, some nurses, medical doctors, and of course dentists. This creates an abundance of potential expert witnesses to testify either for or against the dentist.

Having discussed briefly the more important judicial concepts that govern the outcome of every lawsuit against a dentist, we now turn to an evaluation of the legal duty owed or not owed by dentists in anticipating and preventing or in treating medical emergencies.

FORESEEABILITY OF THE EMERGENCY

One of the underlying principles of our legal system is the concept of foreseeability. If the consequences of an act are foreseeable and result in harm, liability may be imposed. It is arguable that a cardiac arrest or an idiosyncratic reaction to medication or anesthesia in a dental office are not foreseeable events, unless the dentist has a crystal ball in the office. However, experience tells us that, although it is impossible to predict when a particular medical emergency will arise, they do occur and therefore are foreseeable. It is probably for this reason that companies with a great number of employees and large companies that have direct contact with the public, such as department stores, hotels, and restaurants, are in the process of upgrading and maintaining higher standards for responding to medical emergencies. More and more employees of such organizations are learning how to correctly administer such procedures as CPR. At the time of publication of the fourth edition of this book, it remains questionable whether or not a person could bring a successful lawsuit against department store personnel for failing to respond properly to his or her cardiac arrest. However, as the community standard in responding to cardiac arrests is upgraded and as expectations rise as to how department store personnel or those from similar enterprises should respond to medical emergencies, it is arguable that in years to come a department store employee may be considered negligent if he or she does not have the wherewithal to respond to a cardiac arrest.

There is little doubt that the expectations and therefore the anticipated standards of care in responding to a medical emergency are higher in medical facilities, including dental offices. We might ask why this is so. It is common knowledge, as has been borne out in cases that I have defended, that there are circumstances and practices within a dental office that are much more likely to precipitate a medical emergency than those within, for example, a department store. This higher likelihood of emergency, then, helps to explain higher expectations of care.

What are some of the foreseeable circumstances or factors that are likely to give rise to medical emergencies in a dental office?

Many people experience fear and anxiety at the mere thought of having to see a dentist in a day or two. By the time these people find themselves in the dentist's office and are waiting for the dentist to see them, their fear and anxiety may cause measurable metabolic changes. Sometimes, anger and frustration about having to wait for a long time to see the dentist are added, and many of these patients become prone to medical emergencies precipitated by metabolic changes. However, even patients who are seen immediately will probably be substantially more stressed than they would be in most other environments.

A highly stressed patient is not the ideal patient for administration of anesthetics or medications. Furthermore, once treatment begins, the chance of a medical emergency increases for anxious and nonanxious patients alike with the administration of anesthetics and medications, virtually all of which are known to have adverse reactions, idiosyncratic reactions, and side effects. The *Physicians' Desk Reference (PDR)* or the drug package insert accompanying each anesthetic or medication lists reactions that have been reported to be associated with all anesthetics and medications used in the dental office. Virtually every anesthetic agent and medication that a dentist uses can be shown to have been associated with a bizarre medical reaction. It must be kept in mind that those reactions published in the drug package insert and the *PDR*, which are generally identical, are *associated with* the use of a particular anesthestic or medication; in fact, the use of the anesthetic or medication may have absolutely nothing to do with the ensuing medical emergency, whether or not it be cardiac arrest or some other life-threatening reaction that is reported and included in the *PDR*. However, there stands the description of the reaction, in print, for an expert witness to refer to at trial. The witness can say to the jury, "The adverse reaction to the anesthetic is something the dentist knew about or should have known about; it is listed as a known side effect in the pharmaceutical bible, the *PDR*, which every prescriber and administrator of medication has or should have. The same information is included with every vial and every package of medication that is opened in the dentist's office." The *PDR* excerpt for that medication will go into evidence for the jury to read during its deliberations. It can be used as evidence of notice to the dentist—that is, evidence that the dentist used the anesthetic or medication daily with many patients and therefore had a duty to know all of its reported side effects and adverse reactions. Consequently, the argument goes, the dentist should have anticipated and treated correctly the adverse reaction or side effect experienced by his or her patient. Of course, the defense attorney can counter through his or her own expert witnesses, through witnesses from pharmaceutical companies or the FDA, or even

from the *PDR* itself that the side effects, adverse reactions, and incidents reported in association with use of the medication are based on reports made by health care providers, many of which are never investigated and verified. However, this kind of evidence can seem to the jury to be a rationalization. The dentist's attorney must anticipate this and prepare to respond successfully. However, the reader can begin to see that the *PDR*, in presenting information that offers protection to the pharmaceutical companies, also contains information that the dentist should know and use as a tool in his or her practice. Keeping abreast of the *PDR* avoids being painfully confronted with it in a lawsuit. Plaintiffs' attorneys experienced in dental malpractice know that there should be a *PDR* in every dental office or, failing that, that every container of anesthetic or medication in a dental office contains a drug package insert with the very same information. If the *PDR* is not used in the dental office, the plaintiff's attorney will attempt to prove that an emergency occurred because the dentist failed to keep up with medication literature.

Therefore, know the drugs you use. Stay current with them by consulting the *PDR* and its updates throughout the year. Identify patients for whom special precautions may have to be taken. Make a note in patients' charts if reevaluation of medications or further history from the patient is required. These follow-up notations reflect excellent dentistry, and just as important at trial, they are convincing evidence of excellent dentistry.

DEALING WITH THE MEDICAL EMERGENCY

In the preface to this book, Dr. Malamed has said that with proper patient management virtually all medical emergency situations can be prevented. Frankly, I believe that, within a legal and perhaps medical context, this is a rather severe standard to which the dentist is expected to adhere. I would rather say that all medical emergencies are *foreseeable* and that a dentist and his or her staff should therefore be properly trained and equipped to confront the medical emergency as well as can be reasonable anticipated in a dental office. A dentist can probably increase the chances of a medical emergency with poor "bedside" (actually chairside) manner, including keeping a patient waiting. A dentist and his or her staff can increase the chances of a medical emergency by failure to identify genuine anxiety and stress, failure to allay it, or (perhaps) failure to postpone treatment until a patient's anxiety has been allayed. As far as adverse and idiosyncratic reactions to medications are concerned, there are other preventive measures that can and probably should be taken based on the current national standard of dental practice.

HISTORY TAKING

As has been discussed in Chapter 2 and stressed elsewhere in this book, it is imperative that dentists obtain a full and complete medical history from patients before treating them. Even if the patient is in severe pain and presents what can be termed a dental emergency, there are few dental emergencies that cannot wait a few additional minutes while a thorough medical history is obtained from the patient or a person familiar with the patient, such as a spouse or parent. Knowledge of such problems as liver disorders, food and drug allergies, and heart problems is indispensable in the proper care and treatment of a patient. Failure to gather such information can be the most damaging evidence of all if an anesthetic or medication, which would have been contraindicated by a satisfactory medical history, is administered and results in a serious medical emergency. Several excellent medical history questionnaires have been presented in Chapter 2.

It is urged that, to protect himself or herself and more importantly to protect his or her patient, the dentist should have each patient complete such a questionnaire before initial treatment. Because the history of some categories of patients, particularly the young and the elderly, may change markedly from year to year, dentists are urged to have patients update their medical history forms annually. If a dentist has not treated a patient for several months, it's a good idea for the dentist or an office staff member to ask the patient if he or she has had any medical changes or has been seen by a physician for anything other than common, garden-variety illnesses; this rules out any major problems before treatment. It is particularly imporant these days to note on a patient's chart that he or she was asked about any such medical changes or treatment since the last visit. A notation of the patient's response should also be made. To demonstrate how important this is, let us say that a patient suffers a serious adverse reaction from a medication in a dentist's office during treatment, and a lawsuit is brought and subsequently is tried. There is no way in the world that a jury will believe a dentist and his or her staff members if they testify that they specifically recall a patient's verbal statement that nothing of any medical consequence had happened to the patient since his or her last visit—

unless that statement was noted in writing. To discredit a verbal statement, a skilled plaintiff's attorney simply has to establish the fact that, in the months and years that have passed since that particular visit, the dentist has had several thousand dental visits from many patients. Thus, the jury will be asked to view the dentist's recall of the statement with great suspicion. If in fact a significant medical event *has* occurred that the patient has not related to the dentist, and if the dentist records the question and negative response in the patient's chart, this information will support the dentist years later; it will be very difficult evidence for the patient and his or her attorney to rebut at trial.

If a patient's medical history requires clarification, the dentist should contact the patient's primary physician, making a notation in the patient's chart about the consultation and what was discussed. Patients' charts should include the names and phone numbers of their regular physicians for this purpose. When the dentist calls, he should indicate to the physician that he is making a note and would appreciate the physician making a notation of the same discussion in her chart for the patient. These notations may prove to be extremely important at trial.

INFORMED CONSENT

In the past two decades, a national standard pertaining to informed consent has developed. The courts of each state may vary the requirements of obtaining informed consent somewhat, but in essence informed consent requires that a dentist explain the following to a patient in sufficient detail so that the patient understands:

1. Reasons for care and treatment
2. Diagnosis
3. Prognosis
4. Alternatives
5. Nature of care and treatment
6. The risks involved (inherent risks included)
7. Expectations of success
8. Possible results if care and treatment are not undertaken or if instructions are not followed

As with other topics discussed in this chapter, informed consent could be the subject of many chapters or of an entire book. However, a brief overview indicates that within the context of a discussion of medical emergencies, the concept of informed consent has an interesting twist. It is arguable that the more thorough a dentist is in explaining the risks involved and in documenting the risks discussed with the patient, the stronger the evidence may be against the dentist if a medical emergency arises out of the treatment. For instance, let us say that an oral surgeon warns a patient that cardiac arrest is a known reaction to an anesthetic and that the patient subsequently experiences cardiac arrest under that anesthetic. It will be difficult for the oral surgeon to attempt to defend himself by saying that that reaction was an unforeseeable emergency and therefore impossible to prepare for. Consequently, the more thorough a dentist is in informing the patient of risks, the more prepared he or she should be to prevent or treat those risks.

To the extent that it can be shown that medical emergencies will occur with higher frequency in a dentist's office than in many other places, a dentist will be expected to be that much more prepared to prevent or treat such emergencies.

Throughout this text, Dr. Malamed has discussed what kinds of emergencies dentists should anticipate and how they should be treated; therefore that discussion need not be repeated here. It should be emphasized, however, that proper response to a medical emergency often requires effective and efficient teamwork. This is particularly true in a situation in which CPR is administered, especially on the part of the team member administering CPR. Therefore, each dental office should be staffed by appropriately trained personnel who know what their assigned tasks will be in case of a medical emergency. For example, who will telephone for an ambulance? Where will the emergency response equipment, including oxygen, be kept, and whose responsibility will it be to bring that equipment to the patient? In many circumstances, CPR cannot be administered effectively by only one person; therefore, it may be no excuse that the dentist alone knows CPR. Because CPR is forseeable and will probably have to be administered at some time, it may be well for all dental office employees to be familiar with and well-rehearsed in CPR technique and to have current CPR certification. In addition, dentists ought to hold occasional CPR drills in their offices and keep records of these drills, including which staff members participated. Such records will refute very effectively the contention that a patient died during cardiac arrest because of lack of CPR training of office personnel. Cardiopulmonary resuscitation will not always save a patient, and it would be sad for a dentist to be held liable in such instances simply because he or she failed to document the training of employees, as well as practice drills held in the office.

As soon as possible after an emergency, the dentist should thoroughly note what happened to the patient in the patient's chart—from the initiation of treatment to the conclusion of the emergency, or until the patient's care has been undertaken by paramedics or a physician. If the emergency was handled correctly, these notes will be invaluable in the defense at trial.

Because the dentist is responsible for job-related negligence of associates and employees, he or she must be sure that the dental team is well trained so that an employee's act or omission will not create liability for the dentist. Although the dentist may respond superbly to a medical emergency, problems will arise if the staff is untrained.

Often, paramedics may be more expert in handling medical emergencies than dentists; they may not wish to have the dentist accompany them and the patient to the hospital. A dentist should offer assistance to the paramedics before they leave for the hospital. Whatever the paramedics decide, the dentist's offer to continue assistance on the way to the hospital and the paramedics' response to that offer should be clearly documented by the dentist.

A LOWER STANDARD IN AN EMERGENCY?

The law does not require the dentist or any other health care practitioner to respond to an emergency and a nonemergency in the same manner. In other words, the standard of care expected of a dentist in the emergency is not as high as the standard of care expected in a nonemergency. However, as discussed previously, whether or not a dentist is negligent in an emergency situation will ultimately be decided by the jury on the basis of the answer to this question: Did the dentist and his or her staff respond as would an ordinarily prudent dentist and staff in the same or similar circumstances? The dentist and the staff will be held to the standard of the ordinarily prudent dentist and staff to the extent that the medical emergency can be shown to have been foreseeable and to the extent that evidence shows that the dentist and staff should have been prepared. Although the standard of care in emergency situations may not be as high as the nonemergency standard, there are expected standards of conduct in emergencies. If the dentist and staff meet these standards, there will be no liability; if they fail to meet them, there will be liability.

It should be remembered that medical emergencies resulting from dental treatment may occur after the patient has left the office. If a patient begins to experience an adverse reaction to a medication at home and calls the dental office, or if a call is placed on the patient's behalf, the dentist and staff should be prepared to meet these emergencies also. A preplanned response to such a situation should be discussed among staff members so that the patient or his or her family can be given proper and immediate instructions. A dentist's failure to respond in such a circumstance may itself precipitate a lawsuit. If a patient cannot get your attention at the time of the phone call, he certainly will with a lawsuit!

GOOD SAMARITAN CONSIDERATIONS

Good Samaritan statutes differ somewhat from state to state. However, they usually say that health care providers should not be held liable for death or injury (except for gross negligence) in cases in which they render emergency life-and-death treatment, in good faith, to people who are not their patients (that is, people for whose treatment they do not expect to be compensated). The medical emergency of a patient in a dental office probably does not constitute a situation in which a Good Samaritan defense is applicable. Because the victim of the emergency is the patient of the dentist, the dentist has an obligation to treat the patient. However, if a nonpatient of the dentist, such as a family member, happens to be in the waiting room and requires an emergency response to a medical situation, a Good Samaritan defense may well apply.

•   •   •

Establish a relationship with a good, experienced malpractice defense attorney before you ever need one. Additionally, keep in touch with that attorney and seek his or her advice, much as you would recommend to your patients that they have periodic checkups as a preventive measure. Urge your community dental association or society to invite attorneys who specialize in dental malpractice cases to meetings; they will be able to familiarize you with informed consent requirements and other peculiarities of the law in your state. You should know of the statutes and cases that affect your practice so that you can tailor your practice to meet the requirements of the law. Learn how other dentists are equipping and preparing their office and staffs for medical emergencies. Make certain that your preparedness is comparable to what appears to be the standard. Remember that the standard of care is not perfection, particularly when the caregiver is responding to a medical emergency.

Although today's health care professionals are defending themselves against more lawsuits than ever, lawsuits can be prevented; what's more, if they do occur, they can be defended successfully. The prevention or successful defense of lawsuits depends on how you and your staff meet the challenges of increased litigation. Don't let yourself, your staff, or your colleagues down. By preventing lawsuits or providing information leading to a successful defense, you not only protect yourself but also maintain the presumption that dentists care about their patients and take prudent precautions to protect them. If you follow the suggestions in this chapter, practice within the standard of reasonableness, maintain your continuing dental education, and document office procedures and your patient's charts, the law will support you.

One last word: courage. If you have competent, experienced counsel and a strong defense, have the courage to go through with a trial, if necessary. Settling claims or lawsuits out of court, if you should and can win in court, will only encourage additional lawsuits. By going through with a trial and winning the suit, you will not only vindicate yourself and your staff, and discourage similar lawsuits—you will also become a better dentist.

5 *Unconsciousness: General Considerations*

In the recent past the loss of consciousness was not an uncommon occurrence in dental situations. In surveys by Fast[1] and Malamed,[2] vasodepressor syncope (common faint) was the most often reported medical emergency. Although the loss of consciousness may be produced by any number of other causes (Schultz[3] presents 33 potential causes to be considered in a differential diagnosis of syncope [see accompanying box]), the initial steps in the management of unconsciousness from any cause will be essentially the same and are primarily directed toward certain basic, life-sustaining procedures (**A**irway, **B**reathing, **C**irculation).

In most instances in dentistry the loss of consciousness will prove to be transient, and carrying out the aforementioned basic, yet crucial, procedures will be all that is required initially for proper management. However, there are still other causes of unconsciousness that will require significant additional attention once these steps have been taken.

This section will cover several of the more common emergency situations that may result in the loss of consciousness. Definitions of relevant terms follow:

anoxia. Absence or lack of oxygen

coma. From the Greek *koma,* meaning deep sleep; it is most often used to designate a state of unconsciousness from which the patient cannot be aroused, even by powerful stimulation. Huff[4] defines coma as "that altered state that exists in a patient manifesting inappropriate responses to environmental stimuli who maintains eye closure throughout the stimuli."

consciousness. From the Latin *conscius,* meaning aware; the term *consciousness* implies the capability of responding appropriately to question or command and the presence of intact protective reflexes,

---

DIFFERENTIAL DIAGNOSIS OF SYNCOPE

Neurogenic causes
  Breath holding
  Carotid sinus disease
  Vasovagal syncope
  Vasodepressor syncope
  Orthostatic hypotension
  Glossopharyngeal neuralgia
  Seizure disorders
Vascular causes
  Cerebrovascular disease
    Tussive (cough) syncope
    Cerebrovascular accidents
  Pulmonary embolism
  Aortic arch syndromes
Endocrineopathies
  Hypoglycemia
  Addisonian crisis
  Pheochromocytoma
  Hypothyroidism
Exposure to toxins and drugs
Psychogenic problems
Cardiogenic causes
  Valvular heart disease
  Dysrhythmias
  Myocardial infarction
  Certain congenital heart anomalies
  Hypertrophic cardiomyopathy
  Pacemaker syndrome
Disorders of oxygenation
  Anemia
  High altitude exposure
  Barotrauma
  Decompression sickness

Modified from Schultz KE: Vertigo and syncope. In Rosen P (editor): *Emergency medicine: concepts and clinical practice,* ed 2, St Louis, 1988, Mosby–Year Book.

Table 5-1. Possible causes of unconsciousness in the dental office

Cause	Frequency	Where covered in text
Vasodepressor syncope	Most common	Unconsciousness (Section Two)
Drug administration/ingestion	Common	Drug-related emergencies (Section Six)
Orthostatic hypotension	Less common	Unconsciousness (Section Two)
Epilepsy	Less common	Seizures (Section Five)
Hypoglycemic reaction	Less common	Altered consciousness (Section Four)
Acute adrenal insufficiency	Rare	Unconsciousness (Section Two)
Acute allergic reaction	Rare	Drug-related emergencies (Section Six)
Acute myocardial infarction	Rare	Chest pain (Section Seven)
Cerebrovascular accident	Rare	Altered consciousness (Section Four)
Hyperglycemic reaction	Rare	Altered consciousness (Section Four)
Hyperventilation	Rare	Altered consciousness (Section Four)

including the ability to independently maintain a patent airway.[5]

faint. Sudden, transient loss of consciousness

hypoxia. Low oxygen content

syncope. From the Greek *synkope;* a sudden, transient loss of consciousness without prodromal symptoms followed within seconds to minutes (less than 30 minutes) by resumption of consciousness usually with the premorbid status intact.[6]

unconsciousness. A lack of response to sensory stimulation[7]

The terms *syncope* and *faint* are commonly used interchangeably to describe the transient loss of consciousness caused by reversible disturbances in cerebral function. Throughout this text the term *syncope* will be employed to describe this occurrence.

It must be remembered that syncope is only a symptom and that although syncopal episodes may occur in healthy individuals, they may also be indicative of serious medical disorders. It must also be remembered that any loss of consciousness, however brief, represents a potentially life-threatening situation. Prompt recognition and effective management will be required whenever the loss of consciousness occurs.

PREDISPOSING FACTORS

Some of the possible causes of the loss of consciousness in the dental office setting are presented in Table 5-1 along with their relative frequency of occurence. Review of this list will provide the reader with the impression that there are many possible causes of unconsciousness. Although this is relatively accurate, a closer examination will reveal three factors that, when present, increase the chances that alterations of consciousness or loss of consciousness will occur. These factors are (1) stress, (2) impaired physical status, and (3) the administration or ingestion of drugs.

In the dental setting stress will be the primary cause for most cases of unconsciousness. Vasodepressor syncope, the most common cause of unconsciousness, may be regarded as a manifestation of unusual stress. Syncope occurring during venipuncture or during an intraoral injection of local anesthetic are typical examples of vasodepressor syncope.[8,9]

Impaired physical status (ASA III or IV) is a second factor that increases the incidence of syncope. Many of the causes listed in Table 5-1 are not usually associated at the onset with syncope but may progress to this state if the primary problem is not promptly recognized or if the patient is debilitated. If a patient with impaired physical status must be exposed to undue physiologic or psychologic stress, the chances are even greater that this patient will react adversely to the situation. Individuals with underlying cardiac disease may respond by sudden death occurring secondary to cardiac dysrhythmias precipitated by the same physiologic stress that would cause vasodepressor syncope in the normal individual.[10]

A third factor potentially associated with the loss of consciousness is the administration or ingestion of drugs. The three major categories of drugs employed in dentistry are analgesics (nonnarcotics, including NSAID's; narcotics, and local anesthetics), antianxiety agents (sedative-hypnotics and tranquilizers), and antibiotics. Drugs in the first two categories are all potent central nervous system (CNS) depressants and may therefore readily induce alterations in consciousness (e.g., sedation) or the loss of consciousness. Some of these drugs, primarily the narcotic agonists, will predispose the ambulatory dental patient to orthostatic (postural) hypotension (Chapter 7), whereas narcotics and drugs such as barbiturates and other sedative-hypnotics, if administered in larger doses, may induce the loss of consciousness through entry into the second or third stages of anesthesia (Guedel's classification).*

Local anesthetics are the most commonly employed drugs in dentistry, and because they are injected, they are a major predisposing factor for syncope. It is conservatively estimated that in excess of 1 million cartridges of local anesthetics are injected each day by dentists in the United States alone, yet morbidity and mortality rates from these agents are incredibly low.[12] However, life-threatening situations can develop in conjuction with the use of local anesthetics. The overwhelming majority of adverse reactions to local anesthetics will be precipitated by stress (fear and anxiety)[13]; however, reactions can develop that are directly related to the agents themselves. These include the overdose (toxic) reaction and allergy. Adverse reactions to local anesthetics and other common dental drugs will be discussed more fully in Section VI.

PREVENTION

Loss of consciousness can be prevented in many instances by a thorough pretreatment medical and dental evaluation of the prospective patient. Important elements in this evaluation include a determination of the patient's ability to tolerate, both physiologically and psychologically, the stress associated with the planned dental treatment. Use of a medical history questionnaire and physical examination of the patient, followed by the dialogue history may uncover medical and/or psychological disabilities that might predispose a patient toward syncope. Detection of these disabilities permits the doctor to modify the planned treatment to better accommodate the impaired physical or psychologic status of the patient. Determination of fear and anxiety related to dentistry is often more difficult to uncover as patients frequently seek to keep their fears hidden. A method of determining the presence of dental fears has been employed successfully at the University of Southern California School of Dentistry since 1973. It consists of a short anxiety questionnaire (p. 13), which is included in the medical history that each patient is required to complete prior to the start of dental care. This has been patterned after the questionnaire devised by Corah,[14] which presents the patient with a series of questions related to his or her attitudes toward various aspects of dental treatment.

Once it has been determined that a fear of dentistry is present, the dentist can use any of the techniques of conscious sedation to reduce the patient's stress during treatment. These include nondrug techniques, such as iatrosedation and hypnosis; pharmacosedative procedures, including oral, rectal, and intramuscular sedation; inhalation sedation with nitrous oxide and oxygen; and intravenous sedation. When employed properly, conscious sedation can greatly reduce the medical and psychological risks associated with dental care. However, as mentioned, the use of drugs will always have associated risk factors that the doctor administering the agents must be aware of and be capable of managing. According to McCarthy,[15] 90% of potential emergency situations may be prevented through the proper use of preliminary patient evaluation and the appropriate use of conscious sedation and pain control.

Another major factor in preventing the loss of consciousness in dentistry was the introduction of sit-down dentistry with patients treated while they lie in a supine or somewhat recumbent position. The supine position (ideally with feet elevated about 10° to 15°) prevents the development of cerebral anoxia, the most common mechanism producing syncope. Use of the supine position for patients during treatment has been responsible for a dramatic decrease in the number of episodes of syncope occurring in dental offices.

CLINICAL MANIFESTATIONS

An unconscious patient is incapable of responding to sensory stimulation and has lost protective reflexes (swallowing, coughing) along with an at-

---

*The stages of anesthesia may best be understood by explaining the basic pattern of action of general anesthetics (and all other CNS depressant drugs). This pattern consists of a progressive depression of the central nervous system. Central nervous system depressants (general anesthetics, tranquilizers, sedative-hypnotics, and alcohol) first depress the cerebral cortex, producing a loss of sensory function, followed by loss of motor function. Then the basal ganglia and cerebellum are depressed, followed by the spinal cord, and lastly, the medulla. Medullary depression leads to depression of the respiratory and cardiovascular systems and is the usual cause of death from drug overdose. Guedel[11] described four stages of anesthesia based on this information. Stage 1, analgesia or altered consciousness, corresponds to the action of these drugs on the higher cortical centers (sensory). The various techniques encompassing the concept of psychosedation are found in this stage. Stage 2, delirium or excitement, corresponds to the increasing depressant action of these drugs on higher motor centers. The patient is unconsciousness during this stage. Stages 1 and 2 comprise the induction phase of anesthesia. In stage 3, surgical anesthesia, spinal reflexes are depressed, producing skeletal muscle relaxation. Stage 4, medullary paralysis, corresponds to the depression of the respiratory and cardiovascular centers of the medulla, producing first respiratory and then cardiovascular arrest.

Table 5-2. Classification of causes of unconsciousness by mechanism

Mechanism	Clinical example
Inadequate delivery of blood or oxygen to the brain	Acute adrenal insufficiency Orthostatic hypotension Vasodepressor syncope
Systemic or local metabolic deficiencies	Acute allergic reaction Drug ingestion and administration: 　Nitrites and nitrates 　Diuretics 　Sedatives-narcotics 　Local anesthetics Hyperglycemia Hyperventilation Hypoglycemia
Direct or reflex effects on nervous system	Cerebrovascular accident Convulsive episodes
Psychic mechanisms	Emotional disturbances Hyperventilation Vasodepressor syncope

tendant lack of ability to maintain a patent airway. Primary management of unconsciousness is directed at reversing these clinical manifestations.

Clinical signs and symptoms associated with the impending loss of consciousness (presyncope) and the actual state of unconsciousness (syncope) will vary somewhat according to the primary cause of the situation. For this reason the precise clinical manifestations of presyncope and syncope will be discussed in greater detail under specific situations (see Chapters 6 through 9).

PATHOPHYSIOLOGY
Mechanisms of Unconsciousness

Engle,[16] in his classic test on fainting, classified the mechanisms that produce syncope into four categories: (1) reduced cerebral metabolism resulting from inadequate delivery of blood or oxygen to the brain, (2) reduced cerebral metabolism resulting from general or local metabolic deficiencies, (3) direct or reflex effects on that part of the central nervous system concerned with regulation of consciousness and equilibrium, and (4) psychic mechanisms affecting levels of consciousness with their respective mechanism or mechanisms (categories 1 to 3) of action (Table 5-2). Lack of oxygen (hypoxia/anoxia) and lack of adequate blood sugar (hypoglycemia) are the two most often noted causes of syncope in both adult and pediatric patients.

Inadequate Cerebral Circulation

The most common mechanism of syncope is a sudden decrease in the supply of blood to the brain. Vasodepressor syncope (common faint) and orthostatic hypotension will be the most frequently encountered clinical examples of this. Physiologic disturbances that result in a decrease in blood supply to the brain include (1) dilation of the peripheral arterioles, (2) failure of normal peripheral vasoconstrictor activity (orthostatic hypotension), (3) a sharp fall in cardiac output (from heart disease, dysrhythmias, or decreased blood volume), (4) constriction of cerebral vessels as CO_2 is lost through hyperventilation, (5) occlusion or narrowing of the internal carotid or other arteries to the brain, and (6) ventricular asystole. The first four factors rarely produce unconsciousness when the patient is in the supine position. Management of these factors will be directed at increasing the supply of well-oxygenated blood to the brain.

General or Local Metabolic Change

Changes in the quality of blood perfusing the brain that are caused by chemical or metabolic derangements may also be associated with unconsciousness or may predispose an individual to its occurrence. Clinical situations most frequently encountered that may lead to syncope through this mechanism include hyperventilation, hyperglycemia, the administration or ingestion of drugs, and an acute allergic reaction. In these cases consciousness will not return until the underlying chemical or metabolic cause is corrected.

Actions on the Central Nervous System

Loss of consciousness associated with alterations within the brain itself or through reflex effects on the central nervous system are manifested clinically as convulsions and cerebrovascular accident.

Psychic Mechanisms

Psychic mechanisms such as emotional disturbances are the most common causes of unconsciousness in the dental environment and include several of the clinical situations discussed previously. Vasodepressor syncope and hyperventilation are in this category.

Oxygen Deprivation

With loss of consciousness there is a generalized decrease in skeletal muscle tone in the body equivalent to that occurring in Guedel's stage 3 of anesthesia. The tongue, a muscle mass, loses tone, and because of the effect of gravity, falls back into the hypopharynx, producing either a complete or a partial airway obstruction (Fig. 5-1). In the unconscious patient hypopharyngeal obstruction by the base of the relaxed tongue always occurs when the head is flexed and almost always when the head is maintained in the mid-position.[17,18] Relief of this obstruction will thus become the primary objective of resuscitation of the unconscious patient. Until this obstruction is removed, the patient will receive hypoxic levels of oxygen (partial obstruction) or will be anoxic (total obstruction) and will therefore remain unconscious with a decreased likelihood of successful resuscitation.[19] The vital importance of oxygen in the maintenance of consciousness may be explained as follows. Under normal conditions the brain derives most of its energy from the oxidation of glucose. To maintain this energy source, a continuous supply of glucose and oxygen must be delivered to the brain. Without oxygen some glucose can still be metabolized to lactic acid to provide some energy, but this source will not fulfill the brain's requirements for more than a few seconds, rapidly leading to the loss of consciousness.

The human brain, which accounts for only 2% of the total body mass, uses approximately 20% of the total oxygen and 65% of the total glucose consumed by the body. To do this, approximately 20% of the total blood circulation per minute must reach the brain. When the supply of either of these fuels is diminished, brain functioning is rapidly affected. It is estimated that the cerebral blood flow of a normal human in the supine position is 750 mL per minute. At any moment then, the blood circulating through the brain contains 7 mL of oxygen, an amount sufficient to supply the brain's requirements for less than 10 seconds. Rossen and coworkers[20] carried out experiments in which the human brain was deprived of oxygen by sudden and complete arrest of cerebral circulation. Consciousness was lost in 6 seconds.

Complete airway obstruction, with the victim anoxic, will lead to permanent brain damage within 4 to 6 minutes and to cardiac arrest within 5 to 10 minutes. In a study of dogs asphyxiated for 5 minutes, 50% of survivors sustained gross brain damage; after 10 minutes of asphyxiation all had significant brain damage.[19] Some authorities contend that anoxic periods of as little as 3 minutes' duration will cause permanent brain damage.[21] Partial airway obstruction in which the victim receives hypoxic levels of oxygen may lead to the same result, although more slowly and through other, more complex pathways. In either case it is quite evident that the doctor and staff must be able to rapidly and effectively institute the steps of basic life support. Adequate ventilation has been termed the

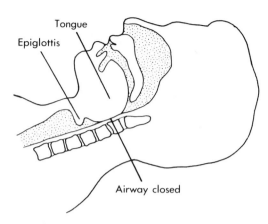

Fig. 5-1. Unconscious victim. Tongue falls backward against wall of pharynx, producing airway obstruction.

sine qua non of resuscitation.[22] Once a patent airway has been secured, and only then, can the doctor proceed to more definitive life support measures (chest compression or drug administration).

MANAGEMENT—BASIC LIFE SUPPORT

Immediate management of the unconscious victim will be predicated on two objectives: (1) the recognition of unconsciousness, and (2) the management of the unconscious victim, which will include the recognition of possible airway obstruction and its management.

Recognition of Unconsciousness

Step 1: Assessment of consciousness. Determine that the patient is either conscious or unconscious. It is critical to be able to distinguish between consciousness and unconsciousness because many of the steps of basic life support that follow should not be carried out on a conscious person. For this reason, we set certain criteria for unconsciousness based upon our prior definition of unconsciousness. Thus we have three criteria to aid us in the recognition of unconsciousness: (1) a lack of response to sensory stimulation, (2) the loss of protective reflexes, and (3) an inability to maintain a patent airway.

The first of these criteria, the lack of response to sensory stimulation, is the most useful to the rescuer who must rapidly assess a victim's state of consciousness. Criteria 2 and 3, loss of protective reflexes and the inability to maintain a patent airway, are also clinical manifestations of unconsciousness but are less frequently employed as determining factors than is the lack of response to sensory stimulation.

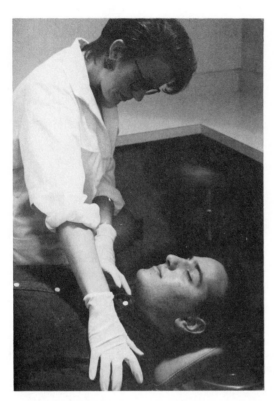

Fig. 5-2. Unconsciousness is determined by gently shaking shoulders and calling victim's name; the "shake and shout" technique.

To determine the lack of response to sensory stimulation, the American Heart Association[23] recommends that the rescuer gently shake the patient's shoulder and shout loudly, "Are you all right?" to arouse him. If the patient does not respond to this shake and shout maneuver (Fig. 5-2), the rescuer works with the assumption that the patient is unconscious and immediately proceeds to the steps of basic life support.

Pain is another stimulus that may be used as an aid in determining the level of consciousness. Peripheral pain (such as pinching the suprascapular region) will usually evoke a motor response from the patient such as deep inhalation, the movement of a limb, furrowing of the forehead, or an auditory response. Absence of a response to this stimulus is yet another indicator of unconsciousness. If the patient does not respond, the doctor should begin basic life support procedures.

Step 2: Call for help. If the victim does not respond to peripheral stimulation (step 1), the rescuer immediately calls for assistance by activating the dental office emergency system.

Management of the Unconsciousness Patient

Loss of consciousness depresses many of the vital functions of the body, including the protective reflexes—choking, coughing, sneezing, and swallowing—and the ability of the patient to maintain an open or patent airway. The steps to be followed next permit the rescuer to maintain these vital functions until the victim either recovers spontaneously or is transported to a hospital where more definitive treatment is available.

Step 3: Position patient. As soon as unconsciousness is recognized the patient should be placed in the supine (horizontal) position with the brain at the same level as the heart and the feet elevated slightly (at 10° to 15° angle). The head-down (Trendelenburg) postion should be avoided because gravity will act to push the abdominal viscera superiorly into the diaphragm, thus restricting respiratory movements and diminishing the effectiveness of breathing.[24] A primary objective in the management of unconsciousness is the delivery of oxygenated blood to the brain, and the supine position enables the heart to more readily accomplish this. A slight elevation of the feet to approximately 10° to 15° will further increase the return of blood to the heart. With a contoured dental chair the patient may easily be placed in this position (Fig. 5-3).

One situation requiring modification of basic positioning is the loss of consciousness in a pregnant woman near term. Positioning a woman who is in

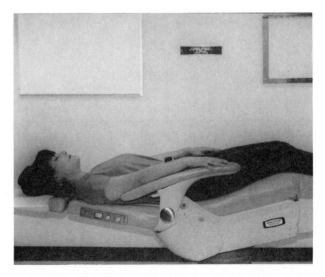

Fig. 5-3. Positioning of unconscious victim. Thorax and brain are at same level with feet elevated slightly (by 10 degrees), aiding return of venous blood to heart.

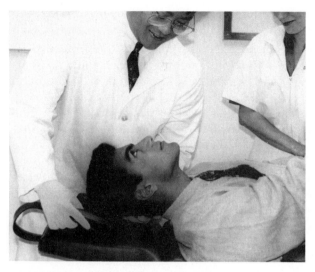

Fig. 5-4. Remove any extra head support, such as pillow or donut, from headrest of chair.

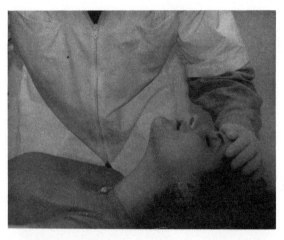

Fig. 5-5. Head tilt. Place one hand on victim's forehead and apply firm, backward pressure with the palm to tilt the head back.

the later stages of pregnancy in the supine position may actually produce a decrease in the return of venous blood to the heart, thereby decreasing the supply of blood available to be delivered to the brain. The gravid uterus may actually obstruct blood flow through the inferior vena cava on the right side of the abdomen, thereby trapping large volumes of blood in the legs. Normal, healthy, pregnant women have actually lost consciousness by simply lying on their backs on a hard surface. Should a pregnant woman in the third trimester lose consciousness while in a dental chair, the back of the chair should be quickly lowered to the supine position and the patient turned toward her right side, with a blanket or pillow under her back on her left side to help maintain that position.[25] The uterus will no longer lie directly over the vena cava, and the return of blood from the legs will be unimpeded.

Step 4: Assess and open airway. In all cases of unconsciousness, some degree of airway obstruction will be present. For this reason, the first maneuver to be employed after positioning the patient will be the establishment of a patent airway. Opening of the airway and the restoration of breathing constitute the most basic and important steps of basic life support. They may be performed quickly under most circumstances and without adjunctive equipment or assistance from other persons.

Any type of head support on the dental chair, such as a pillow or donut-shaped support, should be removed because such supports flex the neck,

thus making airway maintenance more difficult to perform (Fig. 5-4).

Head tilt. The initial and most imporant step in providing a patent airway is the head-tilt procedure. This technique is usually augmented with the chin-lift technique. The technique of head tilt–neck lift has been abandoned since it was demonstrated that head tilt–chin lift is more effective.[26]

The head-tilt procedure is accomplished by placing the (rescuer's) hand on the victim's forehead and applying a firm, backward pressure with the palm (Fig. 5-5). In situations in which some degree of muscle tone remains, head tilt by itself may provide a patent airway. When a lesser degree of muscle tone is present, the use of chin-lift or jaw-thrust techniques in conjunction with the head-tilt technique will be necessary.

Jaw thrust (if needed). Although head tilt will be effective in reestablishing airway patency in most cases, on occasion an airway may remain obstructed and additional procedures may be required. In most instances additional displacement of the mandible will be adequate to remove the obstruction. This may be accomplished by the jaw-thrust maneuver (Fig. 5-6), in which the rescuer places his or her fingers behind the posterior border of the ramus of the mandible and (1) displaces the mandible forward, dislocating it, while (2) tilting the head backward and (3) using the thumbs to retract the lower lip to allow breathing through the mouth, as well as the nose. To properly carry out the jaw-thrust maneuver, it will be necessary for the rescuer to stand behind the top of the supine victim's head.

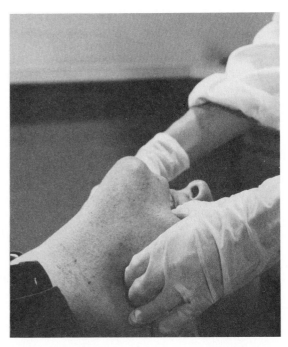

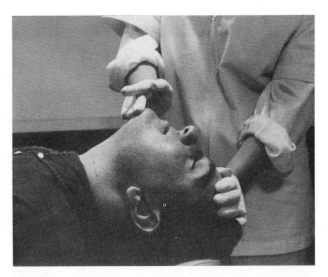

Fig. 5-7. Head tilt, chin lift. Rescuer places fingers of one hand on bony anterior portion of victim's mandible; other hand is placed on victim's forehead and rotates the head back. This is the preferred airway maintenance technique.

Fig. 5-6. Jaw thrust—forward displacement of the mandible by grasping the angles of the mandible with both hands and displacing the mandible forward. When possible neck injury is present, jaw-thrust without head tilt is the most effective air management technique.

The rescuer's elbows should rest on the surface on which the victim is lying.

Carrying out the jaw-thrust maneuver also provides the rescuer with a gauge of the depth of unconsciousness. As previously mentioned, pain is a potent sensory stimulus, and dislocation of the mandible is a painful procedure. Thus, the response of the victim to this procedure will aid the rescuer in determining the level of unconsciousness. A victim's movement and audible response are considered positive signs, whereas lack of response is an indication of a deeper level of unconsciousness. In addition, it has been the author's experience that the ease with which the mandible is dislocated is yet another gauge of depth of unconsciousness. With profound unconsciousness there is a marked loss of muscle tone throughout the body, and dislocation of the mandible may be easily carried out. This is in sharp contrast to attempts at dislocation of the mandible in a conscious patient or in one with a lesser degree of unconsciousness. In these instances some degree of muscle tone remains, making it difficult (and painful) to carry out this procedure.

The modified jaw-thrust technique (without head tilt) is the safest initial approach to opening the airway of a victim with a suspected neck injury (an unlikely occurrence in the dental environment) because it can be accomplished without extending the neck. The neck must be carefully supported without tilting it backward or turning it from side to side.

Head tilt—chin lift. To maintain an airway using the head tilt—chin lift technique (Fig. 5-7), the fingers of one hand are placed under the bony symphysis region of the mandible to lift the tip of the mandible up, bringing the chin forward. Because the tongue is attached to the mandible, it is thereby pulled forward and off of the posterior pharyngeal wall. Lifting the mandible forward also tilts the head backward, aiding in head tilt.

It is vitally important to remember that the tips of the rescuer's fingers should only be placed *on bone,* not on the soft tissues of the chin. Compressing these soft tissues will increase airway obstruction by pushing the tongue farther upward into the oral cavity. The chin should be lifted so that the teeth are almost brought into contact with each other. Try to avoid completely closing the mouth.

Research conducted during the past 15 years has provided evidence that the head tilt—chin lift technique of airway management provides the most consistently reliable airway.[26] The head tilt—neck lift technique offered no advantage over this technique yet was potentially dangerous, as will be described shortly. For this reason, in 1986 the American Heart Association (AHA) changed its guidelines for teaching airway management to state that the head tilt—chin lift technique was preferred.[23]

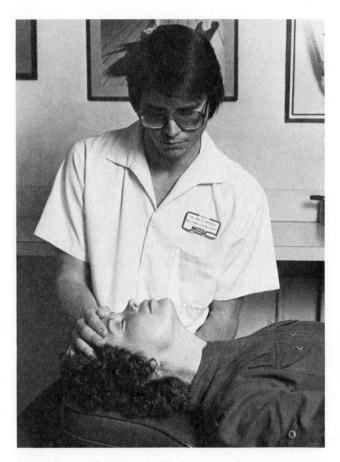

Fig. 5-8. Head tilt, neck lift. Rescuer places one hand beneath victim's neck; other hand is placed on forehead and rotates the head back.

Head tilt–neck lift. Until 1980 the head tilt–neck lift technique of airway maintenance was the technique recommended by the AHA. In 1980, after evidence surfaced that head tilt–chin lift technique was at least equally effective, the AHA suggested that these two procedures could be used interchangeably.[27] In 1986 the recommendation was changed to read that head tilt–chin lift was to be the preferred method.[23]

In the head tilt–neck lift procedure, one hand of the rescuer is placed on the forehead of the victim, and the other hand is placed beneath the victim's neck to lift and support it (Fig. 5-8). If excessive force is applied to the neck in this technique (as has occurred on too many occasions), injury to the cervical spine can occur. Because the desired movement in this technique is a rotation of the victim's head backward rather than the neck being lifted, the rescuer's hand supporting the neck should be placed as close to the base of the skull as possible to minimize any risk of hyperextenstion. Gentleness is very important when performing the

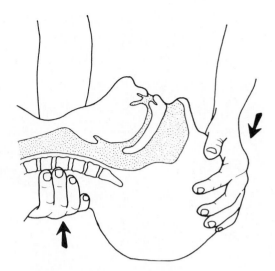

Fig. 5-9. Head tilt. Head tilt stretches soft tissues of the neck, lifting the victim's tongue off the pharynx and opening the airway.

head tilt–neck life procedure. Because the head tilt–chin lift technique of airway management is more effective and less hazardous, it has become the preferred technique of airway management.

In summary, at the present time, recommendations for airway management techniques overwhelmingly favor the head tilt–chin lift procedure.

All of the aforementioned head-tilt maneuvers stretch the tissues between the larynx and the mandible, lifting the base of the tongue and/or the epiglottis from the posterior pharyngeal wall (Fig. 5-9). Anatomic obstruction of the airway caused by soft tissues is relieved by these maneuvers in approximately 80% of unconscious patients.[28] The head of the patient must be maintained in this position at all times until consciousness returns.

To what degree should the head of the victim be extended during airway management techniques? It is important to extend the head sufficiently to elevate the tongue, thus establishing a patent airway, but it is equally important that the head not be overextended (possibly producing damage to vertebrae and the spinal cord). One method of gauging this in the adult is to examine the relationship of the tip of the chin to the earlobes of the victim. When the head is not extended, the unconscious victim's airway is obstructed and the tip of the chin will lie well below the earlobes (Fig. 5-10). When the head is properly extended this relationship is altered so that the tip of the chin is pointing up in the air and is in line with the earlobes. This line should be perpendicular to the surface on which the victim is lying (Fig. 5-11).

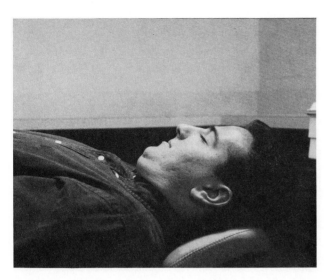

Fig. 5-10. Obstructed airway. Chin, mandible, and tongue are forced into airway, producing obstruction.

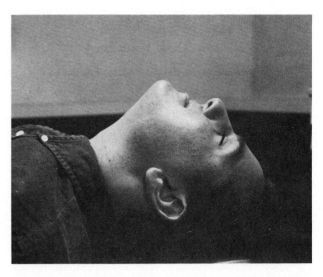

Fig. 5-11. Adequate extension of adult airway. Tip of chin extended, lifting mandible and tongue off wall of pharynx.

In the unconscious adult it is unlikely that the head will be overextended; the problem is usually the opposite—failure to extend the head far enough. In the infant or child, however, overextension of the head may produce or worsen airway obstruction. Because of anatomic differences in the size of the upper airway and trachea in children and adults (Table 5-3), extension of a child's head in head tilt need not be quite as great as in an adult. Extension of the child's head to the same degree as that of an adult may lead to airway obstruction as the narrowest portion of the trachea is compressed. Although the degree of extension suggested earlier will usually produce a patent airway in a child, it is not an absolute guideline and must be modified as the need arises.

Step 5: Assess airway patency and breathing*. Following head tilt–chin lift, the rescuer must assess the patency of the airway (Table 5-4). The victim may breathe spontaneously, may be breathing inadequately, or may not be breathing at all. During this assessment the victim's head must be maintained in the extended position previously established by head tilt–chin lift. To properly carry out this step, the rescuer leans over the victim and puts his or her ear about 1 inch from the victim's nose and mouth, while at the same time looking toward the

---

*Breathing, as discussed in this section, refers to the actual exchange of air through the mouth and nose of the victim. This must be distinguished from the movement of the chest, which occurs during attempts at breathing. Chest movement may be present in the absence of adequate air exchange through the victim's mouth and nose.

victim's chest (Fig. 5-12). Whether or not the victim is breathing is determined by *looking, listening,* and *feeling.* Looking at the chest and seeing it and/or the abdomen move is an indication that the victim is attempting to breathe but is not necessarily an indication that he or she is exchanging air; feeling and hearing air at the nose and mouth of the victim are also necessary to confirm airway patency. In addition, it is possible that chest and abdominal movement will not be noticed if the victim is fully clothed. However, if the victim's breath can be felt and heard, visual signs of chest movement are not necessary to determine adequacy of ventilation.

If the unconscious victim is exchanging air adequately, the airway is maintained (via head tilt–chin lift), and the dental team should proceed with additional therapy, including the administration of oxygen and the monitoring of vital signs (blood pressure, heart rate, and respiratory rate). If no air can be felt or heard at the mouth and nose and there is no evidence of chest or abdominal movement, a tentative diagnosis of respiratory arrest is made and artificial ventilation is started immediately (step 8).

If, in the presence of labored chest or abdominal movements, no air flow can be felt or heard at the mouth and nose or if minimal air exchange is detected along with noisy air flow, airway obstruction, either complete or partial, is present. Repeat head tilt–chin lift (step 4) and recheck for effectiveness (step 5). If airway obstruction is still present, the rescuer must proceed to the next step of airway maintenance with utmost speed. The various

Table 5-3. Anatomic differences between adult and infant airways and their significance

Difference	Significance
Infant head is larger than adult head	Do not need to elevate infant head to align axes
Infant mouth and nose are smaller	Infant requires mouth-to-mouth *and* nose resuscitation
Infant tongue is larger relative to oral cavity	Increases potential for obstruction
At 1 year of age tracheal diameter is less than the width of a pencil	Increases potential for obstruction
At 2 years of age the glottic opening is only 6.5 mm	Increases potential for obstruction
Cricoid cartilage ring is narrowest segment of the infant airway, whereas glottic closure is the narrowest in the adult	Precludes use of cuffed endotracheal tubes at less than 12 years of age
Infant cricothyroid membrane is not palpable	Precludes cricothyrotomy
Air passages in infants are smaller than adults	Decreases airway reserve and increases vulnerability to obstruction; finger swep contraindicated because it can increase obstruction

Modified from Kastendieck JG: Airway management. In *Emergency medicine: concepts and clinical practice,* ed 2, Rosen P (editor): St Louis, 1988, Mosby–Year Book.

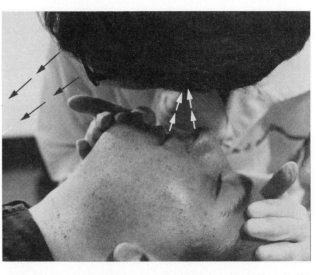

Fig. 5-12. Look, listen, and feel. Maintaining head tilt, rescuer assesses airway patency by placing ear approximately 1 inch from victim's nose and mouth while looking toward the victim's chest for spontaneous respiratory movements.

Table 5-4. Determination of airway patency and breathing

Clinical signs	Diagnosis	Management
Can feel and hear air at nose and mouth *and* see chest and abdominal movement	Airway patent; patient is breathing	Maintain airway
Can feel and hear air at nose and mouth *but see no* chest and abdominal movement	Airway patent; patient is breathing	Maintain airway
Cannot feel or hear air at mouth and nose *and* chest and abdominal movements are heaving and erratic	Patient is attempting to breathe, but airway obstruction is still present	Repeat head tilt, then if necessary proceed to step 6 of airway maintenance
Cannot feel or hear air at mouth and nose *and* no chest and abdominal movements are evident	Respiratory arrest has occurred	Proceed to step 8, begin artificial ventilation

Table 5-5. Causes of partial airway obstruction

Sound heard	Probable cause	Management
Snoring	Hypopharyngeal obstruction by the tongue	Repeat head tilt, then proceed to triple airway maneuver, if necessary
Gurgling	Foreign matter (blood, water, vomitus) in airway	Suction airway
Wheezing	Bronchial obstruction (asthma)	Administer bronchodilator (via inhalation, only if conscious; IM or IV if unconscious)
Crowing	Laryngospasm (partial)	Suction airway; positive pressure O_2

causes of partial or complete airway obstruction are associated with sounds that may prove to be diagnostic (Table 5-5).

Remove foreign material in the airway. If there is evidence of foreign matter in the airway following a check for airway patency, the rescuer should immediately take steps to remove the material before attempting to perform artificial ventilation (if necessary). Partial airway obstruction produces noise; complete airway obstruction produces silence, an ominous "sound."

The presence of foreign matter, primarily liquid, in the hypopharynx produces a gurgling sound similar to that produced when air bubbles through water. Most commonly the materials present are saliva, blood, water, or vomitus. Regardless of the nature of this material, it must be removed from the airway as quickly as possible. If present in large volume, it may lead to complete airway obstruction. In addition, if particulate material is present (vomitus), it may enter the trachea, creating complete obstruction of the respiratory tract, which can lead to asphyxiation and death of the patient unless corrected (see Chapter 10).

The unconscious patient should have previously been placed in the supine position. As soon as foreign material is thought to be present in the airway, the dental chair should be tilted back even further so that the patient's head is below the level of the heart (the Trendelenburg position), and the patient's head should be turned to one side (Fig. 5-13).

Lowering the patient's head will allow the foreign material to pool in the upper segments of the airway, which are more readily accessible to the rescuer. Turning the patient's head to the side will place the material in the most dependent side of the mouth, both facilitating its removal and leaving the upper side of the mouth free of material, thus creating a patent airway.

Immediately after carrying out these two steps

the rescuer should place two fingers in the patient's mouth and remove anything in the entire oral cavity that can be removed. The sweeping motion of the fingers should begin in the upper portion of the mouth, move posteriorly and finally downward and anteriorly (Fig. 5-14). A high-volume suction may be used instead of fingers. Suction tips should be rounded so that they may be placed blindly, if necessary, into the posterior areas of the mouth or the hypopharynx without fear of causing bleeding (from the delicate and highly vascular pharyngeal mucosa), which might compound the problem of airway obstruction. Suctioning should continue until all foreign material is removed from the patient's airway. The basic steps of airway maintenance should follow completion of suctioning.

Once airway patency and exchange have been ensured, the rescuer or a member of the team should loosen any constricting clothing, such as belts, ties, or collars, that might interfere with breathing and blood circulation. Vital signs must be monitored and, if available, oxygen administered.

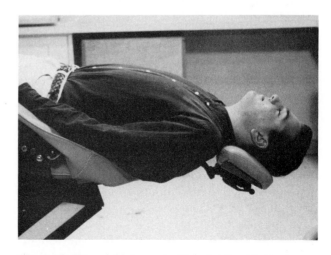

Fig. 5-13. Trendelenberg position for liquids in airway. Head is then turned to side.

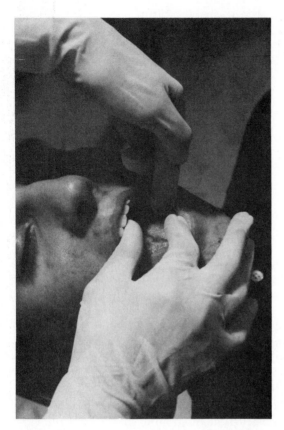

Fig. 5-14. Removal of foreign material from mouth. Fingers of rescuer's hand maintain open mouth while fingers of other sweep through oral cavity, removing any foreign material. Suction may also be used.

Step 6: Artificial ventilation (if needed). If respiratory arrest is present or if spontaneous ventilation is deemed inadequate, the dental team must ventilate the victim so that adequate oxygen is available to the brain. (See Table 5-5 for the criteria to initiate artificial ventilation.) Artificial ventilation may be provided in one of three ways: (1) exhaled air ventilation, (2) atmospheric (ambient) air ventilation, and (3) oxygen-enriched ventilation.

Exhaled air ventilation. Exhaled air from the rescuer may be delivered to the lungs of the victim as one source of oxygen. Exhaled air can deliver 16% to 18% inspired oxygen, yielding a PAO_2 of 88 torr at a tidal volume of 1000 to 1500 cc and maintaining an oxygen saturation of 97% to 100%, which is quite adequate to maintain life.[29,30] Two basic types of exhaled air ventilation are mouth-to-mouth breathing and mouth-to-nose breathing. Because no adjunctive equipment is required for these techniques, they may be carried out in any rescue situation. For this reason they still remain the basic techniques of artifical ventilation. With ever-increasing concerns about the possibility of contagion with infectious diseases during ventila-

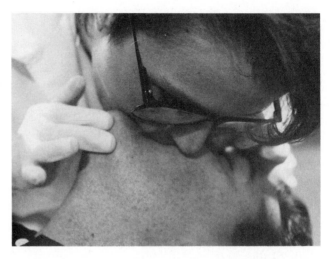

Fig. 5-15. Mouth-to-mouth ventilation. Rescuer maintains head tilt, pinches victim's nostrils closed, and blows into victim's mouth. Adequate ventilation is assessed by watching victim's chest rise with each ventilatory effort.

tion, the use of devices such as the pocket mask has become more popular.

To adequately perform mouth-to-mouth ventilation, the rescuer uses the head-tilt or head tilt–chin lift position (step 4) to maintain the victim's head in an optimal backward tilt. The hand on the forehead continues to maintain a backward tilt; at the same time the thumb and index fingers pinch the victim's nostrils closed (Fig. 5-15). With mouth opened widely, the rescuer takes a deep breath, makes a tight seal around the victim's mouth, and blows into the victim's mouth. A rapid and deeply inhaled breath immediately before blowing delivers expired air with the lowest CO_2 content.[22]

The first ventilatory cycle should consist of two full breaths, allowing 1 to 1.5 seconds per inspiration with the rescuer taking a breath after each ventilation. Exhalation occurs passively when the rescuer's mouth is removed from the victim's, allowing gravity to deflate the lungs. Artificial ventilation in the adult must be repeated once every 5 seconds (12 times per minute) for as long as is necessary. In the child the ventilatory rate is once every 4 seconds (15 times per minute), whereas the infant is ventilated at a rate of once every 3 seconds (20 times per minute).

Adequacy of ventilatory efforts for patients of any size or age may be gauged by the following: (1) feeling air escape as the victim passively exhales, and (2) seeing the rise and fall of the patient's chest. The latter is the more important factor. In most adults the volume of air required to produce chest expansion is 800 mL (0.8L). Adequate ventilation usually does not need to exceed 1200 mL.[31]

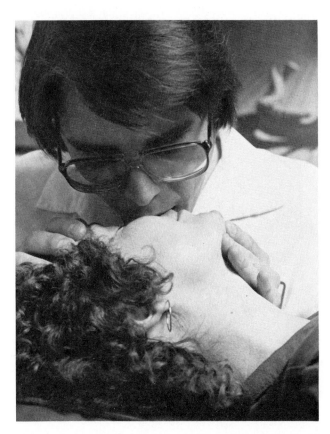

Fig. 5-16. Mouth-to-nose ventilation. Maintaining head tilt, chin lift, rescuer closes victim's mouth, sealing his lips around victim's nose. Adequate ventilation is assessed by watching victim's chest rise with each ventilatory effort.

Gastric distention and the subsequent risk of aspiration are potentially the most serious disadvantages of artificial ventilation. Much more common in children than in adults, the major cause of gastric distention is overinflation during ventilation. Other causes are ventilation against a partially or totally obstructed airway, thereby forcing air into the esophagus and gastrointestinal tract. Gastric distention is dangerous for two reasons: (1) it increases the incidence of regurgitation during resuscitation, and (2) by increasing intraabdominal pressure, it may limit movement of the diaphragm, thereby reducing the ability of the rescuer to ventilate the victim.[32] Gastric distention can be minimized by limiting ventilatory efforts to the point at which the chest rises. Mouth-to-nose ventilation, which will be discussed shortly, may be better in preventing over-ventilation because the greater resistance to the flow of ventilating gases through the nose will decrease the pressure of gases reaching the pharynx.

In some instances mouth-to-nose ventilation is more effective than mouth-to-mouth ventilation.[33]

This is especially true when it is impossible to open a victim's mouth (e.g., as with trismus or fractured mandible), when it is impossible to ventilate through the victim's mouth, or if the rescuer is unable to adequately seal the mouth of the victim. In the mouth-to-nose technique (Fig. 5-16) the rescuer keeps the head tilted backward with one hand on the forehead; the other hand lifts the victim's mandible, sealing the lips. Taking a deep breath, the rescuer seals his or her lips around the victim's nose and blows until he or she feels and sees the victim's lungs expand. Exhalation, as in the mouth-to-mouth technique, is passive. The same rates—12, 15, and 20 breaths per minute—are employed in mouth-to-nose for the adult, child, and infant, respectively, as are employed in mouth-to-mouth ventilation.

Modifications in ventilatory technique must be made if the victim is an infant or a young child (see previous discussion of the head tilt procedure). Opening of the airway and the method of artificial ventilation are essentially the same in children; however, when the victim is smaller, both the mouth and nose may be covered with the rescuer's mouth. The respiratory rate is increased to once every 4 seconds for children aged 1 year through 8 years and once every 3 seconds for infants under 1 year, using smaller breaths with less volume. The same criteria for successful ventilation, (1) feeling air escape as the victim passively exhales and (2) seeing the rise and fall of the chest of the patient with each inhalation, apply as for adults. In addition, the neck of the child is more flexible than that of the adult; therefore, care should be taken not to overextend the neck, thus further increasing airway obstruction. When properly performed, artificial ventilation using either method may be continued for long periods without the rescuer becoming fatigued.

Atmospheric air ventilation. The administration of oxygen will enhance any resuscitative effort. Though exhaled air ventilation, with 16% to 18% oxygen, is adequate to maintain life, the delivery of greater concentrations of oxygen provide greater benefit to the victim. The air we breathe contains approximately 21% oxygen. Devices are available that permit the rescuer to deliver atmospheric air to the lungs of the victim. However, all such devices will be effective only if basic airway procedures are continually carried out.

Self-inflating bag-valve-mask devices (Fig. 5-17). Bag-valve-mask (BVM) devices such as the Ambu-Bag and Pulmonary Manual Resuscitator (PMR) usually provide less ventilatory volume than mouth-to-mouth or mouth-to-nose ventilation be-

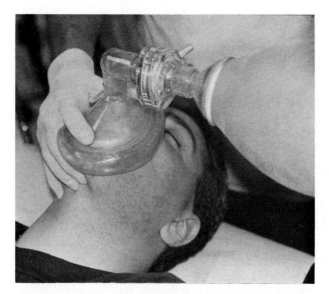

Fig. 5-17. Atmospheric air ventilation. Head tilt is maintained, and face mask is held securely in place with one hand. Chest of victim must rise with each compression of self-inflating bag-valve-mask device.

cause of the difficulty in maintaining an airtight seal. For this reason, the American Heart Association recommends that manually operated, self-inflating bag-valve-mask devices be used only by well-trained and experienced personnel.[34] To use these units properly, the rescuer must be positioned near the top of the victim's head, making it virtually impossible to perform single-rescuer CPR (see Section VIII).

To be considered adequate, a bag-valve-mask unit must[35-37]:

1. Be self-refilling, but without sponge rubber inside
2. Have a transparent, plastic face mask with an air-filled or contoured resilient cuff
3. Provide a system for delivery of high concentrations of oxygen through an ancillary oxygen inlet at the back of the bag or by means of an oxygen reservoir
4. Have a nonrebreathing valve
5. Be available in adult and pediatric sizes
6. Have standard 15 mm/22 mm fittings (for endotracheal tubes)
7. Be easy to clean
8. Have minimal dead space

Before purchasing this device the doctor should enroll in a program of advanced airway maintenance and become thoroughly trained in the proper use of this and other adjunctive equipment.

Artifical airways. Artificial airways (e.g., oropharyngeal, nasopharyngeal), as seen in Fig. 5-18, may

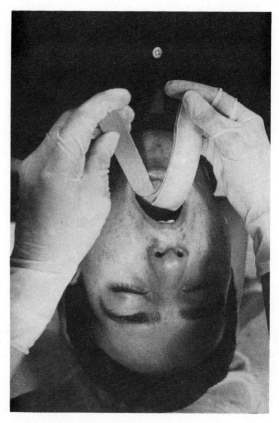

Fig. 5-18. Insertion of oropharyngeal airway. It is recommended that oropharyngeal airways not be employed without advanced training.

be used whenever a bag-valve-mask device is employed but only by an individual well trained in their use. Artificial airways should be used only on deeply unconscious persons when it is difficult to manage the airway with conventional (manual) techniques. If used on a conscious or stuporous patient, artificial airways, especially the oropharyngeal airway, may provoke gagging, vomiting, or larynospasm, causing a delay in obtaining adequate ventilation.[38] An orophyarngeal airway must be carefully placed because, if it is improperly positioned, it may displace the tongue further back into the pharynx and add to the airway obstruction. The nasopharyngeal airway is of use when it is difficult to enter the patient's mouth. In addition, the nasopharyngeal airway is less likely to stimulate gagging or vomiting in the unconscious patient than is the oropharyngeal airway.[39] Nasopharyngeal airways are much better tolerated in semiconscious and even conscious patients than are oropharyngeal airways. However, insertion of the nasopharyngeal airway is more likely to produce bleeding, because the delicate and highly vascular nasal mucosa is traumatized.

A variation of the oropharyngeal airway is the S tube. Advantages of the S tube are that it overcomes certain aesthetic considerations of direct mouth-to-mouth contact, assists in maintaining a patent airway, and helps to maintain the mouth in an open position. Disadvantages include the fact that it does not provide as effective a seal as does direct mouth-to-mouth or mouth-to-mask ventilation, it may induce vomiting if used improperly (similar to the oropharyngeal airway),[40] it prevents effective single rescuer CPR, and it requires training for safe and effective use.

Several studies have demonstrated that direct mouth-to-mouth ventilation provides more effective artificial ventilation than that obtained through the use of adjunctive devices such as those already mentioned.[41,42] Other devices and techniques of airway maintenance, including the esophageal obturator airway and endotracheal intubation,[43,44] are recommended for use only by well-trained personnel. A pocket mask should always be available so that initial efforts at ventilation need not be through direct mouth-to-mouth contact.[45] Dentists who are properly trained through advanced cardiac life support courses or who have training in anesthesiology are capable of using such devices safely and effectively.

Enriched-oxygen ventilation. Wherever possible, artificial ventilation with supplemental oxygen should be employed. Exhaled air ventilation delivers 16% to 18% oxygen, whereas atmospheric air provides 21% oxygen. Because the object of basic life support is to provide the brain with oxygen, the use of supplemental oxygen ($>21\%$ O_2) should be considered as soon as it becomes available. However, artificial ventilation must never be delayed until supplemental oxygen becomes available. As suggested in Chapter 3, every doctor's office should have available a size "E" compressed oxygen cylinder. In situations in which artificial ventilation is required, the E cylinder will provide approximately 30 minutes of oxygen; smaller cylinders will provide lesser amounts and are entirely inadequate. Sources of oxygen in the dental office may include the portable E cylinder with adjustable oxygen flow (10 to 15 L per minute) and face mask, an E cylinder with demand-valve mask unit (Fig. 5-19), or the inhalation sedation unit. If the inhalation sedation unit is to be used for artificial ventilation, the nasal hood must be removed and replaced with a full face mask. The reservoir bag on the inhalation sedation unit will be pressed to deliver oxygen to the victim's lungs. Sources of oxygen from other than compressed gas cylinders (such as from can-

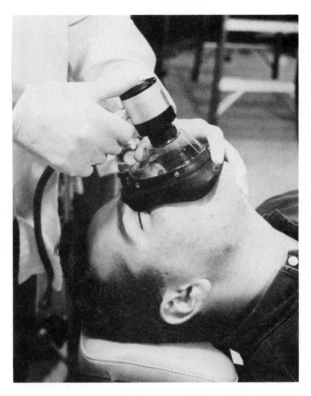

Fig. 5-19. Enriched oxygen ventilation. Demand-valve mask unit can provide up to 100% oxygen to the conscious or unconscious patient.

isters that produce oxygen via chemical reaction) should not be considered, because they are entirely inadequate for artificial ventilation.

Although oxygen benefits the unconscious patient, it behooves the doctor to receive adequate training in airway maintenance through mouth-to-mouth and mouth-to-mask ventilation, because administration of enriched oxygen will be effective for only as long as oxygen remains in the cylinder. When the cylinder is empty or if one is not available at the onset of the emergency, the rescuer must revert to the basic technique of artificial respiration.

Step 7: Assess circulation. After establishing a patent airway, the rescuer must determine the adequacy of the patient's circulation. This will include monitoring the patient's heart rate and blood pressure. Several sites are available for recording heart rate, including the brachial and radial arteries in the arm and the carotid artery in the neck. In nonemergency situations, either artery in the arm is an adequate indicator of heart rate; however, when a patient is unconscious, and particularly when respiratory movements have ceased, the carotid artery in the adult is the most reliable indicator of cardiovascular function.

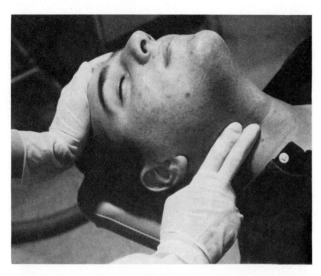

Fig. 5-20. Location of carotid pulse. Rescuer's fingers (not thumb) are placed on thyroid cartilage (Adam's apple), then moved laterally into groove formed by sternocleidomastoid muscle.

MANAGEMENT OF UNCONSCIOUSNESS

Recognition of problem
(assessment of consciousness)
↓
Discontinue dental care
↓
Activate office emergency team
↓
Position patient in supine position with feet elevated
↓
Assess breathing—look, listen, feel
Provide breathing, if necessary, through assisted or controlled ventilation
↓
Assess circulation—palpate carotid pulse for five to ten seconds
Provide circulation, if necessary, through artificial circulation
↓
Activate emergency medical services if recovery not immediate
↓
Provide definitive management of unconsciousness

The ability to properly locate the carotid artery is important (Fig. 5-20). It may be found in the following manner. Place the hand supporting the patient's chin on the thyroid cartilage (Adam's apple). On the side on which the rescuer is positioned, allow the fingers to slide into the groove between the thyroid cartilage and the sternocleidomastoid muscle band in the neck. The carotid artery is located in this groove. Allow 5 to 10 seconds to feel a pulse before initiating external chest compression if the pulse is absent. If a pulse is palpable, however weak, the victim should continue to be maintained (steps 1 to 6) until recovery occurs or until further medical assistance is available. In the child victim (aged 1 through 8 years) the carotid artery is also employed, whereas in the infant (less than 1 year of age) the brachial artery in the upper arm is recommended.[46] In the absence of a palpable pulse, external chest compression should be commenced immediately.

Step 8: Definitive management of unconsciousness. Once a patent airway has been provided and adequacy of circulation is ensured, the dental team may proceed with the definitive management of the unconscious patient. These procedures will be discussed in each of the three chapters to follow. The steps described in this chapter comprise the A and B segments of the ABCs of basic life support. *A* stands for *airway, B* for *breathing,* and *C* for *circulation.*

In every instance in which consciousness is lost, these steps must be carried out in precisely the order in which they were described. In most cases of unconsciousness, fulfillment of segment A alone, or in fewer cases both segments A and B of basic life support will be all the support required to sustain the patient. However, circulatory adequacy, or segment C, must always be determined; if a palpable pulse is not present, external chest compression must begin immediately. This important component of basic life support will be discussed in depth in Chapter 30. The accompanying box summarizes the management of the unconscious patient.

Additional airway management procedures will be discussed in the section on respiratory difficulty. The preceding discussion was based on the fact that hypopharyngeal obstruction by the tongue is the most common cause of airway obstruction in the unconscious patient.[18] The problem of lower airway (tracheal and bronchial) obstruction will be considered in Chapter 10.

REFERENCES

1. Fast TB, Martin MD, Ellis TM: Emergency preparedness: a survey of dental practitioners, *J Amer Dent Assoc* 112:499, 1986.
2. Malamed SF: Survey of emergencies in dental practice, unpublished data, 1992.
3. Schultz KE: Vertigo and syncope. In *Emergency medicine: concepts and clinical practice*, ed 2, Rosen P, editor: St Louis, 1988, Mosby–Year Book.
4. Huff JS: Coma. In *Emergency medicine: concepts and clinical practice*, ed 2, Rosen P, editor: St Louis, 1988, Mosby–Year Book.
5. Council on Dental Education: Guidelines for teaching the comprehensive control of pain and anxiety in dentistry, Chicago, 1987, American Dental Association.
6. Martin GJ, Adals SL, Martin HG, and others: Prospective evaluation of syncope, *Ann Emerg Med* 13:499, 1984.
7. American Dental Association, Council on Dental Education: Guidelines for teaching the comprehensive control of pain and anxiety in dentistry, *J Dent Educ* 36:62, 1972.
8. Reutz PO, and others: Fainting: a review of its mechanisms and a study in blood donors, *Medicine* 46:363, 1967.
9. Tizes R: Cardiac arrest following routine venipuncture, *JAMA* 236:1846, 1976.
10. Engel GL: Psychologic stress, vasodepressor (vasovagal) syncope, and sudden death, *Ann Intern Med* 89:403, 1978.
11. Guedel AE: *Inhalation anesthesia: a fundamental guide*, ed 2, New York, 1952, Macmillan.
12. Malamed SF: Systemic complications. In Malamed SF: *Handbook of local anesthesia*, ed 3, St Louis, 1991, Mosby–Yearbook.
13. Aldrete JA, Johnson DA: Evaluation of intracutaneous testing for investigation of allergy to local anesthetic agents, *Anesth Analg* (Cleve)49:173, 1970.
14. Corah NL, Gale EN, Illig SJ: Assessment of a dental anxiety scale, *J Am Dent Assoc* 97:816, 1981.
15. McCarthy FM: *Emergencies in dental practice*, ed 3, Philadelphia, 1979, WB Saunders.
16. Engel LL: *Fainting*, ed 2, Springfield, Il, 1962, Charles C Thomas.
17. Safar P, Escarraga L, Change F: A study of upper airway obstruction in the unconscious patient, *J Appl Physiol* 14:760, 1961.
18. Boidin MP: Airway patency in the unconscious patient, Br J Anaesth 57:306, 1985.
19. Redding JS, and others: Resuscitation from asphyxia, *JAMA* 182:283, 1962.
20. Rossen R, Kabat H, Anderson JP: Acute arrest of the cerebral circulation in man, *Arch Neurol Psychiatr* 50:510, 1943.
21. Goldberg AH: Cariopulmonary arrest, *N Engl J Med* 290:381, 1974.
22. Safar P: Ventilatory efficacy of mouth-to-mouth artificial respiration, *JAMA* 182:283, 1958.
23. American Heart Association and National Academy of Sciences: National Research Council: standards and guidelines for cardiopulmonary resuscitation (CPR) and emergency cardiac care (ECC), *JAMA* 255:2917, 1986.
24. Erie JK: Effect of position on ventilation. In Faust RJ, editor: *Anesthesiology Review*, New York, 1991, Churchill Livingston.
25. Wright KE Jr., McIntosh HD: Syncope: a review of pathophysiological mechanisms, *Progr Cardiovas Dis* 13:580, 1971.
26. Guildner CW: Resuscitation—opening the airway: a comparative study of techniques for opening an airway obstructed by the tongue, *JACEP* 5:588, 1976.
27. American Heart Association and National Academy of Sciences: National Research Council: standards and guidelines for cardiopulmonary resuscitation (CPR) and emergency cardiac care (ECC), *JAMA* 244:453, 1980.
28. Safar P: Ventilatory efficacy of mouth-to-mouth artificial respiration: airway obstruction during manual and mouth-to-mouth artificial respiration, *JAMA* 167:335, 1958.
29. Gordon AS, and others: Mouth-to-mouth versus manual artificial respiration for children and adults, *JAMA* 167:320, 1958.
30. Safar P, and others: A comparison of the mouth-to-mouth and mouth-to-airway methods of artificial respiration with the chest-pressure arm-lift methods, *N Engl J Med* 258:671, 1958.
31. Melker R: Recommendations for ventilation during cardiopulmonary resuscitation: Time for change? *Crit Care Med* 13:882, 1985.
32. Zwillich CW, and others: Complications of assisted ventilation, *Am J Med* 57:161, 1974.
33. Ruben H, Elam JO, Ruben AM, and others: Investigation of upper airway problems in resuscitation, *Anesthesiology* 22:271, 1961.
34. American Heart Association and National Academy of Sciences: National Research Council: standards and guidelines for cardiopulmonary resuscitation (CPR) and emergency cardiac care (ECC), *JAMA* 255:2841, 1986.
35. American Heart Association and National Academy of Sciences: National Research Council: standards and guidelines for cardiopulmonary resuscitation (CPR) and emergency cardiac care (ECC), *JAMA* 255:2934, 1986.
36. White RD, Gilles BP, Polk BV: Oxygen delivery by hand-operated emergency ventilation devices, *JACEP* 2:105, 1973.
37. Carden E, Friedman D: Further studies of manually operated self-inflating resuscitation bags, *Anesth Analg* 56:202, 1977.
38. Cavallaro D, Grauer K: Management of airway and ventilation. In *ACLS: certification preparation and a comprehensive review*, ed 2, St Louis, 1987, Mosby–Year Book.
39. American Heart Association: Textbook of advanced cardiac life support, ed 2, Dallas, 1987, American Heart Association.
40. Harrison RR, Maull KI, Keenan RI, and others: Mouth-to-mask ventilation: a superior method of rescue breathing, *Ann Emerg Med* 11:74, 1982.
41. American Heart Association and National Academy of Sciences: National Research Council: Standards and guidelines for cardiopulmonary resuscitation (CPR) and emergency cardiac care (ECC), *JAMA* 255:2841-3044, 1986.
42. Elling R, Politis J: An evaluation of emergency technicians' ability to use manual ventilation devices, *Ann Emerg Med* 12:765-768, 1983.
43. Donen N, Tweed WA, Dashfsky S, and others: The esophageal obturator airway: an appraisal, *Can Anaesth Soc J* 30:194, 1983.
44. Uhl RR: *Respirator care in emergencies: subject of the mouth/trauma/emergency medicine*, San Diego, 1976, University of California at San Diego.
45. Safar P: Pocket mask for emergency artificial ventilation and oxygen inhalation, *Crit Care Med* 2:273, 1974.
46. Cavallaro D, Melker R: Comparison of two techniques for determining cardiac activity in infants, *Crit Care Med* 14:397, 1983.

6 Vasodepressor Syncope

Vasodepressor syncope, also known as vasovagal syncope, but more often referred to as common faint, is a frequently observed, usually benign, and self-limiting process, which however is potentially life threatening. In two surveys of emergencies occuring in dentistry, vasodepressor syncope appeared as the most common emergency situation observed.[1,2] Patients have fainted during all phases of dental care: during tooth extraction and other surgical procedures, during local anesthetic injections, or during procedures such as venipuncture, on being seated in the dental chair, and even on first entering the dental office.[3-5] As described in the preceding chapter, *syncope* is a general term that refers to a sudden, transient loss of consciousness that is usually secondary to a period of cerebral ischemia. There are many synonyms that are used to describe this situation, a number of which are listed in Table 6-1. *Vasodepressor syncope*, the most descriptive and accurate of these terms, will be the name applied to this situation throughout this discussion.

Vasodepressor syncope is ordinarily a relatively harmless situation during which the victim either falls gently to the floor or is laid down by a second party. Consciousness returns almost immediately, and within a short period of time the victim appears to be completely recovered. The relative benignity of this situation was borne out by statistics from Great Britain.[6] During World War II, over 25,000 blood donors fainted and all recovered. Yet despite its seemingly innocuous nature, vasodepressor syncope does lead to the loss of consciousness, and any loss of consciousness, however brief, produces physiologic changes in the victim that are deleterious to the continuation of life.[7] Examples of these are cardiopulmonary changes occurring secondary to hypoxia or anoxia that are produced by airway obstruction in the unconscious patient. Although

Table 6-1. Synonyms for vasodepressor syncope

Atrial bradycardia
Benign faint
Neurogenic syncope
Psychogenic syncope
Simple faint
Swoon
Vasodepressor syncope
Vasovagal syncope

vasodepressor syncope is a fairly common emergency situation, it is one that can usually be prevented. When promptly recognized and properly managed, this type of emergency is associated with exceptionally low morbidity and mortality rates.

PREDISPOSING FACTORS

Factors that can precipitate vasodepressor syncope may be divided into two groups. The first group consists of psychogenic factors such as fright, anxiety, emotional stress, and receipt of unwelcome news. Two other factors that may be included in this group are pain, especially of a sudden and unexpected nature, and the sight of blood or of surgical or other dental instruments (such as a local anesthetic syringe). As will be seen, these factors lead to the developement of the fight-or-flight response and, in the absence of muscular activity by the patient, are manifest clinically as the transient loss of consciousness, termed *vasodepressor syncope*.

The second group consists of nonpsychogenic factors. These include sitting in an upright position or standing, which permits blood to pool in the periphery, thereby decreasing cerebral blood flow below critical levels; hunger from dieting or a missed meal, which decreases the glucose supply to the brain below critical levels; exhaustion; poor physical condition; and a hot, humid, crowded environment.

Vasodepressor syncope is more common in young adults, but by no means is exclusive to this group. In addition, men have a higher incidence of vasodepressor syncope than do women. Indeed, men between the ages of 16 and 35 may be the most likely candidates for vasodepressor syncope. This is probably due to the male image as someone who can "take it," that is, can tolerate pain or anxiety without exhibiting emotion.[8] The fear of injury coupled with the expectation by one's peers to act courageously sets the scene for the escape mechanism of fainting. In a prospective study of patients who fainted, Martin and others demonstrated an average age of 35.5 years.[9] It is for precisely this reason that vasodepressor syncope is such a rare finding in pediatric patients. Children do not hide their fears—they yell, cry, and move about, unlike the more mature and usually more inhibited typical adult male. A diagnosis of vasodepressor syncope should be seriously questioned in pediatric patients or in adults above the age of 40 years in whom syncope develops (especially if it develops without prodromal symptoms, as will be explained shortly).[9]

Within the dental setting, the most common precipitating factors of vasodepressor syncope will be those of a psychogenic nature. If any one common dental situation had to be selected as the most likely cause of vasodepressor syncope, it would be the administration of a local anesthetic to an anxious male patient under the age of 35, who is seated upright in the dental chair. Table 6-2 summarizes predisposing factors to vasodepressor syncope.

PREVENTION

Prevention of vasodepressor syncope is directed at the elimination of any predisposing factors that may be present. Most dental offices are not hot, humid, or crowded, and they are usually air conditioned, so that factor is eliminated. Hunger, the result of dieting or missing a meal before the dental appointment must be considered. Especially with an anxious patient, the dentist should request that the patient eat a light snack or meal before a dental appointment to minimize the risk of hypoglycemia developing in addition to a psychogenic response. (Hypoglycemia will be discussed further in Chapter 17.) Impaired physical status (ASA III or greater) will increase the possibility of life-threatening situations developing. The term *irreversible syncope* has been used when patients collapse and die suddenly. Psychological stress, which in non–cardiovascularly

Table 6-2. Vasodepressor syncope: predisposing factors

Psychogenic factors

Fright
Anxiety
Emotional stress
Receipt of unwelcome news
Pain, especially of a sudden and unexpected nature
The sight of blood or of surgical or other dental instruments (such as a local anesthetic syringe)

Nonpsychogenic factors

Sitting in an upright position or standing
Hunger from dieting or a missed meal
Exhaustion
Poor physical condition
Hot, humid, crowded environment
Male sex
Age between 16 and 35 years

impaired persons might precipitate a simple faint, may induce sudden death secondary to life-threatening dysrhythmias in persons with underlying cardiac disorders.[8] Serious consideration to dental treatment modification is an essential part of treatment planning for the more medically compromised patient.

Proper Positioning of the Patient

An important contributing factor in most cases of vasodepressor syncope is the position of the patient in the dental chair. If the apprehensive patient is standing or is seated upright in the dental chair, the risk of vasodepressor syncope is greatly increased. With the introduction of the contoured dental chair and the advent of sit-down dentistry, most patients are no longer treated in a seated upright position. More common today, the patient will be in a supine or semisupine (30° to 45°) position, a practice that has greatly reduced the incidence of vasodepressor syncope in the dental chair.

For the dentist who seats patients in the upright position and is unable to make the change to sit-down dentistry, it might still be possible to minimize the risk of this cause of vasodepressor syncope. The act of injecting local anesthetics is *the* dental procedure that most often precipitates vasodepressor syncope. If the dentist is able to administer local anesthetics to patients while they are in a supine position, vasodepressor syncope (the actual loss of consciousness) will rarely, if ever, occur. Following completion of the local anesthetic administration, the patient may be repositioned and dental care resumed in the usual manner.

Relief of Anxiety

The most frequently encountered factors that lead to vasodepressor syncope in dental settings are psychogenic. For this reason every potential patient must be evaluated for the presence of dental anxiety. If anxiety is present, dental care should be modified to minimize or eliminate it. The recognition of anxiety will not always be as easy. Women, as well as men, do not consider admitting fear to be the "adult" thing to do. The anxiety questionnaire developed by Corah[10] has proved to be a great asset in the recognition of anxiety (p. 39). Although many patients will not admit to being fearful in an oral interview, experience with the anxiety questionnaire has shown that they will more honestly express their feelings in writing. Therefore, the inclusion of this short survey or several questions in the medical history questionnaire is worthwhile. Conversely, the presence of anxiety and fear in children is usually not difficult to recognize. As already mentioned, children, not having the inhibitions of adults, usually make their feelings quite well known to the doctor and to all others present. For this reason, vasodepressor syncope is rarely observed in children.

Medical History Questionnaire

The University of Southern California (USC) medical history questionnaire (see Figs. 2-1 and 2-2) provides the doctor with some information concerning patient anxiety:

Question 2: *Do you feel very nervous about having dentistry treatment?*

Question 3: *Have you ever had a bad experience in the dentistry office?*

Such questions permit a patient to voluntarily provide information concerning his or her dental attitudes. An affirmative response to either or both questions should result in a thorough dialogue history and possible treatment modifications aimed at decreasing the patient's dental fears.

DENTAL THERAPY CONSIDERATIONS

After anxiety has been recognized it must be managed. Along with the more appropriate positioning of the patient in the dental chair (supine or reclining), the increased use of various modalities of psychosedation has been responsible for greatly decreasing the incidence of vasodepressor syncope. Routes of drug administration include oral, rectal, and intramuscular sedation; inhalation sedation with nitrous oxide and oxygen; and intravenous sedation. The intraoperative use of psychosedation is but one of a number of stress-reducing factors discussed in Chapter 2. The concept of total patient care has led to the development of

the stress reduction protocols and has been responsible for the decreasing number of stress-related, life-threatening situations arising in dental practices. Use of these protocols will virtually eliminate the occurrence of vasodepressor syncope in dentistry.

CLINICAL MANIFESTATIONS

Clinical signs and symptoms of vasodepressor syncope usually develop rapidly in the presence of an appropriate stimulus; however, the actual loss of consciousness does not usually occur for a period of time. It is for this reason that persons who experience vasodepressor syncope while alone are rarely seriously injured. There is usually sufficient time for them to sit or lie down before losing consciousness.

The clinical manifestations of vasodepressor syncope may be grouped into three definite phases: presyncope, syncope, and postsyncope (the recovery period).

Presyncope

The prodromal manifestations of vasodepressor syncope are well known. The patient in the erect or sitting position complains of a feeling of warmth in the neck and face, loses color (becomes pale or ashen-gray), and is bathed in a cold sweat (noted primarily on the forehead). During this time the patient will usually complain of "feeling bad" or "feeling faint." Nausea may also be present. Blood pressure monitored at this time is at the baseline or slightly lower than baseline level, while the heart rate increases significantly (for example, to 120, or more, beats per minute).

As the process continues, pupillary dilation, yawning, hyperpnea (increased depth of respiration), and a coldness in the hands and feet are noted. The blood pressure and the heart rate become acutely depressed (hypotension and bradycardia) just before loss of consciousness.[4,7,11] At this time vision will become disturbed, the patient feels dizzy, and syncope occurs.

Patients developing syncope usually have several minutes of warning symptoms before the loss of consciousness.[9] If the patient is erect, presyncope may lead to unconsciousness in a relatively short time (approximately 30 seconds), whereas if the patient is supine, the presyncopal phase may not pass into the syncopal phase at all. Table 6-3 summarizes presyncopal signs and symptoms.

Syncope

With the onset of syncope, breathing may become irregular, jerky, and gasping; it may be quiet,

Table 6-3. Clinical manifestations of vasodepressor syncope: presyncopal signs and symptoms

Early

Feeling of warmth
Loss of color: pale or ashen-gray skin tone
Heavy perspiration
Complaints of feeling "bad" or "faint"
Nausea
Blood pressure approximately at baseline
Tachycardia

Late

Pupillary dilation
Yawning
Hyperpnea
Coldness in hands and feet
Hypotension
Bradycardia
Visual disturbances
Dizziness
Loss of consciousness

shallow, and scarcely perceptible; or it may cease entirely (respiratory arrest or apnea). The pupils of the eyes dilate, and the patient presents a death-like appearance. Convulsive movements or muscular twitching of the hands, legs, or facial muscles are common when consciousness is lost and the brain is hypoxic, even for as short a period as 10 seconds.

Bradycardia, which developed during the late presyncopal phase, continues. A heart rate of less than 50 beats per minute is not uncommon during syncope. In a severe episode, periods of complete ventricular asystole have been recorded even in normal healthy persons. The blood pressure, which falls precipitously to an extremely low level (30/15 mmHg is not uncommon), also remains low during this phase and is often difficult to obtain. The pulse becomes weak and thready. With loss of consciousness there is a generalized muscular relaxation that quite commonly produces partial or complete airway obstruction. Fecal incontinence may occur, particularly with a systolic blood pressure below 70 mmHg.

The duration of syncope will be extremely brief once the patient is placed in the supine position, ranging from seconds to several minutes. If unconsciousness persists for more than 5 minutes after positioning and management, or if complete clinical recovery is not evident in 15 to 20 minutes,

causes other than syncope must be considered, especially if the patient is over 40 years and does not report prodromal symptoms prior to the loss of consciousness.[9]

Postsyncope (Recovery)

With proper positioning of the patient, recovery (the return of consciousness) is rapid. In the postsyncopal phase the patient may exhibit pallor, nausea, weakness, and sweating, which may last for a few minutes to many hours. Occasionally, symptoms persist for 24 hours.[12] During the immediate postsyncopal phase there may be a short period of mental confusion or disorientation. The arterial blood pressure begins to rise during this time; however, its return to baseline levels may not occur for several hours following the episode. The heart rate, which is depressed, also returns slowly toward baseline, and the quality of the pulse becomes stronger. It is important to bear in mind that once the loss of consciousness has occurred, the tendency for the patient to faint again if raised into the sitting position or if allowed to stand too soon, may persist for hours.

PATHOPHYSIOLOGY

Vasodepressor syncope is most commonly caused by a decrease in cerebral blood flow below a critical level and is usually characterized by a sudden fall in blood pressure and a slowing of the heart rate. In the presence of predisposing factors, the following pattern of events usually develops.

Presyncope

Stress, whether emotionally triggered (as with fear) or sensorially triggered (as with unexpected pain), causes the body to release increased amounts of the catecholamines epinephrine and norepinephrine into the circulatory system. This is a part of the body's adaptation to stress, commonly called the fight-or-flight response. This results in changes in tissue blood perfusion designed to prepare the individual for increased muscular activity. Among the many responses to catecholamine release are a decrease in peripheral vascular resistance and an increase in the blood flow to many tissues, particularly the peripheral skeletal muscles. In situations in which this anticipated muscular activity occurs, the blood volume that has been diverted to the muscles in preparation for this movement is pumped by the muscles back to the heart. No pooling of blood occurs in the periphery in these cases. The blood pressure remains at or above baseline level, and signs and symptoms of vasodepressor syncope do not develop.

By contrast, in situations in which the prepared for muscle activity does not take place (such as sitting still in the dental chair and "taking it like a man"), the diversion of large volumes of blood into skeletal muscle causes a significant pooling of blood in these muscles and a lack of return of this blood to the heart. This leads to a relative decrease in circulating blood volume, a drop in arterial blood pressure, and a decrease in cerbral blood flow. Presyncopal signs and symptoms are related to decreased cardiac output, diminished cerebral blood flow, and other physiologic alterations that are taking place.[4]

As blood pools in peripheral vessels and the arterial blood pressure begins to fall, compensatory mechanisms are activated that attempt to maintain cerebral blood flow. These mechanisms include the baroreceptors, which reflexly constrict peripheral blood vessels, and the carotid and aortic arch reflexes, which increase the heart rate. These mechanisms act to increase venous return to the heart, increase cardiac output, and are responsible for the increase in heart rate and the maintenance of a near-normal blood pressure that are noted during the early presyncopal period. However, these compensatory mechanisms soon fatigue (decompensate), which is noted by development of a reflex bradycardia. It is not uncommon for the heart rate to slow to less than 50 beats per minute. Slowing of the heart rate leads to a significant drop in cardiac output, which is associated with a precipitous fall in blood pressure to levels below the critical level for consciousness (see text that follows). Cerebral ischemia results and consciousness is lost.

Syncope

It has been estimated that the critical level of cerebral blood flow to maintain consciousness is about 30 mL of blood per 100 g of brain tissue per minute. The human adult brain weighs approximately 1360 g (for a young adult male of medium stature). The normal value of cerebral blood flow is 50 to 55 mL per 100 g per minute. In a fight-or-flight situation in which muscular movement is absent and the patient is maintained in the upright position, the ability of the heart to pump this critical supply of blood to the brain is impaired and this minimal blood flow is not reached, leading to syncope. In a normotensive individual (systolic blood pressure below 140 mmHg), this minimal blood flow would be approximately equivalent to a systolic blood pressure of 70 mmHg. In patients with atherosclerosis and/or high blood pressure, this critical level for cerebral blood flow may be reached with a systolic pressure considerably above 70 mmHg. Clinically, systolic blood pressure may be as low as 20 to 30 mmHg during the syncopal episode and periods of asystole may occur.

Convulsive movements, such as tonic or clonic contractions of the arms and legs or turning of the head, can occur with the onset of syncope. Cerebral ischemia of as little as 10 seconds duration may lead to seizure activity in patients with no prior history of seizure disorders. The degree of movement will usually depend on the degree and the duration of cerebral ischemia. When present, these muscular movements are usually of brief duration and are rather mild.

Recovery

Recovery is usually hastened by placing the patient into the supine position with his or her feet slightly elevated, thus improving venous return to the heart and increasing blood flow to the brain so that cerebral blood flow again exceeds the critical level necessary for consciousness. Signs and symptoms such as weakness, sweating, and pallor may persist for hours. The body is fatigued and will require as long as 24 hours to return to its normal functioning state after the syncopal episode.[13] An additional factor that speeds recovery is the removal of the precipitating factor (for example, a syringe or blood-soaked gauze).

MANAGEMENT
Presyncope

As soon as presyncopal signs and symptoms are noted, the procedure should be stopped and the patient placed into the supine position with the legs elevated slightly. This will usually halt the progression of the episode short of syncope. Muscular movement can also aid the return of blood from the periphery. If the patient can move his or her legs vigorously, significant peripheral pooling of blood will be less likely, thus minimizing the severity of the reaction.

The fairly common practice (outside of medical/dental offices) of placing the victim's head between his or her legs when presyncopal signs and symptoms develop should be discontinued. Bending over to such an extreme degree may actually further impede the return of blood from the legs by partially obstructing the inferior vena cava, thereby causing a greater decrease of blood flow to the brain. In addition, should consciousness be lost with this technique, the victim will be in a rather awkward position for proper airway management (i.e., face down or prone).

If thought to be necessary, oxygen may be administered to the patient using a full-face mask or nasal hood. An ammonia ampule may be crushed and held under the patient's nose to aid recovery (Fig. 6-1).

Following management of presyncope the pa-

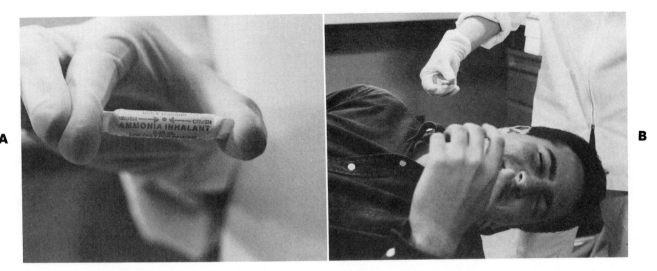

Fig. 6-1. A, Aromatic ammonia vaporole respiratory stimulant. **B,** Aromatic ammonia vaporole is crushed between fingers and held near victim's nose stimulating movement.

tient should be permitted to recover and the doctor should determine the cause of the episode. Modifications in further dental care should be considered to minimize the risk of another episode arising. Dental care may proceed if both the doctor and the patient feel it is appropriate. Should any doubt be present, postponement of dental care is recommended.

Syncope

Proper management of vasodepressor syncope will follow the basic management for all unconscious patients (see Chapter 5). A summary is presented here.

Step 1: Assess consciousness. Patient shows lack of response to sensory stimulation.

Step 2: Call for assistance. Activate the dental office emergency system.

Step 3: Position the patient. Placing the patient in the supine position is the first and most important step in the management of syncope. In addition, a slight elevation of the legs will increase the return of blood from the periphery. This step is of the utmost importance because the majority of the clinical manifestations noted in this situation are a product of inadequate cerebral blood flow. Failure to lower the patient into this position may lead to death or to permanent neurologic damage caused by cerebral ischemia and may occur in as little as 2 to 3 minutes if the patient is seated upright. The ancient Roman practice of crucifixion is an example of death from vasodepressor syncope when the upright position is forcibly maintained.

The supine position is therefore the preferred position for management of the unconscious patient (Fig. 6-2). An important exception to this po-

sition would be the unconscious female patient who is in the later stages of pregnancy (see Chapter 5). Other possible modifications of this positioning will be discussed in later sections of this textbook.

Step 4: Assess and open airway. A patent airway must immediately be established. In most instances of vasodepressor syncope, head tilt–chin lift will be the only maneuver necessary to establish a patent airway (Fig. 6-3).

Steps 5 and 6: Assess airway patency and breathing. Adequacy of the airway must then be confirmed by looking at the chest and hearing and feeling exhaled air (Fig. 6-4). Spontaneous respiration will be evident in almost all of these patients; however, artificial ventilation will be necessary on those few occasions when spontaneous respiration has ceased. Positioning of the patient and establishment of a patent airway will commonly lead to the rapid recovery of consciousness.

Step 7: Assess circulation. The carotid pulse should be palpated. Though rare, brief periods of ventricular asystole may develop during syncope. In most circumstances, however, a weak, thready pulse will be palpable in the neck. The heart rate is commonly quite slow.

IF THE PATIENT CONTINUES TO REMAIN UNCONSCIOUS SUMMON MEDICAL ASSISTANCE IMMEDIATELY

It is more common, however, for consciousness to have returned by this time.

Definitive management. After completing steps 1 through 7, members of the emergency team may assist the doctor with several additional procedures that can aid in recovery.

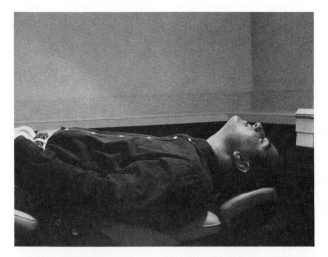

Fig. 6-2. Position of unconscious victim. Patient is placed in supine position with feet elevated slightly.

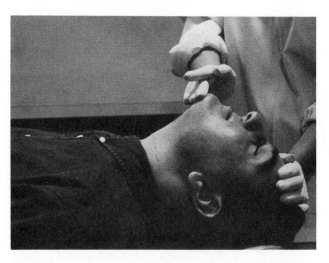

Fig. 6-3. Airway patency using head tilt–chin lift technique.

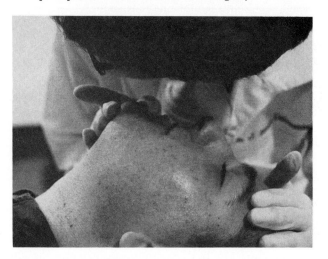

Fig. 6-4. Adequacy of airway is determined by look, listen, and feel technique.

Step 8: Administer oxygen. Oxygen can be administered to the syncopal or postsyncopal patient at any time during the episode.

Step 9: Monitor vital signs. Vital signs, including blood pressure, heart rate, and respiratory rate, should be monitored and evaluated in relation to the preoperative baseline values for the patient, to determine the severity of the reaction and the degree of recovery.

Step 10: Provide definitive management. These procedures include the loosening of binding clothes such as ties and collars (which if tight may decrease blood flow to the brain) and belts (which might

decrease blood flow from the legs). A respiratory stimulant such as aromatic ammonia may be crushed between the rescuer's fingers and the patient allowed to inhale it. Ammonia, which has a noxious odor, stimulates both increased breathing and muscular movement. If the vaporole has previously been taped to the back of the dental unit where the doctor may readily reach it without having to wait for the arrival of the emergency kit, the episode of syncope may be ended before assistance ever arrives. A cold towel can be placed on the patient's forehead, and blankets can be placed over the patient if he or she complains of feeling cold or is shivering. In lieu of blankets, a plastic patient drape of the type commonly found in dental offices may be used. If bradycardia persists, an anticholinergic such as atropine may be administered intravenously or intramuscularly.

Maintain composure. As consciousness returns, it is important for the doctor and the entire emergency team to maintain their composure. In addition, the stimulus that precipitated the episode (syringe, instruments, bloody gauze) must be removed from the patient's field of vision. The presence of a terrified dental staff or of the precipitating agent may very well cause a second episode of syncope.

Step 11: Delay patient recovery. In the event that recovery of consciousness has not occurred after the initial steps of basic life support are employed (steps 1 through 7) or if complete recovery has not occurred in 15 to 20 minutes, another cause for the episode should be considered and the Emergency Medical Services (EMS) system activated. Indeed, EMS should be activated at any time during the episode should the doctor feel it prudent. Basic life support must be continually applied while awaiting the arrival of the emergency team. If another cause of unconsciousness is obvious (such as hypoglycemia or acute adrenal insufficiency), definitive management of the problem may be instituted. In the absence of an obvious cause, however, continued basic life support is indicated. If possible, the doctor should start an intravenous infusion.

Postsyncope

Following recovery from a period of unconsciousness, the patient should not be subjected to additional dental care for the remainder of that day. The possibility of a second episode of syncope is greater during this period of time, and it has been demonstrated that the body requires up to 24 hours to return to its presyncopal state. Prior to dismissal, the doctor should determine from the patient what the primary precipitating event was and what other factors may have been present (such as hunger or fear). With this information the doctor can formulate a plan for future treatment to prevent this event from recurring.

Arrangements should then be made for the patient to be taken home by a friend or family member. It may not be prudent to allow the patient to leave the office unescorted to drive a car because of the possibility of recurrent syncopal episodes. This is especially important where the loss of consciousness occurred.

The accompanying box summarizes the management of vasodepressor syncope.

Drugs used in management: Oxygen, ammonia, and atropine.

Medical assistance required: Assistance is not usually required because consciousness is normally regained rapidly after positioning the patient correctly and assessing the airway, breathing, and circulation. A delayed recovery of consciousness or a delayed return to a normal status dictates activation of EMS.

REFERENCES

1. Fast TB, Martin MD, Ellis TM: Emergency preparedness: a survey of dental practitionners, *J Am Dent Assoc* 112(4):499-501, 1986.
2. Malamed SF: The incidence of medical emergencies in dentistry, *J Am Dent Assoc*, submitted 1992.
3. Graham DT: Prediction of fainting in blood donors, *Circulation* 23:901, 1961.
4. Reutz PP, Johnson SA, Callahan R: Fainting: a reveiw of its mechanism and a study in blood donors, *Medicine* 46:363, 1967.

MANAGEMENT OF VASODEPRESSOR SYNCOPE

Assess consciousness
↓
Activate office emergency team
↓
Position patient in supine position with feet elevated
↓
Assess and open airway
↓
Assess airway patency and breathing
↓
Assess circulation
↓
Activate EMS if recovery is not immediate
↓
Administer oxygen
↓
Monitor vital signs
↓
Provide definitive management of unconsciousness:

Aromatic ammonia
Atropine, if bradycardia persists
Maintain composure

↙   ↘

Postsyncopal recovery   Delayed recovery
↓   ↓
Arrange escort home   Activate EMS

---

5. Tizes R: Cardiac arrest following routine venipuncture, *JAMA* 236:1846, 1976.
6. Ebert RV: Response of normal subjects to acute blood loss, *Arch Int Med* 68:578, 1941.
7. Wright KE, McIntosh HD: Syncope: a review of pathophysiolgical mechanisms, *Prog Cardiovasc Dis* 13:58, 1971.
8. Engel GL: Psychologic stress, vasodepressor (vasovagal) syncope, and sudden death, *Ann Intern Med* 89:403, 1978.
9. Martin GJ, Adams SL, Martin HG, and others: Prospective evaluation of syncope, *Ann Emerg Med* 13:499, 1984.
10. Corah NL: Development of a dental anxiety scale, *J Dent Res* 48:596, 1969.
11. Glick G, Yu PN: Hemodynamic changes during spontaneous vasovagal reactions, *Am J Med* 34:42, 1963.
12. Friedberg CK: Syncope: pathological physiology, differential diagnosis and treatment, *Mod Concepts Cardiovasc Dos* 40:55, 1971.
13. Thomas JE, Rooke ED: Fainting, *Mayo Clin Proc* 38:397, 1963.

7 *Postural Hypotension*

Postural hypotension, also known as orthostatic hypotension, is the second leading cause of transient loss of consciousness in the dental environment. Postural hypotension may be defined as a disorder of the autonomic nervous system in which syncope occurs when the patient assumes an upright position. Postural hypotension is also defined as a fall in systolic pressure of 20 mmHg or more upon standing.[1,2] Postural hypotension results from a failure of the baroreceptor-reflex—mediated increase in peripheral vascular resistance in response to positional changes.[3]

Postural hypotension differs in several important respects from vasodepressor syncope and is only infrequently associated with fear and anxiety. Awareness of predisposing factors will allow the dentist to prevent this situation from developing. Two examples of postural hypotension arising in dental situations are syncope that develops in a 76-year-old woman whose recumbent blood pressure is 180/100, which drops to 100/50 mmHg immediately upon rising from the dental chair, and a 35-year-old male who, following 1 hour of lying in the supine position in the dental chair, stands up and walks to the reception desk to arrange another appointment. On reaching the front desk he stands still, feels faint, and loses consciousness.

PREDISPOSING FACTORS

Many factors have been identified that may be responsible for the development of postural hypotension, including several of importance to the practice of dentistry. They include the administration and ingestion of drugs,[4] prolonged periods of recumbency and convalescence,[5] an inadequate postural reflex, pregnancy (later stages),[6] advanced age,[2,7] venous defects in the legs (varicose veins), postsympathectomy for "essential" hypertension, Addison's disease, physical exhaustion[8] and star-

vation, and chronic postural hypotension (Shy-Drager syndrome).

The incidence of postural hypotension increases with age.[2,7] In a group of 100 ambulatory patients aged 65 years and older, 31% demonstrated a decrease in systolic blood pressure of 20 mmHg or more, whereas 16% had a diastolic drop of 10 mmHg or greater. Twelve percent had a significant drop in both systolic and diastolic blood pressure upon standing.[2] Postural hypotension is uncommon in infants and children.

Drug Administration and Ingestion

Probably the most frequently encountered cause of postural hypotension in the dental office is the use of various drugs that can produce this situation. These drugs may have been given to the patient by the doctor before, during, or after dental therapy, or they may have been prescribed by the patient's physician for the management of specific physical or psychological disorders. These agents fall into the broad categories of antihypertensives, especially the sodium-depleting diuretics, calcium channel blockers, and the ganglionic blocking agents; psychotherapeutics (sedatives and tranquilizers); narcotics; antihistaminics; and L-dopa for Parkinson's disease. In general, these drugs act to produce postural hypotension by diminishing the ability of the body to maintain blood pressure (and adequate cerebral perfusion) in response to the increased influence of gravity that results when the patient rises suddenly. A greatly exaggerated blood pressure response is thus seen. Table 7-1 summarizes the most commonly encountered drugs that may produce postural hypotension.

Medications employed to manage fear and anxiety are capable of producing postural hypotension—especially with parenteral administration (intramuscular, intravenous, or by inhalation).

128

Table 7-1. Drugs producing postural hypotension

Category	Generic name	Proprietary name
Antihypertensives	Guanethidine	Ismelin
Phenothiazines	Chlorpromazine	Thorazine
	Thioridazine	Mellaril
Tricyclic antidepressants	Doxepin	Sinequan
	Amitriptyline	Elavil
	Imipramine	Tofranil
		Presamine
Narcotics	Meperidine	Demerol
	Morphine	Morphine
Antiparkinson drugs	Levodopa (L-dopa)	Dopar
		Larodopa

Those most often used in dentistry include nitrous oxide and oxygen (by inhalation), diazepam, midazolam and pentobarbital (intravenous), and meperidine (intravenous, intramuscular). Positional changes in patients receiving these agents should be made slowly and with care.

Age

The incidence of postural hypotension shows a definite increase with increasing age and proves to be a major problem in the aging population.[1,2,7,9,10] Patients who demonstrated a drop in both diastolic and systolic blood pressures were more likely to have had a fall during the year prior to their evaluation and decreased functional ability compared to those without postural hypotension.[2] Of 761 persons studied prospectively by Campbell[11] who were 70 years of age or older, 507 experienced falls during the preceding year of monitoring. Though multiple risk factors for falls were present in many patients, postural hypotension was frequently present. Macrae[7] evaluated blood pressure changes in elderly patients in the morning and afternoon. In elderly patients a decrease in systolic pressure was greatest in the morning approximately 30 seconds after standing—a decrease of 9.3 mmHg—and returned to normal within two minutes. In contrast, diastolic pressure rose a maximum of 9.7 mmHg by 2 minutes. When measured in the afternoon after lunch, the decrease in blood pressure ($n = 13$) was significantly greater: 20.8 mmHg ± 3.6 against 7.1 ± 2.0 mmHg in the morning ($p = 0.01$).

Prolonged Recumbency and Convalescence

Confinement to bed for as little as 1 week in a normal subject has been shown to predispose a patient to postural hypotension.[5] This is one of the reasons hospitalized patients are encouraged to walk as soon as possible after surgical procedures. Although dental patients are not usually confined for periods up to a week, a recent trend in dental practice has been toward an increase in the length of appointments. It is no longer uncommon for a dental patient to be seated in a dental chair for up to 2 or 3 hours, usually in a reclining position. In these circumstances postural hypotension may develop at the end of the appointment when chair position is returned to the upright posture and/or the patient stands up. The concomitant use of psychosedative agents during the dental appointment will further increase the incidence of postural hypotension.

Inadequate Postural Reflex

Healthy young people may faint when forced to stand motionless for prolonged periods of time, such as during school assemblies, religious services, or parades. Syncope might also develop if a patient is seated upright in the dental chair for prolonged periods of time. This is more likely to occur in a hot environment, which produces a concomitant peripheral vasodilation. The following, excerpted from the *Los Angeles Times*,[12] illustrates one government agency's response to this physiologic occurrence:

How to Faint by the Numbers
VANCOUVER (UPI)—The order has gone out: Canadian troups may no longer faint in a slovenly or unseemly way while on parade. Soldiers disobeying the order will be put on report.

The memo said: "To avoid the possibility of fainting, a soldier should make sure he has had breakfast on the morning of parade day. If worse comes to worst and he must faint, a soldier should fall to the ground under control. To do so, he must turn his body approximately 45°, squat down, roll to the left, and retain control of his weapon to prevent personal injury and minimize damage to the weapon. We must ensure that soldiers who have not complied with the above instructions be charged."

Pregnancy

The pregnant female may demonstrate two forms of hypotension. In the first form, postural hypotension is usually encountered during the first trimester of pregnancy, occurring on arising from bed in the morning but not recurring again during the day. The precise cause of this phenomenon is not known. The second form, known as the supine hypotensive syndrome of pregnancy, occurs late in the third trimester if the patient is allowed to remain in the supine position for more than 3 to 7 minutes.[13] Signs and symptoms of syncope become evident during this period, with consciousness lost shortly thereafter. It has been demonstrated that the flaccid, gravid uterus compresses the inferior vena cava, decreasing venous return from the legs. If the patient is allowed to alter her position to the lateral seated or standing position, the weight of the uterus is taken off the vena cava and the clinical symptoms are rapidly reversed.

Venous Defects in the Legs

Postural hypotension has been noted in patients with varicose veins and other disorders of the vascular system of the legs, which permits excessive pooling of blood in the legs to occur in these patients.

Postsympathectomy for High Blood Pressure

Surgical procedures to lower blood pressure and to improve circulation to the legs may lead to a greater incidence of postural hypotension. This is usually seen in the immediate postsurgical period with the symptoms usually declining spontaneously with time.

Addison's Disease

Postural hypotension is frequently seen in patients with chronic adrenocortical insufficiency. It may be managed through the administration of corticosteroids (see Chapter 8).

Physical Exhaustion, Fatigue, and Starvation

Syncope observed during physical exhaustion, fatigue, and starvation is caused by postural hypotension. This factor is not usually of importance in the dental office.

Chronic Postural Hypotension (Shy-Drager Syndrome)

The Shy-Drager syndrome, also known as idiopathic postural hypotension or multiple systems atrophy, is an uncommon disorder, the cause of which is unknown.[14] Its course is progressive. Severe disability or death usually occurs within 5 to 10 years of onset. Patients are usually in their fifties and initially experience postural hypotension, urinary and fecal incontinence, sexual impotence (males), and anhidrosis (lack of sweating) in the lower trunk.

PREVENTION

The clinical manifestations of postural hypotension may be prevented if the doctor is aware of its causative factors. Prevention is based on three factors: the medical history and physical examination to determine whether or not the potential problem exists, and if it does, making certain dental care considerations to prevent the loss of consciousness.

Medical History Questionnaire

The medical history questionnaire (see Fig. 2-1) is a valuable source of information. Relevant questions include the following:

QUESTION 6. **Have you taken any medicine or drugs during the past 2 years?**

COMMENT. Medications taken by a patient may produce the side effect of postural hypotension. The drug package insert or an appropriate textbook should be consulted. Table 7-1 lists commonly prescribed drugs that may produce postural hypotension.

QUESTION 9. **Do you have fainting spells or seizures?**

COMMENT. A history of frequent fainting spells may indicate the presence of postural hypotension. The ensuing dialogue history should seek to determine the factors involved in these episodes and the presence or absence of prodromal signs and symptoms associated with these syncopal episodes. In patients with postural hypotension, determine any medications the patient may be taking to assist in maintaining adequate blood pressure. Ephedrine, up to 75 mg orally per day, is commonly prescribed. Fludrocortisone acetate in doses of 0.1 mg or more daily is also effective.[15] In the event that the patient does not know the name of a drug being taken, the doctor should have a text available, such as the *Physician's Desk Reference*, in which illustrations of many medications are shown.

Physical Examination

An integral part of the pretreatment evaluation for all potential patients is recording of the vital signs. These include the blood pressure, heart rate and rhythm (pulse), respiratory rate, temperature, height, and weight.

The presence of postural hypotension may be detected if the blood pressure and heart rate of a patient are recorded in the supine and standing positions. The first recording is taken after the patient has been supine for 2 to 3 minutes and then after standing for 1 minute.[16] The normal response of blood pressure when recorded in the supine and then the standing position 1 minute later is a standing systolic blood pressure within 10 mmHg (higher or lower, usually higher) of the supine blood pressure. The heart rate normally accelerates on standing and generally remains about 5 to 20 beats per minute faster than in the supine position.

CLINICAL CRITERIA FOR POSTURAL HYPOTENSION

1. Symptomatology develops upon standing
2. Increase in standing pulse at least 30 beats per minute
3. Decrease in standing systolic blood pressure at least 25 mmHg
4. Decrease in standing diastolic blood pressure at least 10 mmHg

---

If severe clinical symptoms develop (see text that follows), the test for postural hypotension is positive and the patient should lie down immediately. Other criteria for a positive test include a rise in the standing pulse of at least 30 beats per minute or a decrease of systolic blood pressure in excess of 25 mmHg and 10 mmHg diastolic, simultaneous with the appearance of symptoms. The doctor should recheck the blood pressure in each position, and if this differential is still evident, medical consultation should be considered before dental care is initiated. The accompanying box summarizes criteria for postural hypotension.

DENTAL THERAPY CONSIDERATIONS

In the dental patient with a history of postural hypotension, or a patient receiving sedation (inhalation, intravenous, or intramuscular sedation) during dental care, or when at the end of prolonged appointments, certain basic precautions should be observed to prevent hypotensive episodes from developing when positional changes of the patient are made. The patient should be cautioned against rising too rapidly from the supine or semisupine position. When in the dental chair, the patient should be slowly returned to the sitting (upright) position at the conclusion of therapy. This might be accomplished by two or three positional changes over a period of a minute or two to reach the upright position. Allow the patient to remain at each level until any dizziness that might develop has passed. As the patient moves off the chair and stands up it may be prudent for the doctor or an assistant to stand in front of the patient until the patient is standing upright and is determined to be stable. Should the patient become faint or weak on rising, dental personnel may support and assist the patient back into the dental chair, thereby preventing possible injury. These precautions are especially important in patients who have been recumbent for longer periods of time.

CLINICAL MANIFESTATIONS

In patients with chronic postural hypotension, standing or sitting upright leads to a precipitous drop in blood pressure and to loss of consciousness, often without the prodromal signs and symptoms observed with vasodepressor syncope, such as lightheadedness, pallor, dizziness, blurred vision, nausea, and diaphoresis. In postural hypotension the patient may rapidly lose consciousness or may merely develop blurred vision or become lightheaded but not actually lose consciousness. Clinical signs and symptoms are more often seen in patients with other predisposing factors for postural hypotension, such as the administration of drugs, and may include some or all of the usual prodromal signs and symptoms of vasodepressor syncope before consciousness is lost.

Blood pressure during the syncopal period of postural hypotension is quite low, as it is in vasodepressor syncope. Unlike the bradycardia associated with vasodepressor syncope, the heart rate in postural hypotension remains at the baseline level or somewhat higher (>30 beats per minute above baseline). The patient exhibits all of the clinical manifestations of the typical unconscious patient described in Chapters 5 and 6. Minor convulsive movements may be noted if unconsciousness persists for 10 or more seconds. When the patient is returned to the supine position, consciousness rapidly returns.

PATHOPHYSIOLOGY
Normal Regulatory Mechanisms

When a patient's position is changed from the supine to the erect position, the effect of gravity upon the cardiovascular system is intensified. Blood pumped from the patient's heart must now be moved upward, opposite the force of gravity, to reach the cerebral circulation and supply the brain with the oxygen and glucose needed for the maintenance of consciousness. With the patient supine, the force of gravity is distributed equally over the entire body, and blood flows more readily from the heart to the brain. In other positions (e.g., semisupine, Trendelenburg), the effect of gravity is such that systolic blood pressure is decreased by 2 mmHg for every inch the patient's head is above the heart level, while for every inch the head is below the heart level, blood pressure is increased by 2 mmHg (Fig. 7-1).

To protect the brain and to ensure an adequate and continuous supply of oxygen and glucose to the cerebral circulation, a number of intricate mechanisms have evolved that aid in the mainte-

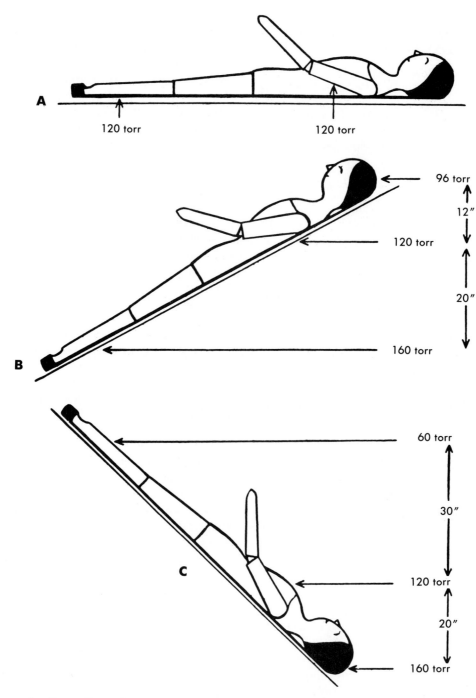

Fig. 7-1. Effect of gravity on blood pressure. **A,** Supine position. Effect of gravity is equalized over entire body. Blood pressure in legs, heart, and brain is approximately equal. **B,** Semiupright position. Blood pressure is decreased by 2 mmHg for every inch above level of heart. **C,** Trendelenburg (head down) position. Blood pressure increases 2 mmHg for every inch below level of heart. (From Enderby GEH: *Lancet* 1:185, 1954.)

nance of an adequate blood pressure when postural changes occur.[17] These include (1) a reflex arteriolar constriction that is mediated through baroreceptors (pressure receptors) located in the carotid sinus and the aortic arch; (2) a reflex increase in heart rate, which occurs simultaneously with the increase in arteriolar tone and is mediated through the same mechanisms; (3) a reflex venous constriction, increasing the return of venous blood to the heart, both intrinsic and sympathetically mediated; (4) an increase in muscle tone and contraction in the legs and abdomen—the so-called venous pump—which facilitates the venous return of blood (of vital importance because at least 60% of circulating blood volume at any one moment is found in the venous circulation); (5) a reflex increase in respiration, which also aids in the return of blood to the right side of the heart via changes in intraabdominal and intrathoracic pressures; and (6) the release into the blood of various neurohumoral substances, such as norepinephrine, antidiuretic hormone, renin, and angiotensin.

The usual (normal) reaction of the cardiovascular system when a person is tilted from the supine to the erect position is an immediate drop in the systolic blood pressure from 5 to 40 mmHg, but an equally rapid rise occurs so that within 30 seconds to 1 minute, the systolic blood pressure is equal to or slightly higher than that recorded in the supine position. Thereafter, the systolic blood pressure tends to remain within 10 mmHg higher or lower (usually higher) of the supine recording. The diastolic blood pressure rises approximately 10 to 20 mmHg. Heart rate (pulse) increases approximately 5 to 20 beats per minute when the patient is standing.

Postural Hypotension

In patients with postural hypotension, one or more of these adaptive mechanisms fails to function properly, so the body is unable to adequately adapt to the effects of gravity and the blood pressure changes dramatically as alterations in position occur. The fall of blood pressure in the standing position is rapid, with the systolic pressure sometimes approaching a level of 60 mmHg in less than 1 minute. The diastolic blood pressure also falls precipitously. Associated with this fall in blood pressure is little or no alteration in the heart rate; the cardiovascular system is unable to react normally to the blood pressure depression. This combination of signs (rapidly decreasing blood pressure, no change in heart rate) is pathognomonic of postural hypotension. In addition, in many patients none of the usual prodromal signs of vasodepressor

syncope is encountered. Consciousness is lost when cerebral blood flow falls below the critical level required for consciousness (approximately 30 mL of blood per minute per 100 g of brain), equivalent to a systolic blood pressure at heart level of approximately 70 mmHg in a normotensive individual. Unconsciousness is short-lived once the patient is placed into the supine position because of reestablishment of adequate cerebral blood flow. Table 7-2 compares postural responses of blood pressure and heart rate in postural hypotensives and normal individuals.

MANAGEMENT

Management of postural hypotension mimics that of vasodepressor syncope.

Step 1: Assess consciousness. The patient demonstrates a lack of response to sensory stimulation.

Step 2: Call for assistance. Activate the dental office emergency system.

Step 3: Position the patient. Place the unresponsive patient into the supine position with feet elevated slightly. Cerebral perfusion is immediately enhanced and in most instances of postural hypotension the patient will regain consciousness within a few seconds.

*Step 4: Assess and open airway. In the unlikely situation in which a patient with postural hypotension has not yet regained consciousness a patent airway must be established immediately. Head tilt–chin lift will usually be the only maneuver necessary to establish a patent airway.

*Steps 5 and 6: Assess airway patency and breathing. Look, listen, and feel for any obstruction in the mouth.

*Step 7: Assess circulation. The carotid pulse is palpated to determine the adequacy of circulation.

Definitive management. After completing steps 1 through 7, members of the emergency team may assist the doctor with several additional procedures that can assist in the recovery process.

Step 8: Administer oxygen. Oxygen can be administered to the syncopal or postsyncopal patient at any time during the episode.

Step 9: Monitor vital signs. Vital signs, including blood pressure, heart rate, and respiratory rate, should be monitored and evaluated in relation to preoperative baseline values for the patient to determine the severity of the hypotensive reaction and the degree of recovery. The position of the patient should be noted with each recording of vital signs.

Step 10: Definitive management. Following an episode of postural hypotension, the now-supine pa-

---

*Optional steps to be employed only when needed.

Table 7-2. Cardiovascular response to positional change in normal and postural hypotensive individuals

Change (at 60 seconds) in response to sudden elevation to upright position from supine	Normal	Postural hypotension
Systolic blood pressure	Baseline or ± 10 mmHg	Decrease of >25 mmHg
Diastolic blood pressure	Increase 10-20 mmHg	Decrease of >10 mmHg
Heart rate	5-20 beats per minute above baseline	Baseline or higher (>30 beats per minute)

tient will usually feel almost normal. There is little or no postsyncopal feeling of exhaustion or malaise as is frequently observed following vasodepressor syncope. It is important that changes in position from supine to the erect be made slowly. Reposition the patient from supine to approximately 22.5°, permit a suitable period of time to elapse for the patient to adjust (no symptoms or signs present), raise the patient to approximately 45°, allow for accommodation, raise the patient to 67.5°, allow for adjustment, and then raise the patient to an upright position (90°), and allow for accommodation. Any signs and symptoms of hypotension should resolve prior to repositioning the patient.

Before allowing the patient to leave the dental chair, recheck the blood pressure and compare it to the preoperative baseline levels. The doctor or an assistant should help the patient out of the chair and be available for support if necessary.

Delayed recovery. In the unlikely event that hypotensive episodes continue to occur with elevation of the patient from the supine position, the doctor should consider seeking outside medical assistance in an effort to definitively manage the problem.

Step 11: Discharge of the patient. Patients with chronic postural hypotension or postural hypotension as a result of a prescribed medication (such as an antihypertensive) may be permitted to leave the dental office and drive a motor vehicle only if the doctor judges that they have sufficiently recovered from the incident. This judgment might be based on a return of the vital signs to approximately the preoperative level and the ability of the patient to walk freely without any clinical signs and symptoms of hypotension developing. When the patient's history suggests that a prescribed drug may be responsible for the episode, the doctor should consider consultation with the patient's physician if episodes recur.

Patients experiencing postural hypotensive episodes with no prior history of such occurrences, or patients who have these episodes following the ad-

ministration of drugs by the doctor should be permitted to recover in the dental office while arrangements are made to have them transported home by a responsible adult or to an acute care facility by paramedical personnel. Medical consultation with the patient's physician should be considered in those cases in which there is no prior history of postural hypotension.

Management of postural hypotension is summarized in the accompanying box.

Drug used in management: Oxygen

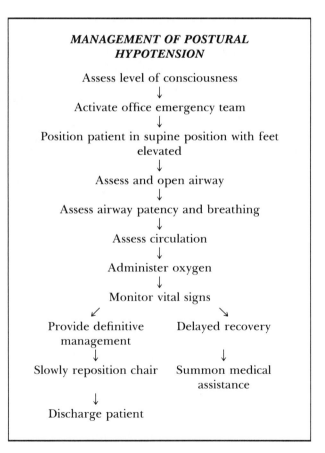

MANAGEMENT OF POSTURAL HYPOTENSION

Assess level of consciousness
↓
Activate office emergency team
↓
Position patient in supine position with feet elevated
↓
Assess and open airway
↓
Assess airway patency and breathing
↓
Assess circulation
↓
Administer oxygen
↓
Monitor vital signs
↙   ↘
Provide definitive   Delayed recovery
management
↓   ↓
Slowly reposition chair   Summon medical
                          assistance
↓
Discharge patient

Medical assistance required: Not usually; with proper positioning, consciousness is quickly regained and assistance is not required. When consciousness is not regained promptly or when recurrent hypotensive episodes develop with repositioning, summoning assistance should be considered.

REFERENCES

1. Six P: Diagnosis and therapy of hypotensive cardiovascular disorders in old age, *Ther Umsch* 46(1):22, 1989.
2. Susman J: Postural hypotension in elderly family practice patients, *J Am Board Fam Pract* 2(4):234, 1989.
3. Hickler RB: Orthostatic hypotension and syncope, *N Engl J Med* 296:336, 1977.
4. Atkins D, Hanusa B, Sefcik T, Kapoor W: Syncope and orthostatic hypotension, *Am J Med* 91(2):179-185, 1991.
5. Akhtar M, Jazayeri M, Sra J: Cardiovascular causes of syncope: identifying and controlling trigger mechanisms, *Postgrad Med* 90(2):87-94, 1991.
6. Ikeda T, Ohbuchi H, Ikenoue T, Mori N: Maternal cerebral hemodynamics in the supine hypotensive syndrome, *Obstetr and Gynecol* 79(1):27-31, 1992.
7. Macrae AD, Bulpitt CJ: Assessment of postural hypotension in elderly patients, *Age Ageing* 18(2):110, 1989.
8. Yang TM, Chang MS: The mechanism of symptomatic postural hypotension in the elderly, *Chung-Hua I Hsueh Tsa Chih* (Chinese Medical Journal) 46(3):147-155, 1990.
9. Mader SL: Aging and postural hypotension: an update, *J Am Geriatr Soc* 37(2):129, 1989.
10. Rosenthal MJ, Naliboff B: Postural hypotension: its meaning and management in the elderly, *Geriatrics* 43(12):31, 1988.
11. Campbell AJ, Borrie MJ, Spears GF: Risk factors for falls in a community-based prospective study of people 70 years and older, *J Gerontol* 44(4):M112, 1989.
12. United Press International: How to faint by the numbers, *Los Angeles Times*, Feb. 23, 1975.
13. Ikeda T, Ohbuchi H, Ikenoue T, Mori N: Maternal cerebral hemodynamics in the supine hypotensive syndrome, *Obstetr and Gynecol* 79(1):27-31, 1992.
14. Mathias CJ, Holly E, Armstrong E, Shareef M, Bannister R: The influence of food on postural hypotension in three groups with chronic autonomic failure—clinical and therapeutic implications, *J Neurol, Neurosurg, Psychiatry* 54(8):726-730, 1991.
15. Ahmad RA, Watson RD: Treatment of postural hypotension: a review, *Drugs* 39(1):74, 1990.
16. Williams TM: Orthostatic hypotension. In Callaham ML, Barton CW, Schumaker HM, editors, *Decision making in emergency medicine*, Philadelphia, 1990, B.C. Decker Inc.
17. Petrella RJ, Cunningham DA, Smith JJ: Influence of age and physical training on postural adaptation, *Can J Sport Sci* 14(1):4, 1989.

8 *Acute Adrenal Insufficiency*

A third potentially life-threatening situation that may result in the loss of consciousness is acute adrenal insufficiency (adrenal crisis). Of the three factors discussed in this section that may result in unconsciousness—vasodepressor syncope, postural hypotension, and adrenal insufficiency—the latter is by far the least often encountered.

Adrenal insufficiency was first recognized in 1844 by Addison. It is an uncommon, potentially life-threatening, and readily treatable condition.

The adrenal gland is an endocrine gland that is actually a combination of two glands, the cortex and the medulla, which are fused together, yet remain as distinct and identifiable entities.

The adrenal cortex produces and secretes over 30 steroid hormones, most of which lack any currently identifiable biologic activity of importance.[1] Cortisol, one of the glucocorticoids, is considered to be the most important product of the adrenal cortex. It helps the body adapt to stress and is thereby extremely vital to survival.

Hypersecretion of cortisol leads to increased fat deposition in certain areas, such as the face and a "buffalo hump" on the back; raises the blood pressure; and produces alterations in blood cell distribution (eosinopenia and lymphopenia).[2] Hypersecretion of cortisol does not usually produce the acute life-threatening situation that is noted with acute cortisol deficiency. Clinically, cortisol hypersecretion is referred to as Cushing's syndrome,[3] a problem that is usually readily corrected through surgical removal of part or all of the adrenal gland.[4] Renal and adrenal surgery today rate as important factors in the development of primary adrenal cortical insufficiency.[5]

Cortisol deficiency, on the other hand, may lead to a relatively rapid onset of clinical symptoms, including the loss of consciousness and, quite possibly, the patient's death. Primary adrenocortical insufficiency is called Addison's disease, an insidious

and usually progresssive disease.[6] The incidence of Addison's disease is estimated to be between 0.3 and 1.0 per 100,000 persons, occurring equally in both sexes and in all age groups, including infants and children.[7] Although all corticosteroids may be deficient in this disease state, it is important to note that the administration of physiologic doses of cortisol will correct most of the pathophysiologic effects associated with Addison's disease.[8]

Clinical manifestations of adrenal insufficiency usually do not develop until at least 90% of the adrenal cortex has been destroyed.[9] Because this destruction usually progresses quite slowly, it may be several months before a diagnosis of adrenal cortical insufficiency is made and therapy (exogenous cortisol) is instituted. During this time the patient will remain in constant jeopardy from possible acute adrenal insufficiency. The patient is capable of maintaining levels of endogenous cortisol adequate to meet the requirements of day-to-day living; however, in stressful situations (e.g., a dental appointment for a fearful patient), the adrenal cortex proves incapable of producing the additional cortisol required, and signs and symptoms of acute insufficiency develop.

A second form of adrenocortical hypofunction may be produced by the administration of exogenous glucocorticosteroids to a patient with functional adrenal cortices. Glucocorticosteroid drugs are widely prescribed in pharmacologic doses for the symptomatic relief of a wide variety of disorders (see Table 8–1). When used in this manner, exogenous glucocorticosteroid administration produces a disuse atrophy of the adrenal cortex, thereby decreasing the ability of the adrenal cortex to provide the required increase in corticosteroid levels in response to stressful situations. This in turn leads to the development of the signs and symptoms of acute adrenal insufficiency. In the development of acute adrenal crisis, secondary adrenal insufficiency is today a much greater potential threat than is Addison's disease.[10]

Acute adrenal insufficiency is a true medical emergency in which the victim is in immediate danger because of glucocorticoid (cortisol) insufficiency. Death is usually the result of peripheral vascular collapse (shock) and ventricular asystole (cardiac arrest).

The dentist is in the unenviable position of being a major stress factor in the lives of many patients. Because of this, all dental office personnel must become capable of recognizing and managing the acute adrenal crisis; even more importantly, they must be capable of preventing this situation from developing.

PREDISPOSING FACTORS

Before the availability of glucocorticosteroid therapy, acute adrenal insufficiency represented the terminal stage of Addison's disease. With such therapy, however, addisonian patients may lead relatively normal lives. Situations involving unusual stress require that the patient modify his or her steroid dosage to prevent the development of acute insufficiency. The major predisposing factor in all cases of acute adrenal insufficiency is the lack of glucocorticosteroid hormones, which develops through the following six mechanisms:

MECHANISM 1. Following the sudden withdrawal of steroid hormones in a patient who has primary adrenal insufficiency (Addison's disease)

MECHANISM 2. Following sudden withdrawal of steroid hormones in a patient with normal adrenal cortices but with a temporary insufficiency as a result of cortical suppression by exogenous corticosteroid administration (secondary insufficiency)

COMMENT. Patients with primary and secondary adrenocortical insufficiency are dependent on exogenous steroids. Abrupt withdrawal from therapy leaves patients with a deficiency of glucocorticoster-

oid hormones, making them unable to adapt normally to stress (they become stress-intolerant). Evidence has indicated that it may take up to 9 months to achieve full recovery of adrenal cortical function following prolonged exogenous steroid therapy in patients with normal cortices.[11] Others have estimated that normal function may not return for as long as 2 years.[12] Patients with Addison's disease will require the administration of glucocorticosteroids for the remainder of their lives. Withdrawal of nonaddisonian patients from exogenous corticosteroid therapy will occur over a long period of time, during which endogenous glucocorticosteroid production by the adrenal glands will increase as the level of exogenously administered steroid decreases. The time required for the return to normal adrenocortical functioning will vary and is influenced by a number of factors (see accompanying box). Protocols have been designed that permit the withdrawal of patients from long-term glucocorticosteroid therapy with minimal symptoms and relative convenience and safety.[13]

The widespread use of glucocorticosteroids in nonaddisonian patients has become the most common cause of adrenal insufficiency. Suppression of the hypothalamic-pituitary-adrenocortical axis generally does not appear unless glucocorticoid therapy has been of long duration, in nonphysiologic doses, or both. For most of the indications for glucocorticosteroids listed in Table 8-1, pharmacologic doses are required that are generally greatly in excess of physiologic doses.*

MECHANISM 3. Following stress, such as physiologic or psychologic stress

COMMENT. Physiologic stress may include traumatic injuries, surgery (including oral, periodontal, or endodontic surgery), extensive dental procedures, infection, acute changes in environmental temperature, severe muscular exercise, and burns. Psychologic stress, such as that seen in the anxious dental patient, may also precipitate adrenal crisis.

In stressful situations there is normally an increased liberation of glucocorticoids from the adrenal cortices. This increase is mediated through the hypothalamic-pituitary-adrenocortical axis and normally results in a rapid elevation of glucocorticosteroids blood levels. If the adrenal gland is unable to meet this increased demand, clinical signs and symptoms of adrenal insufficiency will develop. In dental situations stress will be the most

---

*Physiologic or replacement doses are equal to the normal daily production of a functioning adrenal cortex. This is equivalent to approximately 20 mg cortisol. Pharmacologic doses, on the other hand, are commonly four to five times or more the physiologic dose.

Table 8-1. Clinical indications for adrenocortical steroids

Allergic disease
Angioedema
Asthma, acute and chronic
Dermatitis, contact
Dermatitis venenata
Insect bites
Pollinosis (hay fever)
Rhinitis, allergic
Serum reaction, drug and foreign, acute and delayed
Status asthmaticus
Transfusion reactions
Urticaria

Cardiovascular disease
Postpericardiotomy syndrome
Shock, toxic (septic)

Eye disease
Blepharoconjunctivitis
Burns, chemical and thermal
Conjunctivitis, allergic, catarrhal
Corneal injuries
Glaucoma, secondary
Herpes zoster
Iritis
Keratitis
Neuritis, optic, acute
Retinitis, centralis
Scleritis; episcleritis

Gastrointestinal disease
Colitis, ulcerative
Enteritis, regional
Hepatitis, viral
Sprue

Genitourinary disease
Hunner's ulcer
Nephrotic syndrome

Hemopoietic disorders
Anemia, acquired hemolytic
Leukemia, acute and chronic
Lymphoma
Purpura, idiopathic thrombocytopenic

Infections and inflammation
Meningitis
Thyroiditis, acute
Typhoid fever
Waterhouse-Friderichsen syndrome

Injected locally
Arthritis, traumatic
Bursitis
Osteoarthritis
Tendinitis

Mesenchymal disease
Arthritis, rheumatoid
Dermatomyositis
Lupus erythematosus, systemic
Polyarteritis
Rheumatic fever, acute

Metabolic disease
Arthritis, gouty acute
Thyroid crisis, acute

Miscellaneous conditions
Bell's palsy
Dental surgical procedures

Pulmonary disease
Emphysema, pulmonary
Fibrosis, pulmonary
Sarcoidosis
Silicosis

Skin disease
Dermatitis
Drug eruptions
Eczema, chronic
Erythema multiforme
Herpes zoster
Lichen planus
Pemphigus vulgaris
Pityriasis rosea
Purpura, allergic
Sunburn, severe

common immediate precipitating factor producing acute adrenal insufficiency.

MECHANISM 4. Following bilateral adrenalectomy or removal of a functioning adrenal tumor that had been suppressing the other adrenal gland

MECHANISM 5. Following the sudden destruction of the pituitary gland

MECHANISM 6. Following injury to both adrenal glands by trauma, hemorrhage, infection, thrombosis, or tumor

COMMENT:. These last three causes of adrenal crisis will most commonly be observed in the hospitalized patient and will therefore not be of immediate concern to most dentists. The first three precipitating factors represent major factors in the development of acute adrenal insufficiency in dental situations and will therefore be discussed more fully in the sections to follow.

As noted, stress is a major precipitating factor of acute adrenal insufficiency. Types of acute precipitating stress include: surgery, anesthesia, psychological stress, alcohol intoxication, hypothermia, myocardial infarction, diabetes mellitus, intercurrent infection, asthma, pyrogens, and hypoglycemia.[14-17]

PREVENTION

Acute adrenal insufficiency is best managed by its prevention, which is based on the medical history questionnaire and the ensuing dialogue history between doctor and patient. In many instances specific dental therapy modifications will be necessary for the patient at risk of adrenal insufficiency.

Medical History Questionnaire

QUESTION 6. Have you taken any medicine or drugs during the past 2 years?

COMMENT. The phrase "During the past 2 years" has been added to this question because of the probability of developing varying degrees of adrenocortical suppression following the long-term use of pharmacologic doses of glucocorticosteroids. Table 8-2 lists many of the generic and proprietary names of commonly prescribed corticosteroid drugs. In many instances the patient may only know the proprietary name of the drug. Reference to this list or to the *Physician's Desk Reference* will aid in precise identification of the medication.

QUESTION 9. Circle any of the following that you have had or have at present:

- Rheumatic fever
- Asthma
- Hay fever
- Allergies or hives
- Arthritis
- Rheumatism
- Cortisone medicine

COMMENT. The specific diseases or medication listed in question 9 represent only a small number of the clinical uses of glucocorticosteroids (see Table 8-1). In each of these, pharmacologic doses of the drugs are employed.

Dialogue History

With a positive response to any of the preceding questions, the doctor must vigorously pursue a dialogue history to seek additional relevant information.

1. Drugs used in the management of the disorder
2. Drug dose
3. Route of administration
4. Duration of time that the drug was taken
5. Length of time elapsed since drug therapy was terminated

QUESTION. What drug(s) were used in management of the disorder?

COMMENT. The diseases listed in question 9 are frequently managed in part through the administration of glucocorticosteroids. The doctor must determine the name of the specific agent(s) involved in the patient's treatment. Tables 8-1 and 8-2 may help to obtain this information.

QUESTION. What was the daily dose of the drug?

COMMENT. The specific dose of glucocorticosteroid is important as one measure of the degree of cortical suppression that has occurred. The equivalent therapeutic dose of various glucocorticosteroids varies from agent to agent (Table 8-3). For example, 20 mg of hydrocortisone is equivalent to 5 mg of prednisolone, methylprednisone, and prednisone; to 4 mg of methylprednisolone and triamcinolone; and to 0.75 mg of dexamethasone.

Patients with primary adrenocortical insufficiency (Addison's disease) receive replacement (physiologic) doses of glucocorticosteroids. This usually requires the administration of approximately 15 to 25 mg of hydrocortisone orally daily in two divided doses; two-thirds in the morning and one-third in the late afternoon or early evening. Many patients, however, do not obtain sufficient salt-retaining effect and require fludrocortisone supplementation at a dose of 0.05 to 0.3 mg orally daily or every other day.[18] These doses satisfactorily replace the normal output of the adrenal cortex (approximately 20 mg of cortisol daily).

Patients receiving glucocorticosteroid therapy for symptomatic treatment of their disorders (see Table 8-1) commonly receive large pharmacologic

Table 8-2. Systemic corticosteroids

Generic name	Proprietary name	Generic name	Proprietary name
Hydrocortisone	A-hydroCort Biosone Cortef Fernisone Hydrocortone Lifocoft Solu-Cortef	Methylprednisolone	BayMep-40 Depoject Depo-Medrol Depopred Duralone-80 Medrol Mepred-40 Solu-Medrol
Cortisone	Cortone		
Prednisolone	Articulose Cortalone Deltasone Fernisolone-P Hydeltra Key-Pred-25 Metalone	Triamcinolone	Aristocort, Aristospan Articulose-L.A. Cenocort Kenacort, Kenalog Tracilon Trilog Trilone
	Meticorten Niscort Predaject Predcor-25 Savacort Solupredalone	Paramethasone	Haldrone
		Dexamethasone	Baydex Baycadron Dalalone Decadron Dexone
Prednisone	Cortan Delta-Cortef Hydeltrasol Orasone Panasol Prednicen-M Sterone		Dezone Hexadrol Savacort Solurex
		Betamethasone	Betameth Celestone Selstoject
		Fludrocortisone	Florinef

Table 8-3. Equivalent doses of corticosteroids

Agent	Equivalent dose (mg)
Cortisone	25
Hydrocortisone	20
Prednisolone	5
Prednisone	5
Methylprednisone	5
Methylprednisolone	4
Triamcinolone	4
Dexamethasone	0.75
Betamethasone	0.6

> ***RULE OF TWOS***
>
> Adrenocortical suppression should be suspected if a patient has received glucocorticosteroid therapy:
> 1. In a dose of 20 mg or more of cortisone or its equivalent daily
> 2. Via the oral or parenteral route for a continuous period of 2 weeks or longer
> 3. Within 2 years of dental therapy

or therapeutic doses. In the management of rheumatoid arthritis, a daily oral dose of 10 mg of prednisone is frequently administered.[19] This is equivalent in effect to approximately 50 mg of cortisone. Prednisone is also administered orally to asthmatic patients whose acute episodes do not respond readily to bronchodilator therapy.[20] Divided doses totaling 40 to 60 mg/day are employed. This is equivalent to 200 to 300 mg of cortisone. Doses such as these may readily cause suppression of the normal adrenal cortex if they are continued for a length of time.

The "Rule of Twos" (see accompanying box) though admittedly conservative, is helpful in determining the risk factor of patients who are currently taking or previously have taken glucocorticosteroids.[21] The first of the three factors in the Rule of Twos is the daily administration of 20 mg or more of cortisone or its equivalent.

QUESTION. By what route was the drug administered?

COMMENT. Glucocorticosteroids may be administered by a variety of routes. Parenteral administration (intramuscular, intravenous, and subcutaneous) and enteral administration (oral) may lead to suppression of the normal adrenal cortex with a decrease in the production of endogenous glucocorticosteroids. Drugs administered topically (ophthalmic, dermatologic, intranasal, tracheobronchial, vaginal, or rectal) and by intraarticular application usually do not cause adrenal cortical suppression because of the relatively poor systemic absorption by these routes.

QUESTION. What was the duration of the glucocorticosteroid therapy?

COMMENT. Although the exact length of time required for the development of significant cortical suppression varies from patient to patient, it has been demonstrated that uninterrupted glucocorticosteroid therapy for as little as 2 weeks may produce this phenomenon.[22] Any patient who has received glucocorticosteroid therapy for 2 weeks or longer is at risk of developing adrenal insufficiency. This constitutes the second important factor in the Rule of Twos.

QUESTION. How long has it been since glucocorticosteroid therapy was terminated?

COMMENT. This question is applicable to patients who had normal, functional adrenal cortices at the time of the start of glucocorticosteroid therapy, underwent therapy (probably at pharmacologic dose levels) until the underlying disorder was controlled, and were then gradually withdrawn from it. The atrophic adrenal cortex does not function normally for a variable period of time following withdrawal of exogenous corticosteroids. During this time the cortex is usually capable of producing minimal daily levels of endogenous steroids, but in stressful situations it may prove incapable of meeting the demand, thus inducing signs and symptoms of acute adrenal insufficiency. The length of time required for full regeneration of normal cortical function varies according to the dosage and length of therapy but is normally at least 9 to 12 months.[11] Instances of acute adrenal insufficiency lasting as long as 2 years have been reported following termination of therapy. The third factor in the Rule of Twos relates to patients who have received glucocorticoid therapy with 2 years of dental therapy. The Rule of Twos allows the doctor to predict with a degree of reliability which patients are at increased risk of developing acute adrenal insufficiency.

DENTAL THERAPY CONSIDERATIONS

Possible modification in dental therapy is in order for patients who are currently receiving glucocorticosteroid therapy or have received such therapy and meet the criteria of the Rule of Twos. In such circumstances the following should be considered: medical and dental evaluation should be completed, a provisional treatment plan established, and the patient's physician consulted before dental care is begun. A patient with Addison's disease or a person on long-term pharmacologic dose corticosteroid therapy will usually have ASA II or ASA III level risk.

Glucocorticosteroid Coverage

Because patients with adrenocortical insufficiency are unable to adapt to stress in a normal manner, their blood steroid levels must be increased through the administration of exogenous glucocorticosteroids before, during, and possibly after the stressful situation. The choice of a therapeutic regimen depends on the physician's evaluation of the patient's physical status and on the

---

Card for Patient on Corticosteroid Therapy

Mr.
Mrs.
Miss _____ is being treated for ___(disorder)___
with _(corticosteroid)_ in a dose of ____(dose)____. In the
event of "stress," the steroid dosage should be increased thus:

   1. *Mild "Stress"* (e.g., common cold, single dental extraction, mild trauma): use double doses daily.

   2. *Moderate "Stress"* (e.g., flu, surgery under local anesthesia, several dental extractions): use hydrocortisone, 100 mg, or prednisolone, 20 mg, or dexamethasone, 4 mg daily.

   3. *Severe "Stress"* (e.g., general surgery, pneumonia or other systemic infections, high fever, severe trauma): use hydrocortisone, 200 mg, or prednisolone, 40 mg, or dexamethasone 8 mg daily.

   When vomiting or diarrhea precludes absorption of oral doses, give dexamethasone 1 to 4 mg intramuscularly every 6 hours.

(Signed) _____ M.D.
(Address) _____

Fig. 8-1. Sample corticosteroid coverage protocol for patient receiving corticosteroid therapy. (From Streeten DHP: *JAMA* 232:944, 1975).

---

dentist's evaluation of the stress involved in the planned dental care. Many physicians tend to underestimate the degree of stress associated with nonsurgical dental procedures. The dentist must carefully evaluate this vitally important factor. In extreme instances, such as the patient with Addison's disease who is quite fearful, the patient may be hospitalized and given 200 to 500 mg of cortisone per day. This is equivalent to the maximal response of the normal pituitary-adrenal system to extreme stress. With milder stress, as most dental procedures might be classified, or with moderate anxiety toward dentistry, the needed increase in glucocorticosteroid level is diminished. Usually a two- or fourfold increase in glucocorticoid treatment on the day of the stress (the appointment day) is adequate to prepare the patient. The adrenal cortices of normal adults secrete about 20 mg of cortisol daily, which is the daily maintenance level required by most addisonian patients. Oral medications may be given. Figure 8-1 is a sample of a corticosteroid coverage protocol.

Stress Reduction Protocol

In addition to medical consultation and the possible use of exogenous corticosteroids during the period of dental care, the stress reduction protocol (see Chapter 2) is an extremely valuable adjunct to the proper management of patients with adrenocortical insufficiency.

Additional Considerations

Many patients with Addison's disease wear an identification bracelet stating their name, the name and telephone number of a close relative, and their physician's name and telephone number. The bracelet also states, "I have adrenal insufficiency. In any emergency involving injury, vomiting, or loss of consciousness, the hydrocortisone in my possession should be injected under my skin, and my physician should be notified." Such patients carry small, clearly labeled kits containing 100 mg of hydrocortisone phosphate solution in a sterile syringe ready for use. Even if never needed, this kit is a constant reminder to the patient that survival may depend on the timely administration of this drug.

The kit should be taken from the high-risk patient at the time of the dental appointment and placed on the instrument tray or elsewhere within ready reach of the doctor during treatment.

CLINICAL MANIFESTATIONS

In stressful situations such as might be experienced during dental treatment, the patient with hypofunctioning adrenal cortices may demonstrate clinical signs and symptoms of an acute insufficiency of glucocorticosteroids. The end result of this acute insufficiency may be loss of consciousness and coma. The signs and symptoms of adrenal insufficiency are presented in Table 8-4.

Lethargy, extreme fatigue, and weakness are almost universally present. In extreme cases the weakness may be so pronounced that even speaking can be difficult.[23] Hyperkalemia also develops during adrenal insufficiency, and if severe, can lead to skeletal muscle paralysis.[24]

Mortality and major morbidity noted with adrenal insufficiency are usually secondary to hypotension or hypoglycemia. Hypotension with systolic blood pressure of less than 110 mmHg is found in most addisonian patients. Of 108 addisonian patients studied, only 3% had systolic blood pressure greater than 125 mmHg.[25] Orthostatic hypotension tends to be present and episodes of postural syncope may be noted.

Nausea and vomiting as well as other nonspecific gastrointestinal symptoms are present in more than half of adrenal insufficient patients.[26] Anorexia is almost universally present and leads to the weight loss that always accompanies chronic adrenal insufficiency.[27]

Mucocutaneous hyperpigmentation is present in more than three fourths of addisonian patients.[25,26] Melanin deposits usually occur in areas of trauma or friction, such as the palms and soles, elbows, knees, buccal mucosa, and in old scars.[27]

Two thirds of patients with adrenal insufficiency have hypoglycemia.[25,26] Symptoms are those normally associated with hypoglycemia (see Chapter 17): tachycardia, perspiration, weakness, nausea, vomiting, headache, convulsions, and coma.[28] Electrolyte disturbances are almost always evident in adrenal insufficiency, including hyponatremia in 88% of cases, hyperkalemia in 64% of cases and hypercalcemia in 6% to 33% of cases.[25,26,29,30]

In the dental setting the acute episode will be marked most notably by a progressively severe mental confusion. Intense pain develops in the abdomen, lower back, and legs, and a progressive deterioration of the cardiovascular system is noted. This latter symptom may lead to the loss of

Table 8-4. Clinical presentation of adrenal insufficiency

Symptoms	Frequency (%)
Weakness and fatigue	99-100
Anorexia	98-100
Weight loss	97-100
Hyperpigmentation (skin)	92-97
Hypotension (110/70 mmHg)	82-91
Hyperpigmentation (mucous membranes)	71-82
Nausea, vomiting	56-87
Abdominal pain	34
Salt craving	22
Diarrhea	20
Constipation	19
Syncope	12-16
Musculoskeletal complaints	6
Vitiligo	4-9
Lethargy	—
Confusion	—
Psychosis	—
Auricular calcification	—

Modified from Wogan JM: Endocrine disorders. In Rosen P, editor: *Emergency medicine*, ed 2, St Louis, 1988, Mosby–Year Book.

consciousness and onset of coma. Coma has been defined as a state in which a patient is totally unresponsive or is unresponsive to all except very painful stimuli and immediately returns to the state of unresponsiveness when the stimulus is terminated.

If unmanaged, acute adrenal insufficiency may lead to the death of the patient. Mortality is usually secondary to hypoglycemia or hypotension.

Loss of consciousness does not occur immediately in most instances. The progressive mental confusion and other clinical symptoms will usually permit the prompt recognition of a problem and institution of basic steps of management.

PATHOPHYSIOLOGY
Review of Normal Adrenal Function

The actions of adrenocortical steroid hormones affect all bodily tissues and organs and aid in keeping the internal environment of the body constant (homeostasis) through their actions on the metabolism of carbohydrates, fats, proteins, water, and electrolytes. The body provides a minimal supply of glucocorticosteroid hormones (approximately 20 mg of cortisol daily in the nonstressed adult[31]) through the actions of adrenocorticotrophic hormone (ACTH), which is released by the anterior

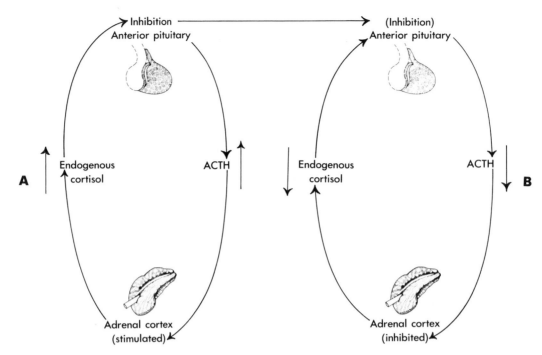

Fig. 8-2. Mechanism of glucocorticosteroid availability (normal adrenal cortex). **A,** Anterior pituitary gland increased production of ACTH, which leads to adrenocortical stimulation and increased adrenal secretion of endogenous glucocorticosteroid. This increased blood level leads to inhibition of the anterior pituitary gland. **B,** Inhibited anterior pituitary produces less ACTH. Decreased blood level of ACTH leads to inhibition of adrenal cortex and decreased production of glucocorticosteroids. Decreased blood level of glucocorticosteroids leads to stimulation of anterior pituitary (see **A**).

portion of the pituitary gland. The ACTH levels in the blood control the adrenal cortex and the production of all steroids except aldosterone.

In nonstressed situations the rate of ACTH secretion is regulated by the level of circulating cortisol; a high level suppresses ACTH secretion, whereas a low circulating cortisol level permits its more rapid secretion (Fig. 8-2, *A* and *B*). The mechanism is relatively slow acting and does not account for the rapid increase in blood ACTH levels observed in more stressful situations. A second factor regulating the secretion of ACTH is an individual's sleep schedule. In persons who sleep at night, plasma ACTH levels begin to rise at 2 AM, reaching their peak at the time of awakening. They fall during the day, reaching their ebb during the evening. This process of fluctuating cortisol blood levels, called diurnal variation, is reversed in persons who work at night and sleep during the day. This factor again is of primary value during nonstressful times.

Under stress, the pituitary gland rapidly increases the release of ACTH into the circulation, and the adrenal cortex responds within minutes by

synthesizing and secreting increased amounts of various steroids. The sum total of this increased steroid production is to prepare the body to successfully manage the stressful situation by increasing the metabolic rate, increasing the retention of sodium (Na^+) and water, and making small blood vessels increasingly responsive to the actions of norepinephrine. In order to rapidly raise the levels of cortical steroids in the blood, a third mechanism must be activated (Fig. 8-2, *C*). When stressful stimuli are received by the central nervous system, they reach the level of the hypothalamus, which releases a substance known as corticotrophin-releasing factor (CRF). This factor is transported by means of the hypothalamic-hypophyseal portal venous system to the anterior lobes of the pituitary gland, where CRF stimulates the secretion of ACTH into the circulation, which then allows the adrenal cortex to increase secretion of corticosteroids. The cortisol secretion begins within minutes and continues as long as the plasma ACTH level is maintained. Once ACTH secretion ceases (e.g., with removal of stress), plasma ACTH concentration has a half-life

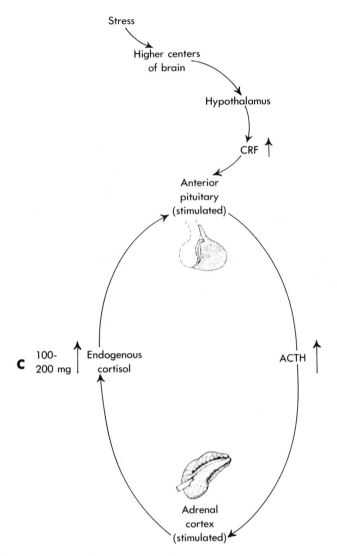

Fig. 8-2, cont'd. C, Mechanism of glucocorticosteroid availability. Normal adrenal cortex (stress situations). In stressful situations the hypothalamus receives stimuli from higher centers of the brain. Corticotrophin-releasing factor (CRF) is released, which stimulates production of ACTH by anterior pituitary. Increased blood levels of ACTH stimulate adrenal cortex to produce increased quantities of endogenous glucocorticosteroids (100 to 200 mg cortisol) required for stress adaptation.

of 10 minutes; once cortisol secretion ceases, the plasma cortisol level falls during a half-life of 1 to 2 hours.

Pathophysiology of Adrenal Insufficiency

In the patient with primary adrenocortical insufficiency (Addison's disease), the adrenal cortex is hypofunctioning and is unable to provide the necessary blood levels of corticosteroids required to maintain life even at nonstressful levels. For this reason, replacement therapy must be provided by means of oral or parenteral corticosteroids. Figure 8-3 shows the feedback mechanisms operating in the addisonian patient. Corticosteroid blood level is fixed, depending on the total milligram dosage administered during the day. As a general rule, a normal adult secretes 20 mg of cortisol per day; thus, replacement therapy in Addison's disease consists of approximately 20 mg of exogenous cortisol (hydrocortisone) daily. It may be administered either orally or parenterally, in single or, more usually, in divided doses. The adrenal cortex is unable to respond to increases or decreases in the blood levels of ACTH, which continues to be secreted by the anterior pituitary.

In the patient with a normal adrenal cortex who is receiving glucocorticosteroid therapy for a non-endocrine disorder, the blood level of cortisol is

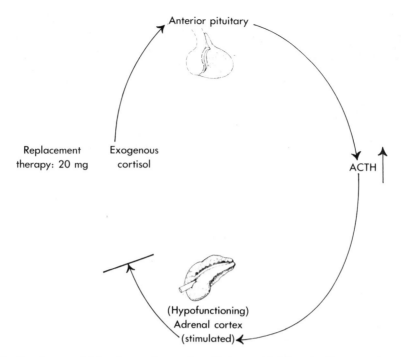

Fig. 8-3. Corticosteroid levels—primary insufficiency (Addison's disease). Anterior pituitary gland secretes ACTH, which stimulates adrenal cortex. Hypofunctioning adrenal cortex is unable to synthesize and secrete required cortisol. Blood levels of glucocorticosteroids do not fluctuate in response to ACTH levels, being fixed by exogenous doses of approximately 20 mg.

determined by the total quantity of endogenous and exogenous glucocorticosteroid. Initially, the adrenal cortex will continue to secrete approximately 20 mg of endogenous cortisol daily, to which may be added doses in excess of 50 mg through the administration of exogenous corticosteroids. The effect of this elevated blood level of glucocorticosteroids is to inhibit the secretion of ACTH by the anterior pituitary gland. This decrease in ACTH inhibits the adrenal cortex from secreting endogenous cortisol. As exogenous steroid therapy continues, the ability of the pituitary gland to secrete ACTH and of the adrenal cortex to produce endogenous glucocorticoids decreases, and a variable degree of disuse atrophy develops (Fig. 8-4, *A*). If exogenous steroid therapy terminates abruptly, or on rare occasions, even after the slow withdrawal of these drugs, the blood level of cortisol falls, thereby stimulating the anterior pituitary to produce higher blood levels of ACTH, which acts to stimulate the adrenal cortex to produce endogenous cortisol. At this time, ACTH and endogenous corticosteroid levels may prove deficient (Fig. 8-4, *B*). The adrenal cortex is unable to produce the required cortisol levels, and the patient is

in a hypoadrenal state. Any increased requirement for cortisol, as in stressful situations, may produce an acute insufficiency. Although the adrenal cortex usually regains normal function within 2 to 4 weeks, it may require longer than a year in other instances.[11] The longer the duration of exogenous therapy and the larger the doses received, the longer the recovery period will be.

In stressful situations the patient with adrenal hypofunction, either primary (Addison's disease) or secondary (exogenous steroids), receives a fixed level of exogenous corticosteroid (Fig. 8-5). The patient is unable to increase this level in response to the increasing ACTH levels present in the blood, produced as a result of CRF released from the hypothalamus, and thus the clinical manifestations of acute adrenal insufficiency develop. Management of this situation requires replacement and augmentation of the low blood levels of steroids.

Hypotension observed in patients with adrenal insufficiency is the result of several mechanisms. A deficiency in cortisol can lead to hypotension even in patients who are normovolemic. This occurs through a direct depression of the myocardial contractility as well as a reduction in responsiveness to catecholamines.[32,33]

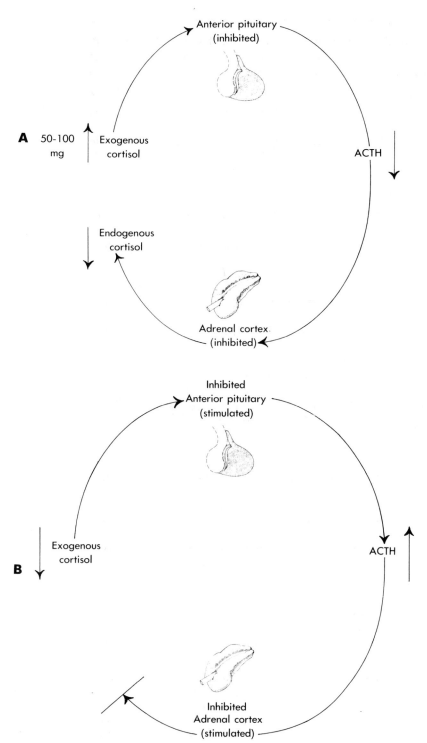

Fig. 8-4. Glucocorticosteroid levels, secondary insufficiency (exogenous therapy). **A,** In presence of normal adrenal cortex and additional exogenous glucocorticosteroid administration, blood levels are greatly increased. ACTH production by anterior pituitary is inhibited, leading to inhibition of adrenal cortical function. Inhibition of both ACTH and glucocorticosteroid production continues for duration of exogenous therapy. **B,** Exogenous therapy. Disuse atrophy of adrenal cortex and anterior pituitary develops with prolonged (2 weeks or longer) glucocorticosteroid therapy. At termination of therapy, blood levels of corticosteroids fall, stimulating anterior pituitary to produce ACTH. ACTH production may be subnormal, or even if normal, response of adrenal cortex may be inadequate. Blood cortisol levels are inadequate with patient in a stress-intolerant state.

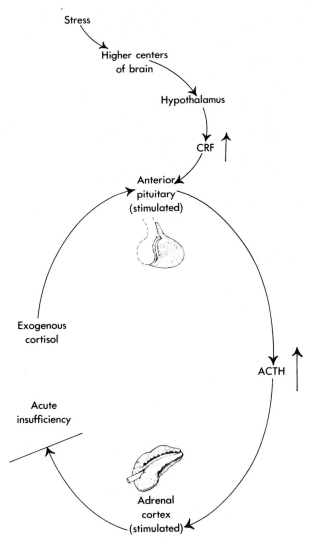

Fig. 8-5. Hypofunctioning adrenal cortex with exogenous cortisol (Addison's disease and nonendocrine cortisol). Blood level of glucocorticosteroid is fixed by exogenous doses. In stressful situation, CRF secreted by hypothalamus induces ACTH secretion by anterior pituitary, which in turn stimulates the adrenal cortex. The anterior pituitary and/or the adrenal cortex may be incapable of proper functioning, leading to cortisol blood levels inadequate to adapt the body to stress. Acute insufficiency results.

Hypoglycemia is noted in about two thirds of adrenal insufficiency cases. Glucose levels are less than 45 mg/dL. Hypoglycemia is produced by a decrease in gluconeogenesis and an increased peripheral use of glucose secondary to lipolysis.[34,35]

Hyperpigmentation is common in patients with chronic adrenal insufficiency and is produced by compensatory secretion of ACTH and MSH (melanin-stimulating hormone).[25,26] It develops over a period of several months when relative adrenal insufficiency is present. Hyperpigmentation is not seen in secondary adrenal insufficiency.

MANAGEMENT

Acute adrenal insufficiency is a life-threatening situation. Effective management of this situation requires the doctor to follow the steps of basic life support and to administer glucocorticosteroids to the patient. The patient with acute adrenal insufficiency is in immediate danger because of glucocorticoid deficiency, depletion of extracellular fluid, and hyperkalemia. Treatment is based on the prompt correction of these conditions.

Conscious Patient
Step 1: Terminate Dental Therapy

As soon as signs and symptoms of possible acute adrenal insufficiency are noted, dental treatment must be interrupted immediately. Acute adrenal insufficiency should be suspected in patients who develop symptoms of mental confusion, nausea, vomiting, and abdominal pain, and who are currently receiving glucocorticosteroids or have received 20 mg or more of cortisone (or its equivalent) by oral or parenteral administration for a period of 2 weeks or longer within the past 2 years (see accompanying box).

CRITERIA FOR DETERMINING ADRENAL INSUFFICIENCY

1. History of current or recent long-term steroid use
2. Mental confusion
3. Nausea and vomiting
4. Abdominal pain
5. Hypotension

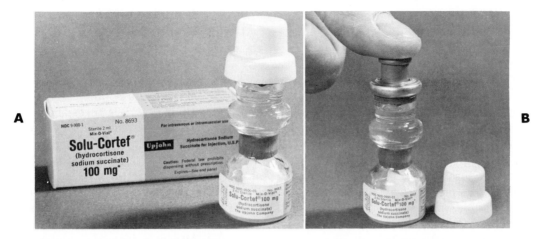

Fig. 8-6. A, Corticosteroid. **B,** Preparation of corticosteroid for use. Depressing plunger mixes powder and liquid so that fresh solution is immediately available for use.

Step 2: Position Patient

If the patient appears mentally confused, wet, and clammy, he or she should be placed into the supine position with the legs elevated slightly. If not, place the patient in a comfortable position.

Step 3: Monitor Vital Signs

Blood pressure and heart rate should be monitored every 5 minutes during the episode. Hypotension will almost always be evident while the heart rate is elevated.

Step 4: Summon Medical Assistance

Medical assistance should be summoned as early as possible. Because the victim is still conscious, it may be wise to also contact the patient's physician. In most cases the patient will be transported immediately to the emergency department of a hospital, where more definitive management may be instituted. If this is required, the doctor should accompany the patient.

Step 5: Emergency Kit and Oxygen

Immediately call for the emergency kit and oxygen. Oxygen may be administered by means of a full face mask or nasal hood. A flow of approximately 5 to 10 L per minute will be adequate.

Step 6: Administer Glucocorticosteroid

If present in the emergency drug kit, remove the corticosteroid and a plastic disposable syringe from the emergency kit. If the patient has a history of chronic adrenal insufficiency, then the doctor may administer the patient's medication that was previously placed on the instrument tray. A corticosteroid is not considered a critical emergency drug because the incidence of this emergency is quite rare and medical assistance can be obtained within a relatively short period of time.

Step 6a. In a patient known to have chronic adrenal insufficiency, the immediate administration of 100 mg of hydrocortisone sodium succinate is suggested and should be readministered every 6 to 8 hours.[36]

Hydrocortisone sodium succinate (Solu-Cortef) is contained as an unmixed powder and liquid in a 2-ml Mix-o-vial (Fig. 8-6). When mixed, each milliliter will contain 50 mg of hydrocortisone. To mix the solution, the top plastic cap is removed and the rubber plunger is depressed. This forces the powder and liquid to combine. Shake the vial until a clear solution has formed. Insert the syringe through the rubber stopper and withdraw the solution.

If possible, the 100 mg of hydrocortisone should be administered intravenously over 30 seconds. The intramuscular route may be employed instead of intravenous administration, with 100 mg (2 mL) injected into the vastus lateralis or mid-deltoid area.

Step 6b. In a patient with no prior history of adrenal insufficiency or corticosteroid use, it is probably most prudent for the dentist to manage the patient as described in steps 1 through 5 and await the arrival of medical assistance.

However, as the immediate diagnosis of acute adrenal insufficiency is empiric (based on presenting signs and symptoms), it is often recommended that corticosteroid therapy be initiated immediately, before the diagnosis is confirmed by laboratory testing (ACTH stimulation test*).

In the office of a doctor with proper training and experience, it is suggested that dexamethasone phosphate be administered in a dose of 4 mg intravenously every 6 to 8 hours while awaiting the ACTH stimulation test.[37] Dexamethasone is approximately 100 times more potent than cortisol.

Step 7: Additional Management

In most cases of adrenal insufficiency in which the patient retains consciousness, the administration of basic life support as needed, oxygen, and corticosteroid will stabilize the patient. Upon arrival of outside assistance, an intravenous line will be established if one is not already in place, and additional drugs will be administered if the diagnosis is confirmed.

Additional drugs include intravenous fluids to counteract the volume depletion and hypotension that are usually present. An addisonian patient may be up to 20% volume depleted.[37] Unless contraindicated by the patient's cardiovascular condition, 1 L of normal saline is infused in the first hour. Dextrose 5% is usually added next to help combat the hypoglycemia. Up to 3 L of fluid may be required over the first 8 hours. Hypoglycemia is also treated immediately and aggressively. If symptomatic or if a finger stick blood glucose test demonstrates low glucose levels (45mg/dL), intravenous glucose in the form of 50 to 100 mL of 50% dextrose in water is administered. In the absence of an intravenous line, 1 to 2 mg glucagon should be administered IM.

Unconscious Patient

When a patient loses consciousness, initially the doctor may not be aware of the patient's medical history of adrenal insufficiency or corticosteroid use.

Step 1: Recognize Unconsciousness

Shake the patient and shout, "Are you all right?" A lack of response will lead to a tentative diagnosis of unconsciousness.

---

*In the ACTH stimulation test 0.25 mg of cosyntropin, a synthetic ACTH, is administered at time zero. For cortisol determination, serum samples are drawn at time zero, 1 hour, and 6 to 8 hours. Normal adrenal glands will respond with an increase in cortisol of at least 10 mg/fl or 3 times baseline level.

Step 2: Position the Patient

The supine position with legs elevated slightly is the preferred position for the unconscious patient.

Step 3: Provide Basic Life Support, as Needed

Immediate institution of the steps of basic life support (see Chapter 5) is necessary. These include the use of head tilt–chin lift, assessment of the airway and of breathing, the jaw thrust maneuver (if necessary), artificial ventilation (if necessary), and assessment of circulation.

In most instances of acute adrenal insufficiency, respiration and blood pressure will be depressed and the heart rate (pulse) will be rapid but weak (thready). Airway maintenance and oxygen administration are required in virtually all cases. In the unlikely occurrence that the pulse is absent, external chest compression should be started immediately and continued until assistance arrives.

Provide definitive management
Step 4: Emergency Kit and Oxygen

Members of the emergency team bring the emergency kit and oxygen to the site of the emergency. Oxygen may be administered through a positive pressure face mask or nose piece. Aromatic spirits of ammonia may be used because it may be difficult, at this time, to differentiate acute adrenal insufficiency from other causes of unconsciousness, including vasodepressor syncope. There will be no response by the patient to the aromatic ammonia.

Positioning the patient, maintaining an adequate airway, and using aromatic ammonia and oxygen will not lead to any noticeable improvement of the patient in acute adrenal insufficiency. If no improvement is noted, the following steps should be considered.

Step 5: Summon Medical Assistance

If unconsciousness continues following the preceding steps, it should be apparent that the cause of this situation is probably not one of those more commonly encountered, such as vasodepressor syncope and orthostatic hypotension. Medical assistance should be summoned.

Step 6: Evaluate the Medical History

While awaiting the arrival of assistance and with the patient maintained by basic life support, a member of the emergency team should review the patient's medical history for evidence of a possible cause of this situation. If no obvious cause is noted, the dental office team should continue to implement the steps of basic life support until assistance

---

MANAGEMENT OF ADRENAL INSUFFICIENCY

Conscious patient

Terminate dental care

↓

Position patient—comfortably, if asymptomatic; supine with feet elevated, if symptomatic

↓

Monitor vital signs

↓

Summon medical assistance

↓

Obtain emergency kit and oxygen

↓

Administer glucocorticosteroid, if available, and if history of adrenal insufficiency

↓

Additional management:
Provide basic life support, as needed
Provide oxygen, as needed
Provide corticosteroid, as needed
Establish IV line

Unconscious patient

Recognize unconsciousness

↓

Postion patient in supine position with feet elevated

↓

Provide basic life support, as needed

↓

Provide definitive management:
Obtain emergency kit and oxygen
Summon medical assistance
Evaluate medical history
Administer corticosteroid
Establish IV line, if possible

↓

Transfer to hospital

---

arrives. If evidence exists that glucocorticosteroid insufficiency is a possible or probable cause of the unconsciousness, proceed to step 7.

Step 7: Administer Glucocorticosteroid

Intravenous or intramuscular administration of 100 mg of hydrocortisone is indicated in cases of suspected adrenal insufficiency. Whenever possible, 100 mg should be injected intravenously over 30 seconds. An intravenous infusion should be started, and an intravenous bottle to which 100 mg of hydrocortisone has been added should be administered over 2 hours. Should the intravenous route be unavailable, 100 mg of hydrocortisone may be administered intramuscularly.

Step 8: Additional Drug Therapy

In the presence of hypotension, an IV infusion of 1 L normal saline or dextrose 5% should be administered in 1 hour while awaiting assistance.

Step 9: Transfer to Hospital

With arrival of medical assistance, the patient will be prepared for transfer to an emergency medical care facility. At this facility blood samples will be taken and any existing electrolyte imbalance, such as hyperkalemia, will be corrected. Definitive therapy is designed to meet the needs of the individual patient but consists initially of large IV doses of glucocorticosteroids, followed by additional doses of oral or IM steroids or both.

It must again be stressed that if there is any possibility that the loss of consciousness is in any way related to a deficiency of glucocorticosteroids, the immediate administration of 100 mg of hydrocortisone succinate may prove to be life saving. In the absence of any such indications the doctor should continue to maintain the patient with basic life support procedures until medical assistance becomes available.

Management of acute adrenal insufficiency is summarized in the accompanying box.

Drugs used in management: Oxygen, corticosteroids

Medical assistance required: Yes, if patient is unconscious; Yes, if conscious patient with history of adrenal insufficiency shows clinical signs and symptoms of acute insufficiency

REFERENCES

1. Guyton AC: The adrenocortical hormones. In *Human Physiology and Mechanisms of Disease*, ed 5, Philadelphia, 1992, W.B. Saunders.
2. Findling JW: Cushing's syndromes: an enlarged clinical spectrum, *N Engl J Med* 321:1677, 1989.
3. Atkinson AB: The treatment of Cushing's syndrome. *Clin Endocrinol* 34(6):507-513, 1991.
4. Zeiger MA, Nieman LK, Cutler GB, Chrousos GP, Doppman JL, Travis WD, Norton JA: Primary bilateral adrenocortical causes of Cushing's syndrome, *Surgery* 1109(6): 1106-1115, 1991.
5. Dahlberg PJ, Goellner MH, Pehling GB: Adrenal insufficiency secondary to adrenal hemorrhage: two case reports and a review of cases confirmed by computed tomography, *Arch Int Med* 150(4):905-909, 1990.
6. Vallotton MB: Endocrine emergencies: disorders of the adrenal cortex, *Baillieres Clin Endocrinol Metabol* 6(1):41-56, 1992.

7. Davenport J, Kellerman C, Reiss D, Harrison L: Addison's disease, *Amer Fam Physic* 43(4):1338-1342, 1991.
8. Streeten DHP: Corticosteroid therapy. I. Pharmacological properties and principles of corticosteroid use, *JAMA* 232:944, 1975.
9. Burke CW: Adrenocortical insufficiency, *Clin Endocrinol Metab* 14:947, 1985.
10. Little JW, Falace DA: Adrenal insufficiency. In *Dental management of the medically compromised patient*, ed 3, St Louis, 1988, Mosby–Year Book.
11. Graber AL, Ney RL, Nicholson WE, and others: Natural history of pituitary-adrenal recovery following long-term suppression with corticosteroids, *J Clin Endocrinol Metab* 25:11, 1965.
12. Streeten DHP: Corticosteroid therapy. II. Complications and therapeutic indications, *JAMA 232:1046*, 1975.
13. Byyny R: Withdrawal from glucocorticoid therapy, *N Engl J Med* 295:30, 1976.
14. von Werder K, Stevens WC, Cromwell TH, and others: Adrenal function during long-term anesthesia in man, *Proc Soc Exp Biol Med* 135: 854, 1970.
15. Sachar EJ: Hormonal changes in stress and mental illness, *Hosp Pract* 10:49, 1970.
16. Bellet S, Kostis J, Roman L, and others: Effect of acute ethanol intake on plasma 11-hydroxy-corticosteroid levels in accidental hypothermia, *Lancet* 1:324, 1970.
17. Jacobs HS, Nabarro JDN: Plasma 11-hydroxycorticosteroid and growth hormone levels in acute medical illnesses, *Br Med J* 2:595, 1969.
18. Fitzgerald PA, Camargo CA: Endocrine disorders. In Schroeder SA, Tierney LM, Jr., McPhee SJ, Papadakis MA, Krupp M editors, *Current Medical Diagnosis & Treatment 1992*, Norwalk, 1992, Appleton & Lange.
19. Hellmann DB: Arthritis and musculoskeletal disorders. In Schroeder SA, Tierney LM, Jr., McPhee SJ, Papadakis MA, Krupp M editors, *Current Medical Diagnosis & Treatment 1992*, Norwalk, 1992, Appleton & Lange.
20. Sertl K, Clark T, Kaliner M editors: Corticosteroids: their biologic mechanisms and application to the treatment of asthma (symposium) *Am Rev Respir Dis* 141(suppl:1S, entire issue), 1990.
21. McCarthy FM: Adrenal insufficiency. In McCarthy FM, editor: *Essentials of safe dentistry for the medically compromised patient;* Philadelphia, 1989, WB Saunders.
22. Melby J: Systemic corticosteroid therapy: pharmacology and endocrine considerations, *Ann Intern Med* 81:505, 1974.
23. Tzagournis M: Acute adrenal insufficiency, *Heart Lung* 7:603, 1978.
24. Bell H, Hayes W, Vosbrugh J: Hyperkalemic paralysis due to adrenal insufficiency, *Arch Intern Med* 115:418, 1965.
25. Nerup J: Addison's disease—clinical studies: a report of 108 cases, *Acta Endocrinol* 76:127, 1974.
26. Dunlop D: Eighty-six cases of Addison's disease, *Br Med J* 2:887, 1963.
27. Kozak G: Primary adrenocortical insufficiency (Addison's disease), *Am Fam Physician* 15(5):124, 1977.
28. Vesely DL: Hypoglycemic coma: don't overlook adrenal crisis, *Geriatrics* 37:71, 1982.
29. Jorgensen H: Hypercalcemia in adrenocortical insufficiency, *Acta Med Scand* 193:175, 1973.
30. Walser M, Robinson BHB, Duckett JWL: The hypercalcemia of adrenal insufficiency, *J Clin Invest* 42:456, 1963.
31. Bondy PK: Disorders of the adrenal cortex. In Wilson JD, Foster DW, editors: *William's textbook of endocrinology*, ed 7, Philadelphia, 1985, WB Saunders.
32. Webb WR, Degerli IV, Hardy JD, and others: Cardiovascular responses in acute adrenal insufficiency, *Surgery* 58:273, 1965.
33. Ramey ER, Goldstein MS: The adrenal cortex and the sympathetic nervous system, *Physiol Rev* 37:155, 1957.
34. Liddle G: The adrenals. In Williams R, editor: *Textbook of endocrinology*, Philadelphia, 1981, WB Saunders.
35. Szwed JJ, White C: Normokalemic nonazotemic adrenal insufficiency, *South Med J* 76:919, 1983.
36. Leshin M: Acute adrenal insufficiency: recognition, management and prevention, *Urol Clin North Am* 9:229, 1982.
37. Wogan JM: Endocrine disorders. In Rose P, editor: *Emergency medicine*, ed 2, St Louis, 1988, Mosby–Year Book.

9 *Unconsciousness: Differential Diagnosis*

Unconsciousness, whatever its cause, must be recognized and managed quickly and effectively. At the onset, the proximate cause may not be obvious, and indeed, at the onset the immediate cause of the problem is not of primary importance.

In all cases in which loss of consciousness has occurred, several basic steps, which have been developed in the preceding chapters on vasodepressor syncope, postural hypotension, and adrenal insufficiency, must be implemented with as little delay as possible. These steps comprise the primary phase of assessment and management and may be summarized as follows:

MANAGEMENT OF UNCONSCIOUSNESS

Recognize unconsciousness
↓
Discontinue dental care
↓
Position patient in supine position with feet elevated
↓
Maintain patent airway with head tilt–chin lift
↓
Assess breathing—look, listen, feel
If necessary, provide breathing through assisted or controlled ventilation
↓
Assess circulation—palpate carotid pulse for 10 seconds
If necessary, provide artificial circulation
↓
Activate EMS, if recovery not immediate

After these steps have been successfully implemented, and while awaiting the arrival of emergency care (if necessary), the team should proceed with the secondary steps of assessment and management. This is also termed the definitive management of the situation. The following information will aid the emergency team in their differential diagnosis of the cause of unconsciousness. Several clinical factors are presented here that will serve as aids in establishing a diagnosis. See Table 5-1 for the various causes of unconsciousness.

AGE OF PATIENT

The age of the patient may assist in the differential diagnosis of unconsciousness. Unconsciousness occurring in the dental office in normal healthy patients in their mid-to-late teens until the late thirties will in almost all instances be related to psychogenic reactions such as vasodepressor syncope. Two other possible causes of unconsciousness in the under-40 age group are hypoglycemia and epilepsy. These are normally easily differentiated from the more common causes of unconsciousness and are discussed fully in other sections of the text.

In patients over the age of 40, unconsciousness is more likely to be precipitated by cardiovascular complications (Section VII) such as acute myocardial infarction, cerebrovascular accident, valvular lesions (such as aortic stenosis), or acute cardiac dysrhythmias. Psychogenic reactions are encountered much less frequently in this age group, because patients are much more likely to have adapted themselves to their dental fears.

Unconsciousness is rarely noted in younger children except in the presence of specific disease states such as diabetes mellitus (hypoglycemia), epilepsy, and congenital heart lesions. Psychogenic reactions

Table 9-1. Causes of unconsciousness

	Age of patient	
Child	*Teens to mid-30s*	*Over 40*
Hypoglycemia Epilepsy	Psychogenic reactions Hypoglycemia Epilepsy	Cardiovascular causes

Table 9-2. Circumstances associated with loss of consciousness

Stress present	*Stress absent*
Vasodepressor syncope	Postural hypotension
Hypoglycemia	Ingestion of drugs
Epilepsy	Allergic reactions
Myocardial infarction	Hyperglycemic reactions
Cerebrovascular accident	
Adrenal insufficiency	

(vasodepressor syncope) are infrequent in this age group because children are extremely vocal in expressing their feelings toward dentistry, releasing their tensions, and producing muscular movement. In short, they act just like children (Table 9-1).

CIRCUMSTANCES ASSOCIATED WITH LOSS OF CONSCIOUSNESS

Stress, whether psychologic (anxiety) or physiologic (pain), is a precipitating factor in most cases of unconsciousness associated with dentistry. Instances in which stress may precipitate unconsciousness include vasodepressor syncope, adrenal insufficiency, cerebrovascular accident, hypoglycemia, epilepsy, and myocardial infarction.

Unconsciousness may also occur in the absence of obvious stress. Postural hypotension will be the most common non–stress-related cause of unconsciousness. Other nonstress factors leading to the loss of consciousness include the administration or ingestion of drugs, allergic reactions, and hyperglycemic reactions (diabetic coma) (Table 9-2).

POSITION OF PATIENT

The position of the patient at the time consciousness is lost may aid in the differential diagnosis of unconsciousness. *Syncope,* defined as the transient loss of consciousness, rarely develops when the patient is in the supine position. There are, however, certain instances in which consciousness may be lost with the patient in the supine position. These include unconsciousness that develops secondary to (1) the administration of drugs, (2) seizures that develop in hypoglycemic or hyperglycemic reactions or with adrenal insufficiency; (3) cardiovascular disorders, including valvular disorders, dysrhythmias, and myocardial infarction; and (4) cerebral vascular accidents. In these circumstances, positioning of the patient in the supine position does not always lead to a restoration of consciousness because the primary factor producing unconsciousness in most of these situations is not related

to a simple deficit in cerebral blood flow. Definitive management is required in all of these cases.

Patients suffering from postural hypotension do not have syncopal episodes when in the supine position; however, signs and symptoms of hypotension develop rapidly when the patient is moved into a more upright position and are reversed just as rapidly when the patient is returned to the supine position.

Hyperventilation only rarely progresses to the loss of consciousness and then only if the patient is permitted to remain untreated in the upright position for long periods of time. More commonly, hyperventilation produces a state of mental confusion (light-headedness and dizziness) (Table 9-3).

PRESYNCOPAL SIGNS AND SYMPTOMS
No Clinical Symptoms

Rapid loss of consciousness without prodromal symptoms leads to a presumptive diagnosis of postural hypotension if the episode occurs immediately following a change in the patient's position (supine to upright). Certain drugs used in dentistry are capable of producing postural hypotension (see Table 7-2). Syncope secondary to cardiac dysrhythmias and heart block is usually of sudden onset and may occur without warning signs or symptoms. It may develop with the patient either sitting or standing. Cardiac arrest, on rare occasion, may lead to unconsciousness without prodromal signs and symptoms. Diagnosis of this situation will be established during implementation of the steps of basic life support.

Pallor and Cold, Clammy Skin

Restlessness, pallor (loss of normal skin color), clammy (moist) skin, nausea, and vomiting are considered classic signs of fainting. They are usually present in vasodepressor syncope; however, these signs may also be present in hypoglycemic reactions, adrenal insufficiency, and myocardial infarction.

Table 9-3. Position of patient at time of syncope

Upright	*Supine into upright*	*Supine*
Vasodepressor syncope Hyperventilation (unlikely)	Postural hypotension	Drug administration Seizures Hypo- or hyperglycemia Adrenal insufficiency Cardiovascular causes

Tingling and Numbness of Extremities

Hyperventilation, although rarely producing syncope, may on occasion do so if the patient is allowed to remain untreated and seated upright for extended periods of time during the episode. Hyperventilation may be readily recognized by the alterations in the rate (increased) and depth (increased) of breathing that accompany it, as well as by the clinical symptoms of tingling and numbness of the fingers, toes, and perioral areas.

Headache

Headache of a very intense nature will often be noted at the outset of a cerebrovascular accident, especially of the hemorrhagic type.

Chest Pain

Chest pain or discomfort may precede the loss of consciousness with angina pectoris (in which unconsciousness rarely occurs), myocardial infarction (in which cardiac arrest and loss of consciousness are more likely), and on occasion with hyperventilation.

Breath Odor

Alcohol is not uncommonly detected on the breath of dental patients and is probably the most frequently self-administered drug for anxiety reduction before dental appointments. The presence of alcohol on the breath should lead the doctor to evaluate the patient for any anxieties or fears concerning dentistry and to be extremely cautious in employing additional drugs during the patient's treatment that are capable of producing further central nervous system (CNS) depression, including local anesthetics. Unconsciousness in these situations might be produced by psychogenic factors or by profound CNS depression produced by one drug or by a combination of various drugs.

The sweet, fruity odor of acetone is present on the breath of patients who are hyperglycemic and have ketoacidosis. In most instances, these patients will be known type I insulin-dependent diabetics.

Tonic-Clonic Movements and Incontinence

All persons who lose consciousness may exhibit tonic-clonic movements of the upper and lower extremities. This is especially likely to occur in patients who are not placed in the supine position, but rather are maintained upright during the period of unconsciousness. Loss of consciousness in this situation is due to decreased cerebral perfusion. Inadequate airway management, regardless of the patient's position, will also produce tonic-clonic movements secondary to cerebral hypoxia (or anoxia). Although tonic-clonic movements are possible during vasodepressor syncope, they are rarely observed if adequate positioning and airway management are provided. Tonic-clonic movements will also be observed in hypoglycemia. In this situation they are secondary to a deficient cerebral blood glucose level. Seizures arising from nonepileptic factors are usually mild and are rarely associated with sphincter muscle relaxation. However, a diagnosis of epilepsy is strongly suggested for seizure activity in which a patient exhibits urinary or fecal incontinence and tongue biting.

Heart Rate and Blood Pressure

In most instances of unconsciousness the heart rate rises above its baseline level while the blood pressure decreases. For example, in a hypoglycemic or hyperglycemic reaction the blood pressure of the patient may be quite low, while the heart, attempting to compensate for the decrease in blood pressure, accelerates its rate of contraction. Exceptions do exist, including vasodepressor syncope, postural hypotension, and cerebrovascular accident.

In vasodepressor syncope it is usual for both blood pressure and heart rate to decrease. A heart rate of 50 beats per minute or less is common during the syncopal phase of vasodepressor syncope. The heart rate during postural hypotension remains at approximately the baseline level, although the blood pressure drops precipitously. The pulse, as monitored in the radial, brachial, or carotid ar-

Table 9-4. Heart rate and blood pressure during unconsciousness

Cause of unconsciousness	Heart rate	Blood pressure
Hypoglycemia/ hyperglycemia	Increases	Decreases
Vasodepressor syncope	Decreases	Decreases
Postural hypo- tension	Baseline	Decreases
Cerebrovascular accident (hemorrhage)	Variable	Increases
Significant dys- rhythmias	Variable	Decreases

Table 9-5. Duration of syncope with basic life support

Short	Prolonged
Postural hypotension	Hypoglycemia
Vasodepressor syncope	Hyperglycemia
Cardiac dysrhythmias	Adrenal insufficiency
	Cardiac dysrhythmias

teries, is usually described as weak or thready in persons whose blood pressure is low. In cerebrovascular accident (hemorrhagic CVA), on the other hand, the blood pressure may be significantly elevated (systolic pressure elevated more than diastolic pressure) with the pulse quite strong, or bounding.

With clinically significant dysrhythmias, the heart rate may be variable (bradycardic, tachycardic, or at baseline), but the functional output of the heart is decreased to a level at which peripheral perfusion is adversely affected. The blood pressure will almost always be depressed in this situation (Table 9-4).

Duration of Unconsciousness and Recovery

Much information of diagnostic importance can be obtained from the response or lack of response of the patient to the basic steps of management outlined here and in Chapter 5. Unconsciousness produced by vasodepressor syncope is usually reversed within a few seconds once the patient is placed in the supine position (Table 9-5). In the recovery period the patient does not rapidly return to a normal state. More frequently, signs and symptoms such as shivering, sweating, headache, and fatigue are present. In patients with postural hypotension, consciousness also returns rapidly after assuming the supine position. Recovery is more

complete and rapid following postural hypotension than after vasodepressor syncope, with residual signs and symptoms being absent or less intense. Syncope secondary to cardiac dysrhythmias also is quickly reversed following correction of the underlying rhythm disturbance, with the patient usually alert on recovery. The duration of syncope is related to the duration of the dysrhythmia.

Syncope produced through mechanisms other than a lack of adequate cerebral blood flow is not readily reversed by positioning the patient. Epileptic patients' seizures usually terminate after a few moments; however, they may remain somnolent and often develop intense headaches during recovery. Significant tonic-clonic seizure activity is not usually observed during vasodepressor syncope or postural hypotension (though this may occur in some isolated instances).

Unconsciousness produced through alterations in the composition of the blood, such as following drug administration, hypoglycemia, hyperglycemia, or adrenal insufficiency, will not be reversed through basic life support procedures alone (Table 9-5). Although proper implementation of these steps is absolutely critical to the patient's survival, in each of these cases definitive management involving specific drug therapy is necessary for the patient to regain consciousness. These situations will be described in subsequent chapters.

10 *Respiratory Distress: General Considerations*

Difficulty in breathing can be very disconcerting to a patient who is conscious yet unable to breathe normally. Several of the more common causes of respiratory distress will be described in this section. These include hyperventilation, bronchospasm (asthma), and pulmonary edema. Because the patient in respiratory distress usually remains conscious throughout the episode, the psychologic aspects of patient management are extremely important.

Definitions of relevant terms follow[1]:

Anoxia. Absence of oxygen

Apnea. Absence of respiratory movements

Dyspnea. A subjective sense of shortness of breath; "air hunger," difficulty in breathing

Hyperpnea. Greater than normal minute ventilation that just meets metabolic demands

Hyperventilation. Ventilation that exceeds metabolic demands; $PaCO_2$ less than 35 torr

Hypoventilation. Ventilation that does not meet metabolic demands; $PaCO_2$ over 45 torr

Hypoxia. Deficiency of oxygen in the inspired air

Orthopnea. Inability to breathe except in the upright position

$PaCO_2$. Arterial carbon dioxide tension (normal is 35 to 45 torr)

PaO_2. Arterial oxygen tension (normal [air] is 75 to 100 torr)

Respiration. Process of gas exchange whereby oxygen is gained and carbon dioxide is lost from the body

Tachypnea. Greater than normal respiratory rate

Torr. Unit of pressure equal to 1 mm Hg (named for Torricelli)

Ventilation, alveolar. Volume of air exchanged per minute (volume/breath − dead space × respiratory rate)

In almost all instances in which unconsciousness occurs, the airway will be obstructed. The primary cause of airway obstruction is the tongue which falls back into the hypopharynx as skeletal muscle tone is lost. The steps of basic life support, airway and breathing, are designed to eliminate this as a factor. Our discussion of the management of airway obstruction continues in Section III.

Respiratory distress will usually not present the dental office staff with an immediately life-threatening situation; however, prompt recognition and management are essential since the patient may not be receiving a normal supply of oxygen during the episode, and may not be eliminating carbon dioxide effectively. It is quite possible that complications resulting from hypoxia or hypercarbia may develop. On the other hand, lower airway obstruction (occurring within the trachea or lungs) is a truly life-threatening situation in which the patient may be receiving little or no oxygen. Recognition must be prompt and management equally prompt and effective.

PREDISPOSING FACTORS

Table 10-1 lists potential causes of acute respiratory distress. In most of these situations the patient does not exhibit respiratory distress unless an underlying medical disorder becomes acutely exacerbated. Examples of this include acute myocardial infarction, anaphylaxis, cerebrovascular accident, hyperglycemia, and hypoglycemia. Awareness of the patient's primary medical disorder allows the doctor to modify the treatment plan to prevent or at least minimize the risk of exacerbating the underlying disorder. However, there are situations, including asthma and heart failure, in

157

Table 10-1. Potential causes of respiratory distress

Cause	Frequency	Where discussed
Hyperventilation	Most common	Respiratory difficulty (Section III)
Vasodepressor syncope	Most common	Unconsciousness (Section II)
Asthma	Common	Respiratory difficulty (Section III)
Heart failure	Common	Respiratory difficulty (Section III)
Hypoglycemia	Common	Altered consciousness (Section IV)
Overdose reaction	Less common	Drug-related emergencies (Section VI)
Acute myocardial infarction	Rare	Chest pain (Section VII)
Anaphylaxis	Rare	Allergy (Chapter 24)
Angioneurotic edema	Rare	Allergy (Chapter 24)
Cerebrovascular accident	Rare	Altered consciousness (Section IV)
Epilepsy	Rare	Seizure disorders (Chapter 21)
Hyperglycemic reaction	Rare	Altered consciousness (Section IV)

which the patient suffers from chronic respiratory problems. Breathing difficulty may be present at all times with these disorders, particularly heart failure, and measures must be taken by the doctor to prevent their exacerbation during dental care.

A major factor that leads to the exacerbation of respiratory disorders is undue stress, either physiologic or psychologic. Indeed, hyperventilation and vasodepressor syncope, which represent the most commonly encountered emergency situations in dentistry, are almost exclusively precipitated by psychologic stress. Psychologic stress in dentistry is *the* primary factor in the exacerbation of preexisting medical problems. Although hyperventilation and vasodepressor syncope are rarely causes of respiratory distress in pediatric patients, children with asthma may exhibit acute episodes of bronchospasm in stressful situations.

PREVENTION

Adequate pretreatment medical and dental evaluation of the prospective patient can often prevent respiratory problems from developing. Once aware of existing medical disorders that may lead to respiratory distress, the doctor can modify patient management to minimize the risk of exacerbating these conditions. When dental anxiety is a major factor, the use of psychosedative procedures and other stress-reduction techniques should also be considered.

CLINICAL MANIFESTATIONS

Clinical manifestations of respiratory distress will vary according to the degree of breathing difficulty present. In most cases the patient will remain conscious throughout the episode. Although retention of consciousness is a positive sign, indicating that

the patient is receiving at least the minimum supply of oxygen required for normal cerebral function, it does create an additional problem: acute anxiety. For this reason it becomes quite important for the doctor managing the situation to remain calm—or at least give the appearance of being calm—and in control of the situation at all times.

The sounds associated with distressed breathing and the clinical symptomatology vary with the cause of the problem. With asthma (bronchospasm), one can usually hear a characteristic wheezing sound that is produced by the turbulent flow of air through partially occluded bronchioles. With heart failure, cough may be present, as well as other sounds that are associated with pulmonary venous congestion. A more detailed discussion and a differential diagnosis of respiratory difficulty follows.

PATHOPHYSIOLOGY

Various portions of the respiratory system are involved in the different syndromes responsible for respiratory distress. For example, with asthma, the bronchioles are the primary site of the disorder. In patients with asthma the bronchi become highly reactive and demonstrate significant smooth muscle reactivity (bronchospasm) in response to various stimuli. The clinical signs and symptoms noted in acute asthmatic attacks are related in large part to the restrictive action of bronchospasm upon the exchange of air into the lungs.

With heart failure, respiratory distress is usually the first sign and symptom noted by the patient. Respiratory distress with heart failure is produced by a chronic inability of the lungs to fully oxygenate venous blood and by the attendant overutilization of that oxygen in the blood that is available to tissues. This type of respiratory distress is related to

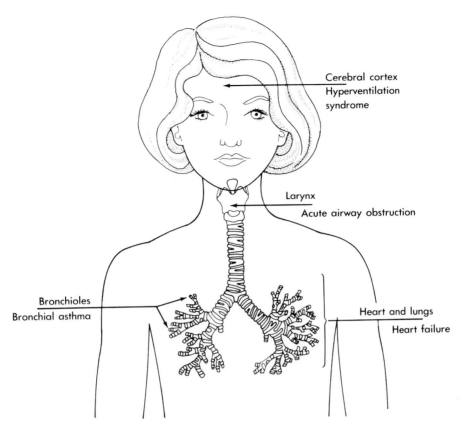

Fig. 10-1. Sites of origin of various respiratory difficulties.

a pulmonary venous engorgement with fluid exuding into the alveolar air sacs. This excess fluid prevents portions of the lung from participating in the ventilatory process (removal of carbon dioxide and absorption of oxygen), producing many of the signs and symptoms associated with heart failure.

Hyperventilation is a more generalized problem. The primary site of the disorder is in the mind of the patient, and its clinical signs and symptoms are produced by an alteration in the chemical makeup of the blood. An excessive amount of carbon dioxide is eliminated as a result of the rapid breathing associated with hyperventilation, which leads to development of respiratory alkalosis. This in turn produces many of the clinical signs and symptoms observed in hyperventilating patients. If managed successfully, hyperventilation produces no residual effects. However, heart failure and asthma, which are chronic disorders, may produce permanent changes in the respiratory system.[2,3] Therefore, patients who are subject to acute exacerbations of asthma (bronchospasm) or heart failure (pulmonary edema) usually require special management considerations during all phases of their dental care.

Acute lower airway obstruction is a life-threatening situation in which a foreign object becomes impacted in the respiratory tract. The level at which the airway is occluded determines the severity of the situation and to some degree the manner in which it may be managed. If an object enters into either the right or left mainstem bronchus, the resulting situation is critical but not immediately life threatening. The chances are excellent that the foreign body will enter the right mainstem bronchus because of the angle at which this bronchus branches off of the trachea.[4] In this situation all or part of the right lung is excluded from the ventilatory process, but the patient is still able to maintain adequate ventilation with the left lung. Hospitalization will be required, but the patient's life is usually not in immediate danger. However, if the foreign object becomes impacted in the trachea, total airway obstruction ensues—an acutely life-threatening situation.[5] Immediate recognition and management are essential to prevent permanent neurologic damage or death. The management of acute airway obstruction will be discussed in Chapter 11. Figure 10-1 illustrates the sites of origin of various respiratory disorders.

MANAGEMENT

The definitive management of respiratory distress is based upon recognition of the problem and a determination of the probable cause of the situation. The following basic steps are common to the management of most cases of respiratory distress:

Step 1: Recognize respiratory distress. Many respiratory disorders are associated with characteristic sounds, such as the wheezing of asthma and the cough and moist respirations of pulmonary edema. There usually is no characteristic sound associated with hyperventilation; however, patients appear to be, and actually are, acutely anxious and unable to control their breathing.

Step 2: Terminate the dental procedure. Dental care should be stopped as soon as the respiratory problem is recognized. Because stress is a primary precipitating factor in most of these situations, the clinical signs and symptoms may greatly improve simply by stopping dental treatment.

Step 3: Position patient. In conscious patients experiencing respiratory distress, positioning should be based upon making the patient as comfortable as possible. In the presence of a near normal blood pressure (as is almost always the case in the situations discussed in this section), most patients will feel more in control of their breathing in an upright (sitting or standing) position. It is important to remember that this position can only be maintained as long as the patient remains conscious.

Step 4: Basic life support as needed. Patients in respiratory distress often experience two major problems: the primary breathing difficulty initially induced by their fear of dentistry and the superimposed problem of increased anxiety produced by their inability to breathe normally. In the unlikely event that a patient in respiratory distress should lose consciousness, he or she must be placed immediately into the supine position and managed like any other unconscious patient. Additional management is based on the patient's response to the steps of basic life support.

Step 5: Monitor vital signs. Measurement of the blood pressure, heart rate (pulse), and respiratory rate should be taken at this time and at intervals throughout the management of this situation. All measurements should be recorded on a permanent record.

Step 6: Definitive management of anxiety. The patient in respiratory distress should be kept as comfortable as possible at this time, and the doctor

---

> **MANAGEMENT OF RESPIRATORY DISTRESS**
>
> Recognize respiratory distress:
> Sounds (wheezing, cough)
> Abnormal rate and/or depth of respiration
> ↓
> Terminate dental procedure
> ↓
> Position patient:
> In supine position if unconscious
> If conscious, depends on patient comfort—
> upright position usually preferred
> ↓
> Provide basic life support, as needed
> ↓
> Monitor vital signs:
> Blood pressure, heart rate (pulse), respiratory rate
> ↓
> Manage patient's symptoms of anxiety
> ↓
> Provide definitive management of respiratory distress

---

should begin to manage anxiety by speaking with the patient in a calm but firm manner. The patient's collar and other tight garments should be loosened because this will enable the patient to breathe (psychologically, if not in reality) more freely.

Step 7: Definitive management of respiratory distress. After assessing the patient's cardiovascular status, the doctor may proceed to the definitive management of the situation. These procedures are described along with the major causes of respiratory difficulty in the chapters that follow.

REFERENCES

1. *Mosby's medical & nursing dictionary*, St Louis, 1983, Mosby–Year Book.
2. Apstein CS, Lorell BH: The physiological basis of left ventricular diastolic dysfunction, *J Card Surg* 3(4):475-485, 1988.
3. Djukanovic R, Roche WR, Wilson JW, Beasley CR, Twentyman OP, Howarth RH, Holgate ST: Mucosal inflammation in asthma, *Amer Rev Respir Dis* 142(2):434-457, 1990.
4. Bhatia PL: Problems in the management of aspirated foreign bodies, *West African J Medicine* 10(2):158-167, 1991.
5. Heimlich HJ, Patrick EA: The Heimlich maneuver: best technique for saving any choking victim's life, *Postgrad Med* 87(6):38-48, 53, 1990.

11 Airway Obstruction

Because of its frequently sudden and critical nature, acute obstruction of the airway must be recognized and managed as quickly as possible. For this reason, an immediate diagnosis of complete or partial airway obstruction must be made and treatment initiated as quickly as possible.

In dentistry the potential is great for objects to fall into the posterior portion of the oral cavity and into the pharynx. Indeed, a great variety of devices and objects is recovered from the throats of patients every year.[1] In the author's experience, items such as the head of a pedodontic handpiece, mouth mirror heads, and gold crowns have been recovered, either orally or from stool specimens, after having been swallowed accidentally. Reports in the literature have documented the retrieval of rubber dam clamps, endodontic instruments, and a post and core.[1-3]

In the conscious dental patient the chances are excellent that any object lost in the pharynx will be swallowed by the patient and enter into the esophagus or will be retrieved after being coughed up, so that the actual incidence of acute airway obstruction or aspiration into the trachea and lung is quite low. There is also a high probability that any dental objects that enter into the airway will be of small enough diameter to pass through the larynx (the narrowest portion of the upper airway) without causing an obstruction. In this situation the object will continue through the trachea (if gravity is assisting), coming to rest in a portion of one of the bronchi or smaller bronchioles of the lung. While an acute life-threatening situation does not exist at this time, certain important steps (see text that follows) must be carried out to ensure the removal of the object within a reasonable period of time to avoid any possible serious sequelae to the patient. However, the possibility that a foreign object will lodge in the larynx and obstruct the trachea does exist, and for this reason all dental office personnel must become familiar with the various techniques of managing acute upper airway obstruction.

The National Safety Council estimated that approximately 3100 persons died from acute airway obstruction in the United States in 1984.[4] More than 90% of deaths from foreign body aspiration in the pediatric age group occur in children younger than 5 years of age, and 65% are in infants.[5] Commonly implicated items include foods such as hot dogs, rounded candies, nuts, and grapes; coins, toys, and other hard, colorful objects.[6,7] Baby aspirin, with a diameter of 7.5 mm, has caused death from an obstructed airway in several younger children.[8] (The diameter of the glottic opening is about 6.5 mm in the 2-year-old child.[9])

After evaluating newer clinical research findings, the American Heart Association[10] implemented changes in the techniques recommended for the management of obstructed airway in infants, children, and adults. These techniques are presented in this chapter.

In most cases the object causing the acute airway obstruction is firmly lodged where it can neither be seen nor felt through the mouth without the aid of special equipment, such as a laryngoscope or Magill forceps, which are not normally available. The doctor must therefore be able to recognize the problem instantly and act rapidly to dislodge the object from the airway.

PREVENTION OF SWALLOWED OBJECTS

In spite of our best efforts at prevention, small objects, such as inlays, alloy, burs, or pieces of debris, may fall into the oropharynx of a patient with subsequent swallowing or aspiration. The introduction of sit-down, four-handed dentistry in which the patient is placed in a semisupine or supine position during treatment has increased the

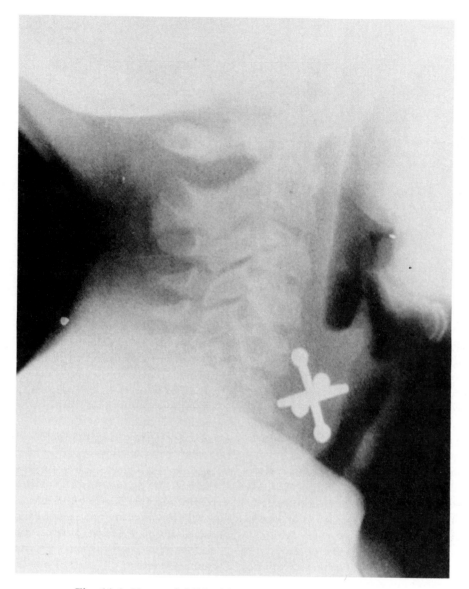

Fig. 11-1. X-ray of child with metal jack in his esophagus.

possibility of this occurrence. Objects that are swallowed will usually enter into the gastrointestinal (GI) tract. This occurs because during the act of swallowing the epiglottis serves to seal the trachea from entry of liquid and solid materials. The most likely site in the gastrointestinal tract for objects to become obstructed will be the esophagus (Fig. 11-1).[11] This is due to the nature of the esophagus, a collapsed tube through which liquids and solids are forced. More than 90% of swallowed foreign objects that successfully pass through the esophagus into the stomach and intestines will pass completely through the GI tract without complication.[12] However, complications are associated with both swallowed and aspirated objects. Swallowed objects en-

tering the gastrointestinal tract have produced GI blockage, peritoneal abscess, perforation, and peritonitis.[13] Objects aspirated into either the right or left bronchus can produce infection, lung abscess, pneumonia, and atelectasis.[14]

In a discussion of prevention of aspiration, Barkmeier[1] stated that two major preventive measures are the use of the rubber dam and oral packing, whenever applicable. Use of these measures will greatly minimize the occurrence of swallowed foreign objects. Other measures that serve to prevent the loss of an object into a patient's GI tract or trachea include: patient positioning in the chair, the dental assistant, suction, Magill intubation forceps, and the use of ligature.

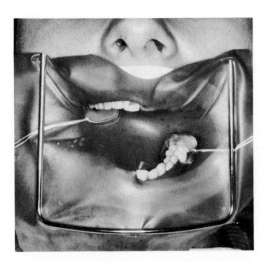

Fig. 11-2. Use of rubber dam, when possible, prevents entry of foreign objects into airway. (From Chasteen J: *Four-handed dentistry in clinical practice,* ed 3, St Louis, 1984, Mosby–Year Book.)

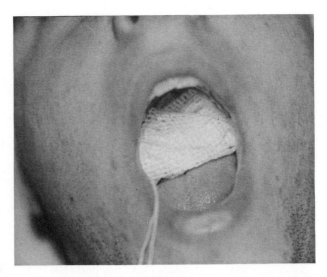

Fig. 11-3. A pharyngeal curtain, created by spreading 3″ × 3″ gauze pads across the posterior portion of the oral cavity effectively prevents small particles or liquids from entering the airway.

Rubber dam: Rubber dam effectively isolates the operative field from the oral cavity and airway and prevents objects from being swallowed (Fig. 11-2). It is suggested that rubber dam be employed whenever possible. Unfortunately, in many dental procedures, such as periodontics and surgery, use of this protective curtain is not possible.

Oral packing: A pharyngeal curtain, created by spreading 3" × 3" gauze pads across the posterior portion of the oral cavity, effectively prevents small particles or liquids from entering the airway (Fig. 11-3). The pharyngeal curtain is of great benefit in patients who are receiving intramuscular or intravenous sedation or general anesthesia, in whom protective airway reflexes might be compromised to varying degrees. Oral packing is not normally tolerated by the nonsedated patient, as it will interfere with swallowing and/or restrict the volume of air being inhaled through the mouth.

Chair position: The supine position, which serves to prevent syncope from occurring, becomes detrimental to the patient when a foreign object is being held tenuously by the body of the tongue against the roof of the mouth. Gravity will act to force the object posteriorly into the pharynx. If equipment is not readily available to aid in retrieving this object, the patient should be asked to turn to the side and bend into a head-down position with the upper body over the side of the dental chair (Fig. 11-4). This position takes advantage of gravity, which might allow the object to fall from the patient's mouth.

Dental assistant: Seated across from the doctor in most situations will be the assistant. In a situation

in which an object becomes free and is in danger of being swallowed, the assistant will have available one or more devices to aid in immediate retrieval. In the absence of a device that can readily grab the object (see text that follows), a high-volume, large-diameter suction tip should be used to remove the object before it can be swallowed. The object will not be lost as there is a trap on the suction line that enables it to be recovered in seconds. Saliva ejectors are not always beneficial in this situation because the force of the suction is not great enough to permit the object to be removed. When it is present, the assistant can quickly pick up a Magill intubation forcep and easily retrieve the object from the posterior part of the oral cavity.

Magill intubation forceps: Included in the basic emergency kit, the Magill intubation forceps (Fig. 11-5) is designed to permit the retrieval of objects both large and small from the distal regions of the oral cavity and pharynx (Fig. 11-6). The right-angled bend permits a comfortable hand position by the user, while the blunt-ended beaks allow for easy attachment to the object. No other device, including pick-up forceps (cotton pliers) or hemostats, are designed for this purpose (Fig. 11-7).

Ligature: The use of ligature or dental floss can aid in both the prevention of loss of objects and in their retrieval in the unlikely event that this becomes necessary. Dental floss should be secured to rubber dam clamps, endodontic instruments, cotton rolls, gauze pads, around the pontics in fixed bridges, and to other small objects that are placed into the oral cavity during dental care (Figs. 11-8

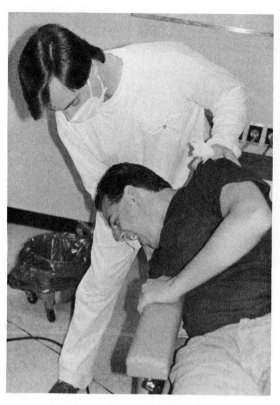

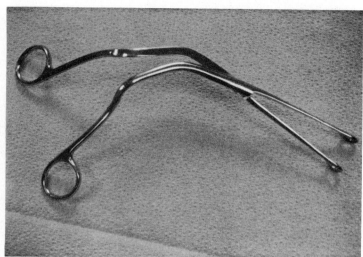

Fig. 11-5. Magill intubation forceps.

Fig. 11-4. The patient should be asked to turn to the side and bend into a head-down position (with the upper body over the side of the dental chair).

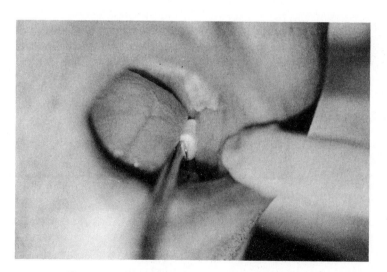

Fig. 11-6. Magill intubation forcep being used.

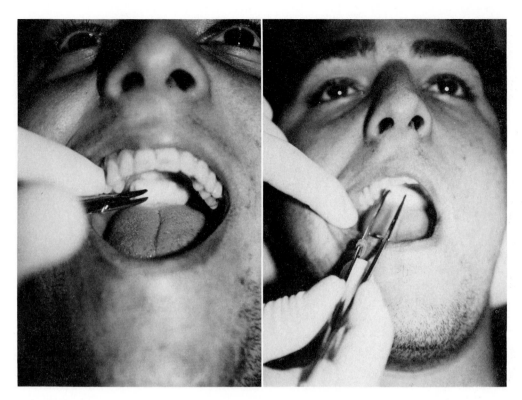

Fig. 11-7. Hemostat and cotton pliers are not designed for easy use in retreiving objects.

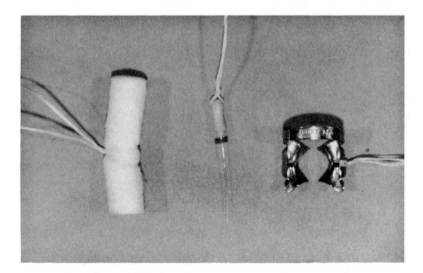

Fig. 11-8. Dental floss tied to object for quick retrieval.

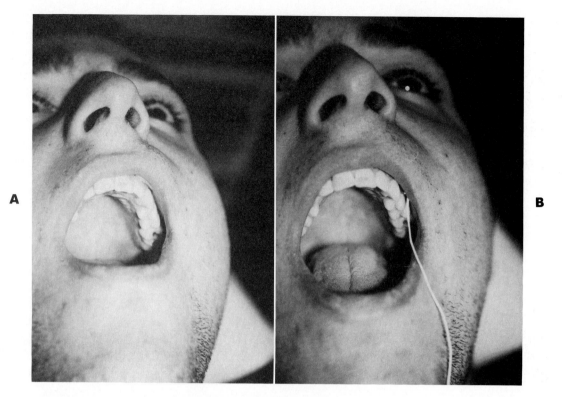

Fig. 11-9. A, Cotton roll—no floss. **B,** Roll with floss.

and 11-9). The presence of dental floss will make it unlikely that a patient will ever swallow an object or inadvertently leave the dental office with a cotton roll still remaining in the buccal fold.

The accompanying box summarizes the steps in prevention of aspiration and loss of objects by swallowing.

MANAGEMENT OF SWALLOWED OBJECTS

When an object is seen to enter the oropharynx of a patient who is in a supine or semisupine position, do not permit the patient to sit up. Instead, place the chair into a more reclined position (Trendelenburg or head-down, if possible) while the assistant gets the Magill intubation forceps. Place-

ment into the Trendelenburg position may allow gravity to bring the object closer to the oral cavity, where it may be more readily visualized and retrieved with the Magill intubation forceps (see accompanying box).

If the object cannot be retrieved, that is, if the patient swallows it, radiographs are warranted to determine its location. These should be obtained prior to dismissing the patient from the office. It is not always possible to determine by clinical signs and symptoms if the object has entered into the gastrointestinal or respiratory tract.

The patient should be taken (by the doctor, if possible) to the emergency department of a local hospital or to a radiology laboratory. In most in-

---

PREVENTION OF ASPIRATION AND
SWALLOWING OF OBJECTS

1. Rubber dam
2. Oral packing
3. Chair position
4. Dental assistant
5. Suction
6. Magill intubation forceps
7. Ligature

MANAGEMENT OF VISIBLE OBJECTS

If assistant is present, place patient in supine
or Trendelenburg position
↓
Use Magill intubation forceps or suction

If assistant is not present, have patient bend
over arm of chair with head down
↓
Encourage patient to cough

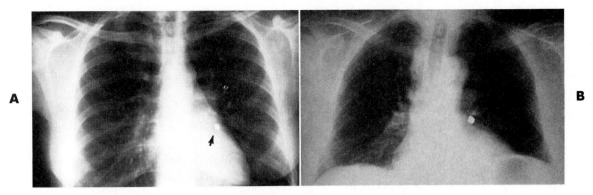

Fig. 11-10. A, Anteroposterior view of chest demonstrating rubber prophylaxis cup (arrow). **B,** Gold crown that had been aspirated into the left lung of patient.

stances the radiologist will recommend the following radiographic series: (1) flat plate of abdomen, and/or (2) anteroposterior (AP) view of chest (Fig. 11-10), or (3) lateral view of chest.

It is hoped that if the object is found, it will be seen on the abdominal radiograph rather than on the chest radiographs within, for example, a bronchus. In any situation in which the foreign object is located within either the GI or respiratory tract, additional assistance will be sought from appropriate medical specialties: gastroenterology, pulmonology, or anesthesiology. Further management of the situation will usually be directed by the physician. If the object cannot be located or if any question exists as to its location or to any potential complications, immediate medical consultation is strongly urged (see accompanying box).

Entry of the object into the trachea will usually, though not always, be noted by the immediate onset of signs and symptoms. These include a sudden onset of coughing, choking, wheezing, and shortness of breath. In over 90% of patients who aspirate, these signs and symptoms will be evident within 1 hour of the aspiration event. A time lag as long as 6 hours may be noted in a few patients.[15] Depending upon the seriousness of the event, this

may be followed by immediate apnea in as many as one third of the patients. These symptoms may progress to cyanosis and other signs of serious hypoxemia.[16]

In situations in which the foreign body presumably enters the patient's trachea, the following management is recommended: Do not allow patient to sit up, as this will, with the aid of gravity, tend to propel the object deeper into the trachea or bronchi. Place the patient into the left lateral decubitus position with the head down (Fig. 11-11). The patient may cough spontaneously; if not, encourage coughing to aid in retrieval of the object. The normal cough reflex is quite powerful and will, in many cases, be adequate to retrieve the aspirated object. Should the patient cease coughing and state that the object has been swallowed, do not permit the

---

MANAGEMENT OF SWALLOWED OBJECTS

Consult with radiologist
↓
Obtain appropriate radiographs to determine location of object
↓
Initiate medical consultation with appropriate specialist

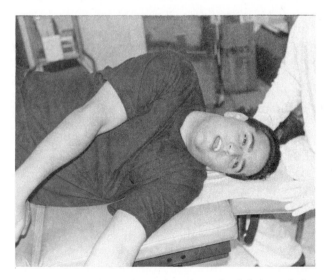

Fig. 11-11. Position the patient into the left lateral decubitus position with their head down.

MANAGEMENT OF ASPIRATED OBJECTS

Place patient in left lateral decubitis position
↓
Encourage patient to cough
↓ ↓
Object is retrieved Object is not retrieved—consult with radiologist or emergency department
↓ ↓
Initiate medical consultation prior to discharge Obtain appropriate radiographs to determine location of object
↓
Perform endoscopy to visualize and retrieve object

---

patient to leave your care until the object has been located by radiograph to ensure it is not in the trachea. Only if the entire object is recovered should the patient be discharged without radiograph. Prior to dismissal it is recommended that medical consultation be obtained with an appropriate medical specialist (i.e., pulmonologist) to discuss possible postaspiration complications, prevention, and management. If the object is not recovered, the doctor should accompany the patient to the emergency department of an acute care facility for definitive diagnosis and management of the aspirant (see accompanying box).

If the object is determined ultimately to be in the tracheobronchial tree, it will most often be located in the right bronchus. This is because the right bronchus takes a more direct path compared to the left bronchus at the bifurcation of the trachea. The right main bronchus comes off of the trachea at an angle of 25°, whereas the left main bronchus comes off at an angle of 45°.

Retrieval of the object from the bronchus may involve the use of a fiberoptic bronchoscope to locate (visualize) the object and bronchoscopy to retrieve it. A surgical procedure, thoracotomy, may be required in the unlikely event that bronchoscopy is unsuccessful.

An immediate life-threatening emergency does not exist in the situations just described. Unless the aspirated object is retrieved, however, the patient should not be dismissed from the dental office. Additional medical management will be necessary in order to prevent possible serious sequelae from developing.

RECOGNITION OF AIRWAY OBSTRUCTION

Acute upper airway obstruction in the conscious patient usually occurs during eating. In adults, meat is the most common cause of the obstruction.[17] Several common factors are identified in cases of the so-called "cafe coronary" syndrome, including: (1) large, poorly chewed pieces of food; (2) elevated blood alcohol levels; (3) laughing or talking while eating; and (4) upper and/or lower dentures.[17] A higher incidence of cafe coronaries has been noted in patients receiving drugs that possess anticholinergic actions.[18] Other causes for airway obstruction include congenital structural abnormalities of the airway[19]; infection, such as acute epiglottitis,[20,21] tonsillitis,[22-24] retropharyngeal abscess,[25] Ludwig's angina,[26] and laryngitis[7]; trauma[27]; tumors and hematomas[28,29]; vocal cord pathologies, including laryngospasm and paralysis; inflammatory processes, such as angioneurotic edema and anaphylaxis,[7] ingestion of corrosives and toxins,[22] and thermal burns[30]; and the sleep apnea syndrome.[7]

Airway obstruction may be divided into complete and partial obstruction. Partial obstruction is additionally subdivided, for management purposes, into two categories: good air exchange or poor air exchange.

Complete Airway Obstruction

The physiological events occurring with asphyxia (complete obstruction) have been documented in the dog.[31] Several phases of physiologic change are noted before death with acute airway obstruction. Initially, sympathetic ouflow is markedly increased, resulting in increases in blood pressure, heart rate, and respiratory rate. As a result of the increased work in breathing, there is a decrease in PaO_2, an increase in $PaCO_2$, and a fall in pH. At 3 to 4 minutes, precipitous drops in blood pressure and heart rate are noted, along with diminished respiratory efforts. Blood gases deteriorate even further. At 8 to 10 minutes, vital signs disappear as the electrocardiogram degenerates from sinus to a nodal bradycardia, then to idioventricular rhythms, and terminates in asystole or ventricular fibrillation.[31]

If the obstruction is relieved within the initial 4 to 5 minutes, all monitored parameters usually return to normal quickly, as well as a return to consciousness. It appears, however, that humans do not tolerate asphyxia as well as the dog model described here. This is especially the case in medically compromised persons.

Dailey[7] has divided the clinical features of acute upper airway obstruction in humans into three phases (Table 11-1). Phase one comprises the first

Table 11-1. Assessment of complete upper airway obstruction*

Phase	Signs and symptoms
First phase (1-3 min)	Conscious; universal choking sign; struggling paradoxical respirations without air movement or voice; increased blood pressure and pulse
Second phase (2-5 min)	Loss of consciousness; decreased respiration, blood pressure, and pulse
Third phase (>4-5 min)	Coma; absent vital signs; pupils dilated

*Modified from Dailey RH: Acute upper airway obstruction, *Emerg Med Clin N Amer* 1:261, 1983.

three minutes: the patient is conscious, in obvious distress with struggling paradoxical respirations, increased blood pressure, and heart rate. The patient often grasps at the throat in the so-called "choking sign" (Fig. 11-12). Though respiratory movements are present, no air is being exchanged and no voice sounds are produced. Supraclavicular and intercostal retractions are evident, breath sounds are absent in the chest, and the victim becomes cyanotic.

Phase two (minutes 2 to 5): The victim becomes unconscious and respiratory efforts cease. Initially, a blood pressure and pulse are present.

Phase three (minutes 4 to 5): Within a short period of time blood pressure and pulse disappear as electromechanical dissociation leads to full cardiac arrest.

The accompanying box lists signs of complete airway obstruction.

Partial Airway Obstruction

In the victim with *good air exchange*, a forceful cough can be elicited. Wheezing may be noted between the coughs. The victim of a partial obstruction with good air exchange should be permitted to continue to cough and breathe without any physical intervention by the rescuer.[32]

With *poor air exchange*, a weak, ineffectual cough reflex is present along with a characteristic "crow-

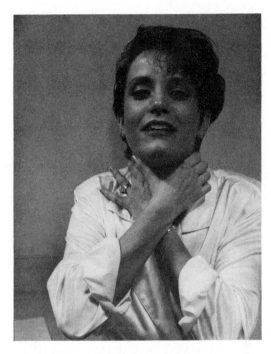

Fig. 11-12. Recommended universal distress signal for obstructed airway; victim clutches neck.

ing" sound that occurs with inspiration. The degree of paradoxical respiration is related to the degree of airway obstruction. Voice sounds may be absent or altered because the vocal cords are unable to appose normally. The inspiratory phase of breathing will be markedly prolonged. The patient will exhibit cyanosis, lethargy, and disorientation if severe hypoxia and hypercarbia are present. The victim with poor air exchange must be treated as though the airway were completely obstructed.[32] The box lists signs of partial airway obstruction.

SIGNS OF COMPLETE AIRWAY OBSTRUCTION

Inability to speak
Inability to breathe
Inability to cough
Universal sign for choking
Panic

SIGNS OF PARTIAL AIRWAY OBSTRUCTION

With good air flow:
Forceful cough
Wheezing between coughs
Ability to breathe

With poor air flow:
Weak, ineffectual cough
Crowing sound on inspiration
Paradoxical respiration
Absent or altered voice sounds
Possible cyanosis
Possible lethargy
Possible disorientation

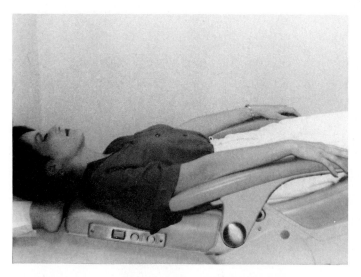

Fig. 11-13. Place patient in the supine position with feet elevated.

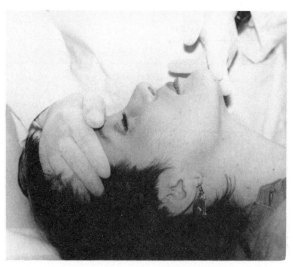

Fig. 11-14. Head tilt-chin lift.

REVIEW OF BASIC AIRWAY MANEUVERS

Once the patient with an obstructed airway loses consciousness, basic life support, including airway maintenance (see Chapter 5) must be applied promptly. These steps are directed at eliminating the most common cause of airway obstruction—the tongue. Performance of these steps permits the rescuer to determine whether the tongue is or is not the cause of the airway problem and whether or not additional steps of airway management will be necessary. In those instances in which a lower airway obstruction is obvious (such as airway obstruction developing immediately after a crown or a dental instrument is swallowed), the basic steps (ABC) are bypassed, with the rescuer proceeding directly to the establishment of an emergency airway.

Step 1: Position patient. Place patient in supine position with the feet elevated slightly (Fig. 11-13).

Step 2: Head tilt. Extension of neck tissues is accomplished by head tilt–chin lift (Fig. 11-14). In 80% of instances in which the tongue is the cause of airway obstruction, the head tilt–chin lift technique effectively clears the airway.[33]

Step 3: Assess airway and breathing. The rescuer's ear is placed 1 inch from the victim's mouth and nose, listening and feeling for the passage of air while looking toward the chest of the victim and watching for respiratory movement (Fig. 11-15).

Step 4: Jaw thrust maneuver (if indicated): Rescuer places fingers behind the posterior border of the ramus of the mandible and displaces the mandible anteriorly while tilting the head backward and

opening the mouth with other fingers (Fig. 11-16). Dislocation of the mandible is a painful procedure. Therefore, the jaw thrust maneuver will give the rescuer a "feel" for the depth of unconsciousness of the victim. When the patient does not respond to this maneuver, the level of consciousness is somewhat deeper, whereas if the victim responds to the jaw thrust technique (i.e., by grimacing, phonating, moving), the level of unconsciousness is not as deep.

Step 5: Assess airway and breathing. Repeat step 3, if needed.

Step 6: Artificial ventilation, if indicated. When the tongue is the cause of the airway obstruction, these steps will usually reestablish a patent airway. When these steps have been carried out properly and the airway remains obstructed (as diagnosed by a continued lack of "hearing and seeing," aphonia, and suprasternal retraction), the rescuer should immediately consider the possibility that the obstruction is located within the larynx or trachea and proceed to establish an emergency airway.

ESTABLISHMENT OF AN EMERGENCY AIRWAY

When a patient's airway is obstructed, establishment of a patent airway becomes the immediate goal of treatment. There are a variety of procedures available for establishing an emergency airway, and there is also a degree of controversy concerning some of them. Two procedures, tracheostomy[34-36] and cricothyrotomy,[37-39] require surgical intervention and therefore considerable

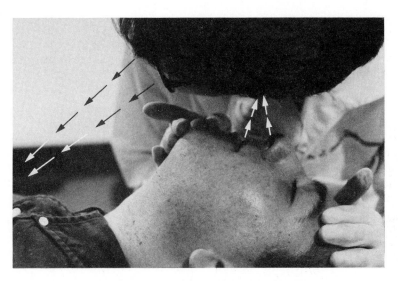

Fig. 11-15. Look, listen, and feel.

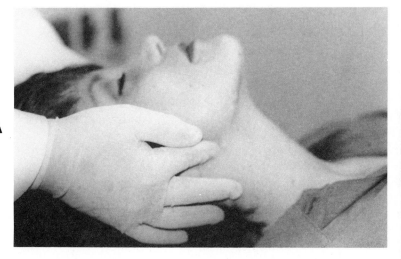

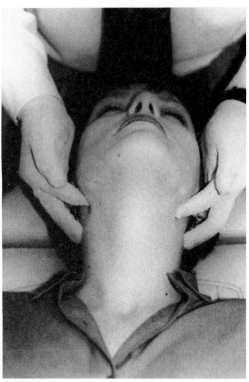

Fig. 11-16. Jaw thrust maneuver: **A,** Side view. **B,** Front view.

knowledge and technical skill in order to be carried out effectively. A third procedure, which is non-surgical, is the procedure of choice for the initial management of all obstructed airways when basic life support techniques for airway management prove inadequate. This is the external subdiaphragmatic compression technique, properly known as the abdominal thrust, or the Heimlich maneuver.[40-46] Because this procedure is nonsurgical, serious complications, though possible, are less

likely to occur, a fact that makes it particularly attractive for the dental office.[47,48] The American Heart Association and the American Red Cross recommend the abdominal thrust as an integral part of the emergency procedures to be followed when lower airway obstruction is a possibility,[32] a situation responsible for 3100 deaths in 1984.[4]

NONINVASIVE PROCEDURES FOR OBSTRUCTED AIRWAY

When foreign objects enter the tracheobronchial tree, a potentially life-threatening situation exists. Airway obstruction may be either partial or complete. Management of the situation will vary according to the degree of obstruction present and the effectiveness of the patient's cough reflex. Manual, noninvasive procedures will be used whenever possible. Surgical procedures, used when all else fails, are also within the doctor's expertise and will be described.

A victim with a *partial obstruction* of the airway who is capable of *forceful coughing* and is breathing adequately (that is, with no evidence of cyanosis or duskiness) should be left alone. Although a degree of wheezing may be evident between coughs, a forceful cough is highly effective in removing foreign objects. *Do not interfere with this victim.*

Should the victim of a *partial airway obstruction* initially demonstrate *poor air exchange* or if previously good air exchange becomes ineffective, the victim must be *managed as if a complete obstruction existed.*

In *complete airway obstruction* the victim is unable to speak or to make any sound, to breathe, or to cough. The victim will retain consciousness as long as the cerebral oxygen level of the blood is sufficiently high. This may range from 10 seconds to 2 minutes, depending upon whether or not the obstruction occurred during inspiration (more oxygen in the blood, therefore consciousness remains longer) or expiration (less oxygen in the blood, more rapid loss of consciousness). Fortunately, most airway obstructions occur during inhalation so that the lungs are somewhat filled with oxygen and are inflated. This increases the duration of consciousness, as well as making the following procedure more effective. The victim may clutch his or her neck (see Fig. 11-12) in the universal distress signal for foreign body airway obstruction. Prompt management is critical, because the victim will lose consciousness and die unless a patent airway is reestablished without delay.

Several manual, noninvasive procedures are available for use in acute airway obstruction. Each technique will be described, followed by the recommended sequencing of these techniques in actual situations. The manual, noninvasive techniques are as follows:

Back blows
Manual thrusts
    Heimlich maneuver (abdominal thrust)
    Chest thrust
Finger sweeps

Back Blows

Back blows formed an integral part of previous regimens for the removal of foreign objects from the airway.[49] However, data presented at the 1985 National Conference on Cardiopulmonary Resuscitation and Emergency Cardiac Care suggested that, as a single method, back blows may not be as effective as the Heimlich maneuver in adults.[42] For this reason, the Heimlich maneuver is the only technique recommended for management of an obstructed airway in adults or children.

Back blows do remain an integral part of the protocol for management of the obstructed airway in the infant. When back blows are performed on an infant, the patient is straddled over the rescuer's arm, with the head lower than the trunk and the head supported by firmly holding the jaw. The rescuer rests his or her hand on his or her thigh and delivers four back blows forcefully with the heel of the hand between the infant's shoulder blades (Fig. 11-17).

Manual Thrusts

Manual thrusts consist of a series of six to ten thrusts to the upper abdomen (Heimlich maneuver or abdominal thrust) or to the lower chest (chest thrust). They function to rapidly increase intrathoracic pressure, acting as an artificial cough that may help to dislodge a foreign body. The objective of each individual thrust should be to relieve the obstruction without having to complete the full series. Studies have demonstrated that there are no significant differences between abdominal and chest thrusts in the amount of air flow, pressure, and volume.[50,51]

There are several special situations in which one technique is preferred over the other. The chest

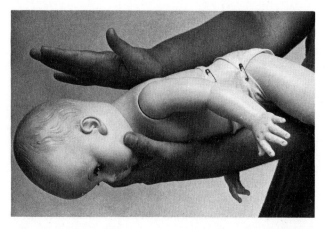

Fig. 11-17. Back blows—four back blows are delivered with heel of hand between shoulder blades of infant victim.

thrust is recommended in advanced stages of pregnancy and in markedly obese individuals. The chest thrust is also less likely to cause regurgitation than the abdominal thrust. Chest thrusts are also recommended in infants because of the greater likelihood of organ damage (e.g., the liver) with abdominal thrusts. The Heimlich maneuver is recommended especially in older patients, whose more brittle ribs are more likely to be fractured in chest thrust, and in children.

Internal injury is always a possibility whenever the abdominal thrust or chest thrust is employed. Injury has been reported to both thoracic and abdominal organs, including the liver, spleen, and stomach.[47,48] Proper hand positioning can minimize these potential side effects. The rescuer's hands must never be located over the xiphoid process or over the lower margins of the rib cage. In the Heimlich maneuver the hands are placed below this area, whereas in chest thrust they are placed above it.

Following the successful application of any manual thrust technique, the patient should be evaluated by medical or paramedical personnel for evidence of any secondary injury, such as abdominal bleeding, before the patient is discharged.

Heimlich Maneuver

The Heimlich maneuver is also known as the subdiaphragmatic abdominal thrust and the abdominal thrust. First described in 1975 by Dr. Henry J. Heimlich,[40] today this maneuver is recommended as the primary technique for relieving foreign body airway obstruction in the adult and child.[41]

TECHNIQUE. Conscious victim—standing or sitting (Figs. 11-18 and 11-19)
1. Stand behind the victim and wrap your arms around the victim's waist and under the victim's arms.
2. Grasp one fist with the other hand, placing the thumb side of the first against the victim's abdomen. The hand is held in the midline slightly above the umbilicus and well below the tip of the xiphoid process (Fig. 11-18).
3. Repeat inward and upward thrusts until either the foreign body is expelled or the victim loses consciousness (Fig. 11-19).

Prior to dismissal of the patient from the office, it is suggested that this patient be evaluated for the possibility of complications by either medical or paramedical personnel.

TECHNIQUE. Unconscious victim
1. Place the victim in the supine position.
2. Open the victim's airway (head tilt–chin lift) and turn the head up into the so-called "neutral"

position. The head is turned up to (1) avoid airway obstruction by kinking the airway, (2) facilitate foreign body movement up the airway, and (3) allow the foreign body to be seen.

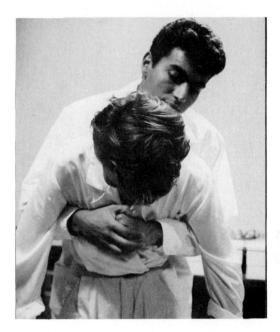

Fig. 11-18. Technique of abdominal thrust.

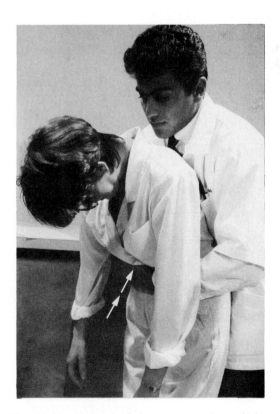

Fig. 11-19. Abdominal thrust—conscious victim.

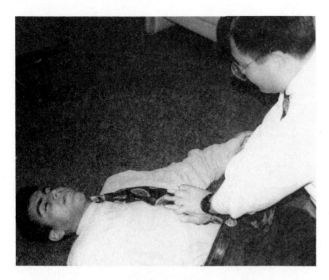

Fig. 11-20. Rescuer straddles victim's legs in Heimlich maneuver on floor.

3. Position of the rescuer: It is recommended that whenever possible the rescuer straddle the victim's legs or thighs (Fig. 11-20) This position will be virtually impossible to achieve with a victim in the dental chair.

   An alternative to the straddle position places the rescuer alongside the victim. The rescuer's knees are placed close to the victim's hips on either the right or left side of the victim (Fig. 11-21). This position, with the rescuer standing astride the victim's hips, is useful when the victim is in the dental chair (Fig. 11-22).

4. Place the heel of one hand against the victim's abdomen in the midline slightly above the umbilicus and well below the tip of the xiphoid process.

5. Place the second hand directly on top of the first hand.

6. Press into the victim's abdomen with a quick inward and upward thrust. Force must *not* be directed laterally.

7. Perform six to ten abdominal thrusts.

8. Open the patient's mouth and perform the finger sweep.

Some final points concerning the Heimlich maneuver: When properly performed, the Heimlich maneuver is exclusively a soft tissue procedure. No bony structures should be involved (ribs or sternum). In all cases the rescuer must apply pressure with the heel of the hand below the rib cage. The maneuver is not a bear hug. If it is carried out as one, injury to intraabdominal organs such as the liver and spleen or to the sternum and ribs could occur. After successful completion of the procedure, the patient should be evaluated by medical or paramedical personnel prior to being discharged from the office.

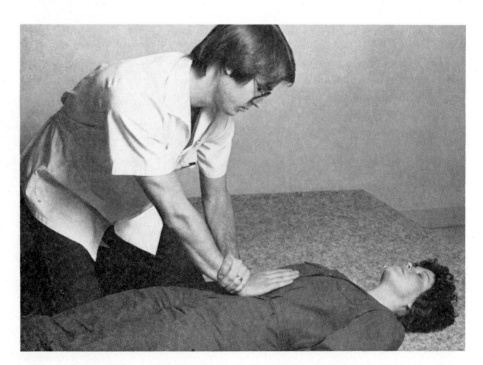

Fig. 11-21. Abdominal thrust. Unconscious victim with rescuer astride victim on floor. Victim's head is in the neutral position.

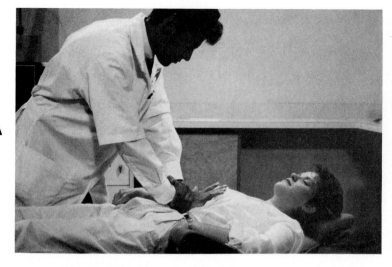

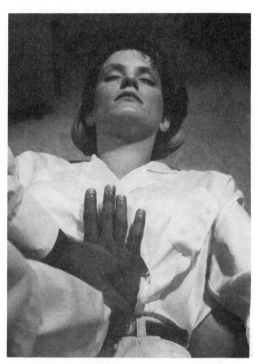

Fig. 11-22. A, Abdominal thrust—unconscious victim in dental chair with rescuer astride victim. **B,** Force of compression must be in upward, not lateral, direction. Victim's head is kept in the neutral position.

Table 11-2. Chest thrust

Indications	*Contraindications*
Infant (<1 year old)	Older victim
Pregnant female	
Extremely obese	

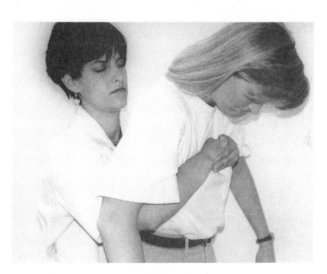

Fig. 11-23. Chest thrust—conscious victim.

Chest Thrust

The chest thrust is an alternative—in special situations only—to the Heimlich maneuver as a technique for opening an obstructed airway. There is no substantial difference in the effectiveness of these techniques when performed properly. Table 11-2 lists the indications and contraindications for the chest thrust.

TECHNIQUE. Conscious victim—standing or sitting

1. Stand behind the victim; place your arms directly under the victim's armpits, encircling the victim's chest (Fig. 11-23).
2. Grasp one fist with the other hand, placing the thumb side of the fist on the middle of the sternum, not on the xiphoid process or on the margins of the rib cage.

3. Perform backward thrusts until the foreign body is expelled or the victim becomes unconscious.

TECHNIQUE. Unconscious victim (Fig. 11-24)

1. Place victim into the supine position.
2. Open the victim's airway (head tilt–chin lift) and place the victim's head into the neutral position.
3. Either straddle or stand astride the victim, as described in the Heimlich maneuver.
4. The hand position and technique for chest thrust are identical to those of closed chest cardiac compression (see Chapter 30). Place the

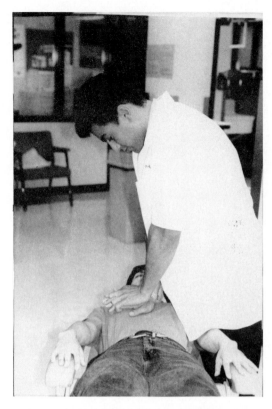

Fig. 11-24. Chest thrust—unconscious victim.

heel of one hand on the lower half of the sternum with the second hand on top of it, but not on xiphoid process.

5. Exert six to ten quick, downward thrusts to compress the chest cavity.

6. Open the patient's mouth and perform the finger sweep.

Finger Sweeps

In the conscious victim it is quite difficult for the rescuer to remove foreign bodies from the airway with his or her fingers. When the victim loses consciousness, the muscles relax and it becomes considerably easier for the rescuer to open the mouth and insert fingers into the oral cavity to seek and remove foreign objects.

Special care must be observed when probing with a finger in an infant or small child's airway so as not to inadvertently force the foreign body deeper into the airway. Therefore, *blind finger sweeps in the infant and child are not recommended.* Foreign bodies may, however, be removed from the airway by this technique if they are located above the level of the epiglottis. Finger sweep is only performed in the unconscious person.

In the dental office it is suggested that a Magill intubation forcep be included as an integral part of the office emergency kit (Fig. 11-25). The Magill intubation forcep may be used, when it is available, to aid in removal of foreign objects from the airway. It is suggested that use of this instrument be limited to situations in which the object can be seen by the rescuer.

TECHNIQUE. Finger sweep

1. Place the victim in the supine position with the head in the neutral position.

2. Grasp the victim's tongue and anterior portion of the mandible. This technique is called the tongue-jaw lift. It pulls the tongue off the posterior wall of the pharynx, away from a foreign object that may be lodged there.

   If the tongue jaw lift is ineffective, the crossed finger technique is used (Fig. 11-26). The mouth is opened by crossing the index finger and thumb between the teeth and forcing the teeth apart.

3. To employ the finger sweep, place the index finger of the other hand along the inside of the victim's cheek, and then advance it deeply into the pharynx at the base of the tongue. Using a hooking movement, attempt to dislodge the foreign body and move it into the mouth where it can be removed by suction or with the Magill

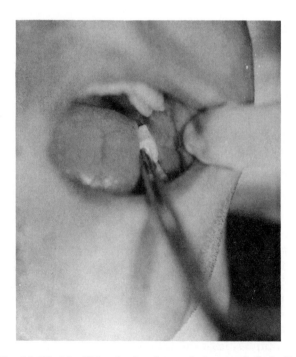

Fig. 11-25. Magill intubation forcep being used clinically.

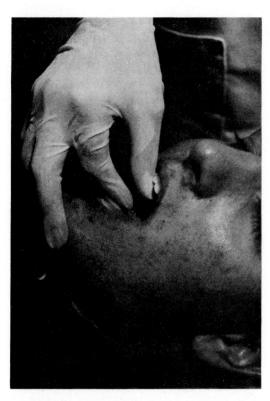

Fig. 11-26. Crossed-finger technique aids in opening mouth of unconscious victim.

intubation forcep. Care must be taken not to force the object more deeply into the airway.

Recommended Sequences

The American Heart Association[32] recommended sequences for removing airway obstruction is outlined in the accompanying boxes.

Procedures for Obstructed Airway in Infants and Children

Foreign body airway obstruction in children ages 1 through 8 years is managed similarly to that of adults: the Heimlich maneuver is the primary technique. However, in the infant victim under the age of 1 year, the combination of back blows and chest thrusts continues to be recommended. The basic rescue procedures for infants and children are reviewed in the accompanying box.

The sequences presented here for infants and children should be repeated until the foreign body has been successfully removed or until the rescuer feels that time has been exhausted. At this time a cricothyrotomy should be seriously considered, *if* the rescuer is well-trained in the procedure and has the necessary equipment available.

RECOMMENDED SEQUENCES FOR REMOVING AIRWAY OBSTRUCTION

For adult conscious victim with obstructed airway

Identify complete airway obstruction: Ask, "Are you choking?"

↓

Identify yourself as someone who will help the victim: Say, "I can help you"

↓

Apply the Heimlich maneuver until foreign body is expelled or the victim becomes unconscious

↓

Have medical or paramedical personnel evaluate patient for complications prior to dismissal

For adult conscious victim with known obstructed airway, who loses consciousness

Place victim in supine position with head in neutral position; call for help

↓

Activate the EMS system (i.e., call 9–1–1) if a second person is available

↓

Open the victim's mouth using tongue-jaw lift

↓

Perform finger sweep

↓

Attempt to ventilate the patient; if ineffective

↓

Perform six to ten abdominal thrusts

↓

Check for foreign body with finger sweep

↓

Attempt to ventilate the patient; if ineffective:

↓

Repeat abdominal thrusts, finger sweeps, and attempted ventilations until effective

↓

Have medical or paramedical personnel evaluate patient for complications prior to dismissal

Continued.

RECOMMENDED SEQUENCES FOR REMOVING AIRWAY OBSTRUCTION—cont'd

For adult unconscious victim, cause unknown

Rescuer manages unconscious victim in usual manner:

Assess unresponsiveness

↓

Position victim in supine position with feet elevated

↓

Call for help (office emergency team)

↓

Open airway (head tilt–chin lift)

↓

Assess breathing (look, listen, feel), and

↓

Attempt to ventilate. If unsuccessful,

↓

Reposition head and attempt to ventilate; if still unsuccessful,

↓

Activate EMS system (call 9–1–1) and

↓

Perform Heimlich maneuver: six to ten abdominal thrusts

↓

Perform foreign body check: finger sweep

↓

Attempt to ventilate; if ineffective,

↓

Repeat Heimlich maneuver, finger sweeps, and ventilation, until successful

---

RESCUE PROCEDURES FOR INFANTS AND CHILDREN

Assess unresponsiveness

↓

Position victim in supine position with feet elevated

↓

Call for help (office emergency team)

↓

Open airway (head tilt–chin lift)

↓

Assess breathing (look, listen, feel), and

↓

Attempt to ventilate; if unsuccessful;

↓

Reposition head and attempt to ventilate, if still unsuccessful,

↓

Activate EMS system (call 9–1–1) and

↓

Manage airway obstruction: (see following section for obstructed airway in infant or child)

↓

Determine presence or absence of pulse

↓

Perform external chest compression, if necessary

Obstructed airway in infants

Back blows:

1. Supporting the head and neck with one hand, place the infant face down with the head lower than the trunk, straddling your forearm and supported on your thigh (Fig. 11-27)

↓

2. Deliver four back blows forcefully between the shoulder blades with the heel of the hand

↓

Chest thrusts:

1. While supporting the head and neck, sandwich the infant between your hands and hold the infant face up with the head lower than the trunk

↓

2. Deliver four thrusts in the midsternal region in the same manner as external chest compressions, but at a slower rate

↓

RESCUE PROCEDURES FOR INFANTS AND CHILDREN—cont'd

Foreign body check:
1. Do a tongue-jaw lift by placing a thumb in the infant's mouth, over the tongue. Lift tongue and jaw with fingers wrapped over lower jaw
↓
2. Remove the foreign body if visualized
↓
Attempt to ventilate:
1. Open airway with head tilt–chin lift
↓
2. Attempt to ventilate, if unsuccessful,
↓
Repeat these steps until successful
↓
Consider surgical airway (cricothyrotomy)

Obstructed airway in children
The following steps are instituted when the basic procedures already presented have proved to be ineffective in reestablishing a patent airway:
Heimlich maneuver:
1. Kneel at victim's feet if on floor, or stand at victim's feet if on a table
↓
2. Place heel of one hand against victim's abdomen in the midline slightly above the navel and well below the tip of the xiphoid process
↓
3. Place second hand directly on top of first hand
↓
4. Press into abdomen with six to ten abdominal thrusts
↓
Foreign body check:
1. Keep victim's face up
↓
2. Use tongue-jaw lift to open mouth
↓
3. Look into mouth and with finger sweep or Magill intubation forceps, remove foreign body, if visualized
↓
Attempt to ventilate:
1. Open airway with head tilt–chin lift
↓
2. Attempt to ventilate. If unsuccessful,
↓
Repeat preceeding steps until successful
↓
Consider surgical airway (for children over 5 years of age)

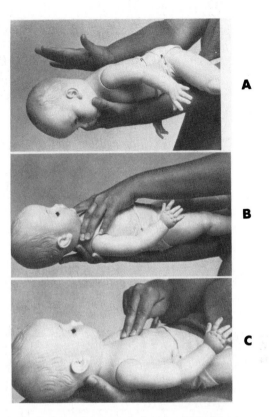

Fig. 11-27. Infant obstructed airway. **A,** Infant is supported by rescuer's forearm. Head lower than rest of body for back blows. **B,** Turning infant over, infant is supported between two arms of rescuer. **C,** Chest thrusts are applied to midsternum of victim with two fingers.

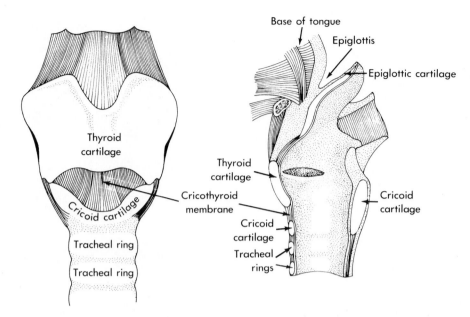

Fig. 11-28. Anatomic relationships of importance in cricothyrotomy.

INVASIVE PROCEDURES FOR OBSTRUCTED AIRWAYS
Tracheostomy versus Cricothyrotomy

The techniques described previously are highly successful in removing foreign objects from the airway of most victims. However, situations have occurred in which these noninvasive techniques were ineffective in removing the object (for example, a dental cotton roll) from a victim's airway. In this situation and in others in which the airway is obstructed by the swelling of tissues, such as laryngeal edema or epiglottitis caused by allergy or illness, invasive procedures may be required if the patient is to survive.

Surgical opening of the airway may be carried out in several ways. Two of the most commonly employed are the tracheostomy[34-36] and the cricothyrotomy.[37-39] Each of these techniques has its adherents and its critics within the medical community but each is of importance, for they both permit the victim's lungs to be oxygenated. These procedures should be performed only by persons trained in these techniques and only if proper equipment is available.

Tracheostomy has been used for more than 2000 years, yet its role in the management of acute airway obstruction has undergone change in recent decades.[52] It was once considered to be the primary technique employed for the relief of acute airway obstruction. For a variety of reasons, cricothyrotomy is now considered by many to be the surgical procedure of choice in sudden airway obstruction.[38,53] In the typical dental situation there is almost no indication for tracheostomy.

Tracheostomy is a surgical procedure now usually employed for long-term airway maintenance and, with few exceptions, such as direct laryngeal fracture[54] and emergency airway management of infants, is not well-suited for emergency airway management. The tracheostomy site contains numerous anatomically important structures, such as the isthmus of the thyroid gland and several large and important blood vessels and nerves.[55] The potential for perforating the esophagus also exists. Complications occur more commonly with tracheostomy even when it is performed slowly and meticulously under controlled conditions, such as in an oxygenated, well-ventilated patient in an operating room, than occur with cricothyrotomy.[54] Hemorrhage and pneumothorax are major complications of tracheostomy, and there is also a risk of penetrating the isthmus of the thyroid gland.[56] In most cases the bleeding that occurs is a major surgical complication that might not be handled satisfactorily in the dental office.

Cricothyroid membrane puncture (cricothyrotomy, cricothyroidotomy) involves establishment of an opening to the airway at the level of the cricothyroid membrane and is readily accepted as a means of obtaining emergency airway access. Cricothyrotomy is carried out more easily and more

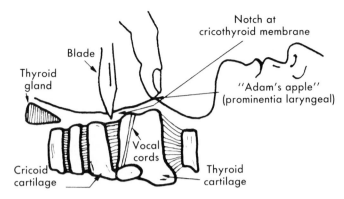

Fig. 11-29. Cricothyrotomy: incision is made inferior to the thyroid cartilage and superior to crocoid cartilage.

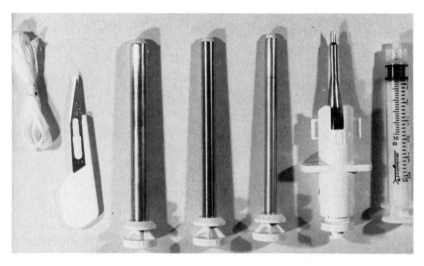

Fig. 11-30. Cricothyrotomy device *(left to right):* cord to secure airway; knifeblade; various size airways (3); puncturing mechanism; and syringe.

quickly than is tracheostomy, and the incidence of complications is significantly lower.[53] Anatomically, no significant structures overlie the cricothyroid membrane. Cricothyrotomy has been said to provide the most accessible point of entry into the respiratory tree inferior to the glottis.[57] The incision is made through skin, adipose tissue, and fascia. Bleeding is seldom encountered in cricothyrotomy (aside from minor bleeding from the skin incision). Inadvertent perforation of the posterior wall of the trachea and laceration of the underlying esophagus are prevented by the fact that the cricoid cartilage has an intact posterior segment (Fig. 11-28). An incision into the cricothyroid membrane begins to heal within a few days of removal of the airway.

Cricothyrotomy
Anatomy

The ability to rapidly locate the proper site for cricothyrotomy is important. The rationale behind any surgical emergency airway procedure is that the opening being made must be *below* the obstruction in order for the procedure to be effective. Where, then, is foreign material most likely to impact in the trachea?

In the adult the narrowest portion of the trachea is located at the larynx. Most objects capable of producing obstruction will come to rest in this area. Objects small enough to pass through the larynx and enter into the trachea will usually pass into one of the mainstem bronchi (usually the right), producing an occlusion of one lung or a significant portion of it. This situation, discussed previously, is not acutely life threatening, although the victim will require hospitalization and perhaps surgery to remove the foreign object.

In children under 3 to 5 years of age, the narrowest portion of the trachea occurs a short distance below the vocal cords at the cricoid cartilage.[58] Obstruction is most likely to occur at this site, making the cricothyrotomy ineffectual. Tracheostomy is the preferred emergency surgical airway in this age group, but it should be undertaken only by practitioners who are experienced performing this procedure on infants and children.[58] Immediate management of this situation in other clinical circumstances rationally requires nonsurgical methods, such as inverting the infant and applying manual thrusts and back blows.

The thyroid cartilage, largest of the tracheal cartilages, and the cricoid cartilage (the second tracheal cartilage) represent the anatomic landmarks for the cricothyrotomy (Figs. 11-28 and 11-29). The thyroid and cricoid cartilages represent the only two tracheal cartilages that are complete rings, the other tracheal rings being open on their posterior aspects. A membranous structure, the cricothyroid membrane forms the anterior connection between these two cartilaginous rings and is the precise site for the cricothyrotomy. The membrane is approximately 10 mm high and 22 mm wide.[59] It may be readily located by placing a finger on the laryngeal prominence (Adam's apple) of the thyroid cartilage and moving the finger inferiorly until a slight depression is located. The cricothyroid membrane is approximately one to one-half fingerbreadths below the laryngeal prominence in the midline of the neck.[37] Inferior to this depression is the prominence of the cricoid cartilage. The cricoid cartilage lies inferior to the incision, whereas the thyroid cartilage and vocal cords are superior to it.

Equipment

A scalpel with a straight (no.11) blade may be employed in an emergency cricothyrotomy for both the skin incision and the membrane incision. Alternatively, it has been suggested that a 13-gauge, ½-inch-long needle be used.

Many devices have been designed to aid in cricothyrotomy. One such device that greatly facilitates the cricothyrotomy procedure is shown in Fig. 11-30.* It contains the following sterile compo-

---

*Nu-Trake, manufactured by International Medical Devices, 19205 Parthenia, Northridge, CA 91324.

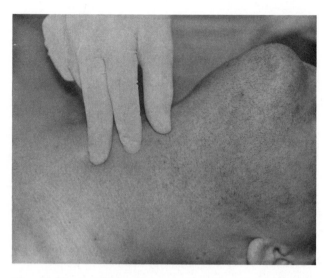

Fig. 11-31. Stabilizing larynx—thumb and middle fingers stabilize cartilage while index finger rests in cricothyroid membrane.

nents: (1) a knife blade, (2) a puncturing mechanism—a two-part needle with a needle stylet, (3) an arcuate point at one end of the stylet to permit initial penetration of the cricothyroid membrane, (4) airways of 4-, 6-, and 8-mm diameters, and (5) obturators for the airways.

Although any of these instruments and devices, when used properly, is effective in creating an emergency airway, it is strongly recommended that only those devices with which the doctor is intimately familiar be considered for inclusion in the emergency kit.

Cricothyrotomy Technique Using a Scalpel

Prepare the neck. In the unlikely event that there is enough time, the neck should be surgically prepared prior to cricothyrotomy. However, in emergency situations antiseptic, if available, should simply be poured over the neck prior to making the incision.

The neck should be hyperextended (head-tilt) to permit easy identification of the thyroid and cricoid cartilages and cricothyroid membrane. A roll of material (e.g., rolled towels) may be placed under the neck to aid hyperextension.

Identify landmarks. The right-handed operator stands on the patient's right side so that his or her left hand may be used to immobilize the larynx and aid in landmark identification while the right hand is used to perform the cricothyrotomy. In clinical practice the right hand is often used to initially

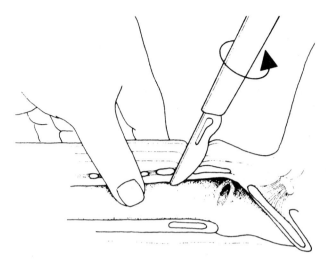

Fig. 11-32. Opening in cricothyroid space is enlarged by rotating scalpel blade 90°.

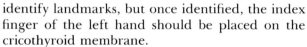

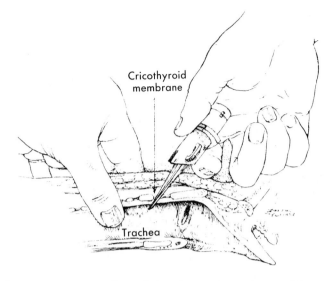

Fig. 11-33. Needle and housing unit are inserted into cricothyroid membrane with a downward thrust toward the chest.

identify landmarks, but once identified, the index finger of the left hand should be placed on the cricothyroid membrane.

Immobilize the larynx. Walls has written that the importance of this step cannot be overstated.[37] The larynx must be immobilized so that the landmarks are not lost during the actual procedure. Immobilization of the larynx is easily accomplished and must be achieved prior to skin incision and maintained until the airway is successfully placed. In the right-handed operator model, the thumb and middle finger of the left hand are used to grasp the upper poles of the thyroid cartilage, permitting the index finger of the left hand to rest on the membrane (Fig. 11-31). Once immobilized, the index finger of the left hand can again be used to palpate the thyroid cartilage, the membrane, and the cricoid cartilage.

Incise the skin. The skin incision must be vertical and in the midline. It should be approximately 2 to 3 cm in length. The vertical incision minimizes the possibility of significant vascular problems during the procedure,[60] whereas a horizontal incision is more likely to lead to bleeding. The vertical incision should be made to the depth of the thyroid cartilage, membrane, and cricoid cartilage. Bleeding that might arise from the skin incision will be minimal and should be ignored. Of primary significance is the establishment of the airway. Once the airway is established, any bleeding can be managed.

Reidentify the membrane. Reinsert the index finger of the left hand into the incision to reidentify the membrane. Quickly move the finger up to the thyroid and down to the cricoid cartilages to ensure proper identification of the cricothyroid membrane. The fingertip may remain in the incision, but should be placed on the most inferior border of the thyroid cartilage to provide a point of reference without interfering with the incision into the membrane.

Incise the membrane. The incision into the membrane should be horizontal, using the no. 11 scalpel blade in the lower third of the cricothyroid space. This is the least vascular part of the membrane. The horizontal incision should be in the midline and at least 1.5 cm long to facilitate placement of the airway,

Upon entering the airway bubbling will be observed. The scalpel is withdrawn and the index finger of the left hand reinserted into the cricothyroid space to identify the incision and verify its correct placement. The finger is again moved to the inferior portion of the thyroid cartilage to be used as a guide for insertion of the airway.

Dilate incision. Enlarge the cricothyroid space by inserting the handle of the scalpel into the horizontal incision and rotating it 90° to open the airway (Fig. 11-32).

Insert tube. If available, a cricothyroid or tracheotomy tube can be inserted temporarily. Prop-

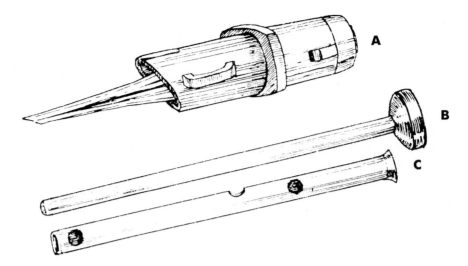

Fig. 11-34. Components of instrument for cricothyrotomy. **A,** Needle and housing unit. **B,** Obturator. **C,** Airway.

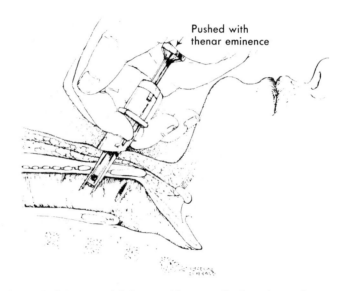

Pushed with
thenar eminence

Fig. 11-35. Obturator/airway unit is inserted into needle/housing unit to open the airway. Obturator is next removed and airway is secured.

erly performed, a cricothyrotomy can be accomplished in 15 to 30 seconds.

Anesthesia is not needed because the patient is unconscious and unable to react to the stimulus of the scalpel incision. It is not unusual for a coughing episode to occur once the trachea is entered.

Cricothyrotomy Technique Using 13-Gauge Needle

When a 13-gauge, ½-inch needle is used, the tissue is prepared and the thyroid cartilage is stablized in the same manner as before, with the index finger identifying the cricothyroid membrane. The needle is inserted through this area in a direction

toward the chest, until the tracheal lumen is entered. Entry into the trachea is confirmed by the sound and feel of air entering and leaving, coughing, and bubbling of fluids. Overinsertion and perforation of the tracheoesophageal wall is prevented by the cartilaginous posterior wall of the cricoid cartilage.

Cricothyrotomy Technique Using a Cricothyrotomy Device[61]

After the 2- to 3-cm vertical skin incision with the scalpel, the needle then punctures the cricothyroid membrane in the midline. This is accomplished with a downward thrust toward the chest (Fig. 11-33). A rush of air indicates successful entry into the trachea, and the obturator/airway unit is inserted (Fig. 11-34). Gently advance the blunt-edged needle farther into the trachea until its plastic hub rests on the skin. Gently rock the instrument; free movement indicates that overpenetration has not occurred. An airway and obturators are now inserted into the distal end of the housing unit (Fig. 11-35). The split end of the needle, within the trachea, is opened by the airway and obturator, after which the obturator is removed, leaving a clear passage for air to reach the lungs. This device is available in both adult and pediatric sizes. Its use, like that of all other emergency airway equipment, is recommended only for those trained in cricothyrotomy technique.

If spontaneous respiratory movements are present, the victim will soon regain consciousness but is still unable to speak because of the continued presence of an obstruction at the larynx. Once consciousness returns it must be remembered that the opening into the trachea cannot be closed until the object producing the obstruction has been removed. In the absence of spontaneous respiratory movements, artificial ventilation should be performed via the cricothyrotomy to ensure adequate oxygenation of the blood. Adequacy of the circulation should next be determined by palpating the carotid artery.

Additional Management

Once a patent airway has been established, oxygen can be administered to the victim. A cannula or face mask can be placed over the tracheal opening. Medical assistance must also be summoned and the patient transferred to an emergency medical care facility for follow-up management (removal of foreign object, closure of tracheal opening) and observation.

Contraindications to Cricothyrotomy

Pediatric age group. Cricothyrotomy should not be undertaken without significant trepidation in children under 10 years old and probably should not be undertaken at all in children under 5 years old.[37] Although tracheostomy is the preferred emergency airway procedure in very young patients,[62] needle cricothyrotomy is more desirable in younger patients.

Preexisting laryngeal pathology. Preexisting pathologies, such as epiglottitis, chronic inflammation, or cancer, make cricothyrotomy more difficult.

Unfamiliarity with the technique. Lack of familiarity with the technique and its complications serve as contraindications to cricothyrotomy. Operator inexperience may be the single largest factor with respect to cricothyrotomy complications.[63]

Anatomic barriers. Anatomic barriers, such as trauma to the neck region, are contraindications to the use of this technique.

Coagulopathies. When uncontrolled hemorrhage is a possibility, the benefits of the procedure must be weighed against its risks.

SUMMARY

Acute, total airway obstruction is a very rare occurrence in the dental environment. However, when it does occur, signs and symptoms must be recognized instantly and management instituted immediately.

Noninvasive procedures for obtaining an emergency airway are preferred in all situations to surgical procedures, which should be held in reserve as last-ditch efforts when all else has failed. All dental personnel should be trained in the management of the obstructed airway via the Heimlich maneuver.

REFERENCES

1. Barkmeier WW, Cooley RL, Abrams H: Prevention of swallowing or aspiration of foreign objects, *J Am Dent Assoc* 97:473, 1978.
2. Alexander RE, Delhom JJ: Rubber dam clamp ingestion: an operative risk, *J Am Dent Assoc*, 82:1387, 1971.
3. Goultschin J, Heling B: Accidental swallowing of an endodontic instrument, *Oral Surg* 32:621, 1971.
4. *Accident facts*, Chicago, 1984, National Safety Council.
5. American Heart Association and National Academy of Sciences, National Research Council: Standards and guidelines for cardiopulmonary resuscitation (CPR) and emergency cardiac care (ECC), *JAMA* 255:2959, 1986.
6. Harris CS, Baker SP, Smith GA, and others: Childhood asphyxiation by food: a national analysis and overview, *JAMA* 251:2231, 1984.
7. Dailey RH: Acute upper airway obstruction, *Emerg Med Clin N Amer* 1:261, 1983.
8. Abman SH, Fan LL, Cotton EK: Emergency treatment of foreign-body obstruction of the upper airway in children, *J Emerg Med* 2:7–12, 1984.
9. Netter FH: Respiratory system, volume 7, *CIBA collection of medical illustrations*, Summit, NJ, 1979, CIBA Pharmaceutical Co.
10. American Heart Association and National Academy of Sciences, National Research Council: Standards and guidelines for cardiopulmonary resuscitation (CPR) and emergency cardiac care (ECC), *JAMA* 255:2905, 1986.
11. Odelowo EO, Komolafe OF: Diagnosis, management and complications of oesophageal and airway foreign bodies, *Internat Surg* 75(3):148-154, 1990.
12. Storey PS: Obstruction of the GI tract, *Amer J Hospice and Palliative Care* 8(3):5, 1991.
13. Weissberg D: Foreign bodies in the gastro-intestinal tract, *South African J Surg* 29(4):150-153, 1991.

14. Mu L, He P, Sun D: The causes and complications of late diangosis of foreign body aspiration in children: report of 210 cases, *Arch Otolaryngol—Head and Neck Surgery* 117(8): 876-879, 1991.

15. Muth D, Scafermeyer RW: All that wheezes, *Pediatric Emerg Care* 6(2):110-112, 1990.

16. Lumpkin J: Airway obstruction, *Top Emerg Med* 2:15, 1990.

17. Hougen RK: The cafe coronary, *JAMA* 186:142, 1963.

18. Craig TJ, Richardson MA: Cafe coronaries in psychiatric patients: Letter to the editors, *JAMA* 248:2114, 1982.

19. Landing BH, Dixon LG: Congenital malformations and genetic disorders of the respiratory tract, *Am Rev Respir Dis* 120:15, 1979.

20. Ossof RH, Wolff AP: Acute epiglottitis in adults, *JAMA* 244:2639, 1980.

21. Kentrell RW: Acute epiglottitis: intubation vs. tracheostomy, *Laryngoscope* 88:994, 1978.

22. Gufferman S, Walker FW: Superglottitis following gasoline ingestion, *Ann Emerg Med* 11:368, 1982.

23. Herzon FS: Peritonsillar abscess: needle aspiration, *Otolaryngol Head Neck Surg* 89:910, 1981.

24. Wolfe JA, Rowe LD: Upper airway obstruction in infectious mononucleosis, *Ann Otol* 89:430, 1980.

25. Hamer R: Tetropharyngeal abscess, *Ann Emerg Med* 11:549, 1982.

26. Oill PA, Rorser SM, Galpin JE: Infectious disease emergencies. Part 3: Patients presenting with respiratory distress syndromes, *West J Med* 125:452, 1976.

27. Miller RD: *Anesthesia*, New York, 1981, Churchill-Livingstone.

28. Rosenbaum L: Upper airway obstruction as a complication of oral anticoagulant therapy, *Arch Intern Med* 139:1151, 1979.

29. Rockswold G, Buran DJ: Inhalation of liquid nitrogen vapor, *Ann Emerg Med* 11:553, 1982.

30. Eliachar I, Moscona R, Joachims HZ, and others: The management of laryngeal tracheal stenosis in burned patients, *Plast Reconstr Surg* 68:11, 1981.

31. Kristoffersen MB, Rattenborg CC, Holaday PA: Asphyxial death: The roles of acute anoxia, hypercarbia, and acidosis, *Anesthesiology* 28:488, 1967.

32. American Heart Association and National Academy of Sciences, National Research Council: Standards and guidelines for cardiopulmonary resuscitation (CPR) and emergency cardiac care (ECC), *JAMA* 255:2923, 1986.

33. Arnold DN: Airway review, *Amer Acad Gnathologic Orthoped* 7(2):4–7, 11, 1990.

34. Piotrowski JJ, Moore EE: Emergency department tracheostomy, *Emerg Med Clin N Amer* 6:737, 1988.

35. *ATLAS Instructors' Manual;* Chicago, 1988, ACS Committee on Trauma.

36. Kirchner JA: Tracheostomy and its problems, *Surg Clin North Am* 60(5):1093, 1980.

37. Walls RM: Cricothroidotomy, *Emerg Med Clin N Amer* 6:725, 1988.

38. Jorden RC: *Cricothyroidotomy*. In Dailey RH, Callahan M, editors: *Controversies in trauma* management, New York, 1985, Churchill-Livingstone.

39. Brantigan CO, Grow JB: Cricothyroidotomy: Elective use in respiratory problems requiring tracheotomy, *J Thorac Cardiovasc Surg* 71:72, 1976.

40. Heimlich HJ: A life-saving maneuver to prevent food-choking, *JAMA* 234:398, 1975.

41. Committee on Emergency Medical Services, Assembly of Life Sciences, National Research Council: *Report of emergency airway management*, Washington, D.C., 1976, National Academy of Sciences.

42. Day RL, Crelin ES, DuBois AB: Choking: The Heimlich abdominal thrust vs back blows: an approach to measurement of inertial and aerodynamic forces, *Pediatrics* 70:113, 1982.

43. Heimlich HJ, Hoffman KA, Canestri FR: Food-choking and drowning deaths prevented by external subdiaphragmatic compression: physiologic basis, *Ann Thorac Surg* 20:188, 1975.

44. Heimlich HJ, Uhtley MH: The Heimlich maneuver, *Clin Symp* 31:22, 1979.

45. Patrick EA: Choking: a questionnaire to find the most effective treatmentt, *Emergency* 12:59, 1980.

46. Heimlich HJ: Pop goes the cafe coronary, *Emerg Med* 6:154, 1979.

47. Visintine RE, Baick CH: Ruptured stomach after Heimlich maneuver, *JAMA* 234:415, 1975.

48. Palmer E: The Heimlich maneuver misused, *Curr Prescribing* 154:155, 1979.

49. American Heart Association and National Academy of Sciences, National Research Council: Standards and guidelines for cardiopulmonary resuscitation (CPR) and emergency cardiac care (ECC), *JAMA* 244:453, 1980.

50. Gordon, AS, Belton, MK, Ridolpho RF: Emergency management of foreign body airway obstruction. In Safar P, Elam J, editors: *Advances in cardiopulmonary resuscitation*, New York, 1977, Springer-Verlag.

51. Guildner CW, Williams D, Subitch T: Airway obstructed by foreign material: The Heimlich maneuver, *JACEP* 5:675, 1976.

52. Frost EAM: Tracing the tracheostomy, *Ann Otol Rhinol* 85:618, 1976.

53. Boyd AD, Romita MC, Conlan AA, and others: A clinical evaluation of cricothyroidotomy, *Surg Gynecol Obstet* 149:365, 1979.

54. Kostendieck JF: Airway management. In Rosen P, editor: *Emergency medicine*, St Louis 1988, Mosby—Year Book.

55. Morris IR: Functional anatomy of the upper airway, *Emerg Med Clin N Amer* 6:639–670, 1988.

56. Gilmore BB, Mickelson SA: Pediatric tracheostomy, *Otolaryngol Clin North Am* 19(1):141, 1986.

57. Weiss S: A new instrument for emergency cricothyrotomy, *JACEP* 23:331, 1973.

58. Barkin RM: Pediatric emergency management, *Emer Med Clin N Am* 6(4):687, 1988.

59. Kress TD, Balasubramaniam S: Cricothyroidotomy, *Ann Emerg Med* 11:197, 1982.

60. Narrod JA, Moore EE, Rosen P: Emergency cricothyrostomy—technique and anatomical considerations, *J Emerg Med* 2:443, 1985.

61. Weiss S: A new emergency cricothyroidotomy instrument, *J Trauma* 23:155, 1983.

62. McLaughlin J, Iserson KV: Emergency pediatric tracheostomy: a usuable technique and model for instruction, *Ann Emerg Med* 15:463, 1986.

63. McGill J, Clinton JE, Ruiz E: Cricothyroidotomy in the emergency department, *Ann Emerg Med* 11:361, 1982.

12 *Hyperventilation*

Hyperventilation is defined as ventilation in excess of that required to maintain normal blood PaO_2 and $PaCO_2$.[1] It may be produced by an increase in either the frequency or the depth of respiration or by a combination of the two. Although the term *hyperventilation* is of relatively recent origin, evidence of the syndrome dates back throughout history.[2] The term *vapors* appeared in eighteenth- and nineteenth-century literature as a phrase for the symptomatic manifestations of anxiety.[3] In Osler's time (the late 1800s), the terms *neurosthenia* or *psychasthenia* were in vogue. During World War I the terms *effort syndrome* and *soldier's heart* were used to describe the symptoms of anxiety encountered in the trenches of Europe.

Hyperventilation is one of the more common emergency situations encountered in dentistry. It almost always occurs as a result of extreme anxiety, although organic causes for hyperventilation do exist. These include pain, metabolic acidosis, drug intoxication, hypercapnia, cirrhosis, and organic central nervous system disorders.[4] In most instances a hyperventilating patient remains conscious throughout the episode. Indeed, unconsciousness produced by hyperventilation is an extremely rare occurrence. Hyperventilation more commonly produces an altered level of consciousness. The patient complains of feeling faint, lightheaded, or both, but does not lose consciousness.

PREDISPOSING FACTORS

The major predisposing factor in hyperventilation is the presence of acute anxiety. In the dental setting hyperventilation most commonly occurs in apprehensive patients who seek to hide their fears from the doctor and to "grin and bear it." Hyperventilation rarely occurs in the adult patient who admits to anxieties concerning dentistry and permits the doctor to employ appropriate stress reduction procedures. Hyperventilation is rarely observed in children, primarily because children usually make no attempt to hide their fears. Instead, apprehensive children voice uncertainties in a manner befitting of their age and the situation: crying, biting, kicking, and so on. If the anxieties of the patient are released, unpleasant situations such as hyperventilation or vasodepressor syncope rarely occur.

Likewise, hyperventilation and vasodepressor syncope are seldom noted in patients over the age of 40 years because these persons are usually more capable of adjusting to the stress imposed by dentistry and are more likely to admit their fears to the doctor. It has been the author's experience that hyperventilation is most likely to be encountered in persons from approximately 15 to 40 years of age.

It has frequently been reported that hyperventilation occurs more commonly in women[5]; however, recent reports and the author's own experiences have demonstrated an almost equal sex incidence of this syndrome.[6]

PREVENTION
Medical History Questionnaire

Prevention of hyperventilation is best accomplished through the recognition and the management of dental anxieties. An anxiety questionnaire (see Chapter 2) might be included as a part of the medical history that the patient completes prior to the start of dental care. The doctor can modify then the planned dental treatment to accommodate the patient's fears. The stress reduction protocol is an invaluable asset in this quest. There are no specific questions on the long- or short-form medical histories that relate to hyperventilation.

Physical Examination

Anxiety about dentistry can usually be detected through a careful examination of the patient. Shaking hands with the patient provides valuable information. Cold, wet (clammy) hands usually are evidence of apprehension. In extreme instances a mild tremor of the hands may be obvious. The patient may appear either quite flushed or pale. In either case, the forehead is usually bathed in perspiration, and the patient may comment on the warmth of the dental office, regardless of its actual temperature.

Fearful patients simply look uncomfortable when seated in the dental chair and will be overly concerned with everything going on around them—their eyes follow every movement made by the doctor, hygienist, or assistant, Such patients appear stiff in the chair and, although seated, seem ready to leave quickly. The hands of apprehensive patients may be firmly attached to the arms of the chair (the "white knuckle" syndrome), or they may be squeezing or tearing at a handkerchief or tissue.

Vital Signs

In the apprehensive patient vital signs will deviate from what is normal or baseline for that individual. Systolic and diastolic blood pressures will be elevated, with a greater elevation noted in systolic pressure. The heart rate (pulse) is rapid, significantly increased above baseline levels for that patient. The rate of respiration in the apprehensive patient increases above the normal adult rate of 14 to 18 breaths per minute, while the depth of respiration will be either deeper or more shallow than normal.

When an apprehensive patient is seen for the first time in the dental office, the vital signs that are recorded will serve as the baseline for all future readings. Therefore, every effort should be made to minimize the anxiety of the patient at this initial visit. Indeed, every effort should be made to reduce the patient's fears at all times during dental care. To do this, and to obtain more realistic baseline vital signs, the patient should be permitted to rest for a few minutes before vital signs are recorded. This is easily accomplished by first starting a review (i.e., dialogue history) of the medical history questionnaire and then, after a 5 minute period, measuring the vital signs.

One other important factor to consider when recording baseline vital signs is that they are most likely to be normal for a given patient if recorded at a visit during which no dental care is undertaken. The patient in this situation is better able to relax, and vital signs will be closer to normal, nondental vital signs. During subsequent visits the monitoring of vital signs may indeed reflect the increased apprehension of the patient toward the impending dental care.

DENTAL THERAPY CONSIDERATIONS

Hyperventilation is prevented primarily through the stress reduction protocol (as outlined in Chapter 2). Care taken by the dental office staff to make every dental visit a pleasant one leads to the reeducation of the fearful patient and to a decrease in dental anxieties. This factor is one of the most important in terms of proper patient management. Through the recognition and management of anxiety, hyperventilation, vasodepressor syncope, and a host of other anxiety-related emergency situations may be prevented.

CLINICAL MANIFESTATIONS
Signs and Symptoms

At the onset of hyperventilation, which is quite commonly precipitated by the fear instilled in a patient by the act of injecting a local anesthetic, the patient may complain of chest tightness and/or suffocation. It is not uncommon for the patient to be entirely unaware of overbreathing at this time.

As hyperventilation continues, the chemical composition of the blood changes and the patient becomes aware of feeling lightheaded or giddy. This may serve to further increase his or her apprehensions. This increase in apprehension leads to an increase in the severity of the situation, and a vicious cycle begins. Hyperventilation caused by anxiety of the dental situation leads to even further increased anxiety when the patient becomes aware of the hyperventilation, and to a further increase in hyperventilation because of the increased anxiety. The goal in management of this situation will be to break this cycle.

At the onset of hyperventilation, symptoms related to the cardiovascular system and gastrointestinal tract often appear. These consist of palpitation (a subjective feeling of a pounding of the heart), precordial discomfort, epigastric discomfort, and globus hystericus (a subjective feeling of a lump in the throat).

Hyperventilation may last for varying lengths of time if untreated. Patients have hyperventilated for 30 minutes or even longer and have had several recurrences a day. In instances in which hyperventilation continues for prolonged periods of time, tingling or paresthesias of the hands, feet, and perioral regions may develop. These are described by the patient as a sensation of numbness or coldness. If hyperventilation is permitted to continue, the patient may develop muscular twitching and carpopedal tetany, a syndrome manifested by flexion of the ankle joints, muscular twitchings and cramps, and convulsions. If the patient's condition is not promptly and precisely managed, syncope may result. Table 12-1 summarizes the signs and symptoms of hyperventilation.

Vital Signs

The primary clinical feature noted during hyperventilation is the change in the rate and depth of the patient's breathing. Normal respiratory rate for an adult is from 14 to 18 breaths per minute. During hyperventilation the respiratory rate may exceed 25 to 30 breaths per minute. Along with this increased rate, an increase in the depth of breathing is usually noted. For the person who has never seen or experienced hyperventilation, the nature of the breathing is similar to that observed at the conclusion of strenuous exercise when an athlete is unable to control his or her breathing. In this situation both the rate and depth of breathing are increased as a normal physiologic response to the increased metabolic rate of the body in an effort to eliminate the excess of carbon dioxide from the body, which has been produced during the exercise. In hyperventilation the nature of the breathing is similar to that of the athlete; however, in this situation it represents an abnormal physiologic response to the presence of anxiety because there is no elevation of carbon dioxide levels in the blood.

As already stated, episodes of hyperventilation are most commonly observed in overtly apprehensive patients; however, many other patients appear outwardly calm and may be totally unaware that they are hyperventilating.

Case Report

A 27-year-old female was scheduled for extraction of two third molars (nonimpacted). She appeared apprehensive when first seen and stated to the dental assistant that she was quite concerned about the procedure, particularly the local anesthetic injections. She was quite flushed and was perspiring. Blood pressure was monitored as 130/90 (baseline, 110/70), heart rate was 110 (baseline, 84), and respirations were 20 (baseline, 18). No preoperative medications were prescribed. The oral surgeon elected to use nitrous oxide and oxygen inhalation sedation during the procedure. The patient was titrated to a concentration of 60% nitrous oxide and 40% oxygen, at which point the patient appeared to be adequately sedated. As the topical anesthetic was applied, the patient became visibly more tense, and her respiratory rate began to increase. During administration of the local anesthetic she began to hyperventilate (rate, 28 breaths per minute and deep), and the administration of the local anesthetic was terminated. The patient was permitted to breathe room air and was calmed by the attending oral surgeon. Slight tingling was noted in the patient's fingers, but the symptom was only of brief duration. Within 10 minutes the patient had relaxed, and her vital signs returned to approximately baseline levels. The contemplated procedure was rescheduled to be managed under intravenous sedation and local anesthetic.

The next week the patient received 30 mg flurazepam orally the evening before the dental procedure and 10 mg diazepam orally 1 hour before the scheduled appointment. The patient was driven to the office by a friend. An intravenous infusion was started in the right forearm with a 21-gauge scalp vein needle, and the patient was titrated to a dose of 17 mg diazepam. Local anesthesia was administered without complication or incident, and the surgical procedure was completed in 25 minutes. The patient tolerated the procedure well, commenting, "With the intravenous (drug) I didn't even need that local injection." She was discharged from the office in the company of an adult companion.

Table 12-1. Clinical manifestations of hyperventilation

Cardiovascular	Palpitations
	Tachycardia
	Precordial pain
Neurologic	Dizziness
	Lightheadedness
	Disturbance of consciousness or vision
	Numbness and tingling of the extremities
	Tetany (rare)
Respiratory	Shortness of breath
	Chest pain
	Dryness of mouth
Gastrointestinal	Globus hystericus
	Epigastric pain
Musculoskeletal	Muscle pains and cramps
	Tremors
	Stiffness
	Tetany
Psychologic	Tension
	Anxiety
	Nightmares

PATHOPHYSIOLOGY

The clinical signs and symptoms of hyperventilation described in the previous section are produced by several distinct causes: anxiety, respiratory alkalosis, increased blood catecholamine levels, and a decrease in the level of ionized calcium in the blood.

Anxiety is responsible for the increased respiratory rate and depth as well as the increase in blood levels of the circulating catecholamines epinephrine and norepinephrine, resulting from the fight-or-flight response. The primary response to these changes in respiration is an increased exchange of oxygen and carbon dioxide by the lungs, which results in an excessive "blowing off" of carbon dioxide. The partial pressure of carbon dioxide decreases from a normal level of 35 to 45 torr to a $PaCO_2$ below 35 torr (hypocapnia or hypocarbia), which results in an increase in the pH of the blood to 7.55 (normal is 7.35 to 7.45), a situation termed *respiratory alkalosis*. This same situation (increased ventilation) occurring at the end of strenuous exercise does not produce respiratory alkalosis because the rate of metabolism of the body has been increased as a result of exercise, producing an increased blood $PaCO_2$. Hyperventilation in this case aids in restoring normal blood levels of carbon dioxide. In the patient who starts with normal levels of carbon dioxide, hyperventilating reduces the $PaCO_2$ to an abnormally low level (hypocapnia).

Hypocapnia and respiratory alkalosis are the result of hyperventilation in the nonexercising individual. Hypocapnia produces vasoconstriction in the cerebral vessels that leads to a degree of cerebral ischemia and helps to explain the observed symptoms of lightheadedness, dizziness, and giddiness.[7] The degree of cerebral ischemia is usually insufficient to produce the loss of consciousness, although this has developed on rare occasion.[8]

Hyperventilation also increases coronary artery vascular resistance. This, combined with the fact that in acute respiratory alkalosis, oxygen becomes more tightly bound to hemoglobin and is less easily released to the tissues, might lead to a reduction in myocardial oxygen supply. In patients with coronary artery disease this may prove to be of great clinical importance. The chest pain often noted in hyperventilating patients is usually described as shooting or stabbing in nature, occurring around the left nipple or under the left breast.[9,10] It may, in certain situations, be difficult to differentiate this chest pain from that of angina pectoris.

Anxiety is also responsible for an increase in the blood levels of catecholamines, which may be responsible for the symptoms of palpitations, precordial oppression, trembling, and sweating frequently observed in spontaneously hyperventilating patients. It is interesting to note that in volunteers asked to hyperventilate, these symptoms, which are thought to be produced by catecholamine release, are not observed, although the symptoms relating to increased breathing rate and depth (e.g., lightheadedness, faintness) are present.[11]

Respiratory alkalosis also has an action on the level of calcium in the blood. As the pH of the blood rises from a normal of 7.4 to approximately 7.55 in hyperventilation, calcium metabolism is disturbed. Although the total serum level of calcium remains approximately normal, the level of ionized calcium in the blood decreases as the pH of the blood increases. Decreases in ionized calcium in the blood result in increased neuromuscular irritability and excitability, which if permitted to progress, lead to the symptoms of tingling and paresthesia of the hands, feet, and perioral regions, carpopedal tetany, cramps, and possible convulsions.

MANAGEMENT

The management of hyperventilation is directed at correcting the respiratory problem and in reducing the anxiety level of the patient.

Anxiety Reduction

Hyperventilation in the dental environment is almost always produced by a fear of dentistry that has been kept well hidden by the patient, a fear that is further increased by the subsequent inability of the patient to control his or her breathing. The doctor must initially attempt to calm the patient. All dental office personnel must remain calm themselves and allow the patient to believe that the situation is well under control.

Step 1: Terminate the dental procedure. Remove the presumed precipitating cause (e.g., syringe, handpiece, forceps) from the patient's line of vision.

Step 2: Position the patient. The patient will remain conscious but will demonstrate varying degrees of difficulty in breathing. The preferred position for this patient is usually upright. The supine position is normally uncomfortable for the patient because of the diminished ventilatory volume usually observed while in this position, caused by the impingement of the abdominal viscera on the diaphragm. Most hyperventilating patients will be

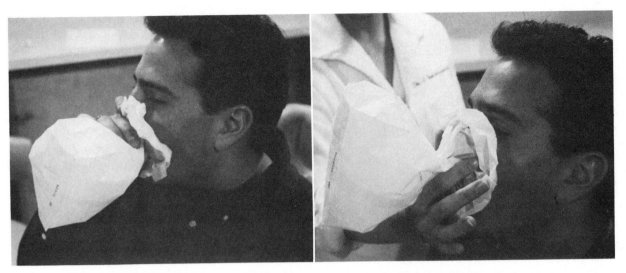

Fig. 12-1. Correction of respiratory alkalosis. Victim rebreathes exhaled air (with increased carbon dioxide content) through paper bag held gently over mouth and nose.

more comfortable if permitted to sit fully or partially upright.

Step 3: Remove materials from patient's mouth. Remove all foreign objects from the patient's mouth, such as the rubber dam, clamp, and partial dentures; if necessary, loosen binding articles of clothing (e.g., tight collar, tie, tight blouse), which may also restrict respiration.

Step 4: Calm patient. Reassure the patient in a calm and relaxed manner that all is well. Attempt to aid the patient to regain control of his or her breathing by speaking calmly. Have the patient breathe slowly and regularly at a rate of about 4 to 6 breaths per minute. This will permit the $Paco_2$ to increase, reducing the pH of the blood to near normal, thereby eliminating any symptoms produced by the respiratory alkalosis. In many cases of hyperventilation this will be all that is necessary to terminate the episode.

Step 5: Basic life support, as indicated. In hyperventilation it is rare that any of the steps of basic life support will be required. The victim is conscious, is breathing quite efficiently (indeed, is overventilating), and the heart is quite functional.

Step 6: Correct respiratory alkalosis. When the preceding steps have not been effective, the next step in management is to aid the patient in increasing the $Paco_2$ level of the blood. This may be accomplished by having the patient breathe in a gaseous mixture of 7% CO_2 and 93% O_2, which is supplied in compressed gas cylinders, but is highly unlikely

to be available in the dental office, or, more realistically, by having the patient rebreathe exhaled air, which contains an increased concentration of carbon dioxide. The second alternative may be accomplished by holding a small paper bag (Fig. 12-1) over the patient's mouth and nose and having the patient breathe into the bag slowly (6 to 10 breaths per minute). (Note: Plastic bags should not be used because they collapse between breaths, making breathing more difficult.) A full face mask from an oxygen delivery unit may also be used. It is important, however, that oxygen *not* be administered to the patient. The patient should breathe into the full face mask, which is held gently but firmly over the face.

Probably the most practical method of increasing $Paco_2$ levels in the blood is to have the hyperventilating victim cup his or her hands together in front of the mouth and nose and breathe in and out of this reservoir of carbon dioxide–enriched exhaled air (Fig. 12-2). In addition to elevating $Paco_2$ levels, the warmth of the exhaled air against the patient's cold palms will serve to warm the patient, thus alleviating one of the frightening symptoms of hyperventilation.

Oxygen is not indicated in the management of this emergency situation because the symptoms of hyperventilation are produced in part by a decrease in the normal blood level of carbon dioxide and not by an increase in the oxygen level. The pH of the blood rises (i.e., respiratory alkalosis), and the

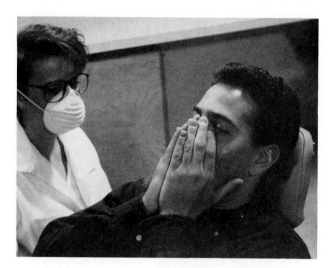

Fig. 12-2. Victim cups hands together in front of the mouth and nose.

symptoms previously discussed are observed. For this reason a major goal of management is to produce an increase, actually a return to normal, in the blood level of carbon dioxide. The administration of 100% O_2 or of any enriched oxygen mixture will act to further decrease the $PaCO_2$ level, thus delaying a return to normal. The administration of oxygen, though not indicated, will not harm the hyperventilating patient. Administration of 100% O_2 will not resolve the clinical problem, but might lead to a further progression of the noted signs and symptoms. A basic rule of thumb in the administration of oxygen is that, *"If ever a patient's condition deteriorates when 100% O_2 is administered, terminate the oxygen flow and permit the patient to breathe ambient air."*

Step 7: Drug management, if needed. In the exceedingly unlikely situation in which the prior steps fail to terminate an episode of hyperventilation, the administration of parenteral drugs may be necessary to reduce the patient's anxiety and slow down the rate of respiration. The drugs of choice in this situation are diazepam or midazolam. If possible, the drug should be administered intravenously, in which case the agent is titrated until the patient's anxiety is visibly reduced and is able to better control his or her breathing. For the average adult this dose will be approximately 10 to 15 mg of diazepam or from 3 to 5 mg of midazolam. When it is not possible to use in intravenous route, 10 mg of diazepam or 3 to 5 mg of midazolam may be admin-

istered intramuscularly. Diazepam, which is not water soluble and does burn when injected intramuscularly, should be injected deeply into the muscle mass and the area then massaged. The oral route could be considered for the administration of diazepam, because the latent period for diazepam is actually somewhat longer following intramuscular administration than following oral administration.[12] An oral dose of 10 to 15 mg of diazepam will usually terminate hyperventilation within 15 to 30 minutes. It must be emphasized that drug therapy to terminate hyperventilation is rarely required. Midazolam is not yet available in the United States for oral administration.

Step 8: Subsequent dental care. Once hyperventilation has been terminated, with the complete resolution of any clinical signs and symptoms, the dentist should determine the cause of the episode. Like vasodepressor syncope, hyperventilation is often the first clinical manifestation of a deep-seated dental fear.

Dental care may continue at this appointment if both the doctor and patient feel comfortable in doing so. However, knowing that hyperventilation has occurred, subsequent dental care should be modified to prevent its recurrence. The stress reduction protocol should be consulted and appropriate steps of treatment modification employed.

Step 9: Discharge. Following termination of hyperventilation and complete resolution of its clinical signs and symptoms, the patient may be discharged from the office as usual. If the doctor is uncertain about the patient's degree of recovery, it might be prudent to have the patient driven home by a relative or friend. An entry should be placed into the dental progress notes concerning the incident and its management. The recommended management of hyperventilation is outlined in the accompanying box.

Drugs used in management: No drugs are usually required in the management of hyperventilation. In the rare patient who does not respond to conservative management, it may be necessary to administer either diazepam or midazolam.

Medical assistance required: None

Hyperventilation, like vasodepressor syncope, ought not occur a second time in the same patient. Proper management of the fearful dental patient through the use of the various techniques of psychosedation eliminates the occurrence of these two anxiety-produced, potentially life-threatening situations.

MANAGEMENT OF HYPERVENTILATION

Terminate the dental procedure
↓
Position the patient
↓
Remove materials from patient's mouth
↓
Calm patient
↓
Provide basic life support, as indicated
↓
Correct respiratory alkalosis
↓
Drug management (if needed)
↓
Subsequent dental care
↓
Discharge patient

REFERENCES

1. *Mosby's medical & nursing dictionary*, St Louis, 1983, Mosby–Year Book.
2. Paulley JW: Hyperventilation, *Recenti Progressi in Medicina* 81(9):594-600, 1990.
3. Dalessio DJ: Hyperventilation: the vapors, effort syndrome, neurasthenia—anxiety by any other name is just as disturbing, *JAMA* 239:1401, 1978.
4. Dailey RH: Difficulty in breathing. In Schwartz GR et al editors: *Principles and practice of emergency medicine*, Philadelphia, 1978, WB Saunders Co.
5. Missri JC, Alexander S: Hyperventilation syndrome: a brief review, *JAMA* 240:2093, 1978.
6. Lum LC: Hyperventilation: the tip and the iceberg, *J Psychosom Res* 19:375, 1975.
7. Luria MN: Syncope. In Schwartz GR et al editors: *Principles and practice of emergency medicine*, Philadelphia, 1978, WB Saunders Co.
8. Edmeads J: Understanding dizziness: how to decipher this nonspecific symptom, *Postgrad Med* 88(5):255-258, 263-268, 1990.
9. Neill WA, Hattenhauer M: Impairment of myocardial oxygen supply due to hyperventilation, *Circulation* 52:854, 1975.
10. Wheatley CE: Hyperventilation syndrome: a frequent cause of chest pain, *Chest* 68:195, 1975.
11. Beck JG, Berisford MA, Taegtmeyer H: The effects of voluntary hyperventilation on patients with chest pain without coronary artery disease, *Behaviour Research and Therapy* 29(6):611-621, 1991.
12. Divoll M, Greenblatt DJ, Ochs HR, Shader RI: Absolute bioavailability of oral and intramuscular diazepam: effect of age and sex, *Anesth Analg* 62:1, 1983.

13 *Asthma*

Asthma was defined in 1830 by Eberle, a Philadelphia physician, as "a paroxysmal affection of the respiratory organs, characterized by great difficulty of breathing, tightness across the breast, and a sense of impending suffocation, without fever or local inflammation."[1] Today, asthma is defined by the American Thoracic Society as "a disease characterized by an increased responsiveness of the trachea and bronchi to varius stimuli and manifested by widespread narrowing of the airways that changes in severity either spontaneously or as a result of therapy."[2]

It is estimated that asthma affects 5% of adults and between 7% and 10% of children in the United States and Australia.[3] A typical asthmatic patient is usually free of symptoms between acute episodes but exhibits varying degrees of respiratory distress during the acute attack. Although the degree of respiratory distress (dyspnea) is usually moderate, death does occur with asthma, with an estimated annual mortality of 1 in 100,000 persons.[4,5] It is estimated that 5000 to 6000 deaths occur from asthma in the United states annually.[6] Asthma is primarily a disease of younger people with one half of all cases developing before the age of 10 years and another third before the age of 40 years.[5] It also represents the most common chronic disease of childhood. Children with asthma represent a significant number of those making visits to emergency rooms and account for up to 8% of all admissions at one large children's hospital.[7] Acute asthmatic episodes are usually self-limiting; however, there is a clinical entity termed *status asthmaticus,* which may be defined as a persistent exacerbation of asthma.[8] It is potentially life threatening and initially is unresponsive to usually successful therapy, such as the administration of adrenergic bronchodilators such as epinephrine and of theophylline.

PREDISPOSING FACTORS

Asthma is usually classified according to etiologic factors into two major categories: extrinsic and intrinsic. In extrinsic asthma a history of allergy exists, whereas in intrinsic asthma there is no history of allergy. One factor, however, characterizes all asthmatics: an extreme sensitivity of the airways characterized not only by an increased contractile response of the airway smooth muscle, but also by an abnormal generation and clearance of secretions and an abnormally sensitive cough reflex.

Extrinsic Asthma

Extrinsic asthma, also known as allergic asthma, accounts for 50% of asthmatics and is more often observed in children and younger adults. Most patients with this form of asthma demonstrate an inherited allergic predisposition. Acute asthmatic episodes may be precipitated in these individuals by the inhalation of specific allergens. These allergens may be airborne, such as house dust, feathers, animal dander, furniture stuffing, fungal spores, and a wide variety of plant pollens.[9] Foods and drugs may also precipitate this form of asthmatic attack. Highly allergenic foods include cow's milk, eggs, fish, chocolate, shellfish, and tomatoes. Penicillin,[10] vaccines, aspirin,[11] and sulfites[12,13] are commonly implicated drugs and chemicals. Bronchospasm usually develops within minutes after exposure to the allergen (antigen). This is a type I hypersensitivity reaction in which immunoglobulin E (IgE) antibodies are produced in response to the allergen. Allergic reactions are discussed in detail in Chapter 24.

Acute episodes of extrinsic asthma usually occur with diminishing frequency and severity during middle and late adolescence and may disappear entirely later in life. Approximately 50% of asthmatic children become asymptomatic before adulthood.[14] It is possible, however, for extrinsic asthma to become chronic. This is apparently much more common when the asthma originally develops in early childhood and when it is associated with eczema.

Intrinsic Asthma

The second major category, accounting for approximately 50% of asthmatics, is intrinsic asthma. Intrinsic asthma usually develops in adults after the age of 35 years. Episodes are precipitated by non-allergic factors, including respiratory infection,[15] physical exertion,[16] environmental and air pollution,[17] and occupational stimuli.[18] Synonyms for this type of asthma include nonallergic asthma, idiopathic asthma, and infective asthma. There is usually a negative history to allergy, and the results of allergy testing (e.g., skin tests) are usually negative. Viral infection of the respiratory tract is the most common causative factor. Viral infections are known to enhance airway reactivity in both asthmatics[19] as well as in nonasthmatics.[20] In exercise-induced asthma (EIA) symptoms begin within 6 to 10 minutes after the start of exercise, followed by a more severe delayed phase of bronchospasm developing at the termination of physical activity. The entire episode classically lasts between 30 to 60 minutes without drug intervention and is seen in all age groups and both sexes.[16]

Psychologic and physiologic stress must not be discounted as important contributory factors in precipitating an asthmatic episode in susceptible individuals.[21] In children with asthma, acute episodes are frequently seen during or after a disciplinary session with a parent.[22] The dental environment is another common site for asthmatic attacks.[23] The asthmatic child may develop an acute episode when escorted into the treatment room. A dramatic resolution of acute signs and symptoms usually occurs by simply removing the child from

---

ETIOLOGIC FACTORS IN ACUTE ASTHMA

Allergy (antigen-antibody reaction)
Respiratory infection
Physical exertion
Environmental and air pollution
Occupational stimuli
Pharmacologic stimuli
Psychologic factors

---

the treatment area.[24] Psychologic factors may also be important in adult asthmatics. Stressful situations, such as dental appointments, produce symptoms in many adult asthmatics. The author has observed asthmatic dental students, who are usually well controlled, experience periods of chronic bronchospasm during final examination week. Fig. 13-1 illustrates a simplified view of the mechanisms involved in asthma.

Acute episodes of intrinsic asthma are usually more fulminant and severe than those of allergic (extrinsic) asthma. The long-term prognosis of infective asthma is also poorer because the disease usually becomes chronic and the patient eventually exhibits clinical signs and symptoms (e.g., cough and sputum production) in the intervals between acute episodes.[25] The accompanying box summarizes the etiologic factors involved in the production of acute episodes of asthma.

Mixed Asthma

Mixed asthma refers to a combination of allergic and infective asthma. In this form the major precipitating factor is the presence of infection, especially of the respiratory tract.

Status Asthmaticus

The most severe clinical form of asthma, with symptoms of wheezing, dyspnea, hypoxia, and

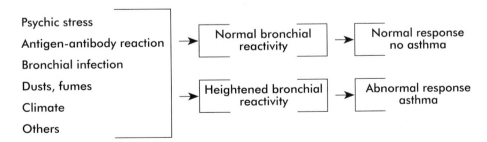

Fig. 13-1. Predisposing factors for asthma. (After Pain MCE: The treatment of asthma, *Drugs* 6:118, 1973.)

Table 13-1. Bronchodilators employed in long-term prophylaxis

Category	Drug generic	Proprietary
Bronchodilators, sympathomimetic	albuterol	Proventil, Ventolin
	metaproterenol	Alupent, Metapent
	pirbuterol	Maxair
	terbutaline	Brethaire, Brethine, Bricanyl
	isoetharine	Bronkometer, Bronkosol
	isoproterenol	Isuprel and others
	epinephrine	many brand names
Anticholinergics	ipratopium bromide	Atrovent
	atropine sulfate	—
Theophyllines	theophylline	many brand names
	aminophylline	—
Antimediators	cromolyn sodium	Intal
Corticosteroids	prednisone	many brands
	methylprednisolone sodium succinate	several brand names
	hydrocortisone sodium succinate	several brand names
	beclomethasone dipropionate	Beclovent, Vanceril
	triamcinolone acetonide	Azmacort

others that are refractory to two to three doses of β-adrenergic agents, is termed *status asthmaticus*.[26] Status asthmaticus is a true medical emergency; if not managed adequately or promptly, the patient may die from the respiratory changes that develop secondary to respiratory distress (e.g., hypotension and respiratory acidosis produced by hypoxemia and hypercapnia).

PREVENTION

The physician's goal in the long-term management of a patient with asthma is to maintain the patient's pulmonary status as close to normal as possible, for as much of the time as is possible. With the advent of newer and longer-acting medications, this goal has become more achievable. A second factor that has helped to achieve this goal is the recognition that the pulmonary status of most asthmatic patients is far from normal in the period between acute episodes.

The goal in dental management of the patient with asthma is prevention of acute episodes of the disease. This is best accomplished with information obtained from the patient's medical history and the dialogue history between doctor and patient.

Medical History Questionnaire

The University of Southern California (USC) medical history questionnaire contains several questions that relate to a prior history of asthma, hay fever, and allergy.

QUESTION 6. Have you taken any medicine or drugs during the past 2 years?

COMMENT. Many patients with asthma, especially children, take oral drugs in the periods between acute episodes in an effort to prevent or to reduce the frequency of recurrences. There are five categories of such drugs commonly employed: β-adrenergic agonists, methylxanthines, chromones, corticosteroids, and anticholinergics. These agents normally will have little effect on the planned dental care. Some of the more commonly prescribed bronchodilating drugs are listed in Table 13-1.

Long-term therapy with corticosteroids is employed in patients for whom acute episodes occur frequently in spite of the therapy already mentioned. Glucocorticosteroids have been used in the treatment of asthma since 1950. Their beneficial effects are probably related to their antiinflammatory actions as they have little or no direct bronchodilating activity.[27] Patients receiving long-term corticosteroid therapy should be carefully evaluated for possible adrenal cortical insufficiency.

A recent addition to the preventive management of acute asthmatic episodes is the chromone, cromolyn sodium (Intal). It is used primarily in patients with allergic (extrinsic) asthma. It is effective only during periods of remission in preventing recurrences and decreasing the patient's requirement for corticosteroids. Cromolyn sodium is administered by inhalation as a micronized powder.

In addition, most asthmatic patients will have in their possession drugs that are used to terminate acute episodes. Most commonly, nebulized epinephrine, isoproterenol, or albuterol are used. These are discussed beginning on p. 204.

QUESTION 9. Circle any of the following that you have had or have at present:

Asthma

Hay fever

Allergy

COMMENT. An affirmative response to any part of this question should lead to an in-depth dialogue history, during which the doctor seeks more information concerning the severity of the patient's asthma.

Dialogue History

QUESTION. **Do you have asthma?**

ANSWER. Yes.

QUESTION. **What type of asthma do you have: allergic (extrinsic) or nonallergic (intrinsic)?**

COMMENT. Patients are usually aware of the type of asthma from which they suffer.

QUESTION. **At what age did you first develop asthma?**

COMMENT. Allergic asthma most often develops in children and younger adults, whereas nonallergic asthma more commonly develops in persons over the age of 35 years.

QUESTION. **How often do you develop acute episodes?**

COMMENT. Determine the frequency of acute asthmatic episodes. The more frequent the occurrence of these episodes, the greater the likelihood that such an episode will develop during dental therapy.

QUESTION. **What precipitates your acute asthmatic attacks?**

COMMENT. Awareness of the factors involved in precipitating a patient's acute attacks is valuable in preventing such episodes during dental care. Of particular importance is the role played by stress. Stress is an important factor in provoking acute attacks in both extrinsic and intrinsic asthma sufferers. Therefore, the patient's outlook toward dentistry must be determined and steps taken to make dental appointments as stress free as possible. The stress reduction protocol should be used (see Chapter 2).

QUESTION. **How do you manage your acute asthmatic attacks?**

COMMENT. Determine which drugs the patient uses to terminate the acute episode. Most patients carry their medications with them at all times. Have the patient show you the medications, make note of them, and direct the patient to have them available at every dental office visit. These medications, usually nebulized β-adrenergic agonists, should be available at each dental appointment and kept within reach throughout the appointment. Frequent reminders to the patient are often necessary as past experience has demonstrated that many asthma sufferers will forget to bring their medication with them to their dental appointments.

QUESTION. **Have you ever required emergency care or hospitalization for your acute asthmatic episodes?**

COMMENT. This question seeks to determine the severity of the acute episodes. Although most episodes are readily terminated following bronchodilator administration, status asthmaticus is refractory to the usual β-adrenergic therapy. Hospitalization of the patient is normally required in these instances. With a history of prior need for emergency medical assistance or hospitalization, the dentist would be more likely to seek out such assistance earlier in an acute episode (see text that follows) than in a situation in which a patient has never required emergency care.

DENTAL THERAPY CONSIDERATIONS

Modifications in dental care depend on the severity of the asthma. Acute episodes precipitated by emotional stress in a patient with many fears of dentistry require judicious handling by the doctor to prevent an acute asthmatic attack. Use of the stress reduction protocol minimizes the likelihood of acute episodes.

There is no contraindication to the use of any conscious sedation technique in the fearful asthmatic patient except for some drug groups such as barbiturates and narcotics, especially meperidine. Barbiturates and narcotics may increase the risk of bronchospasm in a susceptible patient. Narcotics, especially meperidine, may provoke histamine release, which can lead to bronchospasm.[28] Barbiturates may sensitize the respiratory reflexes, increasing the risk of bronchospasms.[29] Both drug groups are therefore relatively contraindicated in asthmatics. Inhalation sedation with nitrous oxide and oxygen, oral sedation with benzodiazepines, and parenteral sedation via the intravenous or intramuscular routes are not contraindicated in the apprehensive asthmatic.

On rare occasion a dentist will be advised by a patient's physician that nitrous oxide administration is contraindicated. This statement is unfounded. Inhalation anesthetic agents, such as ether, that irritate the respiratory mucosa are capable of inducing bronchospasm in these patients.[30] Nitrous oxide is not irritating to the respiratory mucosa, is an excellent antianxiety agent, does not provoke acute asthmatic episodes, and is absolutely indicated for the management of dental fears in this patient population.[31] An asthmatic who also happens to be claustrophobic, might be at increased risk with use of the nasal hood for delivery of anesthetic gases. A nasal cannula, though no longer the preferred means of gas delivery, should be used.

If the patient has extrinsic asthma, care must be taken to eliminate provoking allergens from the dental environment. Drugs that might be implicated in precipitating acute episodes should be avoided in these patients. Aspirin and nonsteroidal antiinflammatory drugs (NSAIDs) and penicillin are the most commonly prescribed drugs that can precipitate acute asthmatic episodes. Bisulfites must also be considered. Bronchospasm induced by aspirin sensitivity is most often noted in adults, but can also develop in children.[11,32] The prevalence of aspirin sensitivity in asthmatics ranges from 3% to 19%.[21] However, in patients with nasal polyps and pansinusitus, the incidence of aspirin sensitivity is 30% to 40%.[33] Substitutes may be prescribed in place of these drugs, but because there is considerable cross-sensitivity between aspirin and other nonsteroidal antiinflammatory compounds, care must be exercised when prescribing analgesics. NSAIDs include indomethacin, fenoprofen, naproxen, ibuprofen, mefenamic acid, sulindac, meclofenamate, tolmetin, piroxicam, oxyphenbutazone, and phenylbutazone.[34]

Sulfur dioxide and other sulfiting agents have been used by the food industry for years to preserve foods. Numerous cases of death and other severe reactions have been reported predominantly among persons with asthma or sensitivity to sulfites following their ingestion at restaurants. These reactions have included urticaria, gastrointestinal upset, bronchospasm, and anaphylactic shock.[12]

Sulfiting agents, such as sodium metabisulfite, are added to certain drugs and chemicals to serve as antioxidants. Asthmatic reactions (bronchospasm) have occurred upon inhalation of isoe-

tharine (Bronkosol)[35] and isoproterenol (Isuprel).[36] Local anesthetics that contain vasopressors (e.g., epinephrine, levonordefrin) have bisulfites added to prevent oxidation of the vasopressor.[37] Though the volume of bisulfite present in the local anesthetic cartridge is minimal, acute asthmatic attacks have been reported following their administration to sensitive patients.[38] The use of local anesthetics containing bisulfites (i.e., vasopressor-containing drugs) is absolutely contraindicated in these patients. Local anesthetics without vasopressors (e.g., lidocaine plain, mepivacaine plain, prilocaine plain) should be used instead in these patients.

Table 13-2 classifies asthmatics by American Society of Anesthesiologists (ASA) physical status. The typical, well-controlled, easily managed asthmatic represents an ASA II risk during dental care. Asthmatics who experience acute episodes precipitated by stress or exercise (i.e., EIA), or who have required emergency care or hospitalization to terminate their acute episodes, may be considered ASA III risks, whereas those very few asthmatics exhibiting clinical symptomatology while at rest are ASA IV risks.

CLINICAL MANIFESTATIONS

Signs and symptoms of an asthmatic attack range in severity from acute episodes consisting of shortness of breath, wheezing, and cough, followed by complete remission (ASA II or III), to a more chronic state in which clinical signs and symptoms are almost continuously present and vary in intensity (ASA IV). An acute asthmatic attack may be an intensely terrifying experience for the patient. There is a large psychologic component in most episodes of asthma because the patient is fearful

Table 13-2. ASA classification: asthma

ASA class	Description	Treatment modifications
II	Typical asthmatic—extrinsic or intrinsic Infrequent episodes Easily managed No need for emergency care or hospitalization	1. Reduce stress, as needed 2. Determine triggering factors 3. Avoid triggering factors 4. Have bronchodilator available during treatment
III	Exercise-induced asthma (EIA) Fearful patient Prior need for emergency care or hospitalization	1. Follow ASA II modifications, 2. Administer sedation—inhalation with N_2O-O_2 or oral benzodiazepines, if indicated
IV	Chronic signs and symptoms of asthma present at rest	1. Obtain medical consultation prior to start of treatment 2. Provide emergency care only in office 3. Defer elective care until respiratory status improves or until patient can be treated in controlled environment

of their inability to breathe normally. Symptoms of acute asthma classically consist of a triad including cough, dyspnea, and wheezing.

Usual Clinical Progression

Signs and symptoms of acute asthma may develop gradually or suddenly. In the typical episode the patient becomes aware of a sensation of thickness or congestion in the chest. This is followed by a spell of coughing, which may or may not be associated with sputum production,[39] and wheezing, which is audible upon both inspiration and expiration. These symptoms tend to increase in intensity as the episode continues. The patient experiences a variable degree of dyspnea, and it is noted that in most episodes the asthmatic patient sits up as if fighting for air. Although the expiratory phase of the respiratory cycle is actually more difficult than the inspiratory phase for the majority of asthmatics, subjectively, many asthmatics feel that inspiration is more difficult and frequently state that they do not know where their next breath is coming from. Air-trapping within the lungs occurs during the acute episode and asthmatics will sit up and use accessory muscles of respiration (i.e., sternocleidomastoid and scalenus muscles) to lift the entire rib cage cephalad and generate high negative intrapleural pressures, thus increasing the work involved in breathing.[40]

Wheezing does not by itself designate the presence, severity, or duration of asthma.[41] The degree of wheezing noted or its absence varies according to the radius of the bronchial tube. Mild wheezing is an audible, low-pitched, coarse, discontinuous noise, whereas with increasing airway obstruction, it becomes more high-pitched and musical, but is still a low-intensity sound. With severe airway obstruction, wheezing vanishes because there is insufficient air movement velocity to produce sound.[42,43]

As the degree of dyspnea increases, so do the levels of patient anxiety and apprehension. Breathing during an acute asthmatic attack is labored, with the respiratory rate increasing to more than 20 breaths per minute in most episodes, but to less than 40 breaths per minute with more severe asthma. This may be the result of apprehension, airway obstruction, or a change in blood chemistry. Blood pressure may remain at approximately the baseline level with milder episodes, although it usually rises, reflecting the increased blood level of catecholamines produced by anxiety. In addition, the heart rate increases. A rate in excess of 120 beats per minute is common in more severe asthma.

Other clinical signs that may be present during an acute episode, which are not diagnostic of asthma but are signs of respiratory distress, include diaphoresis; agitation; somnolence or confusion; cyanosis; soft tissue retraction in the intercostal and supraclavicular regions; and nasal flaring.[44]

If left untreated, the acute asthmatic episode just described may last for a period of minutes to several hours. Termination of the attack is usually heralded by a period of intense coughing with expectoration of a thick, tenacious, mucous plug. This is followed immediately by a sensation of relief and a "clearing" of the air passages. Proper management with an aerosol spray usually aborts the attack within seconds. A summary of the clinical signs and symptoms of acute asthma is found in the box.

Acute asthma, whatever the precipitating cause, is characterized by airway smooth muscle spasm, airway inflammation with edema, and mucous hypersecretion. Smooth muscle spasm probably accounts for the rapidly reversible types of airway obstruction, whereas inflammatory edema and mucous plugging of the airways account for the nonresponsive forms of asthma.[45]

Status Asthmaticus

Status asthmaticus is a clinical state in which a patient with moderate to severe bronchial obstruction fails to respond significantly to the rapid-acting beta-agonist agents administered in the initial treatment protocol. In this situation bronchospasm may

---

SIGNS AND SYMPTOMS OF ACUTE ASTHMA

Feeling of chest congestion
Cough, with or without sputum production
Wheezing
Dyspnea
Patient sits up
Use of accessory muscles of respiration
Increased anxiety and apprehension
Tachypnea (>20 to >40, if severe)
Blood pressure—baseline to elevated
Heart rate—increased (>120 in severe episodes)
Diaphoresis
Agitation
Somnolence
Confusion
Cyanosis
Supraclavicular and/or intercostal retraction
Nasal flaring

continue for hours or even days without remission. Patients in status asthmaticus most commonly exhibit signs of extreme fatigue, dehydration, severe hypoxia, cyanosis, peripheral vascular shock, and drug intoxication from intensive pharmacologic therapy. Blood pressure may be at or below baseline levels, and the heart rate is quite rapid. The patient in status asthmaticus requires hospitalization because the condition is life threatening. Chronic partial airway obstruction may lead to death from fatigue of the muscles of respiration and respiratory acidosis. Status asthmaticus may develop in any asthmatic patient.

PATHOPHYSIOLOGY

Regardless of the type of asthma present, one finding common to all asthmatics is an extreme sensitivity of the airways characterized not only by increased contractile response of the airway smooth muscle, but also by an abnormal generation and clearance of secretions and an abnormally sensitive cough reflex.[43]

Neural Control of Airways

The autonomic nervous system maintains a significant influence upon airway reactivity. Stimulation of the vagus nerve releases acetylcholine, which produces a maximal constriction of airways with an initial diameter of 3 to 5 mm,[46] increases glandular or goblet cell secretion, and dilates pulmonary vessels.[47] This vagally mediated reflex bronchoconstriction may result from stimulation of receptors found in the larynx, lower airways, chemoreceptors, and the subepithelial irritant receptors.[48]

In the adrenergic nervous system, stimulation of beta receptors results in dilation of the airway smooth muscle and bronchial and pulmonary vascular beds. Additionally, ion and water transport into the airway lumen is facilitated, and glandular secretion is likewise stimulated.[48,49] Stimulation of sympathetic nerves innervating the proximal airways has been shown to provide minimal bronchodilation,[47] and it is therefore most likely that the preponderance of the β_2-adrenergic airway receptor stimulation occurs as a result of systemic catecholamine release from the adrenal medulla.[50] Stimulation of α-adrenergic receptors results in bronchial smooth muscle constriction; however, significant α-adrenergic contractile effects are not observed clinically except under conditions of beta-blockade.[51]

The neural component in the pathogenesis of airway hyperreactivity may be summarized as follows.[43] Vagal sensory receptors in airways with increased bronchomotor response (from viral respiratory tract infections and exposure to oxidant air pollutants) are stimulated and produce constriction; there may also be a failure of the normal homeostatic dilator responses (e.g., β_2-blockade provokes bronchoconstriction in asthmatics but not in normal subjects[43]); and other possibilities are currently being investigated.[21]

Airway inflammation is another factor considered important in the production of increased airway responsiveness. This may result from either immunologic or nonimmunologic airway insults, which produce airway edema and the emigration of inflammatory cells into the lumen through the epithelium.[43] Inflammation is associated with an opening of tight cellular junctions and an increase in mucosal permeability, providing access from the lumen to airway smooth muscle, submucosal mast cells, and irritant subepithelial receptors.[52] This could then provide the environment for multiple methods of inducing airway obstruction, including direct effect on smooth muscle, stimulation of mast cells, or vagal reflexes.[43]

Immunologic Responses

It is thought that allergic or presumed allergic factors are involved in the majority of asthma cases.[39] These factors may induce bronchial hyperreactivity, trigger acute episodes, or both. Extrinsic asthma is classified as a type I immune reaction, which is an immediate allergic reaction in which an antigen combines with IgE antibody present on the surface of pulmonary mast cells located in the submucosa of small peripheral airways and in larger central areas at the luminal surface interdigitating with the epithelium.[53] This causes mast cell degranulation and the release or the formation of a number of chemical mediators. These mediators include histamine, prostaglandins, acetylcholine, bradykinin, eosinophilic chemotactic factors, and the leukotrienes (LT).[54] Slow reacting substance of anaphylaxis (SRS-A) has been shown to be composed of leukotrienes LTC, LTD, and LTE. In humans, LTC and LTD are the most potent bronchoconstrictor substances yet described—approximately 1000 times more potent than histamine[55]—with a duration of effect from 15 to 20 minutes.[56]

The physiologic actions of these mediators will be presented in Chapter 24. At this point it is important to note that, once released by the mast cells, the pharmacologic activity of these mediators develops rapidly so that clinical symptoms and signs of the acute asthmatic reaction are readily evident. Type I allergic reactions are characterized by rapidity of reaction time (within 15 to 30 minutes after exposure to the allergen) and are associated with IgE. Clinical examples of the type I immune response include asthma, anaphylaxis, and hay fever.

In intrinsic or nonallergic asthma, although the primary provoking factor may vary (e.g., psychologic stress, physical exertion, cold, irritating inhalants), the chemical mediators and the pathologic conditions seen during the acute episode are similar to those seen in extrinsic asthma. In general, acute episodes of either form of asthma are virtually indistinguishable clinically.

Bronchospasm

Smooth muscle is present throughout the tracheobronchial tree.[57] Bronchial smooth muscle tone is regulated by the vagus nerve, which, when stimulated, causes constriction, and by the sympathetic nervous system, which produces dilation.[43] In nonasthmatic patients bronchial smooth muscle plays a role in protecting the lungs from foreign stimuli. This role involves a degree of narrowing (bronchial smooth muscle constriction) of the airways in response to these foreign stimuli. In the asthmatic patient, however, there is an exaggerated response (more intense constriction), leading to clinical signs and symptoms of respiratory distress. This is most prominent in the small bronchi (0.4 to 0.1 cm in diameter) and bronchioles (0.15 to 0.1 cm in diameter); however, smooth muscle constriction may occur wherever smooth muscle is present. The site of the asthmatic reaction can therefore vary, depending on the anatomic location of the bronchial smooth muscle that is stimulated.

Stimulation of irritant receptors by foreign particles (e.g., gases, pollens, and chemical mediators) initiates an autonomic or vagal reflex. The stimulus is carried by the afferent fibers in the vagus nerve to the central nervous system and then by the efferent fibers, again in the vagus nerve, returning to the lungs; there the efferent fibers terminate on bronchial smooth muscle, producing muscle constriction.

Bronchial Wall Edema and Hypersecretion of Mucous Glands

In gross and microscopic sections of lungs of patients who have died during asthmatic episodes (usually status asthmaticus), the following changes are evident: mucosal and submucosal edema and thickening of the basement membrane, infiltration by leukocytes (primarily eosinophils), intraluminal mucous plugs, and bronchospasm (see Fig. 13-2).[9] When examined in gross section, the lungs appear overdistended, and many of the smaller bronchi

are occluded by mucous plugs. In spite of the overall appearance of overinflation, there are areas of hyperinflation alternating with areas of atelectasis produced by mucous plugs. All of these factors lead to a decrease in the size of the airway lumen, an increase in airway resistance, and clinical manifestations related to the degree of narrowing. Airway resistance varies inversely to the fourth power of the radius. Therefore, halving the radius of an airway leads to a sixteenfold increase in airway resistance (according to Poiseuille's approximation).[58] The result of this increased resistance is increased difficulty in gas exchange and, ultimately, in alterations of blood chemistry and pH.

Breathing
Nonasthmatic Patient

In the nonasthmatic individual breathing is composed of two phases: inspiration and expiration. The inspiratory phase is an active process. Thoracic volume increases as the diaphragm and other inspiratory muscles function. With this increase in volume the intrapleural pressure becomes more negative (going from -2 to -6 torr), and the lungs expand in an attempt to fill the increasing chest volume. Air is then drawn into the lungs until these pressures are equalized.[59]

The expiratory phase of breathing is normally a passive process that does not require the expenditure of muscular energy. As the muscles of respiration relax, the elastic tissues of the lungs, which have been stretched on inspiration, are able to return to their normal unstretched state—a process termed *elastic recoil*. This shortening of fibers forces air out of the lungs, which permits the thorax to return to its normal resting state.

Asthmatic Patient

In the asthmatic patient varying degrees of airway obstruction exist that may produce large increases in airway resistance. As airway resistance increases, air flow during inspiration and expiration is compromised. To accommodate this increased resistance during inspiration, the work of the muscles of respiration is increased in order to produce a greater degree of chest expansion to permit more air to enter the lungs.

It is during the expiratory phase of respiration that the deleterious effects of increased airway resistance occur in the majority of asthmatics. The elastic recoil of the lungs during expiration is no longer adequate to expel air against the increased airway resistance, and air is trapped in the patient's lungs, producing hyperinflation.[60] To minimize this, the normally passive expiratory phase becomes active with both the respiratory and accessory muscles of respiration being used to expel air from the lungs.[61] In addition, ventilation, or the quantity of air exchanged per unit of time, is impaired because of increased resistance. This leads to the commonly observed increase in the rate of breathing (tachypnea).

As the asthmatic episode progresses and the airway obstruction worsens, the expiratory phase of respiration tends to become longer and air becomes increasingly trapped in the lungs. This leads to hyperinflation of alveoli, which tends to produce an increase in airway diameter from increased tension on the one hand, and to cause increased energy utilization on the other. This increase in energy utilization is necessary during the inspiratory phase to overcome the tension of the already stretched elastic tissues of the lungs and to allow air to enter the lungs.

It can therefore be seen that if an acute asthmatic episode is permitted to continue unresolved, a good deal of energy will be expended on the work of respiration. The muscles of respiration will eventually fatigue, further decreasing respiratory efficiency and leading to hypoventilation of alveoli.[62] This will be seen clinically as increased dyspnea, tachypnea, and possibly cyanosis. When severe, alveolar hypoventilation produces carbon dioxide retention or hypercarbia, which is manifested by an increase in the rate and depth of respiration (i.e., hyperventilation) and a further increase in the work of breathing. Sweating or diaphoresis is another clinical sign of hypercarbia.

This process is self-limiting. If the airway obstruction continues to worsen and the work of breathing continues to increase, increasing levels of hypercarbia and hypoxemia lead to a state of acute respiratory acidosis. Table 13-3 lists signs and symptoms associated with hypoxemia and hypercarbia. Respiratory failure may occur, and the patient will require artificial ventilation. The mortality rate in this stage is high.

To conclude this section, let us review the pathophysiology of two degrees of asthmatic episode: mild and severe.

In the mild asthmatic attack, produced primarily by bronchospasm, the moderate airway obstruction present leads to a decrease in blood oxygenation. The ensuing hypoxia and increased respiratory workload lead to a heightened level of anxiety, producing hyperventilation. Hyperventilation leads to a decrease in the carbon dioxide level in the blood (i.e., hypocapnia) and respiratory alkalosis. (Refer to Chapter 12 for a discussion of hyperventilation.)

Table 13-3. Clinical signs and symptoms of hypoxia and hypercarbia

Hypoxia	*Hypercarbia*
Restlessness, confusion, anxiety	Diaphoresis
Cyanosis	Hypertension (converting to hypotension if progressive)
Diaphoresis (sweating)	Hyperventilation
Tachycardia, cardiac arrhythmias	Headache
Hypertension or hypotension	Confusion, somnolence
Coma	Cardiac failure
Cardiac or renal failure	

In the more severe asthmatic episode (greater influence of airway inflammation) or in status asthmaticus, the greater degree of bronchial obstruction present causes a more profound decrease in blood oxgenation. The respiratory workload increases; however, these responses soon become ineffective (the asthmatic becomes fatigued) as the obstruction becomes greater, leading to inadequate ventilation and carbon dioxide retention or hypercapnia. Hypercapnia causes respiratory acidosis and may lead to respiratory failure. These changes that develop in moderate and severe asthma are compared in Table 13-4.

MANAGEMENT
Acute Asthmatic Attack

Management of the acute asthmatic episode requires prompt specific drug therapy as well as symptomatic management.

Step 1: Terminate the dental procedure.

Step 2: Position the patient. Upon recognition of the acute asthmatic episode, the patient should be placed in any comfortable position. This will usually be a sitting position with the arms thrown forward (Fig. 13-2). Other positions are equally acceptable, based upon the comfort of the patient.

Step 3: Remove dental materials from the patient's mouth.

Step 4: Calm the patient. Many asthmatics, especially those who have a history of easily managed bronchospasm, will remain calm throughout the episode. Others, primarily those with acute episodes that have been more difficult to terminate, may exhibit varying degrees of apprehension.

Step 5: Basic life support, as indicated. During an acute asthmatic episode, the patient is conscious, breathes with a partially obstructed airway, and has an increased blood pressure and heart rate.

Step 6: Administer bronchodilator. Before the start

Table 13-4. Physiologic changes developing in moderate and severe asthma*

Severity of airway obstruction	PaO₂	PaCO₂	pH	Base excess
Mild	WNL	L	I	Respiratory alkalosis
Moderate	LL	WNL or L	WNL or I	Normal
Severe	LLL	I	L	Metabolic acidosis
				Respiratory acidosis

From Barkin RM, Rosen P: *Emergency pediatrics*, ed 3, 1990, St Louis, Mosby–Year Book.
*WNL, within normal limits; L, lowered; I, increased.

of dental treatment in an asthmatic patient, the doctor should place the patient's aerosol spray of bronchodilator medication in a place within easy reach. When required, the patient's medication should be used to manage an acute episode.

It is suggested that the patient be reminded prior to each office visit to bring the aerosol inhaler. Experience has demonstrated that too many patients will forget their medication unless they are reminded regularly. (See Fig. 13-3.)

Bronchodilators are the drugs employed to manage the acute asthmatic episode. The most potent and effective dilators of bronchial smooth muscle are the β-adrenergic agonists, such as epinephrine (Adrenalin), isoproterenol (Isuprel), and metaproterenol (Alupent). These are agonists of β₂-receptors in the bronchial smooth muscle and relax bronchial, vascular, and uterine smooth muscle. In addition, β₂-stimulation inhibits histamine release from mast cells, antibody production by lymphocytes, and enzyme release from polymorphonuclear leukocytes.[63] These agents may be administered orally, sublingually, by aerosol inhalation, or by injection. Though the subcutaneous injection of epinephrine provides a rapid onset of relief, it is also associated with many other systemic actions, some of which may be undesirable, such as dysrhythmias, or hypertensive reactions, especially in patients receiving monoamine oxidase (MAO)-in-

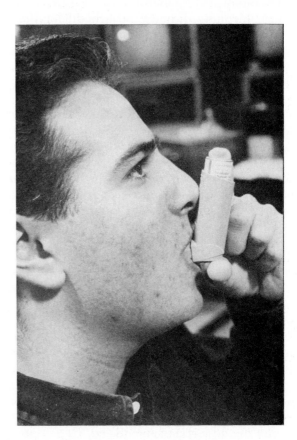

Fig. 13-2. Position for patient having acute asthmatic attack.

Fig. 13-3. Patient using aerosol inhaler.

hibitors or tricyclic antidepressants.[64] Clinically, the best method to achieve the desired result of bronchial smooth muscle dilation is to administer β-adrenergic agonists via the inhalation of aerosolized sprays. This method provides an equally rapid onset of action, but minimizes systemic absorption and side effects.[65] It is stated that aerosolized adrenergic bronchodilators are as effective as those administered intravenously but with much less potential for serious side effects.[66]

The patient should be given the inhaler of medication and be permitted to take the usual dose required to terminate the acute episode. Before administering a bronchodilator, it is important for the patient and doctor to read the package insert accompanying such medication, because there are strict limitations on the maximal quantity that may be safely administered within a given time period. Untoward reactions associated with the use of these drugs relate primarily to the $β_1$- and α-receptor−stimulating actions of epinephrine and isoproterenol. Metaproterenol is a partially selective $β_2$-agonist with little or no $β_1$- and α-stimulating properties. The incidence of side effects (tachycardia 4%) is minimal.[67] Albuterol is a very selective, fast acting, and long duration bronchodilator that is associated with minimal side effects.[68] It was selected by this author as the bronchodilator of choice for inclusion in the office emergency kit, if one chooses to include this category of drug.

Epinephrine and isoproterenol produce palpitation, tachycardia, and disturbances of cardiac rhythm and rate. In addition epinephrine may produce headache and increased anxiety. Epinephrine is contraindicated in asthmatic patients with concomitant high blood pressure; diabetes mellitus (because epinephrine produces hyperglycemia); hyperthyroidism; and ischemic heart disease. Albuterol is much more frequently recommended for use in acute asthma in patients with concomitant medical problems. Another factor to consider when employing these medications is that their use for prolonged periods (from months to years) may produce a state of refractoriness, which will lead to prolonged and not easily terminated episodes of asthma (status asthmaticus). Therefore, these agents, although highly effective in managing the acute asthmatic attack, should be used judiciously.

Aerosolized bronchodilators are usually administered via a Freon-pressurized canister in a metered-dose form. When administered, only about 10% of the dose is actually inhaled.[69] The remaining drug is impacted in the oropharynx, with most swallowed and biotransformed upon passage through the liver.

Proper use of the aerosol inhaler requires a very slow inhalation of the spray—approximately 5 to 6 seconds for the inhalation. This should be done as if sipping hot soup. This is followed by a breath-hold at total lung capacity for 10 seconds and then a slow exhalation through pursed lips.[70] The onset of action of aerosolized bronchodilators is rather rapid, with some improvement often noted within as little as 15 seconds.

Step 7: Subsequent dental care. Once the acute asthmatic episode is terminated, the doctor should determine the cause of the attack. Appropriate steps in the stress reduction protocol should be considered as a means of diminishing the risk of additional episodes arising. The planned dental treatment may continue at this visit if both the patient and the doctor feel it appropriate.

Step 8: Discharge from the office. Following resolution of the acute asthmatic attack, the patient may be discharged from the dental office without escort if, in the opinion of the doctor, the patient is in good condition. This will usually be the case with acute episodes that are readily terminated with bronchodilator therapy.

Severe Acute Asthmatic Attack

Management of the more severe acute asthmatic attack mimics the milder episode initially:

Step 1: Terminate dental therapy.

Step 2: Position patient in the most comfortable position.

Step 3: Remove materials from patient's mouth.

Step 4: Calm patient.

Step 5: Basic life support, as indicated.

Step 6: Administer bronchodilator via inhalation.

In situations in which several administered doses of the aerosolized bronchodilator have failed to terminate the acute episode, consideration should be given to several additional steps of management:

Step 7: Administer oxygen. The administration of oxygen may be considered during any acute asthmatic episode. It may be administered by means of a full face mask, nasal hood, or nasal cannula. The presence of any clinical signs and symptoms of hypoxia and hypercarbia (see Table 13-3) are indications for oxygen administration. With a nasal cannula or nasal hood, a flow of 5 to 7 L per minute should be administered.

Step 8: Summon medical assistance. In situations in which aerosolized bronchodilators have failed to effectively resolve bronchospasm, medical assistance should be summoned.

Step 9: Administer parenteral bronchodilators. For management of the more severe asthmatic episode or in those milder episodes that prove refractory to aerosol medications, the injection of aqueous epinephrine is indicated. For the basic emergency kit, epinephrine is available in a preloaded syringe containing 1 mL of a 1:1000 dilution, whereas for more advanced kits epinephrine might also be available in a 1:10,000 concentration (in a 10-mL syringe). These are equivalent to 1 mg of epinephrine. (See Fig. 13-4).

For the adult patient, the usual subcutaneous or intramuscular dose of epinephrine (1:1000 dilution) is 0.3 mL, or 3 mL of 1:10,000 intravenously, which may be repeated as necessary every 30 to 60 minutes.

Asthmatic children often cease to have acute symptoms when they are removed from the treatment environment. Should this simple measure prove ineffective, the injection of 0.125 to 0.25 mg of aqueous epinephrine is indicated.

Step 10: Administer intravenous medications (optional). Patients who prove refractory to the commonly employed bronchodilators require additional drug therapy to terminate the acute asthmatic episode. Drugs employed in these circumstances include isoproterenol HCl and corticosteroids (i.e., hydrocortisone sodium succinate,

100 to 200 mg intravenously). If the doctor has received advanced training in emergency medicine and is able to start an intravenous infusion, these agents should be considered for inclusion in the office emergency kit.

Isoproterenol is administered when respiratory failure is imminent in spite of prior agressive therapy with aerosols. When isoproterenol is administered, the patient must be monitored closely because it is highly dysrhythmogenic.[71]

Corticosteroids have been considered important drugs in the management of severe acute asthma for over 40 years. Though they have little direct bronchodilating activity, it is felt that their antiinflammatory properties make their early administration during severe acute asthma important. Following intravenous administration, improvements in pulmonary function are noted within 1 hour, usually peaking in 6 to 8 hours.[72] There is a general consensus that "the early administration of steroids is perhaps the most important therapeutic measure to be taken in severe and resistant asthma, and that they should be prescribed early in this situation and in higher doses."[73,74]

Step 11: Additional considerations. Because the asthmatic patient is usually quite anxious during an

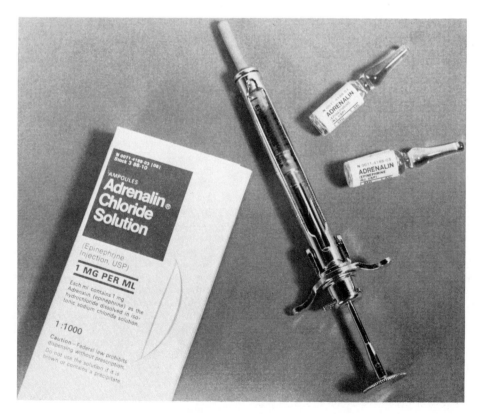

Fig. 13-4. Parenteral bronchodilator. Epinephrine (Adrenalin) is administered intramuscularly or intravenously.

acute attack, the use of sedative medications during acute episodes should be considered. *The more severe the asthmatic attack, however, the more potentially dangerous is the administration of any central nervous system and/or respiratory depressant drugs.* These agents are absolutely contraindicated in status asthmaticus or in very severe asthma when there is any indication of carbon dioxide retention. Potential respiratory depression produced by sedative agents may be accentuated by concurrent hypoxia, and respiratory arrest may occur. In less severe episodes the judicious use of sedatives (such as diazepam, 5 mg IM or IV, titrated) may be indicated to decrease the anxiety component of the problem; however, their administration is rarely indicated. Oxygen may be administered freely at all times during the asthmatic episode.

Step 12:Disposition of patient. Following resolution of the acute episode of bronchospasm that required the administration of parenteral drugs, the patient will most commonly require a period of hospitalization in order to reevaluate long-term therapy. In other situations it may be determined by the emergency medical team that hospitalization is not required. In such cases a decision on how to permit the patient to leave the office (i.e., alone or escorted) should be made before the emergency team departs.

MANAGEMENT OF ACUTE ASTHMA

Terminate the dental procedure
↓
Position the patient comfortably
(usually upright)
↓
Remove materials from patient's mouth
↓
Calm patient
↓
Basic life support, as indicated
↓
Administer bronchodilator via inhalation:
(episode terminates)　(episode continues)
↓　　　　　↓
Subsequent　　Administer oxygen
dental care　　↓
↓　　　Summon medical
Discharge patient　assistance
↓
Administer parenteral
medications
↓
Hospitalize patient or
discharge home

The accompanying box summarizes the steps in management of mild and severe asthmatic episodes.

Drugs used in management: β-adrenergic agonist (epinephrine or albuterol) via aerosol; oxygen; isoproterenol (IV) for severe acute attack; corticosteroids (IV) for severe attack

Medical assistance required: None if mild or terminated by aerosol therapy; yes if refractory to aerosol therapy

REFERENCES

1. Eberle J: *A treatise on the practice of medicine,* vol 2, Philadelphia, 1830, John Grigg.
2. American Thoracic Society: Definitions and classifications of chronic bronchitis, asthma, and pulmonary emphysema, *Am Rev Respir Dis* 85:762, 1962.
3. Gregg I: Epidemiology of asthma. In Clark TJH, Godfrey S, editors: *Asthma,* London, 1977, Chapman & Hall.
4. Senior RM, Lefak SS: Status asthmaticus. In Fishman AP, editor: *Pulmonary diseases and disorders,* New York, 1980, McGraw-Hill.
5. McFadden ER, Austin KF: Asthma. In Thorn GW, and others, editors: *Harrison's principles of internal medicine,* ed 12, New York, 1991, McGraw-Hill.
6. Ford GT: Asthma—prognostic implications in the 1990s re: morbidity-mortality evaluation, Proc Ann Meeting of the Med Section of Amer Council Life Insurance, 1990.
7. Kjellman NI, Croner S, Gustafsson PM: Development of asthma in children, *Allergie et Immunologie* 23(8):351-357, 1991.
8. Bone RC, Burch SG: Management of status asthmaticus, *Ann Allergy* 67(5):461-469, 1991.
9. Daniele RP: Pathophysiology of asthma. In Fishman AP, editor: *Pulmonary diseases,* New York, 1980, McGraw-Hill.
10. Kamada MM, Twang F, Leung DY: Multiple antibiotic sensitivity in a pediatric population, *Allergy Proc,* 12(5):347-350, 1991.
11. Tan Y, Collins-Williams DA: Aspirin-induced asthma in children, *Ann Allergy* 48:1, 1982.
12. Sulfite update, *FDA Drug Bull* 14:24, 1984.
13. Koepke JW, Selner JC, Christopher K, and others: Inhaled metabisulfiite sensitivity, *J Allergy Clin Immunol* 75:135, 1984.
14. Levin RH: Advances in pediatric drug therapy of asthma, *Nursing Clin N Amer* 26(2):263-272, 1991.
15. Hudgel DW, Langston E, Selner JC, and others: Viral and bacterial infetions in adults with chronic asthma, *Am Rev Respir Dis* 120:393, 1979.
16. Scoggin C: Exercise-induced asthma, *Chest* 87:48s, 1985.
17. Salvaggio J. Seabury J, Schoenhardt FA: New Orleans asthma: relationship between Charity Hospital asthma rates, semiquantitative pollen and fungal spore counts, and total particulate aerometric sampling data, *J Allergy Clin Immunol* 48:96, 1971.
18. Murphy RH: Industrial disease with asthma. In Weiss E, Segal MS, editors: *Bronchial asthma: mechanisms and therapeutics,* Boston, 1976, Little, Brown.
19. Busse WW: The precipitation of asthma by upper respiratory infections, *Chest* 87:44s, 1985.
20. Empey DW, Laitinen LA, Jacobs L, and others: Mechanisms of bronchial hyperreactivity in normal subjects after upper respiratory tract infection, *Am Rev Respir Dis* 113:131, 1976.
21. McFadden ER: Pathogenesis of asthma, *J Allergy Clin Immunol* 73:413, 1974.

22. Hamlett KW, Pellegrini DS, Katz KS: Childhood chronic illness as a family stressor, *J Pediatr Psychol* 17(1):33-47, 1992.

23. Fast TB, Martin MD, Ellis TM: Emergency preparedness: a survey of dental practitioners, *J Amer Dent Assoc* 112:499-501, 1986.

24. McCarthy FM: *Essentials of safe dentistry for the medically compromised patient*, Philadelphia, 1989, WB Saunders Co.

25. Ulrik CS, Backer V, Dirksen A: Mortality and decline in lung function in 213 adults with bronchial asthma: a ten-year follow up, *J Asthma* 29(1):29-38, 1992.

26. Soler M, Imhof E, Perruchoud AP: Severe acute asthma: pathophysiology, clinical assessment, and treatment, *Respiration* 57(2):114-121, 1990.

27. Summer WR: Status asthmaticus, *Chest* 87:87s, 1985.

28. Ennis M, Schneider C, Nehring E, Lorenz W: Histamine release indiced by opioid analgesics: a comparative study using procine mast cells, *Agents and Actions* 33(1-2):20-22, 1991.

29. Skidmore-Roth L: *Mosby's 1990 nursing drug reference*, St Louis, 1990, Mosby–Year Book.

30. Tobias JD, Hirshman CA: Attenuation of histamine-induced airway constriction by albuterol during halothane anesthesia, *Anesthesiology* 72(1):105-110, 1990.

31. Little, Fallace: *Dental management of the medically compromised patient*, ed 3, St Louis, 1988, Mosby–Year Book.

32. McDonald JR, Mathison DA, Stevenson DD: Aspirin intolerance in asthma, *J Allergy Clin Immunol* 50:198, 1972.

33. Stevenson DD, Mathison DA, Tan EM, and others: Provoking factors in bronchial asthma, *Arch Intern Med* 135:777, 1975.

34. Mathison DA, Stevenson DD, Simon RA: Precipitating factors in asthma: aspirin, sulfites, and other drugs and chemicals, *Chest* 87:50s, 1985.

35. Twarog FJ, Laung DYM: Anaphylaxis to a component of isoetharine (sodium bisulfite), *JAMA* 249:2030, 1982.

36. Koepke JW, Selner JC, Christopher K, and others: Inhaled metabisulfite sensitivity, *J Allergy Clin Immunol* 75:135, 1984.

37. Ciancio SG: Vasoconstrictors in local anesthetics, *Dental Management* 31(2):49-50, 1991.

38. Wright W, Zhang VG, Salome CM, Woolcock AJ: Effect of inhaled preservatives on asthmatic subjects: i sodium metabisulfite, *Am Rev Respir Dis* 141(6):1400–1404, 1990.

39. Saunders NA, McFadden ER: Asthma: an update, *DM* 24:1, 1978.

40. McFadden ER, Kiser R, DeGroot WJ: Acute bronchial asthma: relationships between clinical and physiologic manifestations, *N Engl J Med* 288:221, 1973.

41. McCombs RP, Lowell FC, Ohman JL: Myths, morbidity and mortality in asthma, *JAMA* 242:1521, 1979.

42. McFadden ER, Feldman NT: Asthma, pathophysiology and clinical correlates, *Med Clin N Am* 61:1229, 1977.

43. Nowak RM: Acute adult asthma. In Rosen P editor: *Emergency medicine*, St Louis, 1988, Mosby–Year Book.

44. Barker RM, Rosen P: *Pulmonary disorders*. In *Emergency pediatric medicine*, ed 3, St Louis, 1990, Mosby–Year Book.

45. Hogg JC: The pathophysiology of asthma, *Chest* 82:8s, 1982.

46. Olsen CR, Colebath HJM, Mebel P, and others: Motor control of pulmonary airways studied by nerve stimulation, *J Appl Physiol Respir Environ Exercise Physiol* 20:202, 1965.

47. Cabezas GA, Graf PD, Nadel JA: Sympathetic versus parasympathetic nervous regulation of airways in dogs, *J Appl Physiol* 31:651, 1971.

48. Nadel JA: Airways: autonomic regulation and airway responsiveness. In Weiss EB, Segal MS, editors: *Bronchial asthma: mechanisms and therapeutics*, Boston, 1976, Little, Brown.

49. Richardson JB: Nerve supply to the lungs, *Am Rev Respir Dis* 119:785, 1979.

50. Leff A: Pathophysiology of asthmatic bronchoconstriction, *Chest* 83:13s, 1982.

51. Leff AR, Munoz MN: Interrelationship between alpha and beta adrenergic agonists and histamine in canine airway, *J Allergy Clin Immunol* 68:300, 1981.

52. Nadel JA: Inflammation and asthma, *J Allergy Clin Immunol* 73:651, 1984.

53. Guerzon GM, Pare PD, Michoud MC, and others: The number and distribution of mast cells in monkey lungs, *Am Rev Respir Dis* 119:59, 1979.

54. Bisgaard H: Leukotrienes and prostaglandins in asthma, *Allergy* 39:413, 1984.

55. Dahlen SE, Hedquist P, Hammarstom S, and others: Leukotrienes are potent constrictors of human bronchi, *Nature* 288:484, 1980.

56. Weiss JW, Drazen JM, McFadden ER, and others: Comparative bronchoconstriction effects of histamine and leukotrienes C and D (LTC and LTD) in normal human volunteers (abstract), *Clin Res* 30:571, 1982.

57. Tortola GJ: The respiratory system. In *Principles of human anatomy*, ed 6, New York, 1992, Harper Collins.

58. Comroe JH: Mechanical factors in breathing. In *Physiology of respiration*, Chicago, 1966, Year Book Medical Publishers.

59. Zamel N: Normal lung mechanics. In Baum GL, Wolinsky E, editors: *Textbook of pulmonary diseases*, ed 3, Boston, 1983, Little, Brown.

60. Mead J: Mechanical prperties of lungs, *Physiol Rev* 41:281–330, 1961.

61. Agostini E: Action of respiratory muscles. In Fenn WO, Rahn H editors: *Handbook of physiology*, sec 3, vol. I, *Respiration*, Washington D.C., 1964, American Physiological Society.

62. McFadden ER Jr., Kiser R, deGroot W: Acute bronchial asthma: relations between clinical and physiologic manifestations, *N Engl J Med* 228:221, 1973.

63. Nelson HS: Beta adrenergic agonists, *Chest* 82:33s, 1982.

64. Adverse reactions of drugs, *Med Lett Drugs Ther* 2:5, 1979.

65. Pliss LB, Gallaher EJ: Aerosol vs. injected epinerine in acute asthma, *Ann Emerg Med* 10:353, 1981.

66. Williams SJ, Winner SJ, Clark TJH: Comparison of inhaled and intravenous terbutaline in acute severe asthma, *Thorax* 36:629, 1981.

67. Shim C, Williams MH: Bronchial response to oral versus aerosol metaproterenol in asthma, *Ann Intern Med* 93:428, 1980.

68. Godfrey S: Worldwide experience with albuterol (salbutamol), *Ann Allergy* 47:423, 1981.

69. Newman SP, Pavia D, Moren F, and others: Deposition of pressurized aerosols in the human respiratory tract, *Thorax* 36:52, 1981.

70. Dolovich M, Ruffin RE, Roberts T, and others: Optimal delivery of aerosols from metered dose inhalers, *Chest* 80:911s, 1991.

71. Klaustermeyer WB, DiBernardo RL, Hale FC: Intravenous isoproterenol: rationale for bronchial asthma, *J Allergy Clin Immunol* 55:325, 1975.

72. Klaustermeyer WB, Hale FC: The physiologic effect of an intravenous glucocorticoid in bronchial asthma, *Ann Allergy* 37:80, 1976.

73. Fanta CH, Rossing TH, McFadden ER: Glucocorticoids in acute asthma: a critical controlled trial, *Am J Med* 74:845, 1983.

74. Leung FW, Santiago SM, Klaustermeyer WB: Corticosteroid therapy and death in cases of acute bronchial asthma, *West J Med* 138:565, 1988.

14 *Heart Failure and Acute Pulmonary Edema*

Heart failure is generally defined as the inability of the heart to supply sufficient oxygenated blood for the metabolic needs of the body.[1] Congestion from fluid accumulation develops in the pulmonary or systemic circulations, or in both. When failure occurs solely in the left ventricle, the observed signs and symptoms are related to congestion of the pulmonary vasculature, whereas right ventricular failure commonly exhibits signs and symptoms of systemic venous and capillary congestion. Left and right ventricular failure may develop as independent entities or they may occur simultaneously. The term *congestive heart failure* or CHF refers to a combination of left and right ventricular failure, in which there is evidence of both systemic and pulmonary congestion. Acute pulmonary edema is a life-threatening condition marked by an excess of serous fluid in the alveolar spaces or interstitial tissues of the lungs and accompanied by extreme difficulty in breathing.

The human heart functions under normal conditions as a pump, supplying the tissues and organs of the body with a supply of blood that contains oxygen and nutrients sufficient to meet their metabolic needs both at rest and during activity. When viewed as a pump, the human heart is remarkable not only for its ability to rapidly adjust to the varying metabolic requirements of the body, but also because of its extreme durability. The heart does last a lifetime—literally. As durable as the heart may be, however, it is also vulnerable to a large number of disorders that may affect its ability to function adequately as a pump. These include congenital, metabolic, inflammatory, and degenerative disorders. Heart dysfunction usually manifests itself clinically in one of two ways. In the first, signs and symptoms of the dysfunction are located directly at the site of the heart. These include chest pain and palpitation, which are represented clinically as angina pectoris (see Chapter 27), myocardial infarction (see Chapter 28), and cardiac dysrhythmias. The second type includes signs and symptoms that are extracardiac and originate in organs of the body that are either hyperperfused (congested) or hypoperfused (ischemic) with blood. Heart failure is a clinical expression of the former.

Under normal circumstances the right ventricle is destined to outperform and outlast the left ventricle. This clinical fact is further accentuated by the fact that the left ventricle is more vulnerable to heart disease and to disorders in its blood supply than is the right ventricle and is therefore where the first expression of heart failure is usually noted. Isolated right ventricular failure is extremely rare. The right ventricle commonly fails soon after left ventricular failure occurs. Cardiac function, both normal and pathologic, is discussed further in the pathophysiology section of this chapter.

Heart failure therefore represents a clinical diagnosis that is applied to a group of signs and symptoms that occur when the heart is unable to handle its load as a pump, thus depriving the various tissues and organs of an adequate supply of oxygen and nutrients. The degree of heart failure varies dramatically, from patients showing only mild clinical signs and symptoms that arise solely on exertion to patients with severe heart failure who demonstrate signs and symptoms in the resting state.

All patients with heart failure represent an increased risk during dental care. Modification of the dental treatment plan may be necessary in order to accommodate their state of cardiac dysfunction. In more advanced heart failure or in patients with moderate degrees of heart failure who are faced with physiologic or psychologic stress or both, the degree of heart failure may become accentuated, producing acute pulmonary edema, in which extreme degrees of respiratory distress are observed. This is a life-threatening medical emergency that must be managed quickly and aggressively.

Heart failure is not an uncommon finding in the general population. Over 2 million Americans have congestive heart failure.[1] In 1984 more than 450,000 patients were discharged from the hospital with a primary diagnosis of congestive heart failure.[2] Unfortunately, the prognosis for patients with CHF is quite poor. Following its initial diagnosis, 52% of males and 34% of females were dead within 4 years.[3] Another study reported an overall mortality of 75% at 6 years after CHF diagnosis.[4] Most persons with progressive cardiovascular disease develop some degree of heart failure at some stage of their lives. Chapter 26 includes a discussion of the etiologic factors found in the majority of these cardiovascular diseases. The dentist is faced with the prospect of managing the dental needs of patients with varying degrees of heart failure. It is important to adequately evaluate this patient before actual dental care begins so that measures may be taken to prevent an acute episode of heart failure, or acute pulmonary edema, from developing during treatment.

PREDISPOSING FACTORS

The tendency of heart failure to begin as left ventricular failure is related to the disproportionate workload of the left ventricle and to the prevalence of cardiac disease in the left ventricle. Disease produces heart failure in one of two basic ways: (1) By increasing the workload of the heart; for example, high blood pressure produces an increased resistance to ejection of blood from the left ventricle, thereby making the myocardium work harder; and (2) by damaging the muscular walls of the heart through coronary artery disease or myocardial infarction.

Other causes of increased cardic workload include: cardiac valvular deficiencies (e.g., stenosis or insufficiency of the aortic, mitral, tricuspid, or pulmonary valves); and increases in the body's requirement for oxygen and nutrients (e.g., pregnancy, hyperthyroidism, anemia, Paget's disease).

Hypertension is responsible for more than 75% of all cases of congestive heart failure.[5]

Failure of the left ventricle is the leading cause of right ventricular failure. Other causes of isolated right ventricular failure include mitral stenosis, pulmonary vascular or parenchymal disease, and pulmonary valvular stenosis, all of which significantly increase the workload of the right ventricle.

Acute worsening of preexisting heart failure leading to acute pulmonary edema may be precipitated by any factor that increases the workload of the heart. Acute pulmonary edema may occur at any time, but is commonly observed at night after the patient has been asleep for a few hours (see the pathophysiology section later in this chapter). Other factors that increase cardiac workload include physical, psychologic, and climatic stress. The dental setting may easily provide these factors.

In pediatric patients heart failure may also be produced by an obstruction to the outflow of blood from the heart, such as coarctation of the aorta or pulmonary stenosis. Of all children who do develop CHF, 90% do so within the first year of life because of congenital heart lesions.[6] Older children may also develop CHF from congenital heart lesions; however, much more common causes are acquired disease from cardiomyopathy, bacterial endocarditis, or rheumatic carditis.

PREVENTION
Medical History Questionnaire

Relevant questions from the medical history questionnaire relating to the presence of cardiovascular disease are presented, with comments added for clarification.

QUESTION 9. Circle any of the following that you have had or have at present:
Heart failure
Heart murmur
Rheumatic fever
Congenital heart lesions
Scarlet fever

COMMENT. An affirmative reply to any of the aforementioned conditions is an indication of the need for further questioning via dialogue history to determine the degree of severity and other relevant factors concerning the disease. All of these conditions can lead to the development of varying degrees of clinical signs and symptoms of heart failure.

QUESTION 10. When you walk up stairs or take a walk, do you ever have to stop because of pain in your chest, or shortness of breath, or because you are very tired?

COMMENT. The ability to negotiate a normal flight of stairs or to walk two level city blocks is an excellent gauge of cardiorespiratory fitness (see section on dialogue history). Shortness of breath that develops after mild exercise is termed *exertional dyspnea* and represents an early sign of left ventricular failure.

QUESTION 11. **Do your ankles swell during the day?**

COMMENT. In response to a "yes" answer, determine at what time of night or day swelling develops. Dependent edema is seen in most patients with right ventricular failure late in the day following many hours of standing. It may be seen in other clinical states as well, such as in the later stages of pregnancy, with varicose veins, and in renal failure.

QUESTION 12. **Do you use more than two pillows to sleep?**

COMMENT. Orthopnea is dyspnea when the patient is supine, and is alleviated by elevation of the trunk.[7] Clinically, the patient is unable to breathe comfortably when lying down, requiring the use of three or more pillows to enable him or her to breathe comfortably. This is termed *three-pillow orthopnea*. When severe, the patient may be able to rest or to sleep only while maintained in an erect or upright position. Orthopnea is a sign of left ventricular failure. Modifications in patient or chair position may be desirable during dental treatment.

QUESTION 13. **Have you lost or gained more than 10 pounds in the past year?**

COMMENT. An affirmative reply to having gained more than 10 pounds—especially if this has occurred relatively rapidly and for no apparent reason—might indicate the development of CHF. Retention of fluid is a significant factor in the development of CHF. The dialogue history must help determine the presence of other reasons for this weight gain aside from CHF.

QUESTION 14. **Do you ever awake from sleep short of breath?**

COMMENT. Termed *paroxysmal nocturnal dyspnea* (PND), this clinical sign is usually related to a more significant degree of left ventricular failure. Patients awaken from sleep with shortness of breath that is relieved by sitting up or standing, especially in front of an open window.

QUESTION 6. **Have you taken any medicine or drugs during the past 2 years?**

COMMENT. Patients diagnosed with heart failure will frequently take one or more of the following: diuretics, vasodilators, medications for high blood pressure, and/or inotropic agents such as digitalis.

Diuretics are often the first line of defense in treating congestive heart failure. Diuretics are used to suppress renal tubular reabsorption of sodium. They are commonly employed in the management

---

DIURETICS USED IN THE MANAGEMENT OF CONGESTIVE HEART FAILURE

Thiazides
Hydrochlorothiazide
Chlorthalidone
Metazolone

Loop diuretics
Furosemide
Bumetanide
Ethacrynic acid

Potassium-sparing diuretics
Spironolactone
Triamterene
Amiloride

---

of diseases associated with excessive sodium and fluid retention. There are several groups of diuretics: thiazide, loop, and potassium-sparing diuretics. The accompanying box lists some of the more commonly employed diuretics used to treat CHF.

Inotropic agents, with the exception of digitalis, have been reserved for the treatment of acute pulmonary edema and refractory CHF in hospitalized patients. These include dopamine,[8] dobutamine,[9] amrinone,[10] milrinone,[10,11] and aminophylline.

The fundamental action of digitalis glycosides is to increase the force and velocity of cardiac contraction, whether or not the heart is failing, through their positive inotropic actions. In CHF, digitalis significantly increases cardiac output, decreases right atrial pressure, decreases venous pressure, and increases the excretion of sodium and water, thus correcting some of the hemodynamic and metabolic alterations that occur in heart failure. The effect of digitalis upon heart rate is to decrease it, whereas it increases the demand of the myocardium for oxygen. Thought digitalis is still considered to be an important therapeutic modality

---

INOTROPIC AGENTS USED IN CONGESTIVE HEART FAILURE

Digoxin
Dopamine
Dobutamine
Amrinone
Milrinone
Aminophylline

> ### *VASODILATORS USED IN CONGESTIVE HEART FAILURE*
>
> #### *Nitrates*
> Nitroglycerin
> Isosorbide
>
> #### *Others*
> Nitroprusside
> Hydralazine
> Minoxidil
> Prazosin
> Phentolamine
> Captopril
> Nifedipine

---

in CHF, more and more frequently, the vasodilators, diuretics, and inotropic agents are replacing it in the treatment of CHF. Inotropic agents are listed in the accompanying box.

High blood pressure represents one of the leading causes of left ventricular failure. Antihypertensive medications are frequently prescribed for CHF patients. Knowledge of which drugs are being taken by the patient will lead the doctor to a better understanding of the degree of cardiovascular dysfunction present, as well as enabling the doctor to prevent certain side effects associated with many of the antihypertensive drugs.

Within the past 10 years, vasodilators have become significantly more popular in managing CHF. Depending upon whether or not a drug is a venodilator, arteriodilator, or possesses mixed properties, treatment of CHF can be tailored for the individual patient after consideration of several factors, including baseline blood pressure, the degree of pulmonary congestion, the degree of peripheral edema, the concomitant presence of angina, renal hypoperfusion, the heart rate, and the likelihood of patient compliance. Vasodilators are listed the the accompanying box.

Dialogue History

Following a review of the medical history questionnaire, the dialogue history is used to gather additional information concerning the severity of the heart failure.

QUESTION. Are you able to carry out your normal daily activities without becoming unduly fatigued?

COMMENT. Related to question 10, this question considers the presence of undue fatigue at rest, not during exercise. Undue fatigue is a common symptom of left or right ventricular failure or both. Fatigue and general weakness usually represent the first clinical manifestations of heart failure.

QUESTION. Can you climb a normal flight of stairs or walk two level city blocks without distress?

COMMENT. As it relates to the preceding question, the inability to climb a normal flight of stairs or walk two level city blocks without distress is an indication of an inefficient cardiorespiratory system. The American Society of Anesthesiologists' (ASA) physical status classification system for CHF (Fig. 14-1) may be linked to the patient's answer to this question.

ASA I patients (i.e., normal, healthy) will be able to climb one flight of stairs or walk two level city blocks without having to pause because of shortness of breath, undue fatigue, or chest pain.

ASA II patients will be able to climb one flight of stairs or walk two level city blocks without distress, but will have to stop once they are finished with either task because of distress. In patients with CHF, the distress seen is most likely to be shortness of breath or undue fatigue.

ASA III patients will be able to climb one flight of stairs or walk two city blocks but will have to stop before completing the task because of distress.

ASA IV patients are unable to negotiate a flight of stairs or to walk two level city blocks because of shortness of breath or undue fatigue that is present at rest.

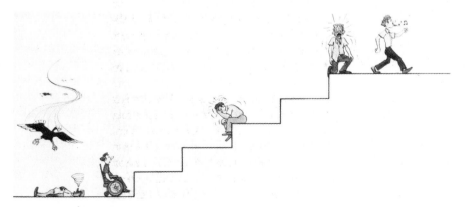

Fig. 14-1. ASA classification for CHF. (Courtesy Dr. Lawrence Day.)

QUESTION. **Have you ever awakened at night short of breath?**

COMMENT. Paroxysmal nocturnal dyspnea (PND), or awakening at night short of breath, is usually noted in more advanced left ventricular failure. When present, medical consultation should be considered before beginning dental therapy.

QUESTION. **What is the cause of your child's congestive heart failure?**

COMMENT. Pediatric patients with CHF secondary to other diseases will have a history of congenital or other heart problems. The parent or guardian will be able to discuss the child's status with the doctor. Consultation with the patient's primary care physician is warranted in cases of pediatric congestive heart failure. In the first year of life 90% of children develop CHF because of congenital heart disease. Older children may also develop CHF from congenital heart disease, but they more commonly suffer from acquired CHF secondary to cardiomyopathy, bacterial endocarditis, or rheumatic carditis.[6]

Additionally, the doctor might encounter patients who appear to have CHF (see the section on physical evaluation that follows), but who provide negative responses to the preceding questions. Always remember that people accommodate their lifestyle rather well to adapt to a degree of physical disability. For example, persons who are unable to climb a flight of stairs or to walk two level city blocks may in fact never try to do so; they may simple use an elevator or motor vehicle instead. The observant doctor will always be on the lookout for clinical clues.

Physical Evaluation

In addition to the steps already outlined, which are used to determine the degree of severity of a patient's heart failure, physical evaluation of the patient will enable the doctor to determine the patient's current state of health more accurately.

Vital Signs

The vital signs of the patient should be recorded. These include the blood pressure, heart rate and rhythm (pulse), respiratory rate, and weight. Patients with congestive heart failure may demonstrate the following:

1. Blood pressure may be elevated, with the diastolic pressure elevated to a greater extent than the systolic pressure. The pulse pressure (the difference between the systolic and diastolic pressure) is narrowed. For example, a normal blood pressure of 130/80 yields a pulse pressure of 50; a blood pressure of 130/ 100, as seen in CHF, yields a pulse pressure of 30. In some situations blood pressure may be decreased.

2. The heart rate (pulse) and the respiratory rate are usually increased. Tachycardia is present because of the increased adrenergic activity, which is a principal compensatory mechanism for support of the circulation in the presence of reduced cardiac output.[12] Tachypnea is evident early in the progression of CHF as dyspnea increases in severity.

3. Any recent, unexplained, large weight gain (more than 3 pounds in a 7-day period) may indicate the onset of acute heart failure. If noted in conjunction with clinical signs of dependent edema, such as ankle swelling, dental care should be withheld until a more extensive medical evaluation is completed.

Physical examination

Physical evaluation should include a careful visual inspection of the following by the doctor.[6]

Skin color. Skin color in the patient with more severe congestive heart failure may appear ashen-gray or grayish-blue. Cyanosis (a bluish tinge) is an indication of underoxygenation of the blood. Its presence should indicate the possibility of heart failure. Although skin color is important, it is perhaps more relevant to examine the patient's mucous membranes, particularly the nailbeds and lips. Nail polish and lipstick may mask these areas, but the color of the intraoral mucous membranes can always be observed.

Neck. Jugular vein distention develops in patients with right ventricular failure, so that when these patients are in the upright or semisupine position, their jugular veins may remain visible. In normal situations jugular vein pressure is negative when the patient is in the upright position and the veins are collapsed and cannot be seen. Jugular veins remain visible with the elevated central venous pressure of CHF.

Prominent jugular veins are normal when patients are placed into a supine position, but these veins will gradually disappear as the patient is slowly raised into a more upright position. At approximately a 30° angle or more, jugular veins should collapse and become undetectable (Fig. 14-2). To determine the presence of increased jugular vein pressure, one measures how far vertically above the sternal angle of Louis the jugular veins are distended and then adds 5 cm for the distance to the atrium. The patient should be placed into a 45° upright position and the right jugular vein should be evaluated.[13] Normally this distance is not

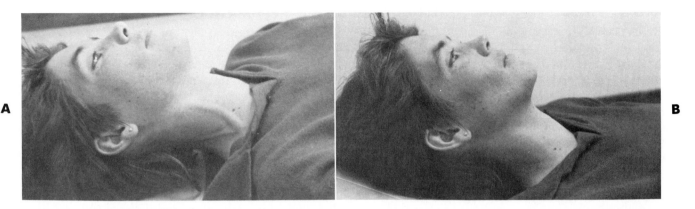

Fig. 14-2. A, Prominent jugular veins. **B,** With upright positioning, jugular vein disappears.

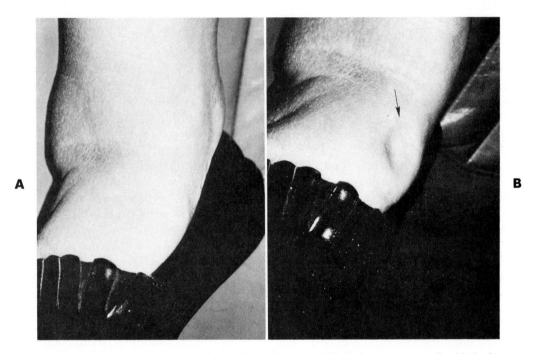

Fig. 14-3. Ankle demonstrating dependent edema. **A,** Clinical appearance of ankle before pressure application with finger. **B,** *Arrows* indicate "pitting" produced by pressure on right side of ankle.

less than 10 cm H_2O (the unit of measurement). The causes of elevated jugular vein pressure (JVP) include right ventricular failure, pulmonic and tricuspid valve stenosis, pulmonary hypertension, right ventricular hypertrophy, and constrictive pericarditis.

Ankles. Ankle edema, also known as pitting or dependent edema, may be noted in patients with right ventricular failure, as well as in pregnant patients, those with varicose veins, and those with renal failure. It occurs in the dependent portions of the body where systemic venous pressures rise to their highest levels. If the patient follows a normal pattern of sleeping at night and being awake during the day, ankle edema develops in the afternoon and disappears overnight. Edematous tissue may be differentiated from adipose tissue by a simple test. Pressure placed on edematous tissue for 30 seconds results in a "pitting" effect as the edema fluid is forced out of the area (Fig. 14-3). This pitting gradually disappears once the pressure is released. In contrast, adipose or normal tissue returns to its original dimension immediately upon release of pressure. As the severity of CHF intensifies, edema progresses, ascending to involve the legs, thighs, genitalia, and abdominal wall.[13]

DENTAL THERAPY CONSIDERATIONS

The information that has been gathered must now be formulated to enable the doctor to determine the degree of risk represented by the CHF patient. The New York Heart Association[14] developed a functional classification of patients with heart disease based on the relation between symptoms and the amount of effort required to provoke them. The classification of the New York Heart Association follows:

Class I—No limitation: Ordinary physical activity does not cause undue fatigue, dyspnea, or palpitation.

Class II—Slight limitation of physical activity: Such patients are comfortable at rest. Ordinary physical activity results in fatigue, palpitation, dyspnea, or angina.

Class III—Marked limitation of physical activity: Although patients are comfortable at rest, less than ordinary activity will lead to symptoms.

Class IV—Inability to carry on any physical activity without discomfort: Symptoms of congestive heart failure are present even at rest. With any physical activity, increased discomfort is experienced.

The ASA physical status classification for CHF, which follows, is similar to the New York Heart Association's categorization.

ASA PHYSICAL STATUS I. No dyspnea or undue fatigue with normal exertion

COMMENT. If all other items of the medical history are negative, this patient may be considered a normal, healthy person. No special modifications in dental therapy are indicated. Patients with heart failure will not be ASA I risks.

ASA PHYSICAL STATUS II. Mild dyspnea or fatigue on exertion

COMMENT. As with the ASA class I patient, this patient may be managed in a normal manner, if the rest of the medical history and physical examination proves to be noncontributory. Use of the stress reduction protocol should be considered if any physical or psychologic stress is evident or anticipated.

ASA PHYSICAL STATUS III. Dyspnea or undue fatigue with normal activities

COMMENT. This patient is comfortable at rest in any position but may demonstrate a tendency toward orthopnea and have a history of paroxysmal nocturnal dyspnea. The ASA class III patient represents an increased risk during dental treatment. Before commencing dental treatment, medical consultation is recommended. The stress reduction protocol and other specific modifications that are thought necessary should be employed for this patient.

ASA PHYSICAL STATUS IV. Dyspnea, orthopnea, and undue fatigue at all times

COMMENT. The ASA class IV patient represents a definite risk. The heart is incapable of meeting the metabolic requirements of the body even when at rest. Any degree of stress, which will further increase metabolic demands, may exacerbate the condition, possibly provoking acute pulmonary edema. Dental care should be withheld for all elective procedures until the cardiovascular disorder is corrected or controlled. Management of dental emergencies (e.g., pain and/or infection) should be handled with medication, and if actual physical intervention is required, the patient should be hospitalized and placed under a physician's care before, during, and immediately following the dental procedure.

General treatment modifications, as per the stress reduction protocol, are indicated for CHF patients.

Supplemental oxygen: In patients with any degree of heart failure, and indeed with any cardiovascular disorder (e.g., angina pectoris and myocardial infarction), there is no contraindication to providing the patient with oxygen during the treatment period. A nasal cannula or nasal hood from an inhalation sedation unit may be used. A flow rate of 3 to 5 L per minute is usually adequate, but the flow rate should be adjusted to patient comfort (Fig. 14-4).

Positioning of the patient: Positioning of the CHF patient in the dental chair may require modification. If the patient finds it difficult to breathe in the supine position, the doctor must modify the chair position until the patient is comfortable again. As noted earlier, this is termed *orthopnea* and usually represents a class III risk, requiring medical consultation before dental therapy. The use of a rubber dam may be contraindicated in this patient, as it may severely restrict an already limited ability to obtain an adequate volume of air.

CLINICAL MANIFESTATIONS

Clinical manifestations of heart failure are related to the specific portion of the heart that is failing. Varying degrees of heart failure may be present so that not all patients exhibit all of the symptoms and signs that will be described shortly. In addition, most patients will exhibit congestive heart failure, which is the combined failure of the left and right ventricles.

Clinical signs and symptoms are presented individually for each ventricle, followed by a description of acute pulmonary edema.

Left ventricular failure is manifested clinically primarily by *symptoms* associated with pulmonary

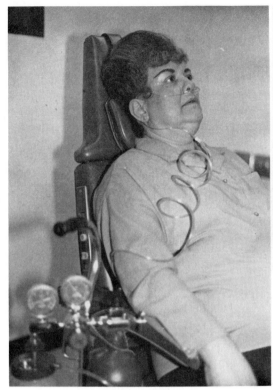

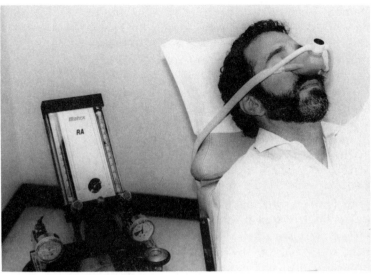

A

B

Fig. 14-4. A, Nasal oxygen or **B,** face mask of inhalation sedation unit used to provide supplemental oxygen to patient with CHF.

congestion, whereas right ventricular failure is dominated by *signs* of systemic venous congestion and peripheral edema. Undue fatigue and weakness are prominent symptoms observed in both types of heart failure.

Left Ventricular Failure
Symptoms

Manifestations of left ventricular failure are primarily associated with respiratory distress, with the severity of the distress related to the degree of heart failure. The pathophysiology of each symptom is discussed here.

Weakness and undue fatigue are usually the first symptoms of left ventricular failure to become evident to the patient. The patient becomes aware of these symptoms when feeling fatigued during a level of exertion that previously caused no fatigue. As the degree of heart failure progresses, fatigue is produced with less and less exertion until it is present even at rest. Dyspnea, or difficulty in breathing, is usually evident with exertion. This is commonly associated with an increase in the rate of breathing (tachypnea). Cough and expectoration are present, and are related to reflexes produced by the congested lungs and bronchi.

The patient with early left ventricular failure may report an increased frequency of urination at night (nocturia), a symptom produced by the rediffusion of edema fluid in the extremities from extracellular sites back into the general circulation.

Orthopnea and paroxysmal nocturnal dyspnea are later, more ominous signs related to more severe failure of the left ventricle. Orthopnea is dyspnea that occurs soon after lying flat and is relieved by sitting up. The patient with orthopnea is able to alleviate the problem by supporting the head and thorax with more than two pillows. As heart failure progresses, this patient may be forced to remain in the upright position (e.g., sitting in a chair) even during sleep. Positioning of this patient for dental care may be difficult. If present, orthopnea and paroxysmal nocturnal dyspnea represent an ASA III medical risk and require specific modifications in dental management. When the condition is severe, this patient may require the use of supplemental oxygen 24 hours a day (ASA IV risk); he or she will carry a portable oxygen cylinder and a nasal cannula. Such a patient is unable to lie down while attempting to sleep, being forced to sleep in a totally upright position.

Paroxysmal nocturnal dyspnea (PND) is an exaggerated form of orthopnea. With PND, the patient is awakened from sleep gasping for breath, with a degree of respiratory difficulty that verges on suffocation. The patient desperately seeks relief from this distress, and usually sits up or rushes to an open window to breathe fresh air. For unknown reasons, such a patient may exhibit inspiratory and expiratory wheezing (cardiac asthma). These episodes usually resolve within a few minutes or they may progress to acute pulmonary edema.

Signs

The patient with moderate to severe left ventricular failure appears pale and is usually diaphoretic (i.e., sweating). The skin is cool to the touch, and it will be obvious to the observer that dyspnea, or difficulty in breathing, is present.

Monitoring of vital signs will almost always demonstrate an increase in the blood pressure, with diastolic pressure elevated to a greater degree than the systolic pressure. The pulse pressure (systolic pressure minus the diastolic pressure) is therefore narrowed. Heart rate is most often increased. It may also be possible to detect pulsus alternans, which is the appearance of alternating strong and weak heart beats even though the basic rhythm of the heart remains normal; it is frequently detected in later stages of heart failure. Tachypnea, or an increased rate of breathing, and hyperventilation, or an increased depth of breathing, are commonly seen in left ventricular failure as a consequence of pulmonary congestion.

Right Ventricular Failure
Signs

Right ventricular failure usually develops after left ventricular failure has been present for a variable length of time, and is characterized primarily by signs indicative of systemic venous congestion. The patient first notices signs of peripheral edema. Swelling of the feet and/or ankles develops during the day in persons with right ventricular failure and subsides overnight. This is referred to as dependent, or pitting, edema. If the patient is bedridden for extended periods, this edema fluid will relocate in the sacral region. Dependent edema is a characteristic feature of right ventricular failure. Pitting refers to the depression or pit left in the tissue following application of finger pressure to the area. This is comparable to the foot impression left in wet sand when walking on the beach. Within several seconds the fluid returns and the pit disappears.

Weakness and undue fatigue are present in right ventricular failure as they are in left ventricular

failure, produced by the deficient supply of oxygen and nutrients to the tissues of the body. Another result of this lack of oxygen is the presence of cyanosis. Especially prominent in mucous membranes (nailbeds and lips), cyanosis is produced by the removal by the tissues of a greater than normal amount of oxygen from the arterial blood in an attempt to compensate for the decreased volume of circulating blood. This decreased blood supply is also a cause of the coolness noted in the extremities.

Other signs of right ventricular failure include the presence of prominent jugular veins in the neck. In normal individuals the jugular veins will not be evident while in the erect position, except during moments of emotional or physical exertion; with failure of the right ventricle, however, systemic venous blood cannot be delivered to the heart normally, and engorgement of the jugular veins occurs.

Engorgement of the liver (hepatomegaly) and spleen (splenomegaly) also occur. On examination, the physician or dentist can palpate an enlarged liver.[13] In normal situations the lower border of the liver is not palpable beneath the right lower costal margin. With hepatomegaly the liver may become palpable from one to four fingerbreadths below the right costal magin. This procedure will evoke a degree of tenderness in the area of palpation. As right ventricular failure progresses, the edematous areas enlarge so that the legs, thighs, and eventually the abdomen (ascites) demonstrate clinical edema. Congestion of the gastrointestinal tract also occurs, and is associated with clinical signs of anorexia, nausea, and vomiting. Signs of edema in the central nervous system include headache, insomnia, and irritability.

In left and right ventricular failure the patient will frequently show considerable anxiety. Once difficulty in breathing manifests itself, the patient, aware of the situation, begins to hyperventilate. Indeed, patients with heart failure may hyperventilate to the point of producing respiratory alkalosis, with clinical symptoms of lightheadedness, cold hands, and tingling fingers (see Chapter 12). In response to anxiety the workload of the heart increases even further, as does the degree of heart failure.

Acute Pulmonary Edema

Acute pulmonary edema is a life-threatening medical emergency in which there is a sudden and rapid transudation of fluid from the pulmonary capillary bed into the alveolar spaces of the lungs.[15] It is often precipitated by stressful situations of either a physical or psychologic nature, although it

Table 14-1. Clinical manifestations of heart failure and acute pulmonary edema

Signs	*Symptoms*
Heart failure	
Pallor, cool skin	Weakness and undue fatigue
Sweating	Dyspnea on exertion
Left ventricular hypertrophy	Hyperventilation
Dependent edema	Nocturia
Hepatomegaly and splenomegaly	Paroxysmal nocturnal dyspnea
Narrow pulse pressure	Wheezing (cardiac asthma)
Pulsus alternans	
Ascites	
Acute pulmonary edema	
All of the signs of heart failure	All of the symptoms of heart failure
Moist rales at the base of the lungs	Increased anxiety
Tachypnea	Dyspnea at rest
Dyspnea	
Cyanosis	
Frothy pink sputum	

may also be induced by a salty meal, noncompliance with medications, or an infection.

The onset of symptoms is usually acute. A slight, dry cough is often the initial symptom; acute pulmonary edema may represent a direct extension of paroxysmal nocturnal dyspnea. Asthmatic-type wheezing may be evident at this state (i.e., cardiac asthma). Dyspnea and orthopnea are commonly present. As the attack progresses, the patient develops a feeling of suffocation and an acute sense of anxiety that further increases the rate and difficulty of breathing. A sense of oppression may be noted in the chest. Physical signs evident at this time include tachypnea, dyspnea, and cough. If auscultated, the lungs demonstrate moist rales at their bases, which progressively extend upward as the episode worsens.

In more severe episodes, pallor, sweating, cyanosis, and a frothy, pink (blood-tinged) sputum are present. Acute pulmonary edema is not uncommon during the period immediately following myocardial infarction if the degree of left ventricular myocardial damage has been great.

Most individuals will resist attempts at recumbency, may panic, and often are quite uncooperative. Table 14-1 summarizes signs and symptoms of heart failure and acute pulmonary edema.

PATHOPHYSIOLOGY

To view heart failure in its proper perspective, it is necessary to first review the normal function of the human heart both at rest and during physical activity. The mechanisms of cardiac dysfunction then become more obvious.

The function of the heart is to propel unoxygenated blood to the lungs and oxygenated blood to the peripheral tissues in accordance with their metabolic requirements.[16] The human heart is comprised of two individual pumps working together (Fig. 14-5). The right side of the heart receives venous (unoxygenated) blood from the sys-

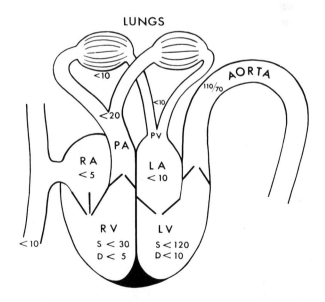

Fig. 14-5. Average blood pressures in various components of circulatory system. *LA,* left atrium; *LV,* left ventricle; *PA,* pulmonary arteries. (From Wylie WD, Churchill-Davidson HC: *A practice of anaesthesia,* ed 3, Chicago, 1972, Mosby–Year Book.)

temic circulation and pumps this blood through the pulmonary arteries to the lungs, where it undergoes oxygenation. From the lungs, the oxygenated (arterial) blood is delivered to the left atrium and then to the left ventricle, where it is pumped to the systemic circulation. The amount of work required by each ventricle to perform its task is considerably different. The right side of the heart may be considered as the low pressure system; an average right ventricular pressure of 24/4–10 torr is required to pump blood out into the pulmonary artery, which, by the way, is the only artery in which unoxygenated blood is normally found. By contrast, the left side of the heart is a high pressure system; the left intraventricular pressure approximates 120/80 torr during systole (contraction). It can therefore be seen that the left ventricle performs the lion's share of the actual work of the heart. Prior to birth, both ventricles are taxed equally because they bear the same pressure loads. Following birth, however, pulmonary arterial pressure falls, the workload of the right ventricle is decreased, and its walls become thin, whereas the workload of the left ventricle increases and its walls enlarge.

The primary function of the heart is to serve as a pump, supplying blood containing oxygen and nutrients to the tissues and cells of the body. Table 14-2 lists minimal oxygen requirements per minute for the average adult performing various activites. Should the heart, for whatever reason, be unable to provide the body with its required oxygen supply, shortness of breath (dyspnea) and undue fatigue are the result. These normally occur when oxygen transport per minute falls below 1000 to 1250 mL per minute. This level usually permits a person to work at a light job and enjoy light recreation and sport without discomfort but does not allow him to put forth more strenuous effort.

Normal Left Ventricular Function

The left ventricle is a thick muscular organ. At rest (diastole), left intraventricular pressure is approximately 6 to 8 torr, whereas the diastolic pres-

Table 14-2. Minimum adult human oxygen requirements

Activity	Oxygen utilization (ml/min)
At rest	250
Standing	375
Walking	400-1000
Light work and exercise	750-1250
Intense exercise	4000 and above

sure in the aorta is approximately 80 torr. For blood to be expelled from the left ventricle into the aorta, the intraventricular pressure must exceed the aortic blood pressure so that the aortic valves will open. The following is the normal sequence of left ventricular function when a person is at rest.

Maximal left ventricular filling, termed the *end diastolic volume*, occurs at the instant just before the start of systole. At this moment, the muscles of the ventricle begin to contract, but no blood is yet being ejected from the ventricle. Instead, the size of the cavity is rapidly decreasing, producing a sharp increase in intraventricular pressure. This interval, termed the *isovolemic period of systole*, normally lasts 50 ms (0.050 second).

In a short time, when the intraventricular pressure exceeds the diastolic aortic blood pressure (80 torr), the aortic valves are forced open and the ejection of blood into the systemic circulation begins. The ventricle continues to contract for a period of time (systole), and then relaxation occurs. The blood pressure within the left ventricle falls rapidly with relaxation. Once the left ventricular blood pressure falls below the aortic blood pressure, the aortic valve closes, signaling the end of systole and the beginning of diastole. During diastole the intraaortic blood pressure exceeds that in the ventricle, permitting filling of the ventricle to occur.

At the time of closure of the aortic valves, the volume of blood in the left ventricle is at its lowest level. The difference in volume between end-diastolic volume (maximal volume) and end-systolic volume (minimal volume) is termed the *ejection fraction*. In a normally functioning heart at rest, this fraction is 0.56 to 0.78; in other words, from 56% to 78% of the blood present in the left ventricle at the end of diastole will be ejected into the aorta during systole. As left ventricular failure develops, the ejection fraction decreases and may be as low as 0.1 to 0.2 in severe heart failure.

Although this mechanism functions in normal situations, it must be remembered that the demands placed on the heart by the body change from second to second. The heart must therefore be capable of responding rapidly to these ever-changing demands by increasing or decreasing the volume of blood ejected per stroke (stroke volume). Three factors—preload, afterload, and contractility—assist in enabling the heart to meet its obligations to the tissues of the body.

Preload is the end-diastolic volume. The greater the preload, the more the myocardial muscle fibers are stretched. According to the Frank-Starling principle,[17] the greater the myocardial muscle is stretched in diastole, the greater it will contract in systole. This may be likened to a rubber band being stretched. This principle is illustrated by the following: With a preload of 100 mL of blood and an ejection fraction of 0.6 (60%), the stroke volume will be 60 mL. Should the preload increase to 140 mL, for example, and the ejection fraction remain 0.6, the stroke volume will increase to 84 mL. In the same manner, decreased preload leads to a diminished stroke volume.

Afterload may be defined as the pressure that resists left ventricular ejection (aortic blood pressure). Increased afterload therefore makes it more difficult for the heart to eject a normal stroke volume. As an example, if the aortic blood pressure rises rapidly (under extreme stress, for example) from 120/80 to 200/120 torr, the intraventricular pressure must rise to 120 torr (the aortic diastolic pressure) before the aortic valve will even open. This valve remains open for only a brief period before the aortic pressure once again exceeds that of the ventricle and closes the aortic valve. The ejection fraction in this instance will be very low (0.1 to 0.2). Such a stroke volume will not be adequate to support the requirements of the body if it is permitted to continue. However, the normal heart is able to compensate for this inadequate stroke volume. The end-systolic volume is larger than normal (because of the nonejected blood). To this will be added the normal blood volume from the left atrium. This increased preload (normal volume plus large end-systolic volume) causes the myocardial fibers to stretch, thereby contracting more forcefully (i.e., the Frank-Starling principle) with the next beat. Within several beats the ventricle is able to adjust the stroke volume to meet the increased blood pressure, from 120/80 to 200/120 torr. There are limits to the Frank-Starling principle in that excessive stretch or a sudden increase in afterload will not be met by an everincreasing contraction of the myocardium.

If the preload and afterload of the heart are permitted to remain the same, it is still possible for the stroke volume to be increased. Contractility is a basic property of cardiac muscle. The sympathetic nervous system can increase the contraction of the heart through the release of epinephrine and norepinephrine. These catecholamines, which are released in increasing amounts under stress, increase the degree of myocardial fiber contraction, thus increasing the ejection fraction (from 0.6 to 0.8), and result in increased stroke volume.

Heart Failure

Heart failure may develop in any patient whose heart has been working for extended periods against an increased peripheral resistance (in-

creased afterload), which is seen in high blood pressure, or in a patient for whom the workload of the heart has increased because of valvular defects (stenosis or insufficiency), or because of prolonged, continuous demands for increased cardiac output (as in hyperthyroidism). These conditions, which demand a chronic increase in cardiac workload, all lead to structural changes in the heart muscle that eventually progress to muscular weakness and the clinical symptoms and signs of heart failure.

Another major cause of myocardial weakness is the presence of disease states that directly attack the muscle, for example, coronary artery disease and myocarditis. In these conditions the myocardium is unable to respond normally to increases in afterload. The increase in fiber length that occurs due to increased ventricular filling will not be met with the usual increase in stroke volume, and clinical heart failure results.

The chronic progression of heart failure may best be illustrated by following the cardiac changes that develop in high blood pressure, one of the leading causes of heart failure. In response to a sustained elevation of the blood pressure (afterload), the myocardium must contract more forcefully for an extended period of time in order to maintain an acceptable stroke volume. As with other muscles doing increased work for periods of time, the myocardial fibers hypertrophy, or increase in diameter and length. This response is seen primarily in the left ventricle and leads to the first sign of heart failure, left ventricular hypertrophy (LVH). A normal heart weighs approximately 250 to 350 g. In mild heart failure the heart may weigh up to 500 g; in more severe heart failure, weights of up to 1000 g have been recorded. Left ventricular hypertrophy may be present for many years before being discovered, generally on a routine electrocardiogram or chest x-rays.

Another important feature of LVH is that, along with the increased size of muscle fibers, there is not a corresponding increase in the number of capillaries delivering blood to them; therefore, the blood supply to the myocardium becomes increasingly compromised as hypertrophy progresses. Because of the compromised blood supply seen in LVH, there comes a point at which hypertrophy alone can no longer maintain an adequate stroke volume in the presence of increased blood pressure. At this point a second mechanism aids in maintaining normal stroke volume. It is called dilation and is an increase in the capacity of the left ventricle, which is brought about by an elongation of myocardial fibers. The force of ventricular contraction of these elongated myocardial fibers increases through the Frank-Starling principle, thereby maintaining a normal stroke volume. It is evident, however, that both the end-diastolic (increased total blood volume) and the end-systolic (increased residual blood) volumes are increased. Therefore, the ejection fraction of the left ventricle is decreased (< 0.56).

As the end-diastolic volume increases, the workload of the heart increases, thereby increasing the myocardial oxygen requirement. In the presence of coronary artery disease or left ventricular hypertrophy, this demand for oxygen may not be met, leading to increasingly severe heart failure, to angina pectoris, or to myocardial infarction. As with left ventricular hypertrophy, dilation is evident on an ECG and chest x-ray.

If the blood pressure continues to rise or if the myocardium weakens, hypertrophy and dilation will be unable to maintain a stroke volume that is adequate to supply peripheral tissues with their required amounts of oxygen and nutrients. As this situation develops the patient first becomes aware of the symptoms of undue fatigue and dyspnea on exertion as the left ventricle becomes unable to increase its output in response to exercise. As left ventricular failure progresses, dyspnea develops with less and less exertion (progressing from ASA II to III to IV risk levels). Left ventricular failure also occurs at night when the patient lies down. At this time the total blood volume is increased as venous return from the lower extremities is improved because of the decreased effects on the legs of gravity in the supine position. A patient must now elevate their head and thorax at night with extra pillows in order to breathe comfortably, because this increased fluid volume begins to produce respiratory distress (e.g., orthopnea) as fluid from the cardiovascular bed enters into the alveolar sacs, thereby preventing the normal exchange of oxygen and carbon dioxide.

Blood volume increases in a second and perhaps more important manner that involves the kidneys. The decrease in stroke volume leads to a decrease in renal blood flow and glomerular filtration rate (GFR), thereby decreasing the excretion of sodium. In fact, tubular reabsorption of sodium is actually stimulated through the increased secretion of renin and its attendant chemical reactions (secondary to a decreased GFR). This increase in sodium retention leads to a decreased secretion of antidiuretic hormone from the pituitary gland, which is responsible for further water retention. These mechanisms result in a further increase in total blood volume (e.g., hypervolemia).

Hypervolemia produces an increased hydrostatic pressure in capillaries, leading at first to interstitial edema and then to an actual transudation of fluid into tissues with decreased tissue pressure. Edema of the ankles and lower extremities develops during the day when the patient is erect because of the downward force of gravity; it develops in the sacral region when the patient is recumbent at night or for long periods during illness or convalescence.

Clinical signs and symptoms of left ventricular failure become more prominent at night when most patients assume the recumbent position. During the day when a patient is in the erect position, the force of gravity causes the excessive fluid volume to be deposited into the subcutaneous tissues of the most dependent portions of the body (e.g.,ankles), producing signs of right ventricular failure.

When the patient assumes a supine position, the edematous fluid in the dependent portions of the body is mobilized, leading to a rapid increase in blood volume and in venous return to the heart. This may lead to overdistention of an already weakened left ventricle, producing an acute reduction in cardiac output and a large increase in the end-diastolic and end-systolic volumes. As a result the end-diastolic pressure may also rise. A normal end-diastolic pressure of 6 to 8 torr may rise to 30 to 40 torr or greater. The increased left ventricular pressure raises the left atrial pressure. The Frank-Starling principle enables the left atrium to accommodate this pressure, and after a few heartbeats the pressure in the left atrium increases to 30 to 40 torr or above, remaining elevated for as long as the left ventricle is failing.

This increased left atrial pressure is next transmitted backward to the pulmonary veins and capillaries so that the pulmonary capillary pressure also increases to 30 to 40 torr. When this occurs, water and solutes diffuse out of the capillaries into the alveolar air sacs, producing paroxysmal nocturnal dyspnea or acute pulmonary edema, or both. In the presence of this fluid in the alveolar air sacs, oxygen and carbon dioxide cannot be exchanged, and dyspnea is the result. Bronchospasm (cardiac asthma) is a common complicating factor of paroxysmal nocturnal dyspnea. Positional changes (e.g., to the upright position) commonly produce dramatic relief from symptoms of left ventricular failure by causing fluid to move from the alveolar sacs and concentrate in the base of the lungs.

Right ventricular and atrial failure occurs shortly after left ventricular failure as the increased pressure in the left heart continue to back up. This results in signs and symptoms of systemic venous and capillary congestion. As this increase in pressure develops, fluid leaves the vessels in the most dependent portions of the body (e.g., ankles and feet). In addition, because of the elevated right atrial pressure, venous return from the head and upper extremities is impaired, and the jugular veins become engorged. Impaired venous return from the lower portion of the body is evident through engorgement of the liver with blood (i.e., hepatomegaly).

Nocturia, or increased frequency of urination at night, is yet another sign of heart failure. During the day with the patient awake, renal function is poor because the patient's activities increase the degree of heart failure. Therefore, the patient produces less urine during the day. At night cardiac function improves, as does renal function. Increased glomerular filtration produces more urine—thus the symptom of nocturia results.

One final sign of heart failure is cyanosis. it is most evident in mucous membranes and is produced by the failure of the heart to provide an adequate stroke volume. In an effort to secure an adequate oxygen supply, the tissues of the body extract more oxygen than normal from the capillary blood. Therefore, the red blood cells within the capillaries and veins are poorly oxygenated and appear a darker color, which is clinically evident as cyanosis.

MANAGEMENT
Acute Pulmonary Edema

The patient with acute pulmonary edema represents a true medical emergency that must be managed quickly. In the dental office the patient who has a prior history of heart failure, be it left or right ventricular failure, or combined (congestive heart failure), and who is experiencing acute respiratory distress should be managed in the following manner:

Step 1: Terminate the dental procedure.

Step 2: Remove dental materials from the patient's mouth.

Step 3: Position the patient. As with patients with other forms of respiratory distress, on most occasions the patient suffering from acute pulmonary edema will remain conscious, although he or she may appear quite panicky and is potentially uncooperative.[1] Position the patient in the most comfortable manner, which will usually be in an upright position. The upright position allows excess fluids within the lung tissues to concentrate at the bases of the lungs, permitting a greater exchange of oxygen to occur. Should such a patient lose consciousness at any time, he or she must be placed in the supine position.

Step 4: Activate emergency medical services (EMS). With the onset of acute respiratory distress in a patient with preexisting congestive heart failure, emergency medical services should be sought immediately. The patient usually requires a period of hospitalization for further medical management. At the earliest opportunity, medical assistance should be sought. Further medical therapy in the hospital may include phlebotomy, an oxygen tent, and drugs such as digitalis and diuretics.

Step 5: Calm the patient. Reassure the patient that you are making an effort to manage the problem and that help has already been summoned.

Step 6: Basic life support, as indicated. In the patient with acute pulmonary edema, the airway, breathing, and circulation will be adequately maintained by the patient.

Step 7: Administer oxygen. Oxygen should be administered to all patients who demonstrate signs of acute pulmonary edema or severe congestive heart failure. High concentrations at high flows should be administered to prevent or alleviate hypoxia. Face masks should be used, with a flow rate of 10L or more of oxygen per minute (see Fig. 14-4).

Step 8: Monitor vital signs. Vital signs should be monitored and recorded, including blood pressure, heart rate and rhythm, and respiratory rate. Increases will be noted in blood pressure, heart rate, and respiratory rate. Such recordings demonstrate the presence of extreme apprehension and cardiac and pulmonary congestion.

Step 9: Alleviate symptoms of respiratory distress. The immediate primary goal in the management of acute pulmonary edema is the alleviation of the patient's breathing difficulties. Proper (upright) positioning of the patient is extremely important. If respiratory distress is still evident, however, additional steps may be taken. In acute pulmonary edema, the heart is unable to adequately handle the quantity of blood being delivered to it.

Step 9a: Bloodless phlebotomy. A procedure that may be carried out in the hospital is phlebotomy. Approximately 350 to 500 mL of blood is removed from the patient. Phlebotomy is sometimes rapidly effective in reducing respiratory symptoms. This effect is achieved through a reduction in venous return to the right side of the heart, while the left side is permitted to drain some of the excess fluid from the lungs.

Phlebotomy in the dental office is not often indicated. A similar effect may be achieved, however, through use of a bloodless phlebotomy. A bloodless phlebotomy temporarily removes approximately 12% of circulating blood volume, or 700 mL out of 6000 mL in the average male, permitting the heart to function more effectively and dyspnea to be alleviated.[18] Tourniquets or blood pressure cuffs are applied to the extremities. Wide, soft, rubber tubing should be used for the tourniquets. The tourniquets are placed approximately 6 inches below the groin and approximately 4 inches below the shoulders. Tourniquets are applied to only three extremities at a time. Every 5 to 10 minutes, one of the tourniquets is released and applied to the free extremity. The tourniquets, (or blood pressure cuffs), should be applied at a pressure less than the systolic blood pressure but greater than the diastolic pressure. An arterial pulse should be palpable distal to each tourniquet or cuff.

Bloodless phlebotomy actually leads to a total reduction in the circulating blood volume. While trapped in the extremities, a protein-poor filtrate is forced out of the capillaries into the tissues, where it remains for a period of time even after the tourniquet is removed.

Step 9b: Administer vasodilator. Within the past few years the administration of vasodilators in the management of congestive heart failure and acute pulmonary edema has become more favored. Venodilators, such as nitroglycerin, reduce the preload (e.g., filling pressure) but not systemic pressures (afterload). Nitrates are predominantly venodilators. Side effects associated with their administration include headache, dizziness, hypotension, and flushing. The administration of 0.8 to 1.2 mg (two to three tablets or sprays) every 5 to 10 minutes is used for the rapid treatment of acute pulmonary edema.[19] Onset of action is within 2 minutes, and duration is about 15 to 30 minutes. When sublingual tablets are used, the patient should be asked if the tablet tingles as it dissolves to ensure potency of the preparation. Nitroglycerin should only be used when the systolic blood pressure is above 100 torr.

Nifedipine, a calcium-channel blocker, has been used sublingually in the place of nitroglycerin in the management of acute pulmonary edema. A 10-mg nifedipine capsule is punctured several times and placed beneath the tongue and the patient instructed to suck on it. If the patient is uncooperative, open the capsule and squeeze the contents out under the tongue. Onset of nifedipine is slower than nitroglycerin, about 10 minutes, with a duration of between 30 and 60 minutes.[20]

Step 10: Alleviate apprehension. Most patients in acute pulmonary edema will be extremely apprehensive, bordering on panic. Increased apprehension leads to increases in cardiac and respiratory workload, which are absolutely contraindicated in these patients. For this reason, anxiety should be reduced.

If the preceding steps diminished the degree of respiratory distress, the patient may no longer be apprehensive. However, in the presence of contin-

ued anxiety and respiratory distress, drug therapy should be considered. A narcotic agonist such as meperidine, 25 to 50 mg IM or IV (titrated slowly), or morphine, 2 to 10 mg IV in 2-mg increments, should be considered for administration, if available (adult doses). Pediatric doses of morphine for pulmonary edema are 0.1 to 0.2 mg IV per kilogram of body weight. These agents act to reduce anxiety and agitation and also to produce vasodilation, thereby decreasing cardiac and pulmonary workloads.[21] An absolute contraindication to these agents in heart failure is the (1) clinical presence of hypoxia (see Table 13-1) with cyanosis, or of (2) mental confusion or delirium. Narcotics further depress respiration in these individuals when they already have severely compromised respiratory function. Naloxone must be available whenever narcotic agonists are employed. Nalbuphine, a narcotic agonist-antagonist, has also been used with considerable success.

Step 11: Discharge from the office. The patient with acute pulmonary edema will be hospitalized for additional management. Once medical assistance becomes available within the dental office, usual emergency treatment for pulmonary edema consists of (in addition to the steps already noted):

1. Continuous cardiac monitoring
2. Intravenous line established
3. Administration of furosemide, 40 mg IV
4. Dopamine infusion administered at 10 μg/kg/min, which increases renal perfusion and elevates blood pressure
5. Intubation, if the patient is in extremely poor condition
6. Emergency transport arranged

Step 12: Subsequent dental care. Once the patient has been stabilized in the hospital and dismissed, future dental care must take into account the event that occurred in the office. The stress reduction protocol must be considered as a means of minimizing future risk. Consultation with the patient's physician is essential in planning a rational dental treatment plan.

Drugs used in management: Oxygen, at high flow; Nitroglycerin, sublingual, or nifedipine; Morphine or meperidine (optional)

Medical assistance required: Yes

The management of congestive heart failure and acute pulmonary edema is summarized in the accompanying box.

MANAGEMENT OF HEART FAILURE AND ACUTE PULMONARY EDEMA

Terminate the dental procedure

↓

Remove dental materials from the patient's mouth

↓

Positon patient

↓

Activate EMS

↓

Calm the patient

↓

Basic life support, as indicated

↓

Administer oxygen

↓

Measure vital signs

↓

Alleviate symptoms of respiratory distress

↓

Bloodless phlebotomy

↓

Administer vasodilator

↓

Alleviate apprehension

↓

Subsequent dental care

REFERENCES

1. Stirling EL: Congestive heart failure. In *Emergency medicine,* ed 2, Rosen P, editor: St Louis, 1988, Mosby–Year Book.
2. Kannel WB, Thom TJ: Incidence, prevalence, and mortality of cardiovascular disease. In Hurst JW, editor: *The heart,* ed 6, New York, 1986, McGraw-Hill.
3. McKee PA, and others: The natural history of congestive heart failure: the Framingham study, *N Engl J Med* 285:1441, 1971.
4. Gibson TC, White KR, Klaimer LM: The prevalence of congestive heart failure in two rural communities, *J Chronic Dis* 19:141, 1966.
5. Hutter AM: Congestive heart failure. In Rubinstein E, Federman D, editors: *Scientific American medicine,* New York, 1985, Scientific American Illustrated Library.
6. Barkin RM, Rosen P: Congestive heart failure. In *Emergency pediatrics,* ed 3, Barkin RM, Rosen P, editors: St Louis, 1990, Mosby–Year Book.
7. Franciosa JA, Dunkman WB: Congestive heart failure. In Rose LF, Kaye D, editors: *Internal medicine for dentistry,* ed 2, St Louis, 1990, Mosby–Year Book.
8. Schulz H: Inotropic drugs and their mechanism of action, *J Am Coll Cardiol* 4:389, 1984.
9. Sonnenblick EH, and others: Dobutamine: a new synthetic cardioactive sympathetic amine, *N Engl J Med* 300:17, 1979.
10. Maskin CS, and others: Long-term amrinone therapy in patients with severe heart failure, *Am J Med* 72:113, 1982.
11. Zelcer AA, LeJemtel TH, Sonnenblick EH: Inotropic therapy in heart failure, *Heart Failure* 1:7, 1985.
12. Chidsey CA, Braunwald E, Morrow AG: Catecholamine excretion and cardiac stores of norepinephrine in congestive heart failure, *Am J Med* 39:442, 1962.
13. Braunwald E: The physical examination. In Braunwald E, editor: *Heart disease,* Philadelphia, 1980, WB Saunders.
14. Criteria Committee, New York Heart Association: *Diseases of the heart and blood vessels, nomenclature and criteria for diagnosis,* ed 6, Boston, 1964, Little, Brown.
15. Visscher MB, Haddy FJ, Stephens G: The physiology and pharmacology of lung edema, *Pharmacol Rev* 8:389, 1956.
16. Braunwald E, Sonnenblick EH, Ross J Jr: Contraction of the normal heart. In Braunwald E, editor: *Heart disease,* Philadelphia, 1980, WB Saunders.
17. Starling EH: *Lecture on the law of the heart (1915);* London, 1918, Longmans, Green.
18. McCarthy FM: Cardiovascular disease. In McCarthy FM: *Essentials of safe dentistry for the medically compromised patient,* Philadelphia, 1989, WB Saunders Co.
19. Cohn JN, Franciosa MD: Vasodilator therapy of cardiac failure, *N Engl J Med* 297:254, 1977.
20. Ludbrook PA, and others: Acute hemodynamic responses to sublingual nifedipine: dependence on left ventricular function, *Circulation* 65:3, 1982.
21. Vismara LA, Leaman DM, Zelis R: The effects of morphine on venous tone in patients with acute pulmonary edema, *Circulation* 54:335, 1976.

15 *Respiratory Distress: Differential Diagnosis*

In most clinical situations the cause of respiratory distress is readily discernible, therefore definitive management of the patient is expedited. However, there may be times in which the precise cause of respiratory distress is not apparent. In these cases consideration of the following factors will assist the doctor in determining the cause of the clinical problem, thereby permitting definitive therapy to proceed.

PRIOR MEDICAL HISTORY

The patient with respiratory distress almost always remains conscious during the episode. The doctor may take advantage of this situation by asking the patient about any previous episodes of respiratory distress. Problems such as asthma, heart failure, or previous episodes of hyperventilation usually are noted on the medical history questionnaire, facilitating the differential diagnosis. Should this patient lose consciousness at any time, management must then proceed as with any unconscious patient (see Section II).

Age of Patient

Respiratory distress in younger patients (under the age of 10) is most commonly related to asthma (usually allergic asthma); hyperventilation and heart failure are less common in this age group. Between the ages of 12 and 40, hyperventilation is the most likely cause of difficulty in breathing. Asthma may also occur in this age group, but in most instances the patient will have indicated a

prior awareness of its presence. Clinically significant heart failure is rarely seen before the age of 40. The peak incidence of heart failure in men is between the ages of 50 and 60 years and in women between the ages of 60 and 70 years.

Sex of Patient

The incidence of hyperventilation, asthma, and heart failure does not differ markedly between males and females, although the incidence of heart failure is somewhat greater in males compared to females under the age of 70 years.

Circumstances Associated with Respiratory Distress

Stress, physiologic or psychologic, is present in most instances of respiratory distress, and increases its severity in all cases. Hyperventilation is precipitated almost exclusively by extreme apprehension. Asthma, especially in children, may be acutely exacerbated in stressful situations regardless of the type of asthma (intrinsic or extrinsic) present. Heart failure patients undergo progressive deterioration of their physical condition when subjected to stress.

Presence of Clinical Symptoms Between Acute Episodes

The patient with heart failure may exhibit clinical signs and symptoms of the problem at all times, either during physical activity or at rest. Orthopnea, dependent edema, peripheral cyanosis, dyspnea, and undue fatigue may be evident at all dental appointments, depending on the degree of pump failure that is present. Asthmatics are usually asymptomatic in the intervals between acute episodes; however, noisy breathing and chronic cough may be present while they are at rest. No clinical signs and symptoms of hyperventilation will be noted between episodes.

Position of Patient

The position of the patient at the onset of clinical symptoms of respiratory distress will be most relevant in heart failure. Respiratory distress becomes progressively more severe as the dental chair is reclined toward the supine position. Dramatic relief of symptoms can often be achieved by permitting the patient to sit upright.

Signs and symptoms of asthma and hyperventilation are not altered by repositioning a patient, although most patients experiencing respiratory distress are better able to breathe when sitting upright.

Sounds Associated with Respiratory Distress

Wheezing is usually present in patients with asthma. It may also be present in paroxysmal nocturnal dyspnea and pulmonary edema (cardiac asthma), although in these circumstances it is associated with other signs and symptoms of heart failure. Partial obstruction of the trachea or bronchi by a foreign object may also produce wheezing. Moist, wet respirations may be evident with heart failure, especially acute pulmonary edema, which is often associated with a frothy, pink-tinged sputum and cough.

With hyperventilation, breathing is usually more rapid and deeper than normal, but no abnormal sound is associated with it.

Symptoms Associated with Respiratory Difficulty

Shortness of breath is observed in most cases of respiratory difficulty. With heart failure, it becomes progressively worse when the patient reclines (orthopnea) and increases with exertion. Shortness of breath seen with hyperventilation is related to anxiety and a feeling of suffocation and is not related to exertion. Hyperventilation is not associated with cough. With asthma, shortness of breath is associated with episodic wheezing during acute periods, and there is an asymptomatic state between episodes.

Peripheral Edema and Cyanosis

Peripheral edema and cyanosis may be present in a patient with heart failure. Other possible causes of peripheral edema are renal disease, varicose veins, and pregnancy, whereas cardiorespiratory disease and polycythemia vera are causes of cyanosis. In severe asthma with hypoxia or hypercarbia, cyanosis may be present; however, peripheral edema is not noted. Hyperventilation is not usually associated with peripheral edema or cyanosis.

Paresthesia of Extremities

Tingling and numbness of the fingers, toes, and perioral region are present with hyperventilation. In milder episodes of acute asthma and heart failure, these symptoms may also be present, produced by hyperventilation secondary to acute anxiety.

Use of Accessory Muscles of Respiration

The patient with acute asthma demonstrates use of the accessory muscles of respiration (abdominal and neck muscles). This may also be noted in patients with acute pulmonary edema.

Chest Pain

Chest pain is commonly experienced by the hyperventilating patient. The pain is often described as a "weight" or a "pressing" sensation, or as "shooting" or "stabbing." Other clinical manifestations of cardiac disease are rarely present, however. The age of the hyperventilating patient (under 35 years) is usually below that at which one normally expects to encounter cardiovascular disease. Asthmatic and heart failure patients usually do not experience chest pain along with their other clinical symptoms.

Heart Rate and Blood Pressure

Measurement of the heart rate and blood pressure during respiratory distress usually demonstrates definite elevations of both of these vital signs. This elevation occurs with hyperventilation and during the acute asthmatic episode because of the presence of anxiety. In these cases blood pressure (systolic and diastolic) and heart rate are elevated.

With heart failure, although both systolic and diastolic pressures are elevated, the diastolic pressure is usually elevated to a greater extent: therefore the pulse pressure (systolic − diastolic) is narrowed (to less than 40). The heart rate increases with heart failure.

Duration of Respiratory Distress

Respiratory distress associated with heart failure often improves dramatically by simply repositioning the patient. However, if pulmonary edema is present, respiratory distress is not improved until definitive management is instituted.

Most asthma attacks will not resolve without drug management for a considerable period of time. Therefore, bronchodilator therapy is employed as soon as it is available in most cases. Status asthmaticus requires more definitive management—possibly a period of hospitalization.

Hyperventilation is usually manageable without drug intervention and rarely, if ever, necessitates the help of additional personnel or hospitalization. The algorithm for the diagnosis and management of respiratory difficulty is found on p. 199.

16 *Altered Consciousness: General Considerations*

A number of systemic medical conditions may present themselves clinically as alterations in the level of consciousness of the victim. Almost every one of the situations listed in Table 16-1 that produce altered consciousness may also lead ultimately to unconsciousness. However, in most cases the prompt recognition of clinical signs and symptoms and the equally prompt institution of corrective measures will permit the victim to retain consciousness until definitive management becomes available.

The following are definitions of relevant terms that are employed in this section:

Confusion. A mental state marked by the mingling of ideas with consequent disturbances of comprehension and understanding, leading to bewilderment.

Delirium. A mental disturbance marked by illusions, delusions, cerebral excitement, physical restlessness, and incoherence.

Dizziness. A disturbed sense of relationship to space; a sensation of unsteadiness with a feeling of movement within the head.

Altered consciousness may be the first clinical sign of a serious medical problem that requires immediate and intensive therapy to maintain life. It is important therefore that the doctor be aware of a patient's medical background in order to promptly recognize a developing problem when it arises and to manage any emergency situation that may develop as a result of it at a later time.

PREDISPOSING FACTORS

The most common cause of altered consciousness in a dental setting is the ingestion or admin-

istration of drugs. With the increasing use of pharmacosedation in dentistry, a dentist is likely to encounter a greater number of reports of inadvertent overadministration of these agents to patients. Knowledge of drug pharmacology and the proper use of these drugs will, however, minimize these incidents.

One particular psychosedative is rarely prescribed by the doctor but may well be the most commonly used drug by dental patients. That drug is alcohol. Most practicing dentists have on occasion been called upon to manage the dental needs of a patient who has taken an accidental (or in some instances, an intentional) overdose; in other words, the patient is intoxicated. Proper patient management at such times is to postpone the planned dental treatment and reschedule the patient for a later date with a strict admonition concerning the self-administration of drugs. It might be important for the doctor to seek out the reasons behind the patient's need for alcohol (or other mood-altering drugs) prior to dental treatment and, if appropriate, to take steps to alleviate the patient's dental anxiety. To administer additional drugs (e.g., local anesthetics or sedatives) that depress the central nervous system (CNS) to a patient who has ingested an unknown quantity of an unknown drug that also possesses CNS-depressant properties is to invite serious consequences.

Hyperventilation is the most common non-drug cause of altered consciousness. Though hyperventilation will rarely lead to the loss of consciousness, with a delay in recognition and management, it may. Fear and anxiety are the primary precipitating factors in almost all cases of hyperventilation, which

Table 16-1. Causes of altered consciousness

Cause	Frequency	Where discussed
Drug overdose (alcohol, barbiturates, insulin)	Most common	Drug-related emergencies (Section VI)
Hyperventilation	Common	Respiratory difficulty (Section III)
Hypoglycemia	Common	Altered consciousness (Section IV)
Hyperglycemia	Less common	Altered consciousness (Section IV)
Cerebrovascular accident, transient ischemic attack	Less common	Altered consciousness (Section IV)
Hyperthyroidism	Rare	Altered consciousness (Section IV)
Hypothyroidism	Rare	Altered consciousness (Section IV)

is seen predominantly in adolescents and young adults (under the age of 40 years). A full discussion of hyperventilation is presented in Chapter 12.

Three additional systemic problems that present with clinical symptoms of altered consciousness—diabetes mellitus, cerebrovascular ischemia and infarction, and thyroid gland dysfunction—are discussed in this section. Diabetes mellitus and its associated acute clinical complications, hypoglycemia and hyperglycemia, are commonly encountered. Inadequate medical management of diabetes and the presence of additional stress may rapidly lead to an altered state of consciousness and possibly to the loss of consciousness. The nondiabetic patient may also be susceptible to episodes of hypoglycemia in certain circumstances.

Cerebrovascular ischemia and infarction (stroke) are less common but potentially more serious causes of altered consciousness. Proper management of the postcerebrovascular accident (CVA) patient greatly reduces the risk of a second incident precipitated during dental treatment. A prodromal form of cerebrovascular ischemia, the transient ischemic attack (TIA), is discussed along with the management of this patient.

Thyroid gland dysfunction is another situation in which states of altered consciousness may develop. Although acute clinical complications from thyroid hypo- or hyperfunction are extremely rare in dental situations, the doctor should be aware of the presence of thyroid gland dysfunction and be able to recognize signs and symptoms of associated complications. Of even more importance to the doctor treating a patient with thyroid dysfunction is the increased incidence of cardiovascular disease, which is observed in these persons.

In all of these situations, an increase in physiological or psychological stress will increase the potential for an acute exacerbation of the patient's underlying medical problem during dental care.

PREVENTION

Recognition of unusually high levels of apprehension in a prospective patient will minimize the occurrence of vasodepressor syncope and hyperventilation, whereas the proper use of pharmacosedative techniques will prevent treatment-related drug overdose. In other situations, awareness of a patient's medical history permits the doctor to modify the treatment plan to minimize any risk to the patient. The health questionnaire, physical examination, and monitoring of vital signs are invaluable in the proper pretreatment assessment of a patient. Specific questions and examinations are referred to as each potential emergency situation is discussed.

CLINICAL MANIFESTATIONS

A spectrum of signs and symptoms may be present in patients with altered consciousness: the cold, wet appearance, mental confusion, and bizarre behavior of the hypoglycemic patient contrasts markedly with the hot, dry, florid appearance of the hyperglycemic diabetic patient. The presence of acetone on the breath further aids in the clinical recognition of hyperglycemia.

Cerebrovascular accident (stroke) may develop with a sudden onset of unconsciousness (presenting an extremely grave prognosis) or with a more gradual onset of symptoms that are related to central nervous system dysfunction. These may include variable degrees of derangement of speech, thought, motion, sensation, or vision. The state of consciousness may be unimpaired (patient is alert) or the patient may demonstrate varying degrees of alteration of consciousness that range from headache, dizziness, and drowsiness to mental confusion.

If untreated, hypothyroidism may cause symptoms of weakness, fatigue, lethargy, and slow speech, as well as many other clinical signs. Untreated hyperthyroidism in contrast causes restlessness, nervousness, irritability, and degrees of motor incoordination ranging from a fine, mild tremulousness to gross tremor. A serious consequence of unmanaged hyperthyroidism is the "thyroid storm" or thyroid crisis. It may arise spontaneously but more commonly follows sudden stress in patients who are clinically hyperthyroid. The death rate associated with this is significant.

PATHOPHYSIOLOGY

In all three situations to be discussed in this section, the clinical manifestations are evident systemically even though a specific factor is responsible for the onset of symptoms and signs. Most clinical complications of diabetes mellitus are caused by a level of blood glucose that is either too high or too low. In addition, diabetes mellitus, although usually considered a disease of impaired carbohydrate utilization, is also a disease of the blood vessels, leading to a much greater incidence of cardiovascular disease in diabetic patients than in nondiabetic patients. A change in the quality of the circulating blood is responsible for most of the acute clinical problems associated with diabetes.

Signs and symptoms of thyroid gland dysfunction are related clinically to the circulating blood level of thyroid hormone (thyroxine) and its pharmacologic actions on other parts of the body.

Inadequate blood flow to the brain also produces signs and symptoms of impaired consciousness. Temporary insufficiency leads to the clinical syndrome called transient ischemic attack; more prolonged insufficiency results in permanent neurologic changes, termed cerebrovascular infarction (stroke).

MANAGEMENT

When altered consciousness is recognized, several basic steps are called for in the immediate care of the patient. Definitive management of each situation is discussed in appropriate chapters.

Step 1: Recognize altered consciousness. Changes in the level of consciousness occurring during dental therapy should be a warning to the doctor to terminate the procedure. Signs and symptoms are described in the following chapters. In most cases of altered consciousness, however, the change in level of consciousness is more gradual (over hours [hypoglycemia] to weeks or longer [thyroid dysfunction]), so the change in level of consciousness will be visible prior to the onset of treatment.

Step 2: Terminate dental procedure.

Step 3: Position the patient. Proper positioning of the patient with an altered state of consciousness varies according to the causative factor. In most instances the patient retains consciousness; therefore, the supine, semisupine, or erect position may be used. Patient comfort and vital signs (particularly blood pressure) are factors that will influence the position to be used. The conscious diabetic or thyroid patient may be most comfortable if permitted to sit up. However, should unconsciousness

occur, the patient must be managed as any other unconscious patient.

Cerebrovascular accidents are often associated with extreme elevations of blood pressure. In such cases a nonrecumbent (supine) position will be important because in an upright position, the cerebral blood pressure will be somewhat reduced. Should a CVA lead to rapid loss of consciousness associated with a high blood pressure level, positioning of the patient is altered slightly. The supine position will cause an increase in cerebral blood pressure that may not be beneficial at this time. Therefore, the patient should be placed in the supine position with the head slightly elevated.

Step 4: Basic life support, as indicated. Institute the steps of basic life support as soon as possible: Assess airway patency and provide an airway if needed; assess spontaneous ventilation and ventilate as needed; assess circulatory adequacy and provide artificial circulation if needed.

Step 5: Monitor vital signs. Blood pressure, heart rate and rhythm, respiratory rate, and temperature should be monitored throughout the crisis period, and a permanent record kept.

Step 6: Manage signs and symptoms. Clinical signs and symptoms should be treated in an effort to increase the patient's comfort. Blankets should be available if the patient is shivering; tight garments should be loosened to allow for ease of breathing.

Step 7: Definitive management. At this point, a decision must be made as to the definitive management of the problem. In-office management will range from basic life support (for the cerebrovascular accident) to the administration of drugs to terminate the episode (for hypoglycemia). The following chapters will describe in detail the therapy recommended for each situation.

MANAGEMENT OF ALTERED CONSCIOUSNESS

Recognize altered consciousness
↓
Terminate dental procedure
↓
Position patient
↓
Provide basic life support, as indicated
↓
Monitor vital signs
↓
Manage signs and symptoms
↓
Definitive management

17 Diabetes Mellitus: Hyperglycemia and Hypoglycemia

Diabetes mellitus represents a syndrome of disordered glucose metabolism and inappropriate hyperglycemia, which result from an absolute deficiency of the secretion of insulin, a reduction in its biologic effectiveness, or both. Approximately 200 million persons worldwide and about 20 million Americans have diabetes mellitus,[1] representing a 50% increase in the incidence of diabetes within the past two decades.[2-5] Only about half of these persons are aware that they have diabetes. Approximately 2% to 4% of the population is estimated to have diabetes. Diabetes is also prevalent in children, with about one in 600 school children having the disease.[6] Statistics indicate that one half of all children currently diagnosed with diabetes will die of renal disease an average of 25 years after the initial diagnosis is made.[2] Diabetes is the third leading cause of death in the United States.[7] Morbidity and mortality from diabetes is most often related to its vascular complications.[8] A study of mortality in diabetics reported 36.8% deaths related to cardiovascular causes, 17.5% to cerebrovascular disorders, 15.5% to diabetic coma, and 12.5% to renal failure.[9]

The incidence of diabetes increases with increasing age.[10] Table 17-1 illustrates the incidence of diabetes with age; approximately 80% of diabetics are over 45 years of age. Little and Falace[11] estimate that a dental practice serving an adult population of 2000 people could expect to encounter about 40 to 70 people with diabetes, about half of whom will be unaware of their condition.

ACUTE COMPLICATIONS

Hyperglycemia, or high blood sugar, and its sequelae represent one of two clinical complications of importance to the doctor who is called upon to treat the diabetic patient. The second and usually more acute life-threatening complication is hypoglycemia, or low blood sugar. Hypoglycemia may be present in diabetic and nondiabetic individuals. Blood glucose levels below 50 mg/100 mL (venous blood) usually indicate hypoglycemia in the adult, whereas blood glucose values of <40 mg/100 mL indicate hypoglycemia in the child.[12] Signs and symptoms of hypoglycemia may become evident within minutes, leading rapidly to the loss of consciousness. Hyperglycemia may also ultimately lead to unconsciousness (diabetic coma), but this occurrence usually represents the end of a much longer process (the time elapsed from the onset of symp-

Table 17-1. Incidence of diabetes by age in the United States

Age group (in years)	Incidence (per 1000 people)
Birth-17	1.3
25-40	17
45-65	45
65 or older	79

Data adapted from Little JW and Falace DA: *Dental management of the medically compromised patient,* ed 3, St Louis, 1988, Mosby–Year Book.

toms to the loss of consciousness is usually at least 48 hours). In either situation the doctor must be able to recognize the clinical problem and proceed to take those steps necessary to manage it properly. The differences between these two conditions are stressed in this chapter to aid in the differential diagnosis of diabetic complications.

CHRONIC COMPLICATIONS

In addition to hyperglycemia and hypoglycemia, there are other, more chronic complications to which the diabetic patient is subject. The importance of these complications is noted by the fact that most morbidity and mortality in diabetic patients occurs from them (Table 17-2).

The three major categories of diabetic complications are large blood vessel disease, small blood vessel disease (microangiopathy), and an increased susceptibility to infection. Large blood vessel disease, such as arteriosclerosis, is seen frequently in the nondiabetic population; however, it is much more common in persons with diabetes and it occurs at an earlier age.[13] The clinical manifestations observed are related to an inadequate blood supply to the heart (angina pectoris, myocardial infarction,

Table 17-2. Chronic complications of diabetes mellitus

Affected part of body or condition	Complication
Vascular system	Atherosclerosis
	Large vessel disease
	Microangiopathy
Kidneys	Diabetic glomerulosclerosis
	Arteriolar nephrosclerosis
	Pyelonephritis
Nervous system	Motor, sensory, and autonomic neuropathy
Eyes	Retinopathy
	Cataract formation
	Glaucoma
	Extraocular muscle palsies
Skin	Xanthoma diabeticorum
	Necrobiosis lipoidica diabeticorum
	Pruritis
	Furunculosis
	Mycosis
Mouth	Gingivitis
	Increased incidence of dental caries and periodontal disease
	Alveolar bone loss
Pregnancy	Increased incidence of large babies, stillbirths, miscarriages, neonatal deaths, and congenital defects

sudden death), the brain (cerebrovascular ischemia or infarction), the kidneys (glomerulosclerosis), and the lower extremities (gangrene). High blood pressure also occurs more frequently and at an earlier age in diabetic patients.[14,15]

Diabetic microangiopathy, or small blood vessel disease, is related to disorders affecting the arterioles, venules, and capillaries. It is thought to be specific, occurring only in patients with diabetes mellitus. Clinical manifestations of microangiopathy are most often noted in the eye (diabetic retinopathy),[16] kidney (arteriolar nephrosclerosis),[17] and lower extremities (gangrene).[18] The cause of diabetic microangiopathy is not yet entirely clear, but two interpretations are most often accepted. The first states that the cause is related to the carbohydrate intolerance associated with diabetes mellitus; however, there are instances in which microangiopathy develops in the absence of carbohydrate intolerance. A second theory links microangiopathy to a genetic factor that also manifests diabetes.

Regardless of the cause, diabetic microangiopathy may represent a more serious disease than the carbohydrate intolerance itself. Studies of the effects of blood glucose level on the progression of microangiopathy have not yet demonstrated that careful control of blood glucose levels decreases or retards small vessel disease. The extent of diabetic microangiopathy is such that approximately 11% to 18% of all diabetics have treatable diabetic retinopathy.[19] Diabetic retinopathy represents the single most common cause of blindness in developed countries for patients between the ages of 36 and 64 years.[20] Diabetic patients have 20 times the incidence of gangrene of the feet as do nondiabetics.[18] It is well known that diabetics are more prone to the development of infection than are nondiabetics. Although the precise cause of this is not known, it is probably related to the combination of vascular lesions and infection.[21] Inflammatory periodontal diseases are also noted with increased frequency in uncontrolled diabetics, though not to any greater extent than in well-controlled diabetics.[22] In order to prevent severe infection, scrupulous personal hygiene must be practiced. Diabetic renal disease, a major cause of illness and death, particularly in female diabetics, may be related to the high glucose levels present in the urine, which serves as an excellent growth medium for microorganisms. Microangiopathy of diabetic renal disease will be observed in two thirds of diabetics after 20 years of the disease and generally will cause proteinuria.[1] Within 5 years of the onset of proteinuria, uremia may ensue.

The doctor who is called upon to treat the dental needs of the diabetic patient must be aware of the acute complications of diabetes (i.e., hyperglycemia and hypoglycemia) and must take measures to avoid their occurrence. He or she must also look for the possible presence of chronic complications of diabetes; their presence increases the medical risk to the patient during dental care. Modifications in the dental treatment plan are likely to be required in these circumstances.

PREDISPOSING FACTORS

Major factors leading to the development of diabetes mellitus are:
1. Genetic disorder
2. Primary destruction of the islets of Langerhans in the pancreas, caused by inflammation, cancer, or surgery
3. An endocrine condition, such as hyperpituitarism or hyperthyroidism
4. Administration of steroids, resulting in iatrogenic diabetes

The most important factor in the development of diabetes mellitus is heredity. It is known that if one identical twin develops diabetes, the other twin will also become diabetic if he or she lives long enough. In addition, the offspring of two diabetic parents have almost a 100% chance of developing the disease. As illustrated in Table 17-3, it is possible to predict a risk factor for the development of diabetes mellitus according to previous family history.

TYPES OF DIABETES

Until recently, the classification of diabetes was based upon the age of onset of the disease. In other words, the classifications were adult-onset and juvenile-onset diabetes (Table 17-4). However, the age of onset is no longer considered to be a criterion for classification of diabetic patients. Instead, in 1979 the National Diabetes Data Group recommended a therapeutic classification, which has been

endorsed by the American Diabetes Association. This classification is presented in Table 17-5 and the types of diabetes are compared in Table 17-6.

The category of impaired glucose tolerance (IGT) is relatively new. It is significant in that it is *not* associated with the complications (chronic and acute) of diabetes mellitus.[23] Many within the IGT group will spontaneously develop a normal glucose tolerance. However, between 1% to 5% of the IGT group will decompensate annually into the diabetes mellitus group.[24]

The primary form of diabetes is genetic or hereditary, of which there are two types, insulin-dependent diabetes mellitus (IDDM) and non–insulin-dependent diabetes mellitus (NIDDM). These forms are described in the following section.

Type I—Insulin-Dependent Diabetes Mellitus (IDDM)

Approximately 5% of diabetic patients develop insulin-dependent diabetes mellitus (IDDM). This is a more severe form of diabetes, characterized in its untreated state by ketoacidosis (DKA—diabetic ketoacidosis). Seen more commonly in adolescents, IDDM may also develop in adults, usually in the nonobese, and in those who are elderly when hyperglycemia first appears. In IDDM, circulating insulin is essentially absent (thus the term *insulinopenic*), glucagon levels in the plasma are elevated, and pancreatic beta cells fail to respond to all insulinogenic stimuli. Exogenous insulin is required to reverse the catabolic state, to prevent DKA, to reduce the hyperglucagonemia, and to reduce the elevated blood glucose level.

Recent studies have demonstrated that the incidence of IDDM is linked to the presence or absence of certain genetically determined cell surface an-

Table 17-3. Prediction of diabetic risk

Relative with diabetes		Diabetic relative on other side of family	Maximum risk (%)
Parent	*plus*	Grandparent and aunt or uncle	85
Parent	*plus*	Grandparent, aunt, or uncle	60
Parent	*plus*	First cousin	40
Parent			22
Grandparent			14
First cousin			9

From Steinberg AG: *Ann NY Acad Sci* 82:197, 1959.

Table 17-4. Prior classification of diabetes by the American Diabetes Association, 1975

Hereditary, primary, or idiopathic diabetes
Prediabetes
Subclinical, latent, or stress diabetes
Chemical diabetes
Overt or clinical diabetes
Juvenile or early-onset diabetes
Maturity-, adult-, or late-onset diabetes

Nonhereditary, secondary diabetes
Damage to or removal of pancreatic islet tissue
Disorders of other endocrine glands
Drugs or chemicals

From National Diabetes Data Group: Classification and diagnosis of diabetes mellitus and other categories of glucose intolerance, *Diabetes* 28:1039-1057, 1979.

Table 17-5. Classification of diabetes mellitus and other categories of glucose intolerance

Diabetes mellitus (DM)

Insulin-dependent diabetes mellitus (IDDM)—Type 1
Non–insulin-dependent diabetes mellitus (NIDDM)—Type 2
    Nonobese
    Obese
Other types—includes diabetes mellitus associated with certain other conditions and syndromes
    Pancreatic disease
    Disease of hormonal etiology
    Drug- or chemical-induced condition
    Insulin receptor abnormalities
    Certain genetic syndromes
    Miscellaneous

Impaired glucose tolerance (IGT)

Nonobese
Obese
Impaired glucose tolerance associated with certain conditions and syndromes
    Pancreatic disease
    Disease of hormonal etiology
    Drug- or chemical-induced condition
    Insulin receptor abnormalities
    Certain genetic syndromes
    Miscellaneous
Gestational diabetes (GDM)
Statistical risk classes (subjects with normal glucose tolerance but statistically increased risk of developing diabetes)
Previous abnormality of glucose tolerance
Potential abnormality of glucose tolerance

From Bennett PH: The diagnosis of diabetes: new international classification and diagnostic criteria, *Ann Rev Med* 34:295, 1983.

Table 17-6. Clinical classification of idiopathic diabetes mellitus syndromes

Type	Ketosis	Islet cell antibodies	HLA association	Treatment
Insulin-dependent (IDDM)	Present	Present at onset	Positive	Insulin (mixtures of rapid-acting and intermediate-acting insulin, at least twice daily) and diet
Non–insulin-dependent (NIDDM)				
Nonobese	Absent	Absent	Negative	1. Eucaloric diet alone 2. Diet plus insulin or sulfonylureas
Obese	Absent	Absent	Negative	1. Weight reduction 2. Hypocaloric diet plus sulfonylureas or insulin for symptomatic control only

From Karam JH: Diabetes mellitus, hypoglycemia and lipoprotein disorders. In Schroeder SA, Tierney LM, editors: *Current medical diagnosis and treatment*, Norwalk, CT, 1992, Appleton & Lange.

tigens found on lymphocytes. Human lymphocyte antigens (HLA) are strongly associated with the development of type I diabetes.[25] They are located on the sixth human chromosome, adjacent to immune response genes. Additionally, an autoimmune cause for type I diabetes is suggested by the discovery of autoantibodies to pancreatic beta cells and other endocrine organs.[26]

Because of the immune factors associated with the development of IDDM, it is felt that IDDM is the result of an infectious or environmental insult to pancreatic beta cells in genetically predisposed persons. These extrinsic factors include damage produced by viruses such as mumps or coxsackievirus B, by toxic chemicals, or by destructive cytotoxins and antibodies released from sensitized immunocytes.[27,28]

Type II—Non–Insulin-Dependent Diabetes Mellitus (NIDDM)

Type II diabetes, non–insulin-dependent diabetes mellitus (NIDDM), represents a heterogeneous group composed of milder forms of diabetes that occur most frequently in adults but are seen occasionally in children. Circulating endogenous insulin blood levels are present and adequate to prevent ketoacidosis (insulinoplethoric), but insulin levels are either subnormal or relatively inadequate in the face of increased needs, caused by insensitivity of the tissues.

Type II diabetes mellitus is a nonketotic form of diabetes that is not linked to HLA markers on the sixth chromosome; it has no islet cell antibodies. Persons with type II diabetes do not depend upon exogenous insulin therapy to sustain life—therefore the name, non–insulin-dependent diabetes mellitus, is appropriate.

Regardless of body weight, the tissues of the NIDDM patient demonstrate a degree of insensitivity to insulin. This is produced by either a lack of insulin receptors in peripheral tissues or by an insensitivity of those insulin receptors that are present.

There are two subcategories of type II diabetes mellitus. These subgroups are based on the presence or absence of obesity.

Nonobese NIDDM

The person with nonobese NIDDM demonstrates either an absent or significantly blunted early phase of insulin release in response to a glucose challenge. This poor insulin release may also be demonstrated in response to other insulinogenic stimuli, such as acute intravenous administration of glucagon or sulfonylureas.

Hyperglycemia noted in nonobese NIDDM often

responds to oral hypoglycemic agents or, on occasion, to dietary therapy alone. On rare occasions, insulin therapy is required to achieve satisfactory control of blood sugar levels, even though it is not required to prevent ketosis.

Obese NIDDM

Obese NIDDM occurs secondary to extrapancreatic factors that produce an insensitivity to endogenous insulin. It is characterized by a nonketotic mild diabetes that occurs primarily in adults but also may be seen in children. The primary problem is a target organ disorder, which results in a lack of sensitivity to insulin. Hyperplasia of pancreatic β cells is often present and probably accounts for the fasting hyperinsulinism and exaggerated insulin responses to glucose and other stimuli seen in the milder forms of this disorder.

Obesity is commonly noted in this disorder because of excess caloric intake, perhaps resulting from hunger caused by mild postprandial hypoglycemia after excess insulin release. In this form of diabetes, insulin insensitivity is correlated with the presence of distended adipocytes. Liver and muscle cells also resist the deposition of additional glycogen and triglycerides in their storage depots.

Two mechanisms have been offered to explain the insensitivity of tissues to insulin in the obese form of diabetes mellitus. It is thought that chronic overfeeding may lead to either (1) sustained pancreatic β cell stimulation and hyperinsulinism, which by itself may induce receptor insensitivity to insulin, or (2) a postreceptor defect associated with overdistended storage depots and a reduced ability to clear nutrients from the circulation. Consequent hyperinsulinism induces receptor insensitivity to insulin.[24]

A reduction in overfeeding can interrupt either cycle regardless of the mechanism. In the first situation, a restricted diet would reduce islet cell stimulation of insulin release, thereby restoring insulin receptor sites and improving tissue sensitivity to insulin. In the second situation, normal tissue sensitivity would return as storage depots became less saturated.

Other possible causes of carbohydrate intolerance and hyperinsulinism in response to glucose include chronic muscle inactivity or disease and liver disease. Secondary causes of carbohydrate intolerance include endocrine disorders (e.g., tumors) associated with excessive production of growth hormone, glucocorticosteroids, catecholamines (e.g., epinephrine), or glucagon. In these latter four cases, the peripheral response to insulin is decreased.

The prognosis for both forms of diabetes mellitus, even in the presence of scrupulous control over blood sugar levels, is still uncertain. The belief that tight glycemic control will limit or reverse diabetic complications has led to more aggressive diabetic therapy and monitoring.[29] Recent research with pancreatic islet transplants[30,31] and improved insulin delivery systems, such as the insulin pump,[32] may make it possible to determine if adequate control can minimize the severity or delay the onset of complications.

In one series of 164 juvenile-onset, insulin-dependent diabetics (median age, 9 years old at onset), data were collected after 25 years. Out of every group of five from the larger group on standard dietary and insulin control, one diabetic had died and one was incapacitated with severe proliferative retinopathy and renal failure. Two others were active, contributing members of society despite mild background retinopathy, mild nephropathy, neuropathy, and some degree of ischemia of the feet. The fifth diabetic was completely free of complications.[33]

It appears that the period between 10 and 20 years after the onset of diabetes is a critical one. If the patient experiences no significant complications during this period, there is a strong likelihood that reasonably good health will continue.

Knowledge of the type of diabetes the patient has will enable the doctor to estimate the risk factor in each case. However, there are other factors, such as infection and pregnancy, that may lead to a diabetic patient's disease going out of control. Table 17-7 compares IDDM and NIDDM.

HYPERGLYCEMIA

Hyperglycemia may be precipitated by the following factors, all of which increase the body's requirements for insulin: weight gain, cessation of exercise, pregnancy, hyperthyroidism or thyroid medication, epinephrine therapy, corticosteroid therapy, acute infection, and fever. Although hyperglycemia is not usually a situation that by itself leads to acute life-threatening emergencies, it may, if untreated, progress to diabetic ketoacidosis (DKA) and diabetic coma, which are life-threatening conditions. Diabetic ketoacidosis most often occurs in the type 1 diabetic and is associated with inadequate administration of insulin or with infection, but it can occur in type 2 diabetics and may be associated with any kind of medication, epinephrine therapy, or stress.[34] Infection and a secondary disease state are also common causes of hyperglycemia in diabetic individuals. Diabetic ketoacidosis is slower in onset, producing in the younger patient, 1 day to 2 weeks of malaise, nausea, polydipsa, polyuria, and polyphagia.[35] It is not uncommon for the patient to be vomiting, and to be short of breath.

HYPOGLYCEMIA

Hypoglycemia, unlike hyperglycemia, may manifest itself rapidly. This is especially true in patients receiving injectable insulin therapy, for whom loss of consciousness may occur within minutes after insulin administration. In patients on oral hypoglycemic agents, the onset of symptoms is slower, usually developing over several hours.

Factors that decrease a patient's requirement for insulin include weight loss, increased physical exercise, termination of pregnancy, termination of other drug therapies (e.g., epinephrine, thyroid, corticosteroid), and recovery from infection and fever. Administration of the usual dose of insulin at this time is associated with an increased risk of development of hypoglycemia. Common causes of

Table 17-7. Comparison of type I (IDDM) and type II (NIDDM) diabetes mellitus

Factors compared	Type I (IDDM)	Type II (NIDDM)
Frequency (percentage of total diabetic population)	5	85
Age at onset (years)	15	40 and over
Body build	Normal or thin	Obese
Severity	Severe	Mild
Use of insulin	Almost all	25%-30%
Oral hypoglycemic agents	Very few respond	50% respond
Ketoacidosis	Common	Uncommon
Complications	90% in 20 years	Less common than with IDDM
Rate of clinical onset	Rapid	Slow
Stability	Unstable	Stable
Family history of diabetes	Common	Less common than with IDDM
HLA* and abnormal autoimmune reactions	Present	Not present
Insulin receptor defects	Usually not found	—

From Little JW, Falace DA: *Dental management of the medically compromised patient*, ed 3, St Louis, 1988, Mosby–Year Book.
*HLA, human lymphocyte antigen.

hypoglycemia are omission or delay of meals, excessive exercise before meals, and overdose of insulin. Table 17-8 lists frequently observed causes of hypoglycemia in known diabetic patients.

Dental treatment is a potential threat to the diabetic patient and to the control of this disease state. First, stress, both physiologic and psychologic, increases the body's requirement for insulin, so that hyperglycemia may occur in the diabetic dental patient. (Both the doctor and the patient must be aware of this so that necessary modifications may be made during dental management and, if necessary, to the insulin dosage to preclude the progression of this state to diabetic coma.) Second, dental treatment may necessitate that the patient alter his or her normal eating habits for varying periods of time. Some patients will purposefully avoid eating before a dental appointment so that their teeth will be clean. A dental patient may out of necessity be treated during a normal lunch or dinner hour, thereby delaying a meal or even missing a meal entirely. Third, the ingestion of food may be altered by the dental procedure itself. Prolonged local anesthesia after therapy and extensive dental procedures (e.g., periodontal or oral surgery, or endodontics), using drugs such as bupivacaine and etidocaine, may cause the patient to avoid eating and thus increase the risk of hypoglycemia.

MANAGEMENT OF DIABETES

Diabetes is a fascinating disease in that it produces a myriad of clinical signs and symptoms. In addition, there are many factors that may affect the control of the disease on a day-to-day basis. For these reasons, diabetic patients are quite unusual in that they must be capable of checking the status of their disease and of initiating modifications in its management as indicated.

Management of diabetes requires the patient to control the disease. Though available evidence does not support a decrease in microangiopathy with good control of blood glucose levels, there is some evidence that this might be the case, thus the need for strict control of blood glucose levels.[36] Diabetes is not cured by treatment; therefore, the patient must continue to monitor and to manage the disease for a lifetime. A problem faced by the diabetic, as well as by patients with other controllable but not curable, problems, such as high blood pressure, is long-term compliance.

When compared to the older methods of testing urinary glucose levels, monitoring of blood glucose by patients at home has permitted a greater flexibility in the management of diabetes while achieving improved glycemic control. The risk of hypo-

Table 17-8. Causes of 240 consecutive cases of hypoglycemia in patients known to have diabetes mellitus*

Cause	Percent
Inadequate food (carbohydrate) intake	66
Excessive insulin dose	12
Sulfonylurea therapy	12
Strenuous exercise	4
Ethanol intake	4
Other (kidney failure, liver failure, decrease in corticosteroid dose)	2

From Davidson JK: Hypoglycemia. In Schwartz GR, and others, editors: *Principles and practice of emergency medicine*, Philadelphia, 1978, WB Saunders.
*At the Grady Memorial Hospital Emergency Clinic, 1973-1975.

glycemic episodes arising with tight control of blood sugar levels has been diminished with these more accurate dipstick and electronic blood glucose monitoring devices.[37,38] The patient must be educated to perform three essential steps. They are as follows (Figs. 17-1 and 17-2).

1. Obtain a drop of capillary blood from a finger prick.
2. Apply the blood sample to a test strip and remove the sample at the proper time.
3. Accurately evaluate the color that develops.

Self-monitoring of blood glucose is especially important for brittle diabetics (that is, those who, despite therapy, are unable to maintain a stable blood sugar level and exhibit extremes of both hyperglycemia and hypoglycemia), those attempting to maintain ideal glycemic control during pregnancy, and patients who have little or no warning of impending hypoglycemic episodes. This type of self-monitoring has proved to be a safe and reliable clinical tool in compliant patients. Diagnostic strips include Visidex and Chemstrip-bG. These permit visual estimations of glucose concentrations when compared to a series of color standards.

Capillary blood glucose levels are closer to arterial levels than are those obtained from venous blood. Normal fasting blood glucose levels for venous blood range from 60 to 100 mg/100 mL (60 to 100 mg %). In 1979 the National Diabetes Data Group[39] stated that a fasting blood glucose level of 140 mg/100 mL on two or more occasions would serve as adequate criteria for the diagnosis of the presence of diabetes mellitus.

Diabetes may be managed by controlling diet and physical activity along with the administration of oral hypoglycemic agents and/or insulin. Many type 2 diabetics may be controlled through the

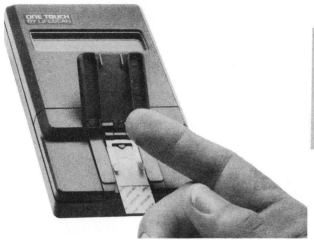

Fig. 17-1. One Touch finger prick for obtaining a drop of capillary blood for blood glucose test.

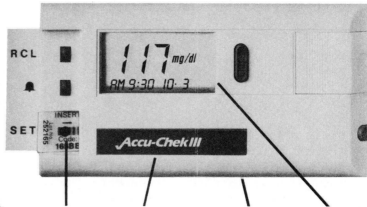

Fig. 17-2. Apply the blood sample to a test strip and remove at the proper time.

combination of weight loss, exercise, and diet control. Where this regimen fails, oral hypoglycemic agents are added. Table 17-9 compares the available oral hypoglycemic agents.

Sulfonylurea agents, such as tolbutamide, tolazamide, and acetohexamide, have been employed for years as oral hypoglycemic agents in controlling the type 2 diabetic. Side effects, such as water retention, gastrointestinal intolerance, prolonged hypoglycemic episodes, and drug interactions (e.g., with aspirin, phenylbutazone, and warfarin) are observed with these sulfonylurea agents. Additionally, a study published in the mid-1970s stated that the sulfonylurea drugs were ineffective in controlling blood glucose levels and additionally that their use was associated with an increased risk of cardiovascular disease.[40-43] Controversy persists about the validity of the conclusions reached by the University Group Diabetes Program (UGDP) because of the heterogeneity of the population studied, with its preponderance of obese subjects and certain features of the experimental design, such as the use of a fixed dose of oral drug.

At present, the Food and Drug Administration requires a warning label inserted in each package of sulfonylureas, but there is no restriction to recommending their use by the American Diabetes Association.

The newer oral hypoglycemic agents, glyburide and glipizide,[44] are significantly more potent than the first-generation oral hypoglycemics, such as tolbutamide, which are members of the sulfonylurea drugs. As such they are used in doses approximately one hundredth as great as the first-generation sulfonylureas. The incidence of adverse side effects, which were commonly seen with sulfonylurea agents, is remarkably diminished with these newer drugs.

The type 1 diabetic requires the administration of insulin in order to control blood glucose levels. Until recently, insulin used by humans was obtained by extraction from the pancreas of the cow and pig. Administration of bovine or porcine insulin was associated with a risk of adverse reaction, including both localized and systemic allergy. Improvements in the purification of beef and pork

Table 17-9. Currently available oral hypoglycemic agents

Generic name	Proprietary name	Daily dose	Duration (hrs)
Tolbutamide	Orinase	250-2000 mg in 6-12 divided doses	
Tolazamide	Tolinase	100-1000 mg as single or divided doses	10-14
Acetohexamide	Dymelor	250-1500 mg as single or divided doses	12-24
Chlorpropamide	Diabinase	100-500 mg as single dose	up to 60
Glyburide	Glucatrol	1.25-20 mg	10-24
Glipizide	DiaBeta, Micronase	5-30 mg	10-20

insulin have minimized the occurrence of serious adverse reactions in most type 1 diabetics. In 1983 genetically designed human insulin became available.[45] This insulin is synthesized in a non–disease-producing special laboratory strain of *Escherichia coli* bacteria that has been genetically altered by the addition of the human gene for insulin production. Though the risk of serious adverse reaction is diminished, reports of such responses still appear.[46]

Insulin is available in several preparations that differ in their onset and duration of action. These are characterized as rapid-acting, intermediate-acting, and long-acting insulin. Regular insulin is rapidly absorbed and is administered before meals, whereas NPH and Lente preparations are intermediate acting and are administered once a day. Long-acting insulin preparations are available, but are rarely required.

Regular insulin can be mixed with either NPH or Lente. By using a morning and early evening injection of NPH and regular insulin, peak insulin levels will be available for breakfast, lunch, and dinner. A few patients may require a separate injection of long-acting insulin to prevent the dawn phenomenon, which represents a rebound hyperglycemia that occurs between 5:00 AM and 8:00 AM in about 75% of IDDM patients and in most NIDDM and normal subjects as well.[47] Insulin preparations are compared in Table 17-10.

PREVENTION

The acute complications of diabetes may be averted through an adequate preliminary evaluation of the diabetic patient. In addition, the dental health professional is in a position to aid in the detection of previously undiagnosed diabetes (there are approximately 10 million undiagnosed individuals with diabetes in the United States). Relevant questions from the medical history questionnaire and the ensuing dialogue history follow.

Medical History Questionnaire

QUESTION 9. Circle any of the following that you have had or have at present:
Diabetes
Cortisone medicine
COMMENT. Knowledge of the presence of diabetes by the patient will lead to a definitive dialogue history. The prolonged use of corticosteroid medications can lead to the onset of diabetes mellitus. Dialogue history must help determine the presence of signs and symptoms.

QUESTION 13. Have you lost or gained more than 10 pounds in the past year?
COMMENT. An affirmative response to unex-

Table 17-10. Currently available injectable insulins

Action	Type of insulin	Peak (hrs)	Duration (hrs)
Rapid	Regular	1-2	5-6
Intermediate	NPH	2-8	24-28
	Lente	2-8	24-28
Long	Protamine	8-12	36

plained weight loss may indicate the presence of undetected diabetes mellitus.

QUESTION 15. Are you on a special diet?
COMMENT. An affirmative response may indicate a patient with NIDDM (type 2). Dietary restrictions in type 2 diabetes will vary from patient to patient, ranging from a strict balance between carbohydrate, protein, and fat intake, to a more liberal diet in which only total caloric intake is controlled.[48]

QUESTION 6. Have you taken any medicine or drugs during the past 2 years?
COMMENT. Table 17-9 lists the oral medications currently being prescribed for the management of NIDDM. It is also important for the doctor to know that other medicines being taken by a patient are capable of producing alterations in the blood sugar level. Table 17-11 lists some of these medications.

Dialogue History

Negative response to question 9: When a patient indicates on question 9 that he or she does not have diabetes mellitus, but answers "yes" to any or all of questions 6, 13, or 15, the following dialogue history should be considered:

QUESTIONS. Are you frequently thirsty? Are you hungry much of the time? Do you have to get up at night to void (urinate) frequently? Have you gained or lost weight recently without dieting; how many pounds?
COMMENT. These signs, although not specific for diabetes mellitus, can lead to a presumptive diagnosis of this disease. The classical triad of symptoms of diabetes, the three Ps: polydipsia (increased thirst), polyphagia (increased appetite), and polyuria (increased frequency of urination), when accompanied by a loss of weight in the absence of dieting, should alert the doctor to the possible presence of diabetes. If the response to question 9 on diabetes in the medical history questionnaire is negative and the questions just mentioned are answered in the affirmative, the doctor should continue with the preliminary medical and dental examination and then consult with the patient's physician before any dental care is begun.

Table 17-11. Commonly used medications that lower blood glucose levels

Potentiate action of sulfonylureas
1. Barbiturates*
2. Bishydroxycoumarin
3. Monoamine oxidase inhibitors
4. Salicylates*
5. Thiazides

Increase insulin production
1. α-Adrenergic blockers
2. β-Adrenergic stimulators
3. Monoamine oxidase inhibitors

Decrease hepatic glycogenolysis
Propranolol

Unknown mechanism
1. Antihistamines
   a. Tripelennamine HCl
2. Morphine*
3. Propylthiouracil
4. Tuberculostatic drugs
   a. Isoniazid
   b. Aminosalicylic acid

*These agents are frequently administered or prescribed in the practice of dentistry.

Positive response to question 9: When a positive history indicates the presence of diabetes mellitus, the doctor should proceed with the following dialogue history.

QUESTION. **How long have you had diabetes, and what type of treatment are you taking to control it?**

COMMENT. As noted earlier, the severity of the diabetes and the potential for the occurrence of its acute complications are greatest in insulin-dependent and brittle non–insulin-dependent diabetics who are managed by injectable insulin plus diet control. Patients successfully controlling their blood glucose levels through diet alone or through diet plus oral hypoglycemic agents (type 2 diabetics) usually have some pancreatic function remaining and are more resistant to diabetic ketoacidosis. Currently available oral hypoglycemic agents are listed in Table 17-9.

QUESTION. **How often do you monitor your urine or blood glucose levels and what have been the results for the past few days?**

COMMENT. For nearly five decades diabetics tested their urine for the presence of glucose. Urine tests for glucose and ketones are still important in the management of some diabetics; however, monitoring of urinary glucose levels is sig-

nificantly less reliable than direct monitoring of blood glucose levels. Indeed, some patients may "spill" sugar into their urine at blood glucose values that are significantly below those for hyperglycemia, whereas others will not demonstrate glucose in their urine with blood glucose levels of 300 to 400 mg/100 mL. More recently, however, most diabetics have turned to self-monitoring of blood glucose levels directly at home, a procedure that is rapidly gaining acceptance.[49] Although a significant departure in appearance from traditional diabetic testing procedures, in reality, blood glucose testing is a more sophisticated and logical extension of tests usually performed by physicians and laboratories. Many of these products are available over the counter. Proprietary names for home blood glucose testing kits include Chemstrip bG (Bio-Dynamics), Dextrostix (Miles Labs), and Glucostix (Miles Labs). Portable, battery-operated devices, such as the Glucometer II or Glucosan II, provide a digital readout of blood glucose levels within 60 seconds, whereas newer devices, such as the One Touch and ExacTech, automatically time the reaction, relieving the patient of possible error in timing. Studies have demonstrated that eight of ten diabetics would rather prick their fingers than use a urine sample.[50] Additionally, these tests are accurate, producing results similar to those obtained by professional laboratories. Sonkson demonstrated that normal blood glucose levels can be maintained by self-assessment of blood rather than urine samples.[51] Levels are recorded in milligrams of glucose per deciliter (100 mL) of whole blood (also read as milligrams %). In children and adults values below 50 mg/dL indicate hypoglycemia. The upper range of values (Chemstrip bG) is 240 mg/dL for a 2-minute reading or 800 mg/dL for a 3-minute reading.

For diabetics who still monitor their urine, the level of blood glucose obtained is less reliable. Readings are 0, trace, 1+, 2+, 3+, and 4+. Patients who are able to keep their glucose levels in the trace or 1+ range may be considered in good control and may be managed in a normal manner in the dental office. Patients with consistently negative (0) readings are more likely to have hypoglycemic reactions.

The diabetic with 2+ readings should be carefully evaluated before dental treatment. Some physicians prefer their patients to remain in the 1+ to 2+ range, where they are less likely to become hypoglycemic. If no clinical signs and symptoms associated with hyperglycemia or hypoglycemia are present, dental treatment may be carried out without modification.

Table 17-12. Optimal physical status classifications of diabetic patients

Type of diabetes	Treatment	Severity	Optimal physical status
Type I—IDDM	Insulin plus diet	Severe	III
Type II—NIDDM			
1. Nonobese	Insulin plus diet	Moderate to severe	II-III
	Oral medication plus diet	Mild to moderate	II
2. Obese	Oral medication plus diet	Mild to moderate	II

Urinary glucose readings of 3+ and 4+ indicate a lack of control of the disease process. Stress (as associated with dental care) further elevates blood sugar and may aid in precipitating ketoacidosis and, potentially, diabetic coma. Medical consultation prior to the start of treatment is indicated so that adjustments may be made in insulin dosages and overall diabetic management.

Table 17-12 summarizes the optimal physical status classification for IDDM and NIDDM patients, whereas Table 17-13 presents modifications in these optimal classifications based upon urinary or blood glucose levels.

QUESTION. **How frequently (if ever) do you have hypoglycemic episodes?**

COMMENT. Awareness of the problem of hypoglycemia better prepares the doctor to manage it. Patients frequently testing negative on urinary glucose or low on blood glucose are more likely to become hypoglycemic.

Physical Examination

Following the medical history questionnaire and dialogue history, the diabetic patient should be carefully evaluated for signs and symptoms of secondary disease, particularly of the cardiovascular system. Vital signs should be recorded before and after all dental treatment.

The skin of a diabetic patient may give an indi-cation to the possible presence of acute complications associated with overly high or low blood sugar levels. Hyperglycemic patients will appear flushed and their skin will be dry (absence of sweating), whereas hypoglycemic patients will have a cold, wet (clammy) appearance. The characteristic smell of acetone, a sweet, fruity odor, on the breath is noticeable in patients with diabetic ketoacidosis. Blood pressure in the hyperglycemic, ketoacidotic patient will be decreased due to hypovolemia, with a compensatory tachycardia. Hypoglycemic patients may demonstrate an increased blood pressure as well as tachycardia (increased sympathetic response).

DENTAL THERAPY CONSIDERATIONS

Following completion of the medical and dental evaluation of the diabetic patient, consideration must be given to proper patient management. If any doubt exists about the patient's medical status, consultation with the patient's physician is indicated.

The type 2, NIDDM patient is less prone to acute fluctuations in blood glucose levels, and is more apt to tolerate, without increased concern, any and all forms of dental treatment, including general anesthesia, parenteral sedation, and local anesthesia.

Basic dental treatment modification considerations with the type 1, IDDM, ketosis-prone diabetic patient include the use of appropriate steps of the

Table 17-13. Physical status classification for diabetes mellitus

Glucose measurement		Change in physical status‡	Comment
Urinary*	Blood†		
0	<50 mg/dL	+1	Acceptable for treatment but more likely to be or become hypoglycemic
Trace, +, ++	80, 120, 180 mg/dL	0	Acceptable for treatment
+++	240 mg/dL	+1	Evaluate carefully prior to treatment
++++	>400 mg/dL	+2	If consistently in this range, medical consultation urged prior to treatment

*Tes-Tape.

†Chemstrip bG.

‡This table lists the change in physical status (PS) from the optimal presented in Table 17-12; thus, if optimally a PS II with a 3+ urinary glucose or 240 mg/dL blood glucose, patient is treated as a PS III.

stress reduction protocol. Additional consideration should be directed toward the maintenance of normal dietary habits. Advise the patient to take the usual insulin dose and to eat a normal breakfast prior to the dental appointment, if at all possible. Scheduling dental appointments earlier in the day will help to minimize episodes of hypoglycemia. The use of appropriate local anesthetics (e.g., shorter acting—mepivacaine plain—versus longer acting—bupivacaine with epinephrine) will minimize posttreatment eating impairment. If the nature of the dental procedure is likely to hamper the patient's normal eating habits either preoperatively (e.g., intravenous sedation) or postoperatively (e.g., surgery), the insulin dosage should be adjusted accordingly. Medical consultation should be considered in the IDDM patient who requires large doses of insulin to maintain blood glucose levels (>40 units daily) or where any doubt remains concerning adjustment of the patient's insulin dosage.

Diabetics are better able to withstand transient periods of hyperglycemia than they are hypoglycemia. After extensive dental procedures (e.g., oral or periodontal surgery), reconstruction, or endodontics, IDDM patients should be instructed to check their blood glucose levels more frequently for the next few days. If glucose or ketone levels are elevated, patients should initiate changes in insulin dosage or contact their physicians. Antibiotic coverage is recommended in ASA III or IV diabetics undergoing extensive surgical procedures to minimize the risk of postoperative infections. Tables 17-12, 17-13, and 17-14 present the physical status classification system and its modifications for diabetic patients.

CLINICAL MANIFESTATIONS
Hyperglycemia

Hyperglycemia, or high blood sugar, may manifest itself in different ways related to the severity of the diabetes. It may be evident in previously undiagnosed diabetic patients or in known diabetics who neglect their therapeutic regimens.

The patient with the milder form of diabetes (NIDDM) may not manifest any clinical signs or symptoms of hyperglycemia. Quite commonly, this form of diabetes is detected during a routine physical examination. Commonly, diabetes mellitus is first diagnosed after a clinical episode brought about by the advanced degree of atherosclerosis associated with the disease. Myocardial infarction in a young man or woman and/or development of peripheral vascular insufficiency at an early age may be events that eventually lead to a clinical diagnosis of diabetes mellitus. Other indicators for

Table 17-14. Diabetes mellitus—dental therapy considerations*

Physical status	Treatment considerations
II	Usual PS II considerations, plus: 1. Eat normal breakfast, take usual insulin dose in morning, if possible 2. Avoid missing meals, pre- and postoperatively 3. If missing meal is unavoidable, either medical consultation or decrease insulin dose by half
III	Usual PS III considerations, plus: 1. Following surgery or extensive procedures, monitor blood glucose levels more frequently for several days and modify insulin dosages accordingly 2. Consider medical consultation
IV	Usual PS IV considerations, plus: 1. Medical consultation prior to dental treatment

*PS, physical status.

further evaluation for the presence of diabetes include: persons with diabetic relatives, obese persons, persons over 40 years of age, women who have delivered large (>10 lb) babies, or who have had spontaneous abortions or stillbirths.[52]

A more severe clinical picture of hyperglycemia is seen in the insulin-dependent diabetic individual. The classic diabetic triad of "P's" or "polys"—polydipsia, polyphagia, and polyuria—with a marked loss of weight is evident for a day or more and is associated with marked fatigue, headache, blurred vision, abdominal pain, nausea and vomiting, constipation, dyspnea, and finally, mental stupor, which can progress to a state of unconsciousness known as diabetic coma.[53]

Clinical signs of hyperglycemia include a florid appearance of the face (bright red color) associated with hot and dry skin, both of which are indicative of dehydration. Respirations are commonly deep and rapid (signs of Kussmaul's respiration), with the fruity-sweet odor of acetone evident if diabetic ketoacidosis is present. The heart rate is rapid and the blood pressure is lower than normal. This combination of tachycardia and hypotension is yet another indication of the presence of dehydration and salt depletion. Table 17-15 presents the clinical signs and symptoms associated with hyperglycemia.

Table 17-15. Clinical manifestations of hyperglycemia*

	Diabetes, type I (IDDM)	Diabetes, type II (NIDDM)
Polyuria	+ +	+
Polydipsia	+ +	+
Polyphagia with weight loss	+ +	−
Recurrent blurred vision	+	+ +
Vulvovaginitis or pruritis	+	+ +
Loss of strength	+ +	+
Nocturnal enuresis	+ +	−
Often asymptomatic	−	+ +

Other symptoms—type I	Other symptoms—type II
Repeated skin infections	Decreased vision
Marked irritability	Paresthesias
Headache	Loss of sensation
Drowsiness	Impotence
Malaise	Postural hypotension
Dry mouth	

* −, not usually present; +, occasionally present; + +, usually present.
From Karam JH: Diabetes mellitus, hypoglycemia, and lipoprotein disorders. In Schroeder SA, Tierney LM, editors: *Current medical diagnosis and treatment*, Norwalk, CT, 1992, Appleton & Lange; and Little JW, Falace DA: *Dental management of the medically compromised patient*, ed 2, St Louis, 1984, Mosby–Year Book.

Hypoglycemia

Hypoglycemia, the second of the acute complications of diabetes mellitus, may rapidly progress to loss of consciousness, or it may be present in a milder form, representing a less ominous clinical picture. Episodes of hypoglycemia usually develop when the patient has not eaten for several hours.

Initially, hypoglycemia is usually evident as a phase of diminished cerebral function, such as an inability to perform simple calculations, decreased spontaneity of conversation, and changes in mood (e.g., lethargy). These have been categorized by this author as altered consciousness. Signs and symptoms of central nervous system involvement follow, including hunger, nausea, and an increase in gastric motility.

Following this is a phase of sympathetic hyperactivity, marked clinically by signs of increased epinephrine activity that includes sweating, tachycardia, piloerection, and increased anxiety. The skin is cold and wet to the touch (in marked distinction to the hot and dry touch of hyperglycemia). The patient is conscious at this time but may exhibit

Table 17-16. Clinical manifestations of hypoglycemia

Early stage—mild reaction
Diminished cerebral function
  Changes in mood
  Decreased spontaneity
Hunger
Nausea

More severe hypoglycemia
Sweating
Tachycardia
Piloerection
Increased anxiety
Bizarre behavioral patterns
  Belligerence
  Poor judgment
  Uncooperativeness

Later severe stage
Unconsciousness
Seizure activity
Hypotension
Hypothermia

bizarre behavioral patterns that often lead to a suspicion of alcohol or drug intoxication. If permitted to progress, the hypoglycemic patient may lose consciousness, and seizures may occur (Table 17-16).

Because hypoglycemia is a much more acute problem than is hyperglycemia, diabetic patients always maintain a readily available source of carbohydrate, such as hard candy. In addition, the state of altered consciousness produced by hypoglycemia may mimic drug intoxication and they may be unable to rationally respond to questioning at this time. For this reason, patients with IDDM will either wear a medical alert bracelet or will carry a card that states that they are not intoxicated but in fact are diabetic and that, if they are found unconscious, a physician should be called (Fig. 17-3).

PATHOPHYSIOLOGY
Insulin and Blood Glucose

Glucose is a major fuel and energy source for all cells of the body. In fact, glucose is the only fuel that can be used by the brain, which requires a continuous supply of it. Too high a level of blood sugar (hyperglycemia) or too low a level (hypoglycemia) produces varying degrees of central nervous system dysfunction (altered consciousness). The homeostatic mechanisms in the body are therefore aimed at maintaining the blood glucose level within a range of 50 to 150 mg/100 mL of blood (milligrams %). The mean blood glucose level in normal

---

I Am a Diabetic and Take Insulin

If I am behaving peculiarly but am conscious and able to swallow, give me sugar or hard candy or orange juice slowly. If I am unconscious, call an ambulance immediately, take me to.a physician or a hospital, and notify my physician. *I am not intoxicated.*

My name _____

Address _____

Telephone _____

Physician's name _____

Physician's address _____

Telephone _____

Fig. 17-3. Card carried by diabetic patients.

persons who fast overnight is 92 mg/100 mL, with a range of from 78 to 115 mg/100 mL. The minimal blood glucose level required by the brain in order to maintain normal cerebral function is 50 mg/100 mL.

When blood glucose levels exceed the saturation point of renal reabsorption (approximately 180 mg/100 mL), glucose "spills" into the urine, resulting in loss of energy (glucose-fuel) and water. Insulin is the most important factor in the regulation of the blood glucose level.

Insulin is synthesized in the beta cells of the pancreas and is rapidly secreted into the blood in response to elevations in blood sugar level (e.g., following a meal). The half-life of insulin in the blood is 3 to 10 minutes, with biotransformation occurring in the liver and kidneys. Insulin promotes the uptake of glucose into the cells of the body and its storage in the liver as glycogen, as well as the uptake of fatty acids and amino acids into cells and their subsequent conversion into storage forms (triglycerides and proteins). In this manner insulin produces a decrease in blood glucose levels, thereby preventing its loss through urinary excretion. In the absence of insulin, cell membranes of many body cells are impermeable to glucose. Cells such as muscle and adipose cells are insulin dependent, requiring its presence to enable glucose to cross the cell membrane, even in hyperglycemic states.[54]

When insulin is absent, these cells break down triglycerides into fatty acids, which may be used as an alternative energy source. This gives rise to the hyperglycemic state known as diabetic ketoacidosis (DKA). Other tissues and organs such as nerve tissue, including the brain, the kidneys, and hepatic tissue are not insulin dependent, because they are capable of glucose transfer across cell membranes even in the absence of insulin.

In the fasting stage decreased blood sugar levels (hypoglycemia) inhibit the secretion of insulin. The cells of the body continue to require glucose, however, and there are several mechanisms through which it is made available. The primary goal of these mechanisms is to provide the central nervous system with the minimal glucose level required to maintain its normal function.

Glycogen stored in the liver is broken down into glucose through a process called glycogenolysis, whereas amino acids are converted into glucose through a process called gluconeogenesis. This newly formed glucose is available principally to the central nervous system; in fact, insulin-dependent cells actually demonstrate a decreased uptake of glucose at this time. Fuel for these cells (e.g., muscle and adipose) is provided through the breakdown of triglycerides, the storage form of fat, into free fatty acids.

In summary, insulin may be described as the body's "fed" signal, and as a means of maintaining glucose homeostasis. After a meal the high blood level of insulin tells the cells of the body to take up and store any fuel that is not immediately required for metabolic needs. In the fasting state low insulin levels tell the body that no food is entering and that storage forms of nutrients should be utilized for fuel.

Hyperglycemia, Ketosis, and Acidosis

After the diabetic patient eats a meal, hyperglycemia occurs, as it does in the nondiabetic individual, but the blood glucose level remains elevated for a prolonged period because of a lack of insulin (as in type I diabetes) or because of a lack of response by tissues to circulating insulin (type II diabetes). Other factors leading to increased blood glucose levels are an increase in the hepatic production of glucose from glycogenolysis, as well as decreased glucose uptake by the peripheral insulin-dependent tissues (muscle and fat).

Glucose is found in the urine when the blood glucose level exceeds the renal reabsorption threshold of approximately 180 mg/100 mL. The presence of glucose in the urine is called glycosuria. Because of its large molecular size, urinary glucose takes with it, by means of osmosis, large quantities of water and the electrolytes sodium and potassium. This, in addition to the presence of ketones, which also increase the secretion of sodium and potassium in the urine, leads to clinical symptoms of polyuria (an increased frequency of urination) and to the dehydrated state of the hyperglycemic patient, as evidenced clinically by a florid appearance and dry skin and polydipsia (increased thirst).

Weight loss despite normal or increased appetite is a common feature of IDDM. Weight loss is initially due to depletion of water, glycogen, and triglyceride stores. In addition, there is a loss of muscle mass as amino acids are diverted to form glucose and ketone bodies.

In the absence of insulin, the cells of the body are unable to utilize the large quantities of glucose present in the blood. Fasting state mechanisms, described earlier, respond to the call for required energy. Liver and muscle glycogen are converted to glucose via glycogenolysis while proteins are broken down into their component amino acids, which are then converted into glucose through the process of gluconeogenesis in the liver. Triglycerides are converted into free fatty acids in the liver. These free fatty acids, primarily acetoacetate and beta-hydroxybutyrate (ketone bodies), are used as fuel by the muscles in the absence of glucose. Acetone, evident on the breath of this patient because of its fruity, sweet odor, is a by-product of the metabolism of acetoacetate. This stage is referred to as diabetic ketoacidosis.

If the insulin deficiency is severe, gluconeogenesis and ketogenesis continue to increase in rate, regardless of the blood glucose level. Tissue utilization of ketones, however, decreases over time so that blood levels of acetoacetate and beta-hydroxybutyrate increase. This leads to a decrease in the pH of the blood, a condition called metabolic acidosis (ketoacidosis). With increasing blood levels of ketones, the renal threshold is soon exceeded and ketones will be detected in the urine. Ketoacidosis depresses cardiac contractility as well as decreasing the response of arterioles to the catecholamines, epinephrine and norepinephrine. More significant perhaps is the effect of metabolic acidosis on blood pH and respiration. As the blood level of the ketoacids rises, the pH of the blood falls below 7.3. This induces hyperventilation, the body's attempt to raise the pH by means of respiratory alkalosis (see Chapter 12). When severe, this type of breathing is called Kussmaul's respirations (deep respirations that may be either slow or rapid). If unmanaged, this may progress to the loss of consciousness as in hyperglycemic or diabetic coma.

Hyperglycemic coma is associated with either severe insulin deficiency (diabetic ketoacidosis) or mild to moderate insulin deficiency (hyperglycemic nonketotic hyperosmolar coma). Poor patient compliance is one of the most common causes of ketoacidosis, particularly when episodes are recurrent.

Hypoglycemia

Hypoglycemia is the most commonly encountered acute complication of diabetes mellitus. It may also be seen in nondiabetic individuals. Approximately 70% of nondiabetic hypoglycemia is caused by functional hyperinsulinism. This is related to an oversecretion of insulin by beta cells of the pancreas because of an exaggerated response to glucose absorption, muscular exertion, pregnancy, or anorexia nervosa, factors that increase insulin requirements. Whatever its cause, diabetic or nondiabetic, the clinical manifestations of hypoglycemia are the same.

By arbitrary definition, hypoglycemia in adults is equated with blood glucose values below 50 mg/100 mL, whereas in children hypoglycemia is defined by a blood sugar of <40 mg/100 mL.[12] It is characterized by varying degrees of neurologic dysfunction, may occur with or without signs of epinephrine overactivity, and is responsive to the administration of glucose.

Although the definition of hypoglycemia indicates a blood glucose level of less than 50 mg/100 mL, hypoglycemic reactions can occur in the presence of normal or higher than normal blood glucose levels. Indeed, reports have been published of hypoglycemic reactions in diabetic patients with blood sugar levels ranging from 82 to 472 mg/100 mL, the reactions developing within 40 minutes of intravenous insulin administration.[55] On the other hand, blood glucose levels of 25 to 30 mg/100 mL have been reported in patients without clinical evidence of hypoglycemia.[56]

It appears that one of the most important factors in precipitating clinical hypoglycemia is the rate at which the blood glucose level falls. After the administration of insulin, the signs and symptoms of hypoglycemia may develop within a few minutes, rapidly progressing to the loss of consciousness. In patients taking oral hypoglycemics the onset of signs and symptoms is normally more gradual, developing over a period of hours. Clinical signs and symptoms of hypoglycemia are similar to those seen in acute anxiety states or after the administration of excessive doses of epinephrine (the so-called epinephrine reactions).

Lack of adequate blood glucose levels alters the

normal functioning of the cerebral cortex, represented clinically as mental confusion and lethargy. This lack of adequate glucose further manifests itself in increased activity of the parasympathetic and sympathetic nervous systems. A part of this response is mediated by an increase in the secretion of epinephrine, which produces an increase in the systolic and the mean blood pressures, increases sweating, and produces tachycardia.

When the blood sugar level declines even more, the patient may lose consciousness and go into a state of hypoglycemic coma, or insulin shock. During this stage, tonic and clonic convulsions are frequently noted, which, if not treated promptly and effectively, may lead to permanent cerebral dysfunction.

MANAGEMENT

Prompt recognition of diabetes-related complications is important. Equally important is the ability to differentiate between hyperglycemia and hypoglycemia. Because of the differing rates of onset of these acute complications, it is usually stressed that diabetic patients who behave in a bizarre manner or who lose consciousness should be managed as if they were hypoglycemic until proved otherwise.

Hyperglycemia and ketoacidosis usually develop over a period of many hours or days, and the patient will appear and behave chronically ill. Other important factors in a differential diagnosis include the hot and dry appearance of the hyperglycemic patient in contrast to the cold and wet look of the hypoglycemic patient. The presence of acetone odor on the breath further confirms a diagnosis of hyperglycemia. When doubt remains in the doctor's mind as to the cause of the clinical problem, supportive therapy is indicated until additional medical assistance becomes available.

Hyperglycemia

Definitive management of hyperglycemia, ketosis, and acidosis consists of the administration of insulin to normalize body metabolism, restoration of fluid and electrolyte deficiencies, a search for the precipitating cause, and avoidance of complications. Dental office management of the hyperglycemic or ketoacidotic patient will usually be of a supportive nature.

Diagnostic clues to the presence of hyperglycemia and its emergency situation, diabetic ketoacidosis and diabetic coma, are the following:

Dry, warm skin
Kussmaul's respirations
Fruity or sweat breath odor

Rapid, weak pulse
Normal to low blood pressure
Altered level of consciousness

Conscious Patient

In the dental office the patient with clinical signs and symptoms of hyperglycemia represents an ASA IV risk and should not receive any dental therapy until a physician has been consulted. Medical consultation in most cases leads to an immediate appointment with the physician or hospitalization if the situation appears to warrant it.

It is interesting to note that emergency medical technicians (EMTs) are trained to regard any unknown diabetic emergency encountered in the field (e.g., in a dental office) as though it were hypoglycemia.[57] The administration of oral glucose is recommended if the patient is awake and alert, or the use of glucose paste if the patient's level of consciousness is altered, while paying attention to airway management.[57] The reason for this is that if hypoglycemia is not treated rapidly, death or serious damage to the patient is likely. On the other hand, death or permanent disability due to hyperglycemia usually takes a long time to occur.[58]

Unconscious Patient

Step 1: Terminate the dental procedure.

Step 2: Position the patient. The unconscious patient is placed into the supine position with the legs elevated slightly.

Step 3: Basic life support, as indicated. If the diabetic patient loses consciousness in the dental office, the doctor should quickly implement the steps of basic life support (positioning; checking airway, breathing, and vital signs). These steps ensure adequate oxygenation and cerebral blood flow. However, this patient will remain unconscious until the underlying metabolic causes (e.g., hyperglycemia, metabolic acidosis) have been corrected. It is most probable that the only steps of basic life support required in diabetic coma will be management of the patient's airway. Breathing will be spontaneous—deep and either rapid or slow, and may exhibit the sweet, fruity smell of acetone. Adequate circulation will be present.

Step 4: Summon medical assistance. Medical assistance should be sought when any unconscious patient demonstrates no improvement after basic life support procedures have been initiated.

Step 5: Intravenous infusion (if available). An intravenous infusion of 5% dextrose and water or of normal saline may be started, if available, prior to the arrival of the emergency medical team. Availability of a patent vein will facilitate subsequent

---

MANAGEMENT OF HYPERGLYCEMIA

Unconscious patient

Terminate the dental procedure
↓
Position the patient
(supine with legs elevated slightly)
↓
Basic life support, as indicated
↓
If recovery does not occur:
Summon medical assistance
↓
Establish intravenous line, if possible
↓
Administer oxygen
↓
If diagnosis is in doubt:
Administer glucose paste
↓
Transport to hospital for definitive diagnosis
and treatment

---

medical management of this patient.

Insulin has no place in the office emergency kit (unless the doctor or a staff member is an insulin-dependent diabetic). Insulin must be carefully administered and its effect on blood glucose monitored through blood tests. Hospitalization of the patient is required to correct the hyperglycemia and other deficits seen in this patient.

Step 6: Administer oxygen. Oxygen may be administered at any time during this situation. Though oxygen administration will not lead to recovery of the patient, no harm can occur from its administration.

Step 7: Administer glucose paste. If doubt is present about the cause of loss of consciousness in this diabetic patient, assume hypoglycemia, and administer glucose paste into the buccal folds. (See section on hypoglycemia that follows for a discussion on the administration of glucose paste.)

Step 8: Transport patient to hospital for definitive treatment. Upon arrival of emergency medical personnel and stabilization of the patient, the patient will be transported to the emergency department of a local hospital for definitive diagnosis (if in doubt) and treatment.

The management of hyperglycemic emergencies is outlined in the accompanying box.

Hypoglycemia

Management of hypoglycemia in the dental office presents more dramatic results than does management of hyperglycemia because most individuals will experience a dramatic remission of symptoms in a short period of time. Choice of management is based on the patient's level of consciousness.

Diagnostic clues to the presence of hypoglycemia include:

Weakness, dizziness
Pale, moist skin
Shallow respirations
Headache
Altered level of consciousness

Conscious and Alert Patient

Step 1: Recognize hypoglycemia. Bizarre behavior (in the absence of alcohol on the patient's breath) and other clinical signs of possible glucose insufficiency should lead the doctor to suspect the presence of hypoglycemia. This may develop in both diabetic and nondiabetic individuals. If diabetic, determine from the patient how long it has been since his or her last meal or insulin dose.

Step 2: Terminate the dental procedure.

Step 3: Position the patient. As with any conscious individual in an emergency situation, position of the patient will be predicated upon comfort. In most situations the patient will prefer an upright position. Variations in position are acceptable if desired by the patient.

Step 4: Basic life support, as indicated. Assess the adequacy of the airway, breathing, and circulation and implement any steps considered necessary. This patient is conscious and will have adequate control over airway, breathing, and circulation.

Step 5: Administer oral carbohydrates. If the patient is conscious and cooperative but still demonstrating clinical symptoms of hypoglycemia, the therapy of choice is oral carbohydrate. The emergency kit contains sugar, which can be dissolved and ingested by the patient. Other available items might include orange juice, cola beverages, and candy bars. A 6- to 12-oz portion of cola soft drink contains 20 to 40 g of glucose. This should be administered in 3- or 4-oz doses every 5 to 10 minutes until symptoms are no longer present.

Step 6: Permit patient to recover. The patient should be observed for approximately 1 hour before being permitted to leave the dental office. The patient may be permitted to leave the office unescorted, if in the opinion of the treating dentist he or she has recovered completely from the episode. Should any doubt persist in the treating doctor's mind about the degree of recovery, the patient should either remain in the office for a longer period of recovery, or arrangements should be made for an adult relative or friend to escort the patient home. Determine if the patient has eaten before the dental appointment, and reaffirm the importance of the patient's eating shortly before the next dental visit.

Unresponsive Conscious Patient

If the patient has no response to oral glucose or will not cooperate by taking oral glucose, the doctor should take the following steps.

Step 1: Recognize hypoglycemia.
Step 2: Terminate the dental procedure.
Step 3: Position the patient.
Step 4: Basic life support, as indicated.
Step 5: Administer oral carbohydrates.
Step 6: Summon medical assistance. When oral carbohydrates have proved ineffective, additional treatment is needed. Coincident with the consideration of additional therapy, outside medical assistance should be summoned.

Step 7: Administer parenteral carbohydrate. Should the administration of oral carbohydrate prove ineffective in reversing the signs and symptoms of hypoglycemia or should the patient be uncooperative and refuse to take oral carbohydrate, the parenteral administration of drugs should be considered. Glucagon, 1 mg, may be administered intra-

muscularly or intravenously, or if available, 50 mL of 50% dextrose can be administered intravenously over 2 to 3 minutes (Fig. 17-4).

The patient will usually respond within 10 to 15 minutes after intramuscular injection of glucagon and within 5 minutes following intravenous dextrose. Oral carbohydrates should be started as soon as they can be tolerated by the patient. Small amounts of honey, syrup, or decorative icing can be placed into the buccal fold if parenteral administration is unavailable and if the patient will cooperate.

Step 8: Monitor the patient. Vital signs should be monitored at least every 5 minutes during the incident until medical assistance becomes available.

Step 9: Discharge the patient and subsequent dental treatment. Medical personnel will provide definitive care to the patient either in the dental office or after transport to a hospital facility. In most instances this patient will be hospitalized, at least until the blood sugar levels are corrected. Prior to subsequent dental care, discuss with the patient possible reasons for this episode having developed, and seek methods of preventing its recurrence during later treatment.

Unconscious Patient

Step 1: Terminate the dental procedure.
Step 2: Position the patient. The unconscious patient is placed into the supine position with the legs elevated slightly.

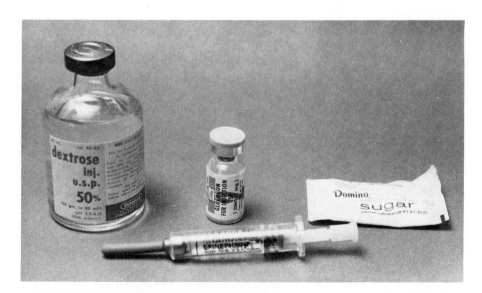

Fig. 17-4. Antihypoglycemic agents. The 50% dextrose solution must be administered IV; glucagon may be administered IM or IV; epinephrine may be administered IV or IM; sugar is administered orally to the conscious patient.

Step 3: Basic life support, as indicated. If the diabetic patient loses consciousness in the dental office, the doctor should quickly implement the steps of basic life support (positioning; checking airway, breathing, and vital signs). These steps ensure adequate oxygenation and cerebral blood flow. However, this patient will remain unconscious until the underlying metabolic cause (e.g., hypoglycemia) has been corrected. It is most probable that the only steps of basic life support required for hypoglycemia or insulin shock will be management of the patient's airway. Breathing will be spontaneous and adequate circulation will be present.

Step 4: Summon medical assistance. If the unconscious patient fails to respond to the steps of basic life support, medical assistance should be sought.

Step 5: Definitive management. An unconscious person with a prior history of diabetes mellitus must always be presumed to be hypoglycemic unless other obvious causes of unconsciousness are present. Definitive management of the unconscious diabetic entails the administration of carbohydrate by the most effective route available. In most instances this will be an intravenous injection of a 50% dextrose solution or an intramuscular injection of glucagon or epinephrine. It must be stressed that the unconscious patient must never be given any liquid or other substance that can run into the throat, because this increases the possibility of airway obstruction and/or pulmonary aspiration.

The intravenous administration of 20 to 50 mL of a 50% dextrose solution over 2 to 3 minutes restores consciousness within 5 to 10 minutes. In children do not exceed 25 mL of 50% dextrose. The usefulness of this drug is such that it is commonly administered to unconscious persons in whom the cause of unconsciousness is unknown. In these instances it serves to rule out hypoglycemia as a possible cause of the unconsciousness, yet its administration does not increase problems if hyperglycemia is present.

Glucagon (1 mg IM or IV) leads to an elevation of blood glucose via the breakdown of glycogen stores in the liver. The response to glucagon is variable,[59] with an onset of action of approximately 10 to 20 minutes, and a peak response in 30 to 60 minutes.[60] If neither glucagon nor 50% dextrose are available, an 0.5-mg dose of a 1:1000 concentration of epinephrine may be administered subcutaneously or intramuscularly and repeated every 15 minutes as needed. Epinephrine increases blood glucose levels. It should be used with extreme caution in patients with known cardiovascular disease. Once consciousness is restored, these patients should receive oral carbohydrates.

Transmucosal application of sugar: In the absence of the parenteral route or of parenteral drugs, the doctor should maintain basic life support until medical assistance arrives. Although it is important that liquids never be placed in the mouth of an

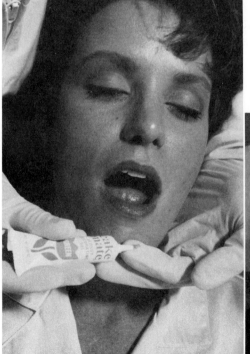
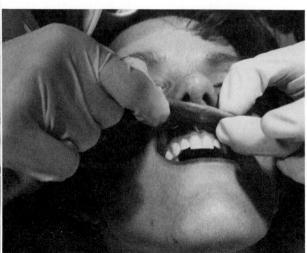

Fig. 17-5. A, B, Sugar icing placed into maxillary and mandibular folds.

unconscious or stuporous patient—the risk of aspiration or airway obstruction is too great—a thick paste of concentrated glucose can be used with a high degree of safety. Recommendations include the placement of a small amount of honey or syrup into the buccal fold.[61] Perhaps even more effective in the dental office situation is a small tube of decorative icing of the kind used for baked goods. Its consistency is similar to or thicker than that of toothpaste. A small, thin strip of this icing can be placed in the maxillary and mandibular buccal folds (Fig. 17-5). Onset will not be rapid, but the blood sugar level will rise slowly—during which time basic life support is continued and the oral cavity is evaluated every 5 minutes and suctioned, if necessary.

Though probably not applicable in many dental office situations, the rectal administration of honey or syrup (30 mL per 500 mL of warm water), the so-called "honey bear enema," has been effective.[61]

Step 6: Recovery and discharge. The unconscious hypoglycemic will recover consciousness when the blood glucose level has been elevated, as long as no additional damage has occurred (e.g., from hypoxia or other causes). Once conscious, oral forms of carbohydrate, such as soft drinks, may be administered.

On arrival, emergency medical personnel will act to ensure basic life support, establish an intravenous line, and administer any drugs considered necessary. Once stabilized, this patient will be transported to a hospital for definitive care and observation.

It must be noted that severe hypoglycemia can be associated with the development of seizures of a generalized tonic-clonic nature. Management of these seizures will follow the guidelines discussed in the section on seizure disorders (see Chapter 21).

The accompanying box reviews management of hypoglycemia.

Drugs used in management: Conscious patient: oral forms of sugar; unconscious patient: 50% dextrose (IV), glucagon (IM or IV), sugar paste (transmucosal), syrup or honey (rectal)

Medical assistance required: None if only mild level of alteration of consciousness; yes for unconscious patient or if unresponsive to administration of sugar.

REFERENCES

1. Graber TW: Diabetes. In Rosen P, editor: *Emergency medicine*, ed 2, St Louis, 1988, Mosby–Year Book.
2. Winter RJ: Recent developments in diabetes research, *Compr Ther* 4:6, 1978.
3. Bingley PJ, Gale EA: Rising incidence of IDDM in Europe, *Diabetes Care* 12(4):289, 1988.
4. Olefsky JM: Diabetes mellitus. In Wyngaarden JB, Smith LH, editors: *Cecil textbook of medicine*, ed 17, Philadelphia, 1985, WB Saunders.
5. Skillman TG: Diabetes mellitus. In Massaferri EL, editor: *Endocrinology*, ed 3, New York, 1986, Medical Examination.
6. Cahill GF: Diabetes mellitus. In Beeson PB, McDermott W, Wyngaarden JB, editors: *Cecil textbook of medicine*, Philadelphia, 1979, WB Saunders.
7. *1992 Heart and Stroke Facts*, American Heart Association, The Association, Dallas, 1991.
8. Skyler JS: Complications of diabetes mellitus: relationship to metabolic dysfunction, *Diabetes Care* 2:499, 1979.
9. Patel JC, Deshpande PS: Diabetes mellitus the cause of death: its ranking, *Indian J Med Sci* 31:150, 1977.
10. Owen OE, and others: Pathogenesis and diagnosis of diabetes mellitus. In Rose LF, Kaye D, editors: *Internal medicine for dentistry*, St Louis, 1983, Mosby–Year Book.

MANAGEMENT OF HYPOGLYCEMIA

Conscious patient

Recognize hypoglycemia
↓
Terminate the dental procedure
↓
Position patient comfortably
↓
Basic life support, as indicated
↓
Administer oral carbohydrates:

Episode terminates	Episode continues
↓	↓
Permit patient to recover	Summon medical assistance
↓	↓
Discharge patient	Administer parenteral carbohydrate
	↓
	Monitor patient
	↓
	Discharge patient

Unconscious patient

Terminate the dental procedure
↓
Position the patient
(supine, legs elevated)
↓
Basic life support, as indicated
↓
Summon medical assistance
↓
Definitive management
50% dextrose IV, 1 mg glucagon IM, transmucosal sugar)
↓
Allow patient to recover and discharge as per medical recommendation

11. Little JW, Falace DA: Diabetes. In Little JW, Falace DA, editors: *Dental management of the medically compromised patient,* ed 3, St Louis, 1988, Mosby—Year Book.

12. Barkin RM, Rosen P: Hypoglycemia. In Barkin RM, Rosen P, editors: *Emergency pediatrics,* ed 3, St Louis, 1990, Mosby—Year Book.

13. Pyoeralae K: Diabetes and coronary heart disease: what a coincidence, *J Cardiovasc Pharmacol* 16(suppl 9):S8, 1990.

14. Douglas JG: Hypertension and diabetes in blacks, *Diabetes Care* 13(11):1191, 1990.

15. Hamilton BP: Diabetes mellitus and hypertension, *Am J Kidney Dis* 16(suppl 4)1:20, 1990.

16. Klein BE, Klein R: Ocular problems in older Americans with diabetes, *Clin Geriatr Med* 6(4):827, 1990.

17. Humphrey LL, Ballard DJ: Renal complications in non—insulin-dependent diabetes mellitus, Clin Geriatr Med 6(4):807, 1990.

18. Fylling CP, Knighton DR: Amputation in the diabetic population: incidence, causes, cost, treatment, and prevention, *J Enterostomal Ther* 16(6):247, 1989.

19. Turner GS, Kohner EM: Diabetic retinopathy, *Practitioner* 228:161, 1984.

20. Frank N: On the pathogenesis of diabetic retinopathy, *Ophthalmology* 91:626, 1984.

21. Rosenberg CS: Wound healing in the patient with diabetes mellitus, *Nurs Clin N Am* 25(1):247, 1990.

22. Wilson TG Jr: Periodontal diseases and diabetes, *Diabetes Educ* 15(4):342, 1989.

23. Al Sayegh H, Jarrett RJ: Oral glucose-tolerance tests and the diagnosis of diabetes: results of a prospective study based on the Whitehall Survey, *Lancet* 2:432, 1979.

24. Keen H, Jarrett RJ, McCartney P: The ten-year follow-up of the Bedford Survey (1962-1972): glucose tolerance and diabetes, *Diabetologia* 22:73, 1982.

25. Goldstein S: Cellular and molecular biological studies on diabetes mellitus, *Pathol Biol* 32:99, 1984.

26. MacDonald MJ: Etiology and classification of diabetes in children: practical genetics and prognosis counseling, *Primary Care* 10:531, 1983.

27. Rayfield EJ, Mento SJ: Viruses may be etiologic agents for non—insulin-dependent (type II) diabetes, *Rev Infect Dis* 5:341, 1983.

28. Bodansky HJ, and others: Which virus causes the initial islet lesion in type 1 diabetes, *Lancet* 1:401, 1984.

29. Hollander P: The case for tight control in diabetes, *Postgrad Med* 75:80, 1984.

30. Sutherland DE: Pancreas and islet transplant registry statistics, *Transplant Proc* 16:593, 1984.

31. McMaster P: What to expect from pancreas transplantation, *Transplant Proc* 16:587, 1984.

32. Raskin P: Treatment of insulin-dependent diabetes mellitus with portable insulin infusion devices, *Med Clin N Am* 66:1269, 1982.

33. Knowles HC Jr: Long-term juvenile diabetes treated with unmeasured diet, *Trans Assoc Am Physicians* 84:95, 1971.

34. Mendoza-Morfin F, and others: Triggering factors of ketoacidosis in 100 diabetic patients, *Rev Invest Clin* 29:99, 1977.

35. Clements RS: Ketoacidosis, *South Med J* 69:217, 1976.

36. Ainslie MB: Why tight diabetes control should be approached with caution, *Postgrad Med* 75:91, 1984.

37. Bell PM, Walshe K: Home blood glucose monitoring: impact on lifestyle and diabetes control, *Practitioner* 228:197, 1984.

38. Aziz S, Hsiang Y: Comparative study of home blood glucose monitoring devices: Visidex, Chemstrip bG, Glucometer, and Accu-Chek bG, *Diabetes Care* 6:529, 1983.

39. National Diabetes Data Group: Classification and diagnosis of diabetes mellitus and other categories of glucose intolerance, *Diabetes* 28:1039, 1979.

40. University Group Diabetes Program: Effects of hypoglycemic agents on vascular complications in patients with adult-onset diabetes. II: Mortality results, *Diabetes* 19(suppl 2):785, 1970.

41. University Group Diabetes Program: Effects of hypoglycemic agents on vascular complications in patients with adult-onset diabetes. V: Evaluation of phenformin therapy, *Diabetes* 24(suppl 1):65, 1975.

42. University Group Diabetes Program: Effects of hypoglycemic agents on vascular complications in patients with adult-onset diabetes. VI: Supplementary report on nonfatal events in patients treated with tolbutamide, *Diabetes* 25:1129, 1976.

43. University Group Diabetes Program: Effects of hypoglycemic agents on vascular complications in patients with adult-onset diabetes. VIII: Mortality and selected nonfatal events with insulin treatment, *JAMA* 240:37, 1978.

44. Glyburide and glipizide, *Med Lett Drugs Ther* 26:79, 1984.

45. Human insulin, *Med Lett Drugs Ther* 25:63, 1983.

46. Grammer LC, Metzger BE, Patterson R: Cutaneous allergy to human (recombinant DNA) insulin, *JAMA* 251:1459, 1984.

47. Stephenson JM, Schernthaner G: Dawn phenomenon and Smogyi effect in IDDM, *Diabetes Care* 12:245, 1989.

48. Bantle JP: The dietary treatment of diabetes mellitus, *Med Clin N Am* 72:1285, 1988.

49. Tomky DM, Clarke DH: A comparison of user accuracy, techniques, and learning time of various systems for self blood glucose monitoring, *Diabetes Educator* 16(6):483-486, 1990.

50. Sonkson PH, Judd S, Lowy C: Home monitoring of blood glucose: new approach to management of insulin-dependent diabetic patients in Great Britain, *Diabetes Care* 3:100, 1980.

51. Sonkson PH, Judd S, Lowy C: Home monitoring of blood glucose, *Lancet* 1:729, 1978.

52. Andreani D, DiMario U, Pozzilli P: Prediction, prevention, and early intervention in insulin-dependent diabetes, *Diabetes/Metabolism Rev* 7(1):61-77, 1991.

53. Nabarro JD: Diabetes in the United Kingdom: a personal series, *Diabetic Med* 8(1):59-68, 1991.

54. Garland PB, Newsholm EA, Randle PJ: Regulation of glucose uptake by muscle, *Biochem K* 93:665, 1964.

55. Hepburn DA, Deary IJ, Frier BM, Patrick AW, Quinn JD, Fisher BM: Symptoms of acute insulin-induced hypoglycemia in humans with and without IDDM: factor-analysis approach, *Diabetes Care* 14(11):949-957, 1991.

56. Arogyasami J, Conlee RK, Booth CL, Diaz R, Gregory T, Sephton S, Wilson GI, Winder WW: Effects of exercise on insulin-induced hypoglycemia, *J Applied Physiol* 69(2):686-693, 1990.

57. Pollakoff J, Pollakoff K: *EMTs guide to treatment,* Los Angeles, 1991, Jeff Gould.

58. Pollakoff J: Diabetes. In *EMT news update,* Pacoima, Calif., 1989, Poicoma Skills Center.

59. Bobzien WF: Suicidal overdoses with hypoglycemic agents, *JACEP* 11:467, 1979.

60. Tchertkoff V, and others: Hyperosmolar nonketotic diabetic coma: vascular complications, *J Am Geriatr Soc* 22:462, 1974.

61. Karam JH: Diabetes mellitus, hypoglycemia, and lipoprotein disorders. In Schroeder SA, Krupp MA, Tierney LM Jr, and others, editors: *Current medical diagnosis and treatment,* Norwalk, 1992, Appleton & Lange.

18 *Thyroid Gland Dysfunction*

The thyroid gland consists of two elongated lobes on either side of the trachea that are joined by a thin isthmus of thyroid tissue located at or below the level of the thyroid cartilage.[1] The thyroid gland produces and secretes three hormones that perform an important function in regulating the level of biochemical activity of most of the tissues of the body. These hormones are thyroxine (T_4), triiodothyronine (T_3), and calcitonin. Proper functioning of the thyroid gland from birth is essential for normal growth and metabolism.

Dysfunction of the thyroid gland may occur through either overproduction of thyroid hormone (hyperthyroidism) or underproduction (hypothyroidism). In both instances the observed clinical manifestations may cover a broad spectrum, ranging from a subclinical dysfunction to acute life-threatening situations. Fortunately, however, most patients with thyroid dysfunction have milder forms of the disease.

Like adrenal insufficiency, thyroid gland hyper- or hypofunction initially present in a slow, insidious fashion, expressing nonspecific signs and symptoms over months to years, and then are acutely precipitated by intercurrent stress. Each are relatively uncommon, and their characteristic symptoms are not easily recognized. All three conditions are potentially lethal if untreated, and in their extreme stages they constitute medical emergencies.[2]

Primary emphasis in the following discussion is on the detection of the clinical signs and symptoms of thyroid gland dysfunction. The life-threatening situations myxedema coma and thyroid "storm" or crisis, both of which are extremely rare, are also considered.

Hypothyroidism is a clinical state in which the tissues of the body do not receive an adequate supply of thyroid hormones. The clinical signs and symptoms of hypothyroidism are related to the age of the patient at the time of onset and to the degree and duration of the hormonal deficiency. Cretinism is a clinical syndrome encountered in infants and children and results from deficiency of thyroid hormone during fetal or early life.[3] Severe hypothyroidism developing in an adult is called myxedema and refers to the appearance of nonpitting, gelatinous, mucinous infiltrates beneath the skin.[4] Severe, unmanaged hypothyroidism may ultimately lead to the loss of consciousness that is called myxedema coma. The mortality rate in myxedema coma is high (up to 50%) even with optimal treatment.[5,6]

Hyperthyroidism is also known by several other names, including thyrotoxicosis, toxic goiter (diffuse or nodular), Basedow's disease,[7] Graves' disease,[8] Parry's disease, and Plummer's disease. It may be defined as a state of heightened thyroid gland activity associated with the production of excessive quantities of the thyroid hormones L-throxine (T_4) and L-triiodothyronine (T_3). Because the thyroid hormones affect the cellular metabolism of virtually all organ systems, the signs and symptoms of hyperthyroidism may be noted in any part of the body. Untreated hyperthyroidism may lead to the acute life-threatening situation known as thyroid storm or thyroid crisis, with manifestations of severe hypermetabolism, including high fever, and cardiovascular, neurologic, and gastrointestinal dysfunction.[9] Although uncommon today, thyroid storm still has a high mortality rate.

PREDISPOSING FACTORS

Dysfunction of the thyroid gland is a relatively common medical disorder. If diabetes mellitus, the most common endocrine disorder, is excluded, thyroid gland dysfunction accounts for 80% of all endocrine disorders.

Hypothyroidism

Thyroid failure usually occurs from disease of the thyroid gland (primary hypothyroidism), pituitary (secondary), or hypothalamus (tertiary).[2] Secondary failure accounts for less than 4% of cases,[10] whereas tertiary failure is even less common. The remainder of the cases are caused by primary thyroid disease. Hypothyroidism in the adult patient usually develops as a result of idiopathic atrophy of the thyroid gland, currently thought to occur through an autoimmune mechanism.[11] Other causes of hypothyroidism include total thyroidectomy, ablation following radioactive iodine therapy, which are procedures frequently employed in the management of hyperfunction of the thyroid gland, and chronic thyroiditis. Thyroid hypofunction is seen 3 to 10 times more frequently in females than males,[12] with its greatest incidence noted in the seventh decade.[13] Myxedema coma, the end stage of untreated hypothyroidism, has a mortality rate of up to 50% but fortunately is infrequently noted clinically.[5,6] It is associated with severe hypothermia,[10] hypoventilation, hypoxia, hypercapnia, and hypotension.[14] Etiologic factors of hypothyroidism are summarized in the accompanying box.

The dental practitioner should be aware of possible hypothyroid patients because, if medically untreated or inadequately managed, they may represent an increased risk in the dental office. The hypothyroid patient is unusually sensitive to most central nervous system (CNS) depressant drugs, including sedatives, narcotics, and antianxiety agents, which are commonly employed by the dental profession. Normal therapeutic doses of these agents may result in extreme overdose reactions in clinically hypothyroid individuals.

Hyperthyroidism

Hyperthyroidism, also called thyrotoxicosis, like hypothyroidism, usually begins insidiously and if left untreated, may progress to a more severe form of the disease called thyroid storm or thyroid crisis. The incidence of thyroid gland hyperfunction is 3 out of 10,000 adults per year, and the disease is found in females in an 8:1 ratio over males.[15] Hyperthyroidism occurs most often in patients between the ages of 20 and 40 years.[16] By far the most common form of thyrotoxicosis is that associated with diffuse enlargement of the gland, and the presence of antibodies against different fractions of the thyroid gland. This autoimmune thyroid disorder is called Graves' disease (Basedow's disease in Europe and Latin America). It has a familial tendency. The accompanying box lists other causes of hyperthyroidism.

Thyroid storm or crisis, although rarely seen today, occurs in patients with untreated or incompletely treated thyrotoxicosis. Not more than 1% to 2% of patients with hyperthyroidism will progress to thyroid storm.[17] On rare occasions, thyroid storm may occur suddenly in a patient in whom hyperthyroidism has not previously been diagnosed. More commonly, thyroid storm supervenes on a long history of uncomplicated hyperthyroidism. Six to eight months of symptoms are usual,

---

CAUSES OF HYPOTHYROIDISM

Primary

Autoimmune hypothyroidism
Idiopathic
Postsurgical thyroidectomy
External radiation therapy
Radioiodine therapy
Inherited enzymatic defect
Iodine deficiency
Antithyroid drugs
Lithium, phenylbutazone

Secondary

Pituitary tumor
Infiltrative disease (sarcoid) of pituitary

From Wogan JM: Endocrine disorders. In Rosen P: *Emergency medicine*, ed 2, St Louis, 1988, Mosby–Year Book.

CAUSES OF HYPERTHYROIDISM

Toxic diffuse goiter (Graves' disease)
Toxic multinodular goiter
Toxic uninodular goiter
Factitious thyrotoxicosis
T_3 thyrotoxicosis
Thyrotoxicosis associated with thyroiditis
    Hashimoto's thyroiditis
    Subacute (deQuervain's) thyroiditis
Jod-Basedow
Metastatic follicular carcinoma
Malignancies with circulating thyroid stimulators
TSH-producing pituitary tumors
Struma ovarii with hyperthyroidism
Hypothalamic hyperthyroidism

From Wogan JM: Endocrine disorders. In Rosen P: *Emergency medicine*, ed 2, St Louis, 1988, Mosby–Year Book.

and hyperthyroidism may have been present for as long as 2½ to 5 years.[17,18] Thyroid storm represents a sudden and severe exacerbation of the signs and symptoms of hyperthyroidism. It is usually accompanied by hyperpyrexia (elevated body temperature), and is precipitated by some form of stress, intercurrent disease, infection, trauma, thyroid surgery, or radioactive iodine administration.

Hyperthyroid patients are unusually sensitive to catecholamines such as epinephrine and may respond to their administration with hypertensive episodes, tachycardias, or significant dysrhythmias. In addition, hyperthyroid patients may appear quite apprehensive, suggesting the need for sedation during their treatment. The use of sedative medications may prove futile in these patients.

Thyroid gland dysfunction, whether hyperfunction or hypofunction, is associated with an increased incidence of cardiovascular disease.[19,20] Milder forms of both types of dysfunction may easily pass unnoticed. Although both hyper- and hypothyroidism lead to an increased risk, it is the more severe, undiagnosed, or untreated individual who represents the greatest potential risk during dental therapy. The doctor must be able to recognize each of these clinical entities and then take steps to decrease the potential risk.

PREVENTION

The goals in management of patients with thyroid dysfunction are (1) to prevent the occurrence of the life-threatening situations myxedema coma and thyroid storm, and (2) to prevent exacerbation of the complications associated with thyroid dysfunction, notably cardiovascular disease.

Only question 9 on the University of Southern California (USC) medical history questionnaire relates to thyroid disease. However, several other questions can provide information about potential thyroid gland dysfunction (questions 4, 5, 6, 13, and 16). Most other medical history questionnaires do not specifically mention thyroid disease.

QUESTION 4. Have you been a patient in the hospital during the past 2 years?

QUESTION 5. Have you been under the care of a medical doctor during the past 2 years?

QUESTION 9. Circle any of the following that you have had or have at present:

Thyroid disease

COMMENT. Patients with a known history of thyroid gland dysfunction will most often mention it in one or more of these three questions.

QUESTION 6. Have you taken any medicine or drugs during the past 2 years?

COMMENT. Patients with thyroid gland hypofunction receive thyroid extract or a synthetic preparation.[21] The most frequently used drug and the agent considered to be the drug of choice is L-thyroxine sodium (Synthroid). Other agents used in management of hypofunction include liotrix (Euthroid, Thyrolar) and dextrothyroxine sodium (Choloxin). The goal in management of thyroid gland hypofunction or hyperfunction is to achieve a normal level of glandular functioning, known as the euthyroid state.

Patients with hyperfunctioning of the thyroid gland undergo treatment aimed at halting the excessive secretion of thyroid hormone. Three methods are available: medical therapy, subtotal thyroidectomy, and radioactive iodine ablation of the gland.[22] Frequently prescribed antithyroid drugs include propylthiouracil and methimazole (Tapazole).[23] Propranolol (Inderal), dexamethasone, and lithium are also employed in management of thyrotoxicosis.[23] Table 18-1 lists common medications taken by the hypothyroid and hyperthyroid patient.

QUESTION 13. Have you lost or gained more than 10 pounds in the past year?

COMMENT. Unexplained weight loss in a patient with a ravenous appetite should alert the doctor to the possible presence of a hyperthyroid state. Conversely, an unexplained increase in weight along with other clinical signs and symptoms might indicate the possible presence of hypothyroidism.

QUESTION 16. Has your medical doctor ever said you have a cancer or a tumor?

COMMENT. Thyroid dysfunction is frequently discovered on routine examination of a patient's

Table 18-1. Medications used to manage hypothyroidism and hyperthyroidism

Hypothyroidism	Hyperthyroidism
Desiccated thyroid (Proloid, S-P-T)	Propylthiouracil
Levothyroxine (Levotroid, Levoxine, Synthroid)	Methimazole (Tapazole)
Liothyronine (T$_3$, Cytomel, Thyrar)	Carbimazole*
Liotrix (Euthroid, Thyrolar)	Propranolol (Inderal)

*As of July 1992, available in Europe, not in United States.

neck, manifesting itself as a lump or bump. This question will lead to an explanation of the type of dysfunction that was present and the mode of treatment. Subtotal thyroidectomy is a common mode of therapy for thyroid hyperfunction. Surgical intervention is especially common in those glands that develop benign or malignant thyroid nodules. Irradiation with radioactive iodine (iodine-131) is another commonly employed technique for destroying hyperfunctioning thyroid tissue.

QUESTION 7. **Are you allergic to (i.e., itching, rash, swelling of hands, feet, or eyes) or made sick by penicillin, aspirin, codeine, or any drugs or medications?**

COMMENT. Patients who are clinically hypothyroid are unusually sensitive to the pharmacologic actions of narcotics and other CNS depressants. Any adverse response to a strong analgesic, such as codeine, or central nervous system (CNS) depressant should be carefully evaluated for precise description of the nature of the response. Overdose reactions (see Chapter 23) that develop after average doses of these agents may indicate thyroid gland hypofunction.

Dialogue History

In the presence of a positive history of thyroid disease (question 9), the following dialogue history is indicated.

QUESTION. **What is (was) the nature of the thyroid dysfunction: hypofunction or hyperfunction?**

QUESTION. **How is it being managed?**

COMMENT. These questions seek to determine general information concerning the disease state. Following the dialogue history, the physical examination should help to provide clinical evidence of the continued presence of the dysfunction. In most instances the patient is euthyroid and will represent a normal risk during dental therapy.

When there is no prior history of thyroid dysfunction but clinical evidence leads to a suspicion of its presence, the following dialogue history is recommended.

QUESTION. **Have you lost or gained weight recently without dieting?**

COMMENT. Recent weight gain (10 or more pounds) is commonly noted in clinical hypothyroidism, whereas weight loss in the presence of an increasing appetite is frequently noted in hyperthyroidism. Note that other medical conditions may also produce weight gain or loss, for example, diabetes, congestive heart failure, or malignancy.

QUESTION. **Are you unusually sensitive to cold temperature or pain-relieving medications?**

COMMENT. These represent commonly seen symptoms of a hypofunctioning thyroid gland.

QUESTION. **Are you unusually sensitive to heat?**
QUESTION. **Have you become increasingly irritable or tense?**

COMMENT. These represent frequently seen signs and symptoms of a hyperfunctioning thyroid gland. The patient may be more aware of changes in temperature tolerance and less aware of changes in temperament; a close acquaintance is more likely to notice such changes.

Physical Examination

In most cases the patient who reports a prior history of thyroid gland dysfunction has received therapy or is currently undergoing therapy. These persons are usually in a euthyroid state (*eu* = "well, good", therefore a condition of normal function) and do not represent an increased risk during dental treatment.

On the other hand the patient with undetected thyroid gland dysfunction represents a possible significantly elevated risk during dental therapy. Clinical signs and symptoms enable the doctor to recognize these dysfunctions of the thyroid gland.

The clinically hypothyroid patient has a large, thick tongue with atrophic papillae, and thick edematous skin with puffy hands and face. The skin is dry and sweating is usually absent. The blood pressure is approximately normal (a possible slight elevation of the diastolic blood pressure), and the heart rate is slow (bradycardia). The patient appears lethargic and slow of speech.

Clinically, the hyperthyroid patient appears nervous, with warm, sweaty hands that may exhibit a mild tremor. Blood pressure is elevated (systolic more than diastolic), and the heart rate is markedly increased (tachycardia). A very difficult differential diagnosis to make is between hyperthyroidism and acute anxiety. One possible clue is that the patient with hyperthyroidism has palms that are warm and sweaty as distinguished from the cold and sweaty palms of the fearful individual. Other signs and symptoms of thyroid dysfunction are discussed in the section on clinical manifestations.

DENTAL THERAPY CONSIDERATIONS
Euthyroid

Patients with thyroid gland dysfunction who are receiving or have received therapy (e.g., surgery, medication, or irradiation), who have a normal level of circulating thyroid hormone, and who are asymptomatic are considered to be euthyroid. These patients represent an ASA II risk and may be managed in a normal manner in the dental environment.

In the presence of mild clinical manifestations, elective dental care may also proceed, although certain possible modifications should be considered. These patients represent ASA III risks.

Hypothyroid

If hypothyroidism is suspected, the following measures should be taken:

1. Medical consultation should be considered before initiating any dental treatment.
2. Any CNS depressant must be used with caution. Of particular concern are the sedative-hypnotics (barbiturates), narcotic analgesics, and the antianxiety drugs. Hypothyroid patients are extremely sensitive to the depressant actions of these drugs, and administration of a normal dose of these agents may prove to be an overdose, leading to respiratory or cardiovascular depression, or both.[24]
3. There is an increased incidence of cardiovascular disease associated with the hypothyroid state. Barnes and Barnes[25] have theorized that most instances of cardiovascular disease are produced by hypofunction of the thyroid gland and that correction of the thyroid deficiency leads to elimination of the cardiovascular disease. Although controversial, this theory is intriguing.

A history of thyroid gland hypofunction should lead the doctor to seek other possible signs and symptoms of cardiovascular disease. With more intense signs and symptoms of thyroid hypofunction (e.g., mental apathy, drowsiness, or slow speech), dental care should be withheld until medical consultation or definitive management of the clinical disorder is accomplished.

Hyperthyroid

Mild degrees of thyroid hyperfunction may pass for acute anxiety, with little increase in clinical risk. It must be noted that various cardiovascular disorders, primarily angina pectoris, are exaggerated in hyperthyroidism. Should these develop, management ought to proceed in the manner prescribed for such situations (see Section Seven). Severe hyperfunction should lead to immediate medical consultation. Dental care should not take place until the underlying metabolic disturbance has been corrected. It should always be remembered that thyroid crisis, although rare, may be precipitated by psychologic or physiologic stresses in untreated or incompletely treated hyperthyroid individuals.

There are additional dental therapy considerations for clinically hyperthyroid individuals. The drug atropine should not be administered. Atropine is a vagolytic agent (i.e., inhibits the vagus nerve, which decelerates the heart); atropine there-

fore increases the heart rate and may be a factor in precipitating thyroid storm. In addition, epinephrine should be used with extreme caution in these patients. Vasopressors act as cardiovascular stimulants, and when the cardiovascular system is already stimulated by the hyperthyroid state, they may precipitate cardiac dysrhythmias, tachycardia, and thyroid storm. Local anesthetics with vasoconstrictors may be used if the following precautions are followed:

- The least concentrated solution that is effective should be employed.
- The smallest effective volume of anesthetic agent should be injected.
- Aspiration should be performed before every injection.

(Injection technique is reviewed more thoroughly in Chapter 23.) Of greater potential risk, however, is the use of racemic epinephrine for gingival retraction. This agent is much more likely to precipitate unwanted side effects, especially in the presence of a preexisting hyperthyroid state. Its use should be absolutely avoided in these patients.

Patients who are mildly hyperthyroid might readily be mistaken for apprehensive persons. The use of conscious sedation techniques in these individuals is not contraindicated. However, because the apparent nervousness is not truly of dental origin but is hormonally induced, the effectiveness of sedative drugs may be less than ideal. Physical status classifications for thyroid gland dysfunction are presented in Table 18-2. Hypothyroid or hyperthyroid patients who have been treated and are presently euthyroid are considered to be ASA II risks, whereas patients exhibiting clinical manifestations of the hypothyroid or hyperthyroid state are ASA III risks.

CLINICAL MANIFESTATIONS
Hypothyroidism

Hypothyroidism may be described as a state in which all bodily functions undergo a progressive slowing caused by an insufficient supply of thyroid hormones. When this deficiency occurs during childhood, alterations are noted in both growth and development, and the syndrome is termed *cretinism*. In cretinism there has been a lack of thyroid hormone in utero or shortly after birth. The entire physical and mental development of the individual is retarded. Ossification of bone is delayed, tooth development is poor and eruption is delayed, and permanent neurologic damage is evident. Clinically, the infant is dull and apathetic, usually displaying a subnormal temperature. The tongue is enlarged, the skin and lips are thick, the face is broad and puffy, and the nose is flat (Fig. 18-1).

Table 18-2. Physical status classifications of thyroid gland dysfunction

Degree of dysfunction	Physical status (ASA)	Considerations
Hypofunction or hyperfunction patient receiving medical therapy; no signs or symptoms of dysfunction evident	II	Usual ASA II considerations
Hypofunction or hyperfunction; signs and symptoms of dysfunction evident	III	Usual ASA III considerations: Avoidance of vasopressors (hyperfunction) or CNS depressants (hypofunction) Evaluation for cardiovascular disease

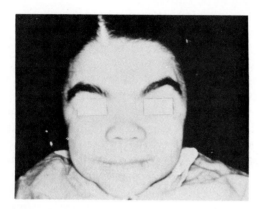

Fig. 18-1. Cretinism—clinical picture includes flat nose and broad, puffy face.

When hypothyroidism occurs in adults, its onset is usually insidious. The patient is often persuaded by a spouse or friends to seek medical assistance because of noticeably increased weakness and fatigue, sudden weight gain usually in the range of 7 to 8 pounds but not associated with an increased appetite,[26] or cold intolerance, present in half of the cases.[27] The patient is usually unaware of these changes.

Later in the course of the disease there may be evidence of slowing of speech, hoarseness, the absence of sweating, moderate weight gain, constipation in 25% of the patients, decreased sense of taste and smell, peripheral nonpitting edema, dyspnea, and anginal pains. Clinical signs include a puffiness of the face and eyelids,[28] a carotenemic (orange-red) skin color with rosy cheeks, thickened tongue, and thickened edematous skin (nonpitting). Blood pressure remains approximately normal (with perhaps a slight elevation in the diastolic pressure)[13]; however, the heart rate decreases (sinus bradycardia is the most common dysrhythmia). Congestive heart failure with pulmonary conges-

tion may also occur in severe, untreated hypothyroidism.

Pseudomyotonic deep tendon reflexes and paresthesias are extremely common in hypothyroid patients. Pseudomyotonic deep tendon reflexes, noted in almost 100% of hypothyroid patients, are characterized by a prolonged relaxation phase noted by testing the Achilles reflex while the patient kneels on a chair. The relaxation phase is at least twice as long as the contraction phase in these patients.[29] Paresthesias are seen in about 80% of the cases,[30] that most commonly observed being the median nerve in carpal tunnel syndrome. Indeed, 5% of patients with carpal tunnel syndrome have hypothyroidism.[31]

The most severe complication of hypothyroidism is myxedema coma. Myxedema coma has a high mortality rate and is marked by hypothermia (29.5° C to 30° C), bradycardia, hypotension, and intense cerebral obtundation (loss of consciousness). Myxedema coma is rare, occurring in only 0.1% of all cases of hypothyroidism and is extremely rare under 50 years of age, being most common in elderly women.[28] Hypothermia is noted in 80% of patients with myxedema, with recorded temperatures as low as 24° C.[10]

Symptoms that are essential to diagnose hypothyroidism include weakness, fatigue, cold intolerance, constipation, menorrhagia, and hoarseness.[32] Signs necessary for diagnosis include dry, cold, yellow, puffy skin; scant eyebrows; thick tongue; bradycardia; and a delayed return of deep tendon reflexes.[32] Table 18-3 summarizes the clinical manifestations of thyroid hypofunction.

Hyperthyroidism

Hyperthyroidism, like hypothyroidism, is rarely severe at onset. In most cases questioning of the patient reveals clinical evidence of the dysfunction over a period of months before its "discovery." As with hypofunction, the person discovering the disease frequently is not the patient but a spouse or

Table 18-3. Clinical manifestations of hypothyroidism

Symptoms (10% or greater incidence)	Percent manifestation
Paresthesias	92%
Loss of energy	79%
Intolerance to cold	51%
Muscular weakness	34%
Muscle and joint pain	31%
Inability to concentrate	31%
Drowsiness	30%
Constipation	27%
Forgetfulness	23%
Depressed auditory acuity	15%
Emotional lability	15%
Headaches	14%
Dysarthria	14%
Signs	
"Pseudomyotonic" reflexes	95%
Change in menstrual pattern	86%
Hypothermia	80%
Dry, scaly skin	79%
Puffy eyelids	70%
Hoarse voice	56%
Weight gain	41%
Dependent edema	30%
Sparse axillary and pubic hair	30%
Pallor	24%
Thinning of eyebrows	24%
Yellow skin	23%
Loss of scalp hair	18%
Abdominal distension	18%
Goiter	16%
Decreased sweating	10%

Modified from Wogan JM: Endocrine disorders. In Rosen P: *Emergency medicine,* ed 2, St Louis, 1988, Mosby—Year Book.

friend who notices changes in the habits and personality of the patient. Nervousness, increasing irritability, and insomnia are usually the first clinical symptoms noted. Other clinical manifestations include an increasing intolerance to heat; hyperhidrosis (marked increase in sweating); overactivity, including quick, uncoordinated movements ranging from mild to gross tremor; and rapid speech. An important sign is unexplained weight loss associated with an increased appetite. Up to half of all patients with thyroid storm seen in emergency departments have a weight loss greater than 40 pounds.[18] Hyperthyroid patients fatigue easily and may be aware of heart palpitation.

Clinical signs include extreme sweating, and the skin appears warm and moist. The extremities, especially the hands, exhibit varying degrees of trem-

ulousness. When hyperthyroidism results from Graves' disease, ophthalmopathy may be noted. The severity of the ophthalmopathy does not parallel the severity of the thyroid dysfunction. The clinical manifestations of ophthalmopathy observed in hyperthyroidism were categorized by Werner[33-35] and include upper lid retraction, staring, lid lag, proptosis, exophthalmos (Fig. 18-2), and extraocular muscle palsies. Cardiovascular manifestations vary from an increase in blood pressure (systolic pressure to a greater extent than diastolic pressure), widening of the pulse pressure, sinus tachycardia (more common during sleep), and on occasion, paroxysmal atrial fibrillation and congestive heart failure. Mitral valve prolapse is seen much more often than in the general population.[16]

Untreated hyperthyroidism may progress to the life-threatening situation called thyroid storm. Although extremely rare today, thyroid storm is essentially an acute exacerbation of the signs and symptoms of hyperthyroidism manifested by signs of severe hypermetabolism. Clinical manifestations include hyperpyrexia (highly elevated body temperature); profuse sweating; nausea, vomiting, and abdominal pains; and cardiovascular disturbances such as tachycardia and atrial fibrillation, as well as congestive heart failure with possible pulmonary edema. Central nervous system manifestations usually progress from mild tremulousness to severe agitation and disorientation to frankly psychotic behavior, stupor (partial unconsciousness), and finally coma. Without management, or in many instances,

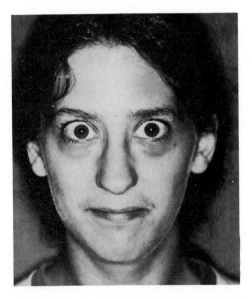

Fig. 18-2. Hyperthyroid patient exhibiting exophthalmos.

even with management, thyroid storm has a high mortality rate.

Symptoms necessary for the diagnosis of hyperthyroidism include weakness, sweating, weight loss, nervousness, loose stools, and heat intolerance.[32] Signs include warm, thin, soft, moist skin; exophthalmos, staring, and tremors.[32] Table 18-4 summarizes the signs and symptoms of thyroid hyperfunction.

PATHOPHYSIOLOGY
Hypothyroidism

The clinical signs and symptoms of hypothyroidism are produced by insufficient levels of circulating thyroid hormone. There is, in effect, a slowing down of all body functions. In addition, with chronic hypofunction there is a progressive infiltration of the skin by mucopolysaccharides and mucoproteins, giving the skin its characteristic puffy appearance. This hard, nonpitting, mucinous edema has been called myxedema and is characteristic of hypothyroidism. Initially, this edema is not found in dependent areas.[28]

Myxedema may also cause significant cardiac enlargement, which leads to pericardial and pleural effusions and to the cardiovascular and respiratory difficulties associated with hypothyroidism.[25,36] Coronary artery disease has been demonstrated to be accelerated in clinically hypothyroid patients.[19]

Myxedema coma is the end point in the progression of severe hypothyroidism. The actual cause of the loss of consciousness may be hypothermia, hypoglycemia, or carbon dioxide retention, all of which are present in this clinical situation.

Hyperthyroidism

Hyperthyroidism results from the excessive production of endogenous thyroid hormone by the thyroid gland or from the excessive administration of exogenous thyroid hormone (as in therapy for hypothyroid states). Clinical signs and symptoms are related to the level of these hormones in the blood.

Thyroid hormones produce an increase in energy consumption by the body and an elevation of the basal metabolic rate (BMR). Fatigue and weight loss result from this increased utilization of energy. Cardiovascular findings in hyperthyroid patients are related to the direct action of thyroid hormones on the myocardium. They are characterized by a hyperdynamic, electrically excitable state. These findings include increased heart rate and increased cardiac irritability. This increased cardiac workload is probably responsible for the increased incidence of cardiac problems (e.g., angina pectoris and

Table 18-4. Clinical manifestations of hyperthyroidism

Symptoms	Percent manifestation
Weight loss	72%-100%
<20 lb	Up to 14%
20 to 40 lb	27%-36%
>40 lb	23%-45%
Palpitations	
Dyspnea	
Edema	
Chest pain	
Nervousness	
Weakness	
Tremor	
Psychosis	
Diarrhea	
Hyperdefecation	
Abdominal pain	
Myalgias	
Disorientation	

Signs	Percent manifestation
Fever	100%
<103°F	57%-70%
>103°F	30%-43%
Tachycardia	100%
100-139	24%
140-169	62%
170-200	14%
Sinus tachycardia	67%
Dysrhythmias	37%
Thyromegaly	100%
Wide pulse pressure	86%-100%
40-59 torr (mmHg)	38%
60-100 torr	62%
Tremor	73%
Thyrotoxic stare/lid retraction	60%
Hyperkinesis	55%
Congestive heart failure	50%
Weakness	23%
Coma	18%-23%
Tender liver	17%
Infiltrative ophthalmopathy	17%
Somnolent/obtundent	14%-46%
Psychosis	9%-29%
Jaundice	9%-24%

Modified from Wogan JM: Endocrine disorders. In Rosen P: *Emergency medicine*, ed 2, St Louis, 1988, Mosby–Year Book.

congestive heart failure), and of cardiac symptoms noted (e.g., palpitations, dyspnea, chest pain) in hyperthyroid individuals.[18,20] Subclinical cardiac disease may have been present before the onset of the hyperthyroid state or in the hypothyroid state before therapy, but with the addition of thyroid hormone, the workload and myocardial oxygen requirement of the heart are increased to the point that clinically significant cardiac disease becomes evident.

Liver function is diminished in hyperthyroidism.[37] Jaundice may appear, but is readily eliminated by treating the thyrotoxicosis.[37] Because of the variable degree of liver dysfunction associated with thyrotoxicosis, all drugs and medications metabolized primarily in the liver should be employed judiciously and in smaller than normal doses. Because of the effects of atropine and epinephrine on the heart and cardiovascular systems, use of these agents should be avoided in severely hyperthyroid individuals.

Thyroid storm or crisis is the end point of untreated hyperthyroidism. The primary difference between thyroid storm and severe hyperthyroidism is the presence of hyperpyrexia, which if allowed to progress may reach lethal body temperatures (105° F or higher) within 24 to 48 hours. In this severe hypermetabolic state, the body's demand for energy overworks the cardiovascular system, leading to clinical signs and symptoms of cardiac dysrhythmia, congestive heart failure, and acute pulmonary edema. The patient will also exhibit profound delirium, vomiting, diarrhea, and dehydration.

MANAGEMENT

Acute thyroid-related emergencies are unlikely to develop during dental care of patients with thyroid disease. When the loss of consciousness occurs, management will prove to be supportive in nature.

Hypothyroidism

No special management is necessary for most patients who exhibit clinical evidence of thyroid hypofunction. If doubt or concern is present in the doctor's mind following complete medical and dental evaluation, medical consultation prior to beginning dental treatment is warranted.

It must always be remembered that hypothyroid patients are unusually sensitive to the following categories of drugs—sedatives (e.g., barbiturates), narcotics (e.g., meperidine, codeine), antianxiety drugs (e.g., diazepam), and most other CNS depressants, such as antihistamines. Severe drug overdose responses may develop following normal doses of these agents.

Effective management of a hypothyroid individual is usually easily achieved through oral administration of desiccated thyroid hormone. In almost all cases therapy must continue for the lifetime of the patient. Within 30 days of the start of therapy, the patient has usually returned to a normal body weight, and all clinical signs and symptoms have disappeared. On the whole the prognosis for treated hypothyroidism is a return to normal health.

Diagnostic clues to the presence of hypothyroidism include:

- Cold intolerance
- Weakness
- Fatigue
- Dry, cold, yellow, puffy skin
- Thick tongue

Unconscious Patient with History of Hypothyroidism

It is extremely unlikely that the undiagnosed, untreated, clinically hypothyroid patient will lose consciousness and be unrevivable in the dental office. It is more likely that this patient, or any patient for that matter, will lose consciousness due to psychogenic stimuli (fear) associated with impending dental care. In this situation the usual steps of management of the unconscious patient will produce a rapid return of consciousness.

Step 1: Terminate the dental procedure.

Step 2: Position the patient. The unconscious patient is placed into the supine position with the legs elevated slightly.

Step 3: Basic life support, as indicated. In the event that a hypothyroid individual loses consciousness, the possibility of myxedema coma must be considered. Management of this individual includes following the steps of basic life support: establishing a patent airway, checking for breathing, administering oxygen, and assessing the adequacy of circulation, as needed.

Step 4: Summon medical assistance. Because the underlying cause of unconsciousness is not a lack of oxygen, this individual will not regain consciousness following these basic procedures. Medical assistance should be summoned immediately whenever consciousness is not regained following the ABCs of basic life support.

Step 5: Establish an intravenous line, (if available). An intravenous infusion of 5% dextrose and water or normal saline may be started, if available, prior to the arrival of the emergency medical team. Availability of a patent vein will facilitate subsequent medical management of this patient.

Step 6: Administer oxygen. Oxygen may be administered at any time during this situation. Though oxygen administration will not lead to recovery of the patient, no harm can occur from its administration.

Step 7: Definitive management. Definitive management of myxedema coma will include transport to the emergency department of a hospital and the

MANAGEMENT OF THE UNCONSCIOUS
PATIENT WITH THYROID DISEASE

Hypothyroid patient (myxedema coma)
Hyperthyroid patient (thyroid storm)

Terminate the dental procedure
↓
Position the patient
(supine with legs elevated slightly)
↓
Basic life support, as indicated
↓
(if recovery does not occur)
Summon medical assistance
↓
Establish intravenous line, if possible
↓
Administer oxygen
↓
Transport to hospital for definitive diagnosis
and management

administration of massive intravenous doses of thyroid hormones (e.g., triiodothyronine or levothyroxine) for several days and the correction of hypothermia. Additional therapy varies according to the clinical state of the patient. The mortality rate from this illness is quite high (40%) in spite of rigorous therapy. The management of the unconscious hypothyroid patient is outlined in the accompanying box.

Hyperthyroidism

Clinically, hyperthyroid individuals most often appear nervous and apprehensive. If clinical symptoms are intense to the point of creating doubt in the doctor's mind, medical consultation before initiating dental treatment is indicated. Although the risk of precipitating thyroid storm is low, undue stress can induce this acute life-threatening situation. The use of certain drugs, particularly atropine and epinephrine, can precipitate thyroid crisis and therefore should not be administered to clinically hyperthyroid individuals.

Diagnostic clues to the presence of hyperthyroidism include:

• Sweating
• Heat intolerance
• Tachycardia
• Warm, thin, soft, moist skin
• Exophthalmos
• Tremor

Unconscious Patient with History of Hyperthyroidism

As with the hypothyroid patient, it is highly unlikely that the undiagnosed, untreated, clinically hyperthyroid patient will lose consciousness and be unresuscitatable in the dental office. Vasodepressor syncope is a much more likely cause of unconsciousness. In this situation the usual steps of management of the unconscious patient will produce a rapid return of consciousness.

Step 1: Terminate the dental procedure.

Step 2: Position the patient. The unconscious patient is placed into the supine position with the legs elevated slightly.

Step 3: Basic life support, as indicated. In the event that a hyperthyroid individual loses consciousness, the possibility of thyroid storm must be considered, especially if the patient has an elevated temperature. Management of this individual includes following the steps of basic life support: establishing a patent airway, checking for breathing, administering oxygen, and assessing the adequacy of circulation, as needed.

Step 4: Summon medical assistance. Because the underlying cause of unconsciousness is not a lack of oxygen, this individual will not regain consciousness following these basic procedures. Medical assistance should be summoned immediately whenever consciousness is not regained following the ABCs of basic life support.

Step 5: Establish an intravenous line, (if available). An intravenous infusion of 5% dextrose and water or normal saline may be started, if available, prior to the arrival of the emergency medical team. Availability of a patent vein will facilitate subsequent medical management of this patient.

Step 6: Administer oxygen. Oxygen may be administered at any time during this situation. Though oxygen administration will not lead to recovery of the patient, no harm can occur from its administration.

Step 7: Definitive management. Definitive management of thyroid storm includes transport to the emergency department of a hospital and the administration of large doses of antithyroid drugs (e.g., propylthiouracil). Additional therapy includes propranolol to block the adrenergic-mediated effects of thyroid hormones, as well as large doses of glucocorticosteroids to prevent the occurrence of acute adrenal insufficiency. Other measures include administration of oxygen, cold packs, sedation, and careful monitoring of the state of hydration and electrolyte balance. The prognosis of thyroid storm is poor. The management of the unconscious hyperthyroid patient is outlined in the box on p. 260.

Drugs used in management: none

Medical assistance: Yes if unconscious hypo- or hyperthyroid

REFERENCES

1. Nikolai TF: The thyroid gland. In Rose LF, Kaye D, editors: *Internal medicine for dentistry*, St Louis, 1983, Mosby–Year Book.
2. Wogan JM: Endocrine disorders. In Rosen P: *Emergency medicine*, ed 2, St Louis, 1988, Mosby–Year Book.
3. LaFranchi S: Diagnosis and treatment of hypothyroidism in children, *Compr Ther* 13:20, 1987.
4. Ord WM: On myxedema, a term proposed to be applied to an essential condition in the "cretinoid" affection occasionally observed in middle-aged women, *Med Chir Trans London* 61:57, 1877.
5. Forester CF: Coma in myxedema, report of a case and review of the world literature, *Arch Intern Med* 111:734, 1963.
6. Nichols AB, Hunt WB: Is myxedema coma respiratory failure? *South Med J* 69:945, 1976.
7. von Basedow CA: Exophthalmos durch Hypertrophie des Zellgewbes in der Augenhohle, Wochenschrift fur die gesammte Heilkunde, Berlin, 1840. Reprinted in Major RH: *Classic descriptions of disease*, Springfield, Ill., 1978, Charles C Thomas.
8. Graves RJ: Newly observed affection of the thyroid gland in females, *London Med Surg J* 7(2):516. Reprinted in Major RH: *Classic descriptions of disease*, Springfield, Ill., 1978, Charles C Thomas.
9. Roizen M, Becker CE: Thyroid storm: a review of cases at University of California, San Francisco, *Calif Med* 115:5, 1971.
10. Senior RM, Birge SJ, Wessler S, and others: The recognition and management of myxedema coma, *JAMA* 217:61, 1971.
11. Amino N: Autoimmunity and hypothyroidism, *Clin Endocrinol Metab* 2:591, 1988.
12. Swanson JW, Kelly JJ, McConahey WM: Neurologic aspects of thyroid dysfunction, *Mayo Clin Proc* 56:504, 1981.
13. Nickerson JF, Hill SR Jr, McNeil JH, and others: Fatal myxedema, with and without coma, *Ann Intern Med* 53:475, 1960.
14. Wartofsky L: Myxedema coma. In *The thyroid: A fundamental and clinical text*, ed 5, Ingbar SH, Braverman LE, editors: Philadelphia, 1986, Lippincott.
15. Hellman R: The evaluation and management of hyperthyroid crisis, *Crit Care Q* 77, 1980.
16. Toft AD, editor: Hyperthyroidism (symposium), *Clin Endocrinol Metab* 14(2):May, 1985, entire issue.
17. Wartofsky L: Thyrotoxic storm. In *The thyroid: a fundamental and clinical text*, ed 5 Ingbar SH, Braverman LE, editors: Philadelphia, 1986, Lippincott.
18. Mazzaferri EL, Skillman TG: Thyroid storm, *Arch Intern Med* 124:684, 1969.
19. Becker C: Hypothyroidism and atherosclerotic heart disease: pathogenesis, medical management, and the role of coronary artery bypass surgery, *Endocr Rev* 6:432, 1985.
20. Waldstein SS, Slodki SJ, Kaganiec GI, and others: A clinical study of thyroid storm, *Ann Intern Med* 52(3):626, 1960.
21. Fish LH, and others: Replacement dose, metabolism, and bioavailability of levothyroxine in the treatment of hypothyroidism: role of triiodothyronine in pituitary feedback in humans, *N Engl J Med* 316:764, 1987.
22. Becker DV: Choice of therapy for Graves' hyperthyroidism (editorial) *N Engl J Med* 311:464, 1984.
23. Dunn JT: Choice of therapy in young adults with hyperthyroidism of Graves' disease, *Ann Intern Med* 100:891, 1984.
24. Urbanic RC, Mazzaferri EL: Thyrotoxic crisis and myxedema coma, *Heart Lung* 7:435, 1978.
25. Barnes BO, Barnes CW: *Solved: the riddle of heart attacks*, Fort Collins, Colo., 1976, Robinson Press.
26. Klein I, Leey GS: Unusual manifestations of hypothyroidism, *Arch Intern Med* 144:123, 1984.
27. Bloomer H, Kyle LH: Myxedema: a reevaluation of clinical diagnosis based on eighty cases, *Arch Intern Med* 104:234, 1959.
28. Meek JC: Myxedema coma, *Crit Care Q* 3(2):131, 1980.
29. Maclean D, Taig DR, Emslie-Smith D: Achilles tendon reflex in accidental hypothermia and hypothermic myxedema, *Br Med J* 2:87, 1973.
30. Sanders V: Neurologic manifestations of myxedema, *N Engl J Med* 266:547, 1962.
31. Doyle JR, Carroll RE: The carpal tunnel syndrome: a review of 100 patients treated surgically, *Calif Med* 108:263, 1968.
32. Endocrine disorders. In Schroeder SA, Krupp MA, Tierney LM, and others, editors: *Current medical diagnosis & treatment 1990;* Norwalk, 1990, Appleton & Lange.
33. Werner SC: Classification of the eye changes in Graves' disease, *Am J Ophthalmol* 68(4):646, 1969.
34. Werner SC: Modification of the classification of eye changes in Graves' disease, *Am J Ophthalmol* 83(5):725, 1977.
35. Lyle WM: Werner's classification of ocular changes in Graves' disease: a review, *Am J Optom Physiol Opt* 55(2):119, 1978.
36. Barnes BO: Hypertension and the thyroid gland, *Clin Exp Pharmacol Physiol* 2(suppl):167, 1975.
37. Greenberger NJ, Milligan FD, DeGroot LJ and others: Jaundice and thyrotoxicosis in the absence of congestive heart failure, *Am J Med* 38:840, 1964.

19 *Cerebrovascular Accident*

Cerebrovascular accident is a focal neurologic disorder caused by the destruction of brain substance as a result of intracerebral hemorrhage, thrombosis, embolism, or vascular insufficiency. Synonyms for cerebrovascular accident include CVA, stroke, and cerebral apoplexy. Throughout this section CVA will be used to identify this disorder.

Cerebrovascular accidents are fairly common in the adult population. In the United States approximately 500,000 new acute CVAs are reported annually. Although mortality rates for the different forms of CVA vary considerably, the overall rate is relatively high. Approximately 160,000 deaths are reported annually from CVAs,[1] making it the third leading cause of death in this country (heart disease and cancer are first and second).[2] Most stroke victims survive but often with significant disability. The frequency with which CVAs occur is emphasized by the fact that approximately 25% of routine autopsies (death from all causes) demonstrate evidence of CVA, even though there may have been no evidence of stroke while the patient was alive. Cerebrovascular accidents are the most common form of brain disease. The average age of persons at the time of their first CVA is approximately 64 years. Twenty-five percent of all CVAs occur in patients under the age of 65 years.[3] Recent evidence demonstrates that the incidence of CVA is decreasing; in the past 30 years, it has declined 25%.[4] For every 100 first episodes of CVA that occurred in a unit of population between 1945 and 1949, only 55 first episodes of CVA occurred between 1970 and 1974. This decline is noted in both sexes and all age groups, but is most noted in the elderly.[5-7]

In children the incidence of stroke is 2.5 per 100,000 per year. Although stroke can occur at any age between infancy and childhood, it occurs most frequently between the ages of 1 and 5 years.[8-9] Cyanotic heart disease is the most common underlying systemic disorder predisposing to stroke in children.

CLASSIFICATION

Cerebrovascular accidents are usually classified by cause. Two major classes of stroke are hemorrhagic and occlusive, with a third type, lacunar infarcts, a type of occlusive stroke. Table 19-1 presents the various forms of CVA and their relative incidence. In addition to the forms of CVA presented in the table, there is a syndrome variously called transient ischemic attack (TIA), transient cerebral ischemia (TCI), or incipient stroke. It consists of brief episodes of cerebral ischemia that result in no permanent neurologic damage, whereas a CVA almost always results in evidence of some degree of permanent neurologic damage.

Lacunar Infarction

Lacunar infarcts are amongst the most common cerebrovascular lesions. Small in size (<5 mm in diameter), lacunar infarcts are often associated with poorly controlled hypertension or diabetes. Lacunar infarcts involve penetrating cerebral arterial branches lying deep in the cerebrum or brainstem.[10] The prognosis for recovery from the deficits produced by lacunar infarction is usually good, with partial or complete resolution occurring over the following 4 to 6 weeks in many cases.[11]

Cerebral Infarction

The most prevalent form of CVA is the occlusive stroke, accounting for over 85% of all CVAs. Occlusive strokes most commonly result from atherosclerotic disease and cardiac abnormalities. Thrombosis of intracranial and extracranial arteries and cerebral embolization from various origins

Table 19-1. Classification of cerebrovascular disease

Cause	Approximate percentage of all CVAs	Initial mortality rate (%)	Recurrence rate (%)
Cerebral ischemia and infarction	88	30	*
Atherosclerosis and thrombosis	81	*	20
Cerebral embolism	7	*	*
Intracranial hemorrhage	12	80	*
Arterial aneurysms	*	45	33
Hypertensive vascular disease	*	50	Rare

*Unknown.

throughout the body are the primary causes of cerebral infarction. Cerebral infarction may be defined as death of neural (brain) tissue from ischemia. The primary cause of ischemia is a prolonged decrease in blood flow to the brain. This form of CVA is most common between the ages of 60 and 69 years and occurs more frequently in males (2:1).

Cerebral infarction is usually accompanied by abnormalities in the arterial blood supply from the heart to the brain. In most instances this alteration in the arterial blood supply is produced by atherosclerosis, which is commonly found in certain anatomic areas. Emboli most often originate from the heart in atrial fibrillation and following myocardial infarction,[12] and from neck veins, specifically in the internal carotid artery at the carotid bifurcation in the neck and the junction of the vertebral and basilar arteries (Fig. 19-1). By the third decade of a normal adult's life, there is usually significant atherosclerotic plaque in arteries, but in most cases clinical evidence, in the form of acute myocardial infarction or cerebral infarction, is not present until the fifth and sixth decades.

Narrowing of atherosclerotic vessels must be significant (a lumenal reduction of approximately 80%) before blood flow is reduced to clinically significant levels. A second factor of importance in atherosclerotic vessels is the formation of thrombi (blood clots). Thrombus formation is much more likely to occur in atherosclerotic than in nonatherosclerotic vessels.

In either atherosclerosis or thrombosis, the blood supply to the area of brain distal to the vessel narrowing, or occlusion, is severely reduced so that a portion of brain tissue becomes ischemic and its cells become necrotic and shrunken or infarcted, producing signs and symptoms of neurologic deficit. Patients with certain diseases have been shown to be more likely to develop atherosclerosis, to develop it at an earlier age, and to have a greater degree of severity. Foremost among these diseases are high blood pressure and diabetes mellitus.[13,14] Acute episodes of cerebral ischemia and infarction may develop at any time; however, approximately 20% occur during sleep.

Cerebral embolization is a causative factor in approximately 7% of CVAs. A major source of emboli is the heart when there is impaired flow or damaged valves. Rheumatic heart disease with mitral stenosis and atrial fibrillation is the most common cause of cerebral embolization in those under 50 years of age; other causes are prosthetic valves, acute myocardial infarction, atrial fibrillation, bacterial endocarditis, mitral valve prolapse, and thyrotoxicosis with atrial fibrillation.[15] Cerebral embolization occurs throughout the age spectrum of 20 to 70 years; however, it is most frequent after the age of 40 years.

Transient Ischemic Attack (TIA)

The transient ischemic attack (TIA), also termed incipient stroke or transient cerebral ischemia, may be considered a "temporary stroke" in much the same manner that angina pectoris might be considered "temporary heart attack." Transient ischemic attacks are characterized by focal ischemic cerebral neurologic deficits that last for less than 24 hours. These attacks rarely last more than 8 hours and often resolve within 15 to 60 minutes. Attacks may occur many times a day or at weekly or monthly intervals. In the periods between episodes, the patient is asymptomatic. They are usually caused by platelet, fibrin, or other atherosclerotic embolic material from the neck or heart that lodges in a cerebral vessel and interferes transiently with blood flow.[16] The clinical importance of TIAs is that they signal the existence of a significant degree of cerebrovascular disease and clearly demonstrate a potential danger of cerebral infarction.[17] Patients with TIAs that last for more than 1 to 2 hours have a greater risk of stroke.[18]

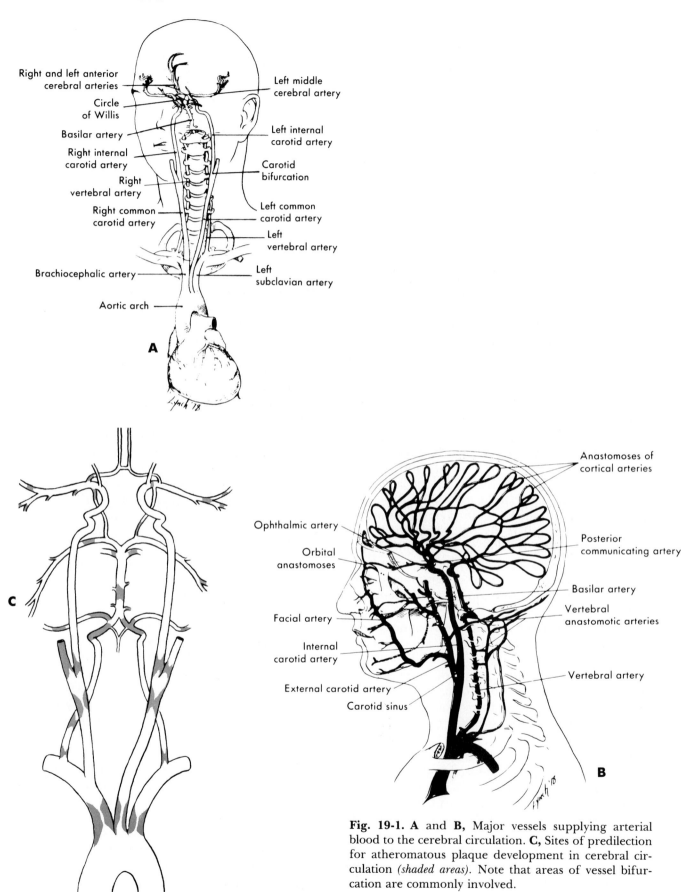

Fig. 19-1. A and **B,** Major vessels supplying arterial blood to the cerebral circulation. **C,** Sites of predilection for atheromatous plaque development in cerebral circulation *(shaded areas)*. Note that areas of vessel bifurcation are commonly involved.

The incidence of TIA in an elderly population is 1 per 1000. The risk of CVA in the elderly is four to ten times that of a control population and may reach as high as 35% incidence of CVA within a 4-year period.[19]

Intracerebral Hemorrhage

The second major category of cerebrovascular accident is intracerebral hemorrhage, also called apoplexy. This category is responsible for approximately 10% of all acute cerebrovascular disease, and regardless of the specific cause, it represents a very serious problem with a high mortality rate. It occurs most commonly in persons over the age of 50 years. Intracerebral hemorrhage may develop from any blood vessel, but the usual source of bleeding is from arteries. Hemorrhagic stroke is categorized by the location of the bleeding. Subarachnoid hemorrhage (SAH) occurs on the surface of the brain within the subarachnoid space, whereas intracerebral hemorrhage (ICH) occurs within the parenchyma.

The two major sources of intracerebral hemorrhage are ruptured arterial aneurysms and hypertensive vascular disease. In both cases the walls of the involved blood vessels are defective—with congenital defects in the former and acquired defects in the latter—producing weakened areas. The cause of the actual rupture of the vessel wall is probably an acute change or elevation in the systolic blood pressure. Subarachnoid hemorrhage most commonly occurs with rupture of an aneurysm resulting from a weakened vessel wall at an arterial bifurcation.[20] Rupture occurs with a sudden increase in local pressure within a critically stretched aneurysm sac. Intracerebral hemorrhages, on the other hand, represent rupture of weakened arterioles caused by chronic systemic hypertension.[16] Clinically, most incidents of intracerebral hemorrhage occur while patients are engaged in their normal activities such as work, heavy lifting, and straining while passing stool—factors categorized as physical stress, all of which are associated with elevations in blood pressure.

With this in mind, it is evident that although intracerebral hemorrhage is responsible for only 10% of all CVAs, it represents more of a potential risk to the dental practitioner dealing with acutely anxious patients and with potentially painful procedures. Both anxiety and pain are associated with potentially significant increases in the heart rate and blood pressure of the patient, making the development of a hemorrhagic CVA more likely.

Survivors of episodes of cerebrovascular disease have a high risk of future recurrences (Table 19-1).

Within 12 to 24 months, 20% of survivors of CVAs from atherosclerotic vascular disease have a subsequent CVA; over 33% of patients with ruptured aneurysms develop recurrences.[21] However, the risk of recurrent CVA is not the major threat to survival of these patients. Cardiovascular disease is the major limiting factor for the post-CVA patient. Over 50% of these individuals die from acute myocardial infarction or heart failure.[22] The post-CVA patient therefore represents a definite increased risk during dental care. Thorough evaluation of this patient before dental treatment and special considerations during treatment reduce the potential risk.

PREDISPOSING FACTORS

A number of factors have been identified that significantly increase the risk of developing cerebrovascular accident. These factors include high blood pressure (hypertension), diabetes mellitus, cardiac enlargement (as determined with electrocardiology), hypercholesterolemia, the use of oral contraceptives, and cigarette smoking. The use of birth control pills has been associated with a ninefold increased risk of thrombotic stroke,[23] although recent analyses suggest this risk is confined to those who smoke cigarettes.[24] Table 19-2 presents the risk factors associated with the various types of stroke.

Consistently elevated blood pressure has been demonstrated to be a major risk factor in the development of both occlusive and hemorrhagic

Table 19-2. Types of stroke and associated risk factors*

Stroke syndrome	Risk factors
Occlusive	
Emboli	Atrial fibrillation
	Acute MI
	Abnormal valves
Thrombi	
TIA	Hypertension
RIND	Smoking
Progressive	Lipids
Completed	Age
	Diabetes
	Prior TIA
Lacunar	Hypertension (90%)
Hemorrhagic	
Subarachnoid	None
Intracerebral	Hypertension (50%)
Cerebellar	Hypertension (50%)

*MI, myocardial infarction; TIA, transient ischemic attack; RIND, reversible ischemic neurologic deficit.

stroke. Evidence from the Framingham study[25] has led to the belief that high blood pressure may well be the major predisposing factor in the development of hemorrhagic CVA. It is estimated that the risk of developing a hemorrhagic CVA increases by 30% for every 10 mmHg elevation of the systolic blood pressure above 160 mmHg.[26] Prolonged periods of elevated blood pressure also produce thickening and fibrinoid degeneration of cerebral arteries. Atherosclerosis develops at an earlier age and to a more severe degree in patients with elevated blood pressure. Yet another mechanism by which high blood pressure leads to an increased incidence of CVA is through the normal response of cerebral arteries to elevations in blood pressure. Cerebral arteries, primarily the smaller cerebral arteries, constrict in response to elevations in blood pressure. This reduces the local cerebral blood flow, leading to ischemia of areas of brain tissue, which if prolonged may produce infarction.

It is worth repeating that high blood pressure represents the single greatest risk factor in the development of all forms of cerebrovascular disease. Fortunately, however, high blood pressure also represents the only major risk factor that if corrected (lowered) is associated with a decreased incidence of CVA. This fact is of particular importance to the dental profession. So much of our dental care is associated with pain, either real or imagined, leading to greatly increased apprehension, that a significant percentage of dental patients exhibit signs of increased cardiovascular system activity. Clinically, this is evident as elevated blood pressure and an increase in heart rate. In patients with evidence of other risk factors of CVA, such as diabetes and atherosclerosis, these increases in cardiovascular activity might well precipitate an acute cerebrovascular accident, most likely of the more ominous hemorrhagic type.

The status post-CVA patient represents an even greater risk in the dental office. Survivors of CVAs have a very good chance of recovering some degree of function. In the Framingham study,[25] 84% of CVA survivors were living at home, 80% were capable of independent mobility, and 69% had total independence in the normal activities of daily living. Yet only 10% exhibited no functional deficit. These CVA survivors might correctly be called "the walking wounded." As McCarthy[27] has stated, they represent "accidents waiting to happen." With independent mobility, the post-CVA patient expects to receive dental care; however, it must always be remembered that the recurrence rate in CVA is high (see Table 19-1) and that factors such as pain and anxiety only add to the risk presented by this patient. Proper management of pain and anxiety are therefore of the greatest importance for the post-CVA patient.

PREVENTION

Prevention of the occurrence or recurrence of CVA is based on the recognition of the risk factors discussed earlier and on possible modifications in dental care to accommodate the diminished ability of the post-CVA patient to handle stress effectively. The medical history questionnaire and dialogue history relating to this disorder follow.

Medical History Questionnaire

QUESTION 6. **Have you taken any medicine or drugs during the past 2 years?**

COMMENT. In the past, all patients who survived a CVA received anticoagulant therapy. Today however, anticoagulants are used much more cautiously because many studies have demonstrated that there is little benefit to be gained from their administration in many forms of stroke, and the risk of hemorrhage is increased.[28,29] Anticoagulant therapy is quite valuable following embolic stroke when there is a cardiac source of embolization, such as atrial fibrillation or valvular disease.[30,31]

Antiplatelet therapy using dipyridamole (Persantine) or aspirin has been successful in reducing recurrences of TIAs, but has not yet demonstrated convincingly decreased long-term stroke risk.[32] This reduction in risk has been limited to males in some studies, but not in all.[33] The range of aspirin dose is from 100 mg/day to over 1 g/day, without notable change in efficacy, but lower doses have shown fewer associated side effects.[33] The currently recommended dose is 325 mg/day.[34]

Antihypertensive medications are prescribed for the 66% of post-CVA patients who have elevated blood pressure. Commonly used drugs for the management of high blood pressure include diuretics (see Chapter 14, Table 14-1), methyldopa (Aldomet), and propranolol (Inderal). The doctor should be aware of the potential side effects of each of these agents and possible drug interactions that might be encountered with drugs used in dentistry. Postural hypotension is a common side effect of many antihypertensive agents. References such as the *Physicians' Desk Reference*,[35] *Facts and Comparisons*,[36] and *AMA Drug Evaluations*[37] are recommended.

QUESTION 9. **Circle any of the following that you have had or have at present:**
- High blood pressure
- Stroke
- Fainting or dizzy spells

COMMENT. High blood pressure is the single most important risk factor in causing CVAs and is the only risk factor that, if altered, results in a decreased risk of CVA. High blood pressure is present in over two thirds of post-CVA patients. The routine screening of blood pressure on all potential dental patients and especially of all medically compromised persons has proved to be a significant means of minimizing the development of CVA and the other major acute sequelae of high blood pressure, such as acute myocardial infarction and renal dysfunction, within the dental environment.

Fainting or dizzy spells might indicate the presence of transient ischemic attacks (TIA). Further evaluation of the patient is warranted through the dialogue history. An affirmative response to "stroke" requires a dialogue history to determine the degree of risk.

Dialogue History

In the presence of a prior history of CVA, the following dialogue history is recommended.

QUESTION. **When did you have your stroke (CVA)?**

QUESTION. **What type of stroke did you have?**

QUESTION. **Were you hospitalized? If so, for how long?**

COMMENT. These questions serve to gather the basic information concerning the nature and severity of the CVA. Following the CVA there is a degree of recovery from neurologic deficit. Although the length of time varies from patient to patient, maximal improvement usually occurs within 6 months. All but emergency dental care should be withheld during this period. The post-CVA patient is routinely classified as an ASA IV for 6 months, then is reevaluated and reclassified as indicated.[38]

QUESTION. **What degree of neurologic deficit (paralysis) occurred as a result of the CVA, and what degree of function has been recovered?**

COMMENT. Although motor deficit (hemiplegia) may be quite obvious to the observer, minor degrees of neurologic deficit may be less obvious. The patient is normally willing to discuss these with the doctor.

QUESTION. **What medication(s) are you now taking?**

COMMENT. Refer to question 6 of the medical history questionnaire for discussion. Antihypertensive and antiplatelet drugs are commonly used for long-term management of the post-CVA patient.

QUESTION. **If high blood pressure was present at the time of CVA, what was your blood pressure when you had your CVA?**

QUESTION. **How often do you measure your blood pressure, and what does it normally read?**

COMMENT. High blood pressure is present in a large percentage of CVA patients. In many instances it is undetected until the CVA develops. Patients who are well motivated in the management of their disease monitor their blood pressure on a regular basis. These blood pressure recordings may serve as a reference point to compare the vital signs that are recorded in the dental office. In general, the blood pressure of a post-CVA patient should not be elevated significantly.

In the absence of a history of prior CVA but with an affirmative response to fainting or dizzy spells, the doctor should suspect the possible presence of transient ischemic episodes. This question may also indicate the presence of anxiety toward dentistry, orthostatic hypotension, or convulsive disorders; a careful evaluation should be carried out.

QUESTION. **Have you ever experienced episodes of unexplained dizziness, numbness of the extremities, or speech defects?**

COMMENT. Transient episodes of cerebral ischemia can produce the aforementioned signs and symptoms. These episodes may occur daily or at more infrequent intervals. In many instances the patient is aware of the existence of TIA and is receiving drug therapy (e.g., anticoagulants, antihypertensives, antiplatelet drugs) to reduce the risk of a CVA developing. These patients should be managed in the dental office as if they have already had a CVA (ASA II or III).

If signs and symptoms of unexplained dizziness, numbness of the extremities, or speech defects appear in a patient who has no prior history of CVA, medical consultation with the patient's physician is indicated before the start of any dental care.

Physical Examination

Physical evaluation of the post-CVA patient should include a thorough visual examination to determine the extent of any residual neurologic deficit. The examination must include recording of vital signs, such as blood pressure, heart rate, and respiratory rate.

Vital Signs

Proper technique is essential to obtain accurate blood pressure recordings (see Chapter 2 for a full description of blood pressure technique). The medical risk presented by elevated blood pressure increases steadily with each elevation in blood pressure (i.e., there is no blood pressure above which an increased risk is present and below which risk is absent). It is therefore necessary to provide guidelines for clinical use. The categorization of blood pressure used in patient screening at the University of Southern California School of Dentistry is presented in Table 2-4. Recommended dental treatment modifications for each category are indicated.

For the doctor managing a post-CVA patient, awareness of the patient's blood pressure at the start of each dental treatment session is vital. Marked elevation in blood pressure is potentially life threatening in this patient, serving to increase the chance of a recurrent CVA. The guidelines indicate that any adult patient with a blood pressure of 200 mmHg systolic and/or 115 mmHg diastolic or above should not receive any dental care until the elevated blood pressure is brought under control (ASA IV). This usually necessitates immediate medical consultation and a delay in dental treatment while antihypertensive therapy is started or corrected. Physical status (ASA) III blood pressure (between 160 and 200 mmHg systolic and/or between 95 and 115 mmHg diastolic) in a post-CVA patient warrants immediate medical consultation prior to the start of any dental treatment.

Other Factors

The presence of unusual apprehension should be determined. The physiologic response to increased anxiety includes higher circulating blood levels of the catecholamines epinephrine and norepinephrine, which increase heart rate and blood pressure.

DENTAL THERAPY CONSIDERATIONS

The post-CVA patient represents a definite risk during dental therapy. Several basic factors are of importance in the management of this patient.

Length of time elapsed since the CVA. No elective dental care should be considered for at least 6 months after a stroke. The risk of recurrence is presumably somewhat greater during this time. Noninvasive emergency care for pain or infection should be managed, if at all possible, with medications. Invasive dental treatment should be delayed, or the patient should be treated in a controlled environment if immediate care is warranted. The hospital dental clinic, or that of a teaching institution (e.g., dental school, hospital training program) might prove to be more appropriate sites for invasive dental care on this patient.

Minimizing stress during dental treatment. The stress reduction protocol should be used for the post-CVA patient. Of particular importance are:

- Short, morning appointments (not to exceed the patient's limit of tolerance)
- Effective pain control: local anesthetics with epinephrine 1:200,000 or 1:100,000 (in judicious volumes)
- Psychosedation during treatment: N_2O-O_2 inhalation sedation or light oral sedation

COMMENT. All central nervous system depressants are relatively contraindicated in the post-CVA patient. Any CNS depressant may produce hypoxia, leading to aggravated confusion, aphasia, and other complications associated with CVA. In the author's experience light levels of sedation, as produced with nitrous oxide and oxygen or the oral benzodiazepines, have proved to be quite safe and highly effective in reducing stress in post-CVA patients. These techniques should be used only if warranted in a particular patient.

Gingival retraction cord impregnated with epinephrine should *never* be employed in a patient with a history of prior CVA.

Determining when the post-CVA patient is too great a risk for dental therapy. The blood pressure and heart rate serve as indicators of the cardiovascular status of the post-CVA patient at the time of dental treatment.

COMMENT. Marked elevations in blood pressure should be viewed with great concern and dental care should be withheld until medical consultation and/or corrective therapy is accomplished. The usual ASA categorizations for adult blood pressure should not be employed in the post-CVA patient. The author recommends that a medical consultation with the patient's primary care physician be obtained whenever there is a significant increase in blood pressure noted compared to prior measurements (thus the importance of baseline values) or when the blood pressure in the post-CVA patient is in excess of 160 mmHg without prior values being available. In addition, post-CVA patients should not receive elective dental care for a period of 6 months following a stroke.

NOTE. **Routine preoperative monitoring of blood pressure in all post-CVA patients is of utmost importance in the prevention of recurrences.**

Bleeding and the post-CVA patient. Most survivors of CVAs and patients with transient ischemic attacks receive antiplatelet (aspirin) or anticoagulant therapy in an effort to reduce the morbidity and mortality associated with recurrences.

COMMENT. If a patient is receiving any of these drugs and dental procedures are contemplated that may produce significant bleeding, medical consultation is indicated before the procedure. Although excessive hemorrhaging in the post-CVA patient is rarely a clinical problem in dentistry, the dentist and the physician must consider the possibility and

Table 19-3. Physical status classifications of CVA and TIA

	Physical status (ASA)	Dental therapy considerations
History of one documented CVA at least 6 months before treatment; no residual neurologic deficit *or* history of TIA	II	ASA II considerations to include: Light levels of sedation only Routine postoperative follow-up by telephone
History of one or more documented CVA at least 6 months before treatment; some degree of neurologic deficit evident	III	ASA III considerations to include: Light levels of sedation only Routine follow-up by telephone
History of documented CVA within 6 months of treatment with or without residual neurologic deficit	IV	ASA IV considerations

take safeguards against it: (1) proceeding with dental therapy without altering the anticoagulant blood level, thereby possibly increasing postoperative bleeding; (2) lowering the prothrombin time (i.e., decreasing anticoagulant levels) before the procedure to decrease the risk of excessive bleeding with a possible increased risk of CVA; or (3) altering the dental treatment plan to avoid excessive bleeding in instances in which the risk of reducing the prothrombin time is too great. In most instances, dental treatment is carried out without alteration in the patient's anticoagulant drug therapy.

Prothrombin time should be determined from the patient or from his or her physician. Considering a prothrombin time (PT) of 11 to 14 seconds as normal, a level of up to 2½ times normal may be considered acceptable for surgical procedures. Prothrombin times greater than 35 seconds demand a delay in dental care, medical consultation, and possible modification of anticoagulant dosages. Bleeding time should be determined for patients receiving antiplatelet therapy with aspirin or dipyridamole.

When dental treatment is carried out in a patient with an elevated prothrombin time, the doctor should consider employing several precautionary steps in order to minimize the chance of significant postoperative bleeding. Among these are advising the patient and physician of the possible need for vitamin K should excessive bleeding occur; the use of hemostatic agents such as oxidized cellulose in extraction sockets; the use of multiple sutures in extraction sites and periodontal surgery; the use of pressure packs for 6 to 12 hours postoperatively (longer if necessary); and the availability of the doctor by telephone for 24 hours following treatment.

In all situations the doctor called on to manage a patient who has previously experienced a CVA should not proceed with the contemplated dental care until there is no doubt about the physical ability of this patient to safely tolerate the planned treatment. Wherever doubt or concern persists, discussion of the contemplated dental procedure and the physical status of the patient with his or her physician is strongly recommended.

The patient with a history of transient ischemic attacks should be managed in the dental office in the same manner as the post-CVA patient. Table 19-3 presents physical status categories for CVA and TIA.

CLINICAL MANIFESTATIONS

Signs and symptoms of cerebrovascular disease vary depending on the area of the brain involved and on the type of CVA experienced. The onset may be violent; the patient may fall to the ground, unmoving, with face flushed and a bounding pulse. Respirations may be slow and one arm and leg flaccid. The onset may also be more gradual, with no alteration in consciousness and only minimal impairment of speech, thought, motor, and sensory functions.

Signs and symptoms commonly observed in CVAs include headache, dizziness and vertigo, drowsiness, sweating and chills, nausea, and vomiting. Loss of consciousness, a particularly ominous sign, and convulsive movements are much less common. Weakness or paralysis occurs in the extremities contralateral to the CVA. Defects in speech may also be noted.

Transient Ischemic Attack

Clinical manifestations of transient ischemic attacks, as with all CVAs, vary according to the area of the brain affected; however, the symptoms in a given individual tend to be constant. Onset is abrupt and without warning and recovery usually occurs rapidly, often within a few minutes. Most TIAs cause transient numbness or weakness of the contralateral extremities (legs, arms, hand), which may be described by the patient as "pins and needles." Transient monocular blindness is a distinctive, common presentation of TIA. A gray-black shade progressively obscures all or part of the vision of one eye. The shade then recedes painlessly as the tiny embolus dislodges from the retinal artery.[16] During the TIA the level of consciousness is usually unimpaired, although the thought process may be dulled.

Transient ischemic episodes normally have a duration of 2 to 10 minutes, although they have been recorded for as long as 1 hour and as briefly as 10 seconds. Their rate of frequency varies from patient to patient.

Cerebral Infarction

In patients in whom cerebral infarction is produced by atherosclerotic changes in cerebral blood vessels or thrombosis, the onset of clinical signs and symptoms is normally much more gradual (neurologic signs and symptoms appearing over a period of hours to days) and is usually preceded by episodes of TIA. Headache, if present, is usually mild and is generally limited to the side of the infarction. Vomiting is rare, and significant obtundation is unusual unless it involves a massive amount of brain, the brainstem or previously diseased brain.

Cerebral Embolism

Cerebrovascular accidents occurring as a result of embolism differ clinically from other CVAs in that the onset of symptoms is usually abrupt. Mild headache is the first symptom, and it normally precedes the onset of neurologic symptoms by several hours. Neurologic symptoms are confined to the contralateral side of the body. Seizures usually herald the onset of a thrombotic stroke, but are not specific for this.[39]

Lacunar strokes are a subset of thrombotic stroke that are seen almost exclusively in patients with high blood pressure. They are small, well-localized infarcts with resultant characteristic neurologic abnormalities. Lacunar strokes are abrupt in onset, stabilize over a few days, and do not affect higher language function or consciousness.[10]

Cerebral Hemorrhage

Because of the stressful nature of dental treatment and its possible effects on cardiovascular function, intracerebral hemorrhage is the most likely form of CVA to develop within the dental environment. The onset of clinical signs and symptoms is usually abrupt, the first manifestation being a sudden, violent headache of maximal intensity at onset and often accompanied by vomiting. Victims have variously described the headache as "excruciating," "intense," and as "the worst headache I have ever experienced." The headache is at first localized but gradually becomes more generalized.

Other clinical signs and symptoms include nausea and vomiting, chills and sweating, dizziness, and vertigo. Signs of neurologic deficit may occur at any time but usually follow in several hours. Severe cases are characterized by confusion, coma, or death.[10]

Hemorrhagic CVAs most commonly occur during periods of exertion, such as sexual intercourse, Valsalva's maneuver, and labor and delivery; or physical and psychologic stress, as in the dental office. Consciousness is lost or impaired in about half of all patients. This is an ominous sign, usually indicating that a large hemorrhage has occurred.[40] Of conscious patients, 50% demonstrate a marked deterioration in consciousness and lose consciousness at a later time. The initial mortality rate from all hemorrhagic CVAs is approximately 50%, but comatose patients have a mortality rate of between 70% and 100%.[41] The accompanying box summarizes the signs and symptoms of CVA.

CLINICAL MANIFESTATIONS OF CVA

Infarction

Gradual onset of signs and symptoms: minutes-hours-days
TIA frequently precedes CVA
Headache, usually mild
Neurologic signs and symptoms*
Transient monocular blindness—TIA

Embolism

Abrupt onset of signs and symptoms (seconds)
Mild headache precedes neurological signs and symptoms* by several hours

Hemorrhage

Abrupt onset of signs and symptoms (seconds)
Sudden, violent headache
Nausea and vomiting
Chills and sweating
Dizziness and vertigo
Neurological signs and symptoms*
Loss of consciousness

*Neurologic signs and symptoms include:
  Paralysis on one side of the body
  Difficulty in breathing and swallowing
  Inability to speak or slurring of speech
  Loss of bladder and bowel control
  Pupils that are unequal in size

PATHOPHYSIOLOGY

Two important factors work together to produce CVA: (1) the brain's continual requirement for large amounts of oxygen and energy substrate, and (2) the inability of the brain to expand within its confining space, the cranium. The brain is unable to store oxygen or glucose in reserve for use in times of increased need or of oxygen deprivation. Acute disruption of the oxygen supply to the brain (e.g., embolism, hemorrhage) produces alterations in brain activity that are detectable by electroencephalogram within 10 to 20 seconds and produces irreversible neurologic death after 5 minutes.[42] Gradual deprivation (atherosclerotic changes) leads to the same result over a longer period of time.

Cerebrovascular Ischemia and Infarction

With the development of ischemia, changes occur in the affected neural tissues. The ischemic tissue becomes soft, and the usually well-demarcated border between the white and gray matter becomes less distinct. Under the microscope, neurons in the ischemic area appear necrotic and shrunken (Fig. 19-2).

A second factor now emerges. Edema is a normal occurrence following cerebral infarction. On a cellular level ischemia results in anaerobic glycolysis with the production of lactate. Mitochondrial dysfunction develops, resulting in membrane and vascular endothelial disruption. Thus, the blood-brain barrier breaks down and edema forms.[43] The degree of edema is related to the size of the infarcted area. Edema increases the mass of tissue within the confined space of the cranium and is responsible for the mild headache noted in atherosclerotic CVA. In more severe CVAs the degree of edema may be great enough to force portions of the cerebral hemisphere down into the tentorium cerebelli, producing a further reduction in blood and cerebrospinal fluid flow to the brain. The degree of ischemia and neurologic deficit therefore increases, leading potentially to ischemia and infarction of the upper brainstem (medulla), which produces loss of consciousness and is invariably fatal.

The clinical importance of edema, and of its management, is noted in the fact that during the first 72 hours following a nonhemorrhagic CVA, a gradual increase in neurologic deficit and a decreasing level of consciousness are commonly observed. These changes are usually brought about by cerebral edema in and around the infarcted area. A gradual return of some neurologic function normally follows, as collateral circulation to the infarcted region improves. Maximal recovery normally occurs within 6 months.

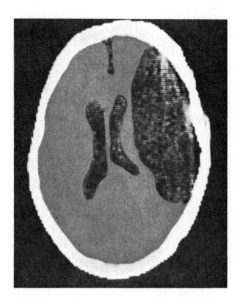

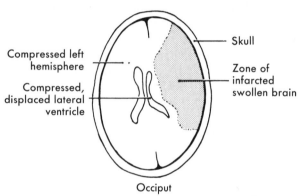

Fig. 19-2. Computerized axial tomography (CAT) scan of cranium in cerebral vascular infarction *(top)*. Explanation of CAT scan *(bottom)*.

Hemorrhagic CVA

Hemorrhagic CVAs differ clinically from nonhemorrhagic CVAs in that they have a more rapid onset, more intense symptoms, and are associated with a greater risk of acute death. The most common source of blood in hemorrhagic CVAs is arterial. There are two primary causes of this type of CVA: subarachnoid hemorrhage (SAH) from ruptured aneurysms and intracranial hemorrhage (ICH) from hypertensive vascular disease. Aneurysms, which are dilations in blood vessels, have weakened muscular walls that may rupture under increased pressure. Hypertensive vascular disease, on the other hand, produces degenerative changes in blood vessel walls, usually smaller arterioles, over a greater length of time, resulting in their weakening and possible rupture. Intracranial hemorrhage may also result from an idiopathic vascular disease of the elderly, known as amyloid angiopathy.[44] Rupture of these vessels invariably occurs during periods of activity that result in elevations in blood pressure.

Once ruptured, the arterial blood rapidly fills the cranium, causing an increase in intracerebral pressure that may produce rapid displacement of the brain into the tentorium cerebelli and ultimately death. Cerebral edema, which always develops, only serves to add to the high mortality rate of this form of CVA (Fig. 19-3).

The intense headache noted with hemorrhagic CVA is related to the irritating effects of blood and its breakdown products on the blood vessels, meninges, and neural tissues of the brain. The headache is localized at first but becomes generalized as meningeal irritation increases because of the spread of blood. The rapid increase in intracranial pressure brought on by hemorrhage and edema is responsible for the significant clinical differences noted between hemorrhagic and nonhemorrhagic CVA. Neurologic deficit can be determined in survivors by the area of neural tissue that has lost its blood supply and become infarcted.

MANAGEMENT

Management of the patient undergoing an acute CVA will be related to the rapidity of onset of clinical signs and to the severity of the situation. In almost all cases supportive therapy and basic life support are indicated.

Cerebrovascular Accident and Transient Ischemic Attack

In most cases of CVA and TIA the patient remains conscious. Indeed, it may initially prove to be quite difficult to differentiate between a TIA and a CVA. The duration of the episode will be important in this regard. Most TIAs are of short duration, lasting approximately 2 to 10 minutes, whereas the signs and symptoms of a CVA do not regress.

Diagnostic clues to the presence of CVA or TIA include[45]:
* Hypertension (blood pressure above 140/90 mmHg)
* Altered level of consciousness
* Hemiparesis, hemiparalysis
* Headache, blurred vision
* Asymmetry of face, pupils of eyes
* Incontinence
* Aphasia

Because of the uncertainty of diagnosis, the initial management of any patient with signs and symptoms of cerebrovascular disease will of necessity be identical, regardless of the ultimate cause, and includes the following:

Step 1: Terminate the dental procedure.

Step 2: Position the patient. A conscious patient complaining of the aforementioned signs and symptoms may be placed in a comfortable position. Most often this will be upright or semiupright.

Step 3: Basic life support, as indicated. Assess the airway, breathing, and circulation and implement any steps that might be necessary. In the situation described here with a conscious patient, rapid assessment will determine the adequacy of airway, breathing, and circulation.

Step 4: Monitor vital signs. Blood pressure is usually markedly elevated during the episode, whereas the heart rate may be normal or elevated. In most cases either the radial or brachial arterial pulses or both are full or bounding. Comparison of vital

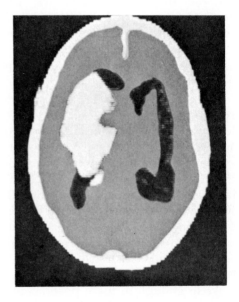

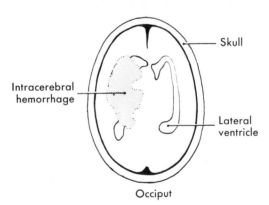

Fig. 19-3. Computerized axial tomography (CAT) scan—hemorrhagic CVA *(top).* Explanation of CAT scan *(bottom).*

signs to baseline values will almost always demonstrate significant elevation of the blood pressure. Monitor and record the heart rate and rhythm and blood pressure at least every 5 minutes during the episode.

Step 5: Summon medical assistance. With the presence of signs and symptoms indicating possible cerebrovascular disease (see diagnostic clues already listed) and an elevation in blood pressure, medical assistance should be obtained immediately. This is true whether or not a history of prior cerebrovascular disease is present.

Step 6: Manage signs and symptoms. Most victims of TIA and CVA remain conscious throughout the episode. Permit the patient to remain in an upright position (45° upright [semi-Fowler's] position is recommended[45]) and attempt to maintain the patient's comfort. The upright or semi-Fowler's position will, to a slight degree, decrease the intracerebral blood pressure, whereas a supine position will increase blood flow to the brain—a situation not desirable during this time of significantly elevated blood pressure.

Oxygen should be administered through a nasal cannula or nasal hood to the patient during this period of time. No CNS-depressant medications should be administered to a patient who is thought to be having a stroke or TIA. Any drug that produces CNS depression (e.g., analgesics, antianxiety agents, narcotics, inhalation sedatives) may adversely affect the patient's condition and make definitive diagnosis of the problem much more difficult by masking neurological signs that might be present.

Transient Ischemic Attack

If the clinical signs and symptoms resolve rapidly prior to the arrival of the emergency medical team, the episode was likely a transient ischemic attack (TIA). With a patient who has had no prior history of cerebrovascular disease, it is probable that the emergency medical team will transport the patient to the hospital for further neurological evaluation. When a history of TIA is present, either hospitalization or immediate referral to the patient's primary care physician is suggested.

Step 7: Follow-up management. Following termination of the TIA episode for which hospitalization is not recommended, the patient's physician should be contacted, with possible medical examination and modifications in future dental care discussed. The patient should not be permitted to operate a motor vehicle and should be dismissed from the dental office in the custody of a responsible adult companion.

Cerebrovascular Accident

In the event that the neurological signs and symptoms do not resolve by the time emergency assistance arrives, stabilization of the patient and transport to a hospital are probable.

Unconscious Patient

The loss of consciousness is associated with a very poor clinical prognosis in CVA (70% to 100% initial mortality rate). The hemorrhagic type of CVA, the most likely to develop during dental treatment, is also the most likely to produce unconsciousness. It is usually preceded by an intense headache, an additional clue to the presence of this problem.

Step 1: Position the patient. Upon losing consciousness, the patient is placed in the supine position. Minor alterations in this position may be indicated later.

Step 2: Basic life support, as indicated. The steps of basic life support are carried out immediately. Airway maintenance and support of respiration are critical. Oxygen should be administered if available. Though it is possible that cardiac arrest has occurred, it is more likely that the patient will require airway management only. Breathing will be spontaneous and the carotid pulse will prove to be strong and bounding (see next step).

Step 3: Monitor vital signs. Vital signs (e.g., blood pressure, heart rate, and respiration) are monitored and recorded. The heart rate in most instances is normal or slow, and the pulse may be full and bounding. Should heart rate, blood pressure, or both be absent, cardiopulmonary resuscitation is immediately initiated. The blood pressure is frequently markedly elevated (systolic pressure in excess of 200 mmHg).

Step 4: Reposition patient, if necessary. When the blood pressure of the unconscious patient is markedly elevated, positioning should be altered slightly from the usual supine position with legs elevated slightly. Because of the increase in cerebral blood flow in the supine position and the markedly elevated blood pressure observed in what is likely a hemorrhagic CVA, the patient should be placed in the supine position with the head and chest elevated slightly. It must still be possible to maintain a patent airway and to ventilate the victim adequately, if necessary. If cardiac arrest ensues and cardiopulmonary resuscitation (CPR) is required in the absence of pulse and blood pressure, the patient must then be repositioned again in the supine position with feet elevated.

Step 5: Establish an intravenous line, if available. An intravenous infusion of 5% dextrose and water or normal saline may be started, if available, prior to the arrival of the emergency medical team. Availability of a patent vein will facilitate subsequent medical management of this patient.

Step 6: Definitive management. Once stabilized at the scene and transported to the hospital, immediate management of the hemorrhagic CVA patient is predicated upon preventing an increase in intracranial pressure by terminating the intracranial bleeding, surgically evacuating the blood from the cranium, and preventing or minimizing edema of the brain.

Management of CVA is summarized in the accompanying box.

Drugs used in management: Oxygen
Medical assistance: Yes

REFERENCES

1. Whisnant JP: The decline of stroke, *Stroke* 15:160, 1984.
2. Silverberg E: Cancer statistics, 1985, *CA* 35:19, 1985.
3. Adelman SM: National survey of stroke: economic impact, *Stroke* 12(suppl 1):69, 1981.
4. Aminoff MJ: Nervous system. In Schroeder SA, Tierney LM, Jr., McPhee SJ, Papadakis MA, Krupp M, editors: *Current medical diagnosis and treatment 1992*, Norwalk, 1992, Appleton & Lange.
5. Garraway WM, and others: The declining incidence of stroke, *N Engl J Med* 300:449, 1979.
6. Levy RI: Stroke decline: implications and prospects, *N Engl J Med* 300:489, 1979.
7. Furlan AJ, and others: Decreasing incidence of primary intracerebral hemorrhage: a population study, *Ann Neurol* 5:367, 1979.
8. Golden GS: Stroke syndromes in childhood, *Neurol Clin* 3:59, 1985.

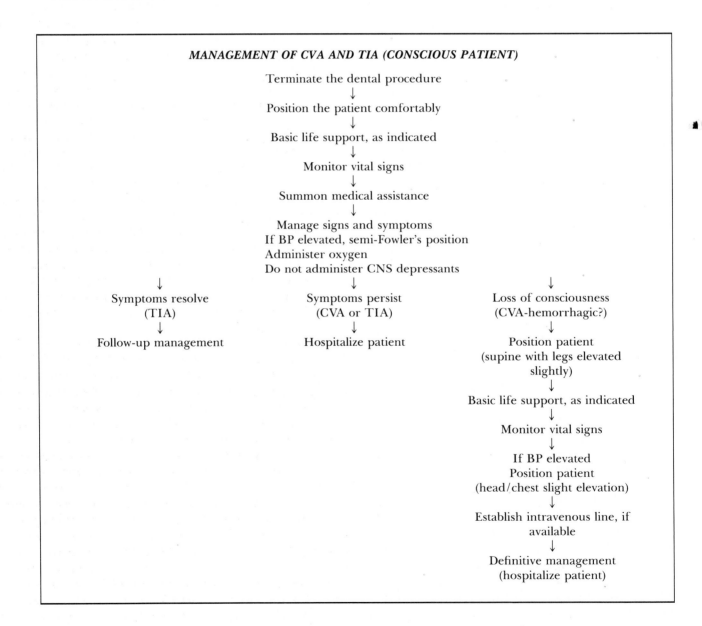

MANAGEMENT OF CVA AND TIA (CONSCIOUS PATIENT)

Terminate the dental procedure
↓
Position the patient comfortably
↓
Basic life support, as indicated
↓
Monitor vital signs
↓
Summon medical assistance
↓
Manage signs and symptoms
If BP elevated, semi-Fowler's position
Administer oxygen
Do not administer CNS depressants

↓	↓	↓
Symptoms resolve (TIA)	Symptoms persist (CVA or TIA)	Loss of consciousness (CVA-hemorrhagic?)
↓	↓	↓
Follow-up management	Hospitalize patient	Position patient (supine with legs elevated slightly)

↓
Basic life support, as indicated
↓
Monitor vital signs
↓
If BP elevated
Position patient
(head/chest slight elevation)
↓
Establish intravenous line, if available
↓
Definitive management
(hospitalize patient)

9. Schoenberg BS, Mellinger JF, Schoenberg DG: Cerebro-vascular disease in infants and children: a study of incidence, clinical features, and survival, *Neurology* 28:763, 1978.

10. Fischer CM: Lacunar strokes and infarcts: a review, *Neurology* 32:871, 1982.

11. Mohr MP: Lacunes, *Neurol Clin* 1:201, 1983.

12. Komrad MS, Coffey CE, Coffey KS, and others: Myocardial infarction and stroke, *Neurology* 34:1403, 1984.

13. Walker AE, Robins M, Weinfeld FD: National survey of stroke: clinical findings, *Stroke* 12(suppl 1):13, 1981.

14. Khaw KT, Barrett-Connor E, Suaret L, and others: Prediction of stroke-associated mortality in the elderly, *Stroke* 15:244, 1984.

15. Easton JD, Sherman DG: Management of cerebral embolism of cardiac origin, *Stroke* 11:433, 1980.

16. Frommer DA: Stroke. In Rosen P, editor: *Emergency medicine*, ed 2, St Louis, 1988, Mosby–Year Book.

17. Earnest MP: Emergency diagnosis and management of brain infarctions and hemorrhages. In Earnest MP, editor: *Neurologic emergencies*, New York, 1983, Churchill Livingstone.

18. Harrison, MJG, Marshall J: Atrial fibrillation, TIAs and completed strokes, *Stroke* 15:441, 1984.

19. Ziegler DK, Hassanein RS: Prognosis in patients with transient ischemic attacks, *Stroke* 4:666, 1973.

20. Wiebers DO, Whisnant JP, O'Fallon WM: The natural history of unruptured intracranial aneurysms, *N Engl J Med* 304:696, 1981.

21. Barrett HJM: Progress toward stroke prevention, *Neurology* 30:1212, 1980.

22. Brown M, Glassenber M: Mortality factor in patients with acute stroke, *JAMA* 224:1493, 1973.

23. Collaborative Group for the Study of Stroke in Young Women: Oral contraceptives and stroke in young women, *JAMA* 231:718, 1975.

24. Longstreth WT, Swanson PD: Oral contraceptives and stroke, *Stroke* 15:747, 1984.

25. Gresham GE, and others: Residual disability in survivors of stroke—the Framingham study, *N Engl J Med* 293:954, 1975.

26. Kannel WB, and others: Systolic blood pressure, arterial rigidity and risk of stroke, *JAMA* 245:1225, 1981.

27. McCarthy FM: Sudden, unexpected death in the dental office, *J Am Dent Assoc* 83:1091, 1971.

28. Duke RJ, Bloch RF, Turpie AC, and others: Intravenous heparin for prevention of stroke progression in acute partial stable stroke: a randomized controlled trial, *Ann Intern Med* 105:825, 1986.

29. Garde A, Samuelsson K, Fahlgren H, and others: Treatment after transient ischemic attacks: a comparison between anticoagulant drug and inhibition of platelet aggregation, *Stroke* 14:677, 681, 1983.

30. Yatsu FM, and others: Anticoagulation of embolic strokes of cardiac origin: an update, *Neurology* 38:314, 1988.

31. Calandre L, Ortega JF, Bermejo F: Anticoagulation and hemorrhagic infarction in cerebral embolism secondary to rheumatic heart disease, *Arch Neurol* 41:1152, 1984.

32. Fields WS, Lemak NA, Frankowski RF, and others: Controlled trial of aspirin in cerebral ischemia, *Circulation* 62:V90, 1980.

33. Hirsh J: Progress review: the relationship between dose of aspirin, side-effects and antithrombotic effectiveness, *Stroke* 16:1, 1985.

34. Grotta JC: Current medical and surgical therapy for cerebrovascular disease, *N Engl J Med* 317:1505, 1987.

35. *Physicians' Desk Reference, 1991*, ed 45, Oradell, N.J., 1991, Medical Economics Data.

36. Olin BR, editor-in-chief: Facts and Comparisons, St Louis, 1992, Facts and Comparisons.

37. American Medical Association: Drug evaluations annual (1992).

38. McCarthy FM: *Essentials of safe dentistry for the medically compromised patient*, Philadelphia, 1989, WB Saunders.

39. Cocito L, Favale E, Reni K: Epileptic seizures in cerebral arterial occlusive disease, *Stroke* 13:189, 1982.

40. Caplan L: Intracerebral hemorrhage revisited: editorial, *Neurology* 38:624, 1988.

41. Sedzimir CB, Robinson J: Intracranial hemorrhage in children and adolescents, *J Neurosurg* 38:269, 1973.

42. White BC, Wiegenstein JG, Winegar CD: Brain ischemic anoxia: mechanisms of injury, *JAMA* 251:1586, 1984.

43. Rehncrona S, Rosen I, Siesjo BK: Brain lactic acidosis and ischemic cell damage: biochemistry and neurophysiology, *J Cereb Blood Flow Metab* 1:297, 1981.

44. Drury I, Whisnant JP, Garraway WM: Primary intracerebral hemorrhage: impact of CT on incidences, *Neurology* 34:653, 1984.

45. Pollakoff J, Pollakoff K: *EMT's guide to treatment*, Los Angeles, 1991, Jeff Gould.

20 Altered Consciousness: Differential Diagnosis

A number of clinical entities are capable of producing a state of altered consciousness (see Table 16-1). In almost all of these situations, the doctor will be required to maintain the life of a patient who is still conscious yet is behaving in an unusual manner. If not recognized and managed promptly, several of these entities can progress to the loss of consciousness. Basic management of these situations is similar and is all that will be required in some cases, yet there are other situations in which definitive management may be undertaken provided that the precise cause of the difficulty is known. The following material is provided to assist in this differential diagnosis.

PAST MEDICAL HISTORY

Several of the clinical entities discussed in this section are normally evident on review of the medical history questionnaire. The patient with diabetes mellitus or thyroid gland dysfunction or the postcerebrovascular accident (post-CVA) patient is usually aware of the presence of the disease and will indicate this on the history. A thorough dialogue history should then enable the doctor to further determine the degree of risk presented by this patient.

Unless it has occurred previously, hyperventilation cannot be diagnosed from data on the medical history, nor can drug overdose.

AGE OF PATIENT

The age of a patient with altered consciousness may assist in the diagnosis of the cause. Hyperventilation is rarely encountered in younger or older age groups; its greatest incidence is between the ages of 15 and 40 years. Hyperthyroidism most commonly occurs between the ages of 20 and 40, whereas more than 80% of diabetics develop the disease after the age of 35. Cerebrovascular disease is extremely rare under the age of 40 years; its incidence increases with age. Drug overdose may occur at any age. In pediatric patients the most likely cause of altered consciousness is hypoglycemia secondary to insulin-dependent diabetes mellitus (IDDM).

SEX OF PATIENT

Hyperthyroidism (thyrotoxicosis) occurs predominantly in females, whereas hyperventilation and the other clinical entities discussed in this section have little or no clinical differentiation between the sexes.

CIRCUMSTANCES ASSOCIATED WITH ALTERED CONSCIOUSNESS

Undue stress from anxiety and pain is an important predisposing factor in hyperventilation. Indeed, this syndrome is primarily a clinical expression of extreme fear. Stress may also be related to the onset of a CVA, particularly of the hemorrhagic type.

Individuals with hyperthyroidism and hypoglycemia may appear clinically to be acutely anxious; however, specific clinical signs and symptoms associated with these problems (see text that follows) usually permit an accurate differential diagnosis to be made.

ONSET OF SIGNS AND SYMPTOMS

Gradual onset of clinical manifestations of altered consciousness occurs in hyperglycemia (many hours to several days), in hyperthyroidism and hypothyroidism (days to months), and in CVAs produced by atherosclerotic changes in blood vessels (days to weeks). A patient will come to the dental office with signs and symptoms of disease already evident. When the patient is known to the dental office staff from prior dental visits, the change in level of consciousness may be readily apparent.

More rapid onset of clinical manifestations (signs and symptoms developing more acutely within the dental office) are evident in hyperventilation, in hypoglycemia, and in CVAs produced by thrombus, embolism, and especially by intracerebral hemorrhage.

PRESENCE OF SYMPTOMS BETWEEN ACUTE EPISODES

The patient with undiagnosed thyroid dysfunction or with known thyroid dysfunction that is inadequately managed has clinical evidence of the disease at all times. Post-CVA patients will usually exhibit a degree of residual neurologic deficit, the severity of which varies from flaccid paralysis to barely perceptible motor or sensory changes. Patients with transient ischemic attacks are clinically free of symptoms between acute episodes. Brittle adult diabetics may manifest signs and symptoms of hyperglycemia at all times.

LOSS OF CONSCIOUSNESS

Although all of the clinical entities discussed in this section manifest themselves primarily as altered states of consciousness, several of them may progress to the loss of consciousness. Cerebrovascular accident, particularly the hemorrhagic type, may be associated with unconsciousness, a particularly ominous clinical sign.

Patients with clinical evidence of thyroid dysfunction may also lose consciousness if the disease is poorly controlled. These two clinical situations, myxedema coma (hypothyroid) and thyroid crisis or storm (hyperthyroid), have significant mortality rates.

Both hyperglycemic and hypoglycemic individuals may also ultimately lose consciousness; however, the hypoglycemic patient is the more likely candidate to develop loss of consciousness much more rapidly. Hyperventilation only rarely leads to unconsciousness.

SIGNS AND SYMPTOMS
Appearance of Skin (Face)

The presence or absence of sweating and the temperature of the skin may assist in the differential diagnosis. The diabetic individual who is clinically hyperglycemic is hot and dry (produced by dehydration) to the touch, whereas the hypoglycemic individual is cold and wet. The clinically hyperthyroid individual is hot and wet, whereas the hypothyroid individual is dry and may have a subnormal body temperature.

Appearance of Nervousness

The clinical signs of agitation, sweating, and possible fine tremor of the extremities (hands) give the appearance of nervousness and are apparent in patients with hyperventilation syndrome, hypoglycemia, and hyperthyroidism, as well as in patients who are simply quite nervous, but otherwise healthy.

Paresthesia

Paresthesia, the feeling of numbness or "pins and needles" in various portions of the body, is noted in several situations. Paresthesia of the perioral region, fingertips, and toes, if occurring in conjunction with a rapid respiratory rate, is diagnostic of hyperventilation.

Patients with transient ischemic attacks (TIA) exhibit unilateral paresthesia or a muscle weakness that is unaccompanied by the respiratory change of hyperventilation and which often develops in the absence of anxiety. An acute CVA also demonstrates the aforementioned signs of TIA but continues to progress, whereas signs and symptoms of TIA commonly subside within 10 minutes.

Headache

Headache may be evident in individuals with hypothyroidism, but is much more likely to develop in the acute CVA. Severe, intense headache, often described as "the worst headache I have ever experienced," is an important clinical finding in intracerebral hemorrhage, a form of CVA.

"Drunken" Appearance

The clinical appearance of inebriation is most commonly produced by a patient overindulging in his or her own premedication—alcohol or other drugs.

Hypoglycemia is another situation that may present a similar clinical picture. The patient exhibits signs of mental confusion and bizarre behavioral patterns that may lead to a suspicion of alcohol or other drug use. A history of diabetes, especially IDDM, or not eating before the dental appointment will assist in this differential diagnosis.

Breath Odor

The telltale odor of alcohol on the breath aids in diagnosing "premedication," whereas patients who are severely hyperglycemic may have the characteristic fruity, sweet smell of acetone on their breath.

VITAL SIGNS
Respirations

The respiratory rate increases with hyperventilation, hyperthyroidism, and hyperglycemia. With hyperglycemia, it is frequently associated with the odor of acetone on the breath. Depressed respiration may be evident with CVA (in the unconscious patient with slow but deep respirations), with an overdose of depressant drugs (alcohol, sedatives, antianxiety drugs, narcotics), and possibly with hypoglycemia.

Blood Pressure

Elevated blood pressure is found with hyperventilation, hyperthyroidism, and in many forms of CVA (intracerebral hemorrhage, subarachnoid hemorrhage, and cerebral thrombosis). The hyperglycemic individual may demonstrate a slight decrease in blood pressure, and the patient with hypothyroidism shows little change in blood pressure.

Heart Rate

Rapid heart rates are noted with hyperventilation, hypoglycemia, hyperglycemia, and hyperthyroidism. A slower than normal heart rate is present in patients with hypothyroidism.

SUMMARY

In conclusion, each of the clinical syndromes of altered consciousness is presented with relevant clinical features.

Hyperventilation: Rapid respiratory rate with deep breaths, acute anxiety, and elevated blood pressure and heart rate; symptoms of paresthesia of the extremities and of the circumoral region; occurs primarily in patients between 15 and 40 years of age; seldom produces unconsciousness

Hypoglycemia: History of diabetes (usually IDDM) or lack of food ingestion; patient appears drunk with a cold and wet appearance; rapid heart rate and possible tremor of the extremities; onset of symptoms may appear rapidly and can quickly lead to loss of consciousness

Hyperglycemia: History of inadequately controlled diabetes; patient appears hot and dry; possible acetone odor on breath; rapid and deep respirations—Kussmaul's respirations; gradual onset of symptoms with lesser likelihood of unconsciousness

Hypothyroidism: Patient is sensitive to cold; speech and mental capabilities appear slower than normal; no sweating—body temperature is lowered; peripheral edema (nonpitting) present, particularly noticeable around face and eyelids, carotenemic skin color; sensitive to CNS-depressant drugs

Hyperthyroidism: Nervousness and hyperactivity present with elevated blood pressure, heart rate, and body temperature; patient appears wet and warm and is sensitive to heat; history of recent unexplained weight loss in spite of increased appetite

CVA: Unusually intense headache with hemorrhagic CVA; onset of unilateral neurologic deficit (flaccid paralysis, speech defects); level of consciousness normally unchanged

The algorithm for the diagnosis and management of altered consciousness is found on p. 229.

21 Seizures

To most persons, witnessing someone having a seizure is a psychologically traumatic experience. The belief persists that a seizure constitutes a life-threatening situation, one requiring prompt intervention by a trained individual to prevent death from occurring. Yet this is normally not the case. Most convulsive episodes, although in no sense benign, are transient alterations in brain function that are characterized clinically by an abrupt onset of symptoms of a motor, sensory, or psychic nature. In these instances the prevention of injury to the victim during the actual seizure and supportive therapy during the postseizure period constitute the essentials of management. With proper management significant morbidity and mortality is rare. A life-threatening medical emergency exists only if seizures follow one another closely of if they become continuous. In these cases prompt action and specific therapy are required to prevent death or significant postseizure morbidity.

The following are definitions of relevant terms:

convulsion, seizure. A seizure, as defined in 1870 by Hughlings Jackson, is: "a symptom . . . an occasional, an excessive and a disorderly discharge of nerve tissue."[1] A more modern definition emphasizes the same essentials, stating that a seizure is "a paroxysmal disorder of cerebral function characterized by an attack involving changes in the state of consciousness, motor activity, or sensory phenomena; a seizure is sudden in onset and usually of brief duration." The terms *convulsion* and *seizure* are synonyms.

epilepsy. From the Greek *epilepsia,* meaning "to take hold of." The World Health Organization[2] defines epilepsy as "a chronic brain disorder of various etiologies characterized by recurrent seizures due to excessive discharge of cerebral neurons." Sutherland and Eadie[3] have updated this definition as follows: "Epilepsy should be regarded as a symptom due to excessive temporary neuronal discharging which results from intracranial or extracranial causes; epilepsy is characterized by discrete episodes, which tend to be recurrent, in which there is a disturbance of movement, sensation, behavior, perception, and/or consciousness."

status epilepticus. A condition in which seizures are so prolonged or so repeated that recovery does not occur between attacks. Status epilepticus is a life-threatening medical emergency.

tonic. A sustained muscular contraction; the patient appears rigid or stiff during the tonic phase of seizure.

clonic. Intermittent muscular contractions and relaxation; the clonic phase is the actual convulsive portion of a seizure.

stertorous. Characterized by snoring; used to describe breathing.

ictus. A seizure.

TYPES OF SEIZURE DISORDERS

The clinical manifestations of paroxysmal excessive neuronal activity in the brain (i.e., seizures) span a wide range of sensory and motor activities that may involve any or all of the following: altered visceral function; sensory, olfactory, auditory, visual, and gustatory phenomena; abnormal motor movements; changes in mental awareness and behavior; and alterations in consciousness. The accompanying box presents the recent classification of the types of epilepsies by the Commission on Classification and Terminology of the International League Against Epilepsy.[4]

The incidence of epilepsy (recurrent seizure activity) in general populations (all age groups) is between 30 to 50 per 100,000 persons per year or about 0.5% of the population of the United States.[5] If isolated, nonrecurrent seizures and febrile convulsions are added to this group, the occurrence rate would be considerably higher. In one study the incidence of epilepsy was 40 per 100,000 persons per year; when isolated, nonrecurrent seizures were added the rate increased to 75 per 100,000, and to 115 per 100,000 persons when febrile convulsions were included.[6] In the United States it is estimated that more than 10 million persons have suffered at least one convulsive episode (isolated, nonrecurrent seizures) and that in excess of 2 million persons have suffered two or more episodes.[7] In addition, it is estimated that more than 200,000 Americans have seizures more than once a month despite medical treatment.[7]

When seizures are examined by age of onset there is a specific pattern observed. Highest rates of incidence occur in the first year of life with a consistent and rapid decline toward adolescence and a gradual leveling off during the remainder of life until the age of 50 years, at which time there is a sharp upswing.[6] More than three quarters of patients with epilepsy experienced their first seizure before 20 years of age.

The chance of having a second seizure after an initial unprovoked seizure is 30%. The chance of remission of seizures in childhood epilepsy is 50%,[8] whereas the recurrence rate in children after withdrawal from drugs is 30%.[9,10]

The seizures that are encountered most frequently and that possess the greatest potential for morbidity and mortality are the generalized seizures. Within this group are the tonic-clonic convulsive episode, which is represented clinically as grand mal epilepsy, and petit mal epilepsy, which is also termed an absence attack.

Partial or focal seizures are those that involve a specific region of the brain. Clinical signs and symptoms of focal seizures relate to the specific area of the brain affected (the ictal focus). As noted in the box, signs and symptoms observed in partial seizures may include specific motor or sensory symptoms or both, therefore they are called simple partial seizures, or they appear as "spells," associated with more complex symptoms involving illusions, hallucinations, or deja vu—called the complex partial seizure. Focal seizures may remain localized, in which case consciousness or the awareness of the victim is normally somewhat disturbed, and variable degrees of amnesia may be evident. On the other hand, a focal seizure can spread and become a generalized seizure producing loss of consciousness. Though all seizures are significant, generalized seizures are of greater clinical importance to the practicing dentist than are focal seizures because of their greater potential for injury and postseizure complications.

Generalized Seizures

The majority of patients with recurrent generalized seizures develop one of three major forms: grand mal, petit mal, or psychomotor seizures. Of all patients with epilepsy, 70% have only one type of seizure disorder, whereas the remaining 30% have two or more types.[11]

Grand mal epilepsy, more properly called generalized tonic-clonic seizure, is the most common form of seizure disorder, present in 90% of epileptics. Approximately 60% of epileptics have this form alone, whereas 30% have other seizure types in addition to grand mal.[11] The tonic-clonic type of seizure disorder is what most persons characteristically think of as epilepsy. Grand mal epilepsy is found equally in both sexes, and may occur in any age group, although over two thirds of cases occur by puberty.[11] The tonic-clonic seizure may be produced by neurologic disorders or it may develop in a neurologically sound brain secondary to a systemic metabolic or toxic disturbance. Causes of tonic-clonic seizures include drug withdrawal, photic stimulation, menstruation, fatigue, alcohol or other intoxications, and falling asleep or awakening.[12] Neurologically induced grand mal seizures usually last from 2 to 3 minutes and seldom more than 5 minutes. The entire seizure, including the immediate postictal period, lasts 5 to 15 minutes with a complete return to normal preictal cerebral function, taking up to 2 hours.[13] This type of seizure forms the basis of our discussion in this section.

Petit mal epilepsy or absence seizures are found in 25% of epileptics.[11] Only 4% have petit mal as the sole form of seizure disorder, the other 21% have it in combination with other forms, most commonly grand mal.[11] Petit mal seizures have an incidence of less than 5% among individuals with childhood epilepsy,[14] almost always occurring in patients between the ages of 3 and 15 years.[15] The incidence of petit mal seizures decreases with increasing age, and its persistence beyond the age of 30 years is rare, however, 40% to 80% of these individuals go on to develop grand mal epilepsy.[16] Petit mal seizures may occur frequently, with multiple daily attacks. Petit mal seizures tend to occur shortly after awakening or when the patient is quiescent. Exercise reduces the incidence of petit mal seizures.[17] Clinically, the petit mal seizure consists of a brief lapse of consciousness, normally lasting from 5 to 10 seconds and only on rare occasions lasting beyond 30 seconds. The patient makes no movement during the episode other than perhaps a cyclic blinking of the eyelids, and the termination of the episode is equally abrupt. If erect at the start of the episode, the victim usually remains standing during the seizure.

A petit mal triad is recognized, consisting of myoclonic jerks, akinetic seizures, and brief absences or blank spells without associated falling and body convulsion. A characteristic electroencephalographic (EEG) pattern consisting of 3 cycles per second is noted in petit mal epilepsy.

With jacksonian epilepsy (simple partial seizure), consciousness is often maintained although there is an impairment of consciousness noted. The focal convulsions of jacksonian epilepsy may be motor, sensory, or autonomic in nature. Commonly, this type of epilepsy begins in a part of a limb as a convulsive jerking or paresthesias or tingling, or on the face as a localized chronic spasm that spreads ("marches") in a more or less orderly manner. For example, it may start in the great toe and extend to the leg, thigh, trunk, and shoulder and may possibly involve the upper limb. If the seizure crosses to the opposite side, consciousness is likely to be lost.[13]

Psychomotor seizures (complex partial seizures, temporal lobe epilepsy) are present in approximately 2% to 25% in children and 15% to 50% in adults[15,18,19] (6% having psychomotor seizures alone, 12% having them in combination with other forms)[11] and involve extensive cortical regions and manifest a variety of psychic symptoms (see text that follows). They are of longer duration than simple partial seizures (1 to 2 minutes), have a more gradual onset and termination, and involve an associated impairment of consciousness.[13] Episodes of psychomotor seizures often progress to generalized seizures.[18] Common causes of psychomotor seizures include birth injury, tumors, and trauma.[20] The usual age of onset extends from late childhood to early adulthood.[15]

The category of psychomotor seizures includes most seizures that do not meet the criteria described previously for grand mal, petit mal, and jacksonian seizures. Automatisms, apparently purposeful movements, incoherent speech, turning of the head, shifting of the eyes, smacking of the lips, twisting and writhing movements of the extremities, clouding of consciousness, and amnesia are commonly observed in psychomotor epilepsy.

Status epilepticus is defined as a seizure that persists for over 1 hour, or repeated seizures that produce a fixed and enduring epileptic condition for more than 1 hour.[21,22] From a clinical perspective, the definition from the Academy of Orthopedic Surgeons appears more practical, defining status epilepticus as a seizure that continues for more than 5 minutes or a repeated seizure that starts before the patient recovers from the initial episode.[23]

The incidence of status epilepticus among epileptic patients appears to be about 5%, although the reported range varies from 1.3% to 10%.[24,25]

Although status epilepticus may occur with any type of seizure, it is usually categorized as convulsive status and nonconvulsive status. Convulsive (tonic-clonic) status is a true medical emergency with an acute mortality rate of 10%[26] and a long-term mortality rate of more than 20%.[27] Seizures of convulsive status are typical generalized tonic-clonic seizures.[28]

The most common factor precipitating status epilepticus is failure of the epileptic patient to take antiepileptic drugs.[29] Status epilepticus is also more common in patients with known causes for their epilepsy.[30] Of 2588 patients with epilepsy, only 1.8% of 1885 with epilepsy of unknown cause (idiopathic) had experienced status epilepticus, whereas 9% of patients with epilepsy of known cause had status epilepticus. The most common causes in the latter group were tumor or trauma.[30]

Petit mal status and psychomotor status are examples of nonconvulsive status and include mild to severe alterations in the level of consciousness and confusion with or without automatisms.[24] Absence status may last from hours to days and is precipitated by hyperventilation, photic stimulation, psychogenic stress, fatigue, and minor trauma. Absence status frequently terminates in a generalized seizure.[31] Nonconvulsive status will not represent a life-threatening medical emergency within the dental environment.

CAUSES

There are many known causes of seizures. In classifying seizures by cause there are two major categories: primary and secondary.[32] Over 65% of persons with recurrent seizures (i.e., epileptics) are said to suffer from idiopathic epilepsy or genetic epilepsy, in which no definite causative factor for the seizures can be found or the seizures are attributed to genetic predisposition. This is called primary epilepsy. Relatives of persons with primary epilepsy have a 3% to 5% incidence rate, which is six to ten times the expected rate. Secondary epilepsy or acquired or symptomatic epilepsy, is present in the remaining 35% of persons with recurrent seizures. The term *secondary* implies that evaluation of the patient demonstrates a probable cause or causes for the seizures.

Secondary or symptomatic epilepsy may be produced by the following:
- Congenital abnormalities
- Perinatal injuries
- Metabolic and toxic disorders
- Head trauma
- Tumors and other space-occupying lesions
- Vascular diseases
- Degenerative disorders
- Infectious diseases

Congenital and perinatal conditions include maternal infection (rubella), trauma, or hypoxia-anoxia during delivery.

Metabolic disorders that may produce seizures include hypocalcemia, hypoglycemia, phenylketonuria, and alcohol or drug withdrawal. Metabolic disorders account for between 10% and 15% of all cases of acute isolated seizures.[33,34] Drugs and toxic substances account for about 4% of acute seizures. Common therapeutic agents that are associated with seizure production include: penicillin, hypoglycemic agents, local anesthetics, physostigmine,[35] and phenothiazines.[36] Withdrawal from drugs such as cocaine can also provoke seizures.[37]

Head trauma is of great importance at any age, but especially in young adults. Posttraumatic epilepsy is more likely when the dura mater was penetrated, with seizures becoming manifest within 2 years following the injury, with 75% occurring within the first year.[38] Epilepsy caused by craniocerebral injuries account for 5% to 15% of all cases of acquired epilepsy[39] with a peak incidence between 20 and 40 years of age.[40]

Tumors and other space-occupying lesions occur at any age, but are especially likely to be noted in middle to later life, when the incidence of neoplastic disease increases. Tumors are uncommon in children (account for 0.5% to 1% of childhood epilepsy[41]), but are the most common acquired cause of seizures between the ages of 35 and 55 years, accounting for 10% of all cases of adult-onset secondary epilepsy.[42] Approximately 35% of cases of cerebral tumors are associated with seizures,[42] which are the initial symptom in 40% of this group.[43]

Vascular diseases increase in importance as seizure producers with aging, and represent the most common cause of seizures with onset after 60 years of age. Any disease that impairs blood flow to the brain can provoke a seizure, the likelihood varying with the severity of cerebral ischemia. Arteriosclerotic cerebrovascular insufficiency and cerebral infarctions are the most common vascular disorders provoking seizures, and their incidence increases with advancing age.[44] In elderly patients they account for 25% to 70% of acquired epilepsy[45] and 10% to 24% of acute isolated seizures.[46]

Infectious disease can occur in all age groups, and are considered to be a reversible cause of seizures. Central nervous system infections, such as bacterial meningitis or herpes encephalitis are frequent causes of seizures. Infections account for 3% of acquired epilepsy[47] and 4% to 12% of acute isolated seizures.[46]

Table 21-1. Causes of seizures—incidence by age

Neonatal (first month)	Infancy (1 to 6 mo.)	Early childhood (6 mo. to 3 yrs)	Childhood and adolescence	Early adult life	Late adult life
1. Birth injury 2. Metabolic disorders 3. Infection 4. Congenital abnormalities	1-4. Same as neonatal 5. Inborn errors of metabolism	1. Febrile convulsions 2. Birth injury 3. Infection 4. Trauma 5. Metabolic disorders 6. Toxins 7. Cerebral degenerative diseases	1. Idiopathic 2. Birth injury 3. Trauma 4. Infection 5. Cerebral degenerative diseases	1. Trauma 2. Tumor 3. Idiopathic 4. Birth injury 5. Infection 6. Cerebral degenerative diseases	1. Vascular disease 2. Trauma 3. Tumor 4. Cerebral degenerative diseases

Data modified from Tomlanovich MC, Yee AS: Seizure. In Rosen P, editor: *Emergency medicine*, ed 2, St Louis, 1988, Mosby–Year Book.

A phenomenon of seizures developing in children and adults exposed to television interference and to the flickering lights and geometric patterns of video games, called photosensitive epilepsy, has been described.[48]

The introduction of new, noninvasive neurodiagnostic techniques, most significantly, computerized axial tomography scans (CAT scans) and nuclear magnetic resonance (NMR) (also called magnetic resonance imaging or MRI), has improved the detection of underlying lesions in persons with epileptic disorders, so that newly diagnosed cases of seizures will increasingly be diagnosed in the secondary category.

Febrile convulsions are usually associated with and are precipitated by marked elevations in temperature. They occur almost exclusively in infants and young children, particularly during the first year of life. Criteria for febrile seizures are:
- Age 3 months to 5 years (most occurring between 6 months and 3 years)
- Fever of 38.8° C (102° F)
- Non-CNS infection

Approximately 2% to 3% of children suffer febrile convulsions. Most febrile convulsions are short, lasting less than 5 minutes. Only 2% to 4% of children with febrile convulsions will develop epilepsy in later childhood or adult life.[49] Febrile convulsions are not a major risk factor in dental practice.

Table 21-1 presents the most common causes of seizures according to the age of the patient.[50] The most likely causes of seizures, of any type or duration, in the dental environment will be:
- Seizures in epileptic patients
- Hypoglycemia
- Anoxia/hypoxia secondary to syncope
- Local anesthetic overdose

PREDISPOSING FACTORS

Management of most patients with a history of epilepsy is based on minimizing or preventing the recurrence of acute seizures. In almost all cases this is accomplished through the use of long-term anticonvulsant drug therapy. In spite of this therapy, acute seizure activity may still develop. In some cases there is no apparent predisposing factor for this occurrence; the seizure episode suddenly develops without warning. There are, however, factors that increase the frequency with which seizure activity develops. It is known, for instance, that the immature brain is much more susceptible to biochemical alteration in cerebral blood flow than is the adult brain. Therefore, convulsions brought about by hypoxia, hypoglycemia, and hypocalcemia are more likely to occur in younger age groups.[50] In the adult patient, a "breakthrough" of seizure activity in a well-managed patient may also occur. In such a patient the onset of the acute episode has been shown in many cases to be correlated with sleep or menstrual cycles.[51]

In a great many instances of seizure activity, there appears to be an acute triggering disturbance. These triggering factors include flashing lights, especially prominent in precipitating petit mal seizures, fatigue or decreased physical health of patient, missed meals, alcohol ingestion, and physical or emotional stress.

Seizures may therefore be said to be precipitated by a combination of several factors. Among these are the genetically determined predisposition to seizures (primary epilepsy) and the presence of a localized brain lesion. One or more of the following factors may also induce acute seizure activity: a generalized metabolic or toxic disturbance that produces an increase in cerebral neuronal excitation; a state of cerebrovascular insufficiency; or an acute triggering disturbance such as sleep, menstrual cycle, fatigue, flickering lights, or physical or psychologic stress. Each of the factors listed may also act individually to produce seizure activity.

PREVENTION
Nonepileptic Causes

The prevention of acute seizure activity in the dental office may be difficult because of the idiopathic nature of most seizures. However, the prevention of seizures produced by metabolic or toxic disturbances can be facilitated by a thorough physical evaluation of the prospective patient before treatment. Refer to Chapter 17 for a discussion of the prevention of the hypoglycemic reaction.

In dentistry a local anesthetic overdose is the most likely nonepileptic cause of seizures. Adequate patient evaluation and preparation and care in selection of a local anesthetic agent go far in preventing this complication. The most important factor in preventing such a toxic reaction is proper technique in administration of the local anesthetic (see Chapter 23).

Epileptic Causes

With most epileptic patients, the goal of the doctor is to determine the probability of an acute seizure developing during the period of dental treatment and to take any necessary steps to minimize that possibility. In addition, the doctor and staff should be prepared to manage any seizure that might arise and attempt to minimize any clinical complications (e.g., soft tissue injury or fractures) associated with seizures.

Medical History Questionnaire

QUESTION 9. Circle any of the following that you have had or have at present:
- Epilepsy or seizures
- Fainting or dizzy spells

COMMENT. Affirmative response to either question indicates a knowledge of the disorder. Most epileptics are aware of their condition and will respond appropriately on the questionnaire.

QUESTION 6. Have you taken any medicine or drugs during the past 2 years?

COMMENT. Most epileptics require long-term drug therapy to minimize recurrent seizure activity. The ideal anticonvulsant is described as long acting, nonsedating, well tolerated, useful in many types of seizures, and without substantive effect on vital organs as it restores the electroencephalogram (EEG) to normal. However, this ideal agent does not exist.

A basic principle followed in the use of anticonvulsants is to select a single drug first (monotherapy), rather than a combination (polytherapy), and use it either until it becomes ineffective or until toxic signs appear.[52] If seizure control proves effective (i.e., no seizures occurring for a period of at least 4 years), the question of terminating drug therapy is normally raised by the patient. Some physicians will gradually withdraw anticonvulsant medications over a period of weeks to months, one drug at a time, if the patient has been free of seizures for 2 to 4 years. However, in many cases recurrences of seizure activity do occur. Sudden withdrawal of anticonvulsant therapy is a common cause of status epilepticus. In a study of 68 children who were seizure free for 4 years, more than two-thirds were successfully withdrawn from drugs without seizure recurrence.[53] Callaghan[10] reported that only 33% of patients—both adults and children—relapsed after being seizure free for 2 years. They were followed for 3 years after discontinuation of drug therapy. Withdrawal is rarely attempted at puberty, especially in females, with whom drug therapy is usually continued through adolescence. Drugs used in long-term management of epilepsy are listed in Table 21-2.

Dialogue History

In response to a positive history of convulsive seizures, the following information should be sought:

QUESTION. What type of seizures (epilepsy) do you have?

QUESTION. How often do you have (acute) seizures? When was your last seizure?

COMMENT. Grand mal epilepsy is effectively controlled in many patients. Proper treatment with drug therapy will prevent seizures in more than 70% of epileptics. These patients may have been seizure free for several years, or seizures may occur only infrequently (i.e., once or twice a year). In other patients the frequency of seizures may be greater, perhaps several times a week or even daily. Petit mal seizures may occur as frequently as every several days, or they may occur frequently in clusters of 100 or more per day. Greater frequency of occurrence (decreased seizure control) implies a greater likelihood of seizures developing during dental therapy.

QUESTION. What signals the onset of your seizure?

COMMENT. Patients with grand mal epilepsy have a specific aura, or premonition, that heralds the onset of a seizure. The aura commonly lasts a few seconds, but in many patients may occur for many

Table 21-2. Drugs used in the long-term management of epilepsy

	Usual adult total daily dose (mg/kg/d)*	Usual pediatric total daily dose (mg/kg/d)*	No. of divided doses/day	Therapeutic blood level (μg/mL)*,†,‡	Side effects*,†,‡
Generalized tonic-clonic (grand mal) or partial (focal) seizures					
Phenytoin (Dilantin)	4-8	5-10	1 a§ 1-2 c‖	10-20	GI distress, ataxia, sedation, gingival hypertrophy, rash, fever
Carbamazepine (Tegretol)	5-25	15-25	2 a 2-4 c	5-12	Nystagmus, ataxia, drowsiness, nausea, rash
Phenobarbital	2-5	3-8	1 a, c	10-40	Sedation, hyperactivity in children, ataxia, confusion, rash, possible learning difficulties
Primidone (Mysoline)	5-20	10-25	3 a 3-4 c	5-15	Sedation, vertigo, GI distress, anorexia, rash, dizziness
Valproic acid (Depakene, Depakote)	10-60	15-60	3 a 2-4 c	50-100	GI distress, sedation, ataxia, weight gain
Absence (petit mal) seizures					
Ethosuximide (Zarontin)	20-35	10-40	2 a 1-2 c	40-100	GI distress, sedation, dizziness, headache
Valproic acid (Depakene, Depakote)	10-60	15-60	3 a 2-4 c	50-100	GI distress, sedation, ataxia, weight gain
Clonazepam (Klonopin)	0.05-0.2	0.1-0.2	2 a 2-3 c	20-80 ng	Sedation, ataxia, behavioral changes, hypotension
Myoclonic seizures					
Valproic acid (Depakene, Depakote)	10-60	15-60	3 a 2-4 c	50-100	GI distress, sedation, ataxia, weight gain
Clonazepam (Klonopin)	0.05-0.2	0.1-0.2	2 a 2-3 c	20-80 ng	Sedation, ataxia, behavioral changes, hypotension

*From Aminoff MJ: Neurologic disorders. In Watts HD, editor: *Handbook of medical treatment*, ed 17, Greenbriar, Calif., 1983, Jones.
†Moe, PG, Seay, A: Seizure disorders. In Hathaway WE, Groothuis JR, Hay WW Jr, and others: editors: *Current pediatric diagnosis & treatment*, ed 10, Norwalk, 1991, Appleton & Lange.
‡Tomlanovich MC, Yee AS: Seizure. In Rosen P, editor: *Emergency medicine*, ed 2, St Louis, 1988, Mosby–Year Book.
§a, adult.
‖c, child.

minutes, and is related to the specific region of the brain in which the abnormal electrical discharge originates. The aura may be stereotyped for an individual patient. Some common auras include an odd sensation in the epigastric region; an unpleasant taste or smell; various visual and/or auditory hallucinations; a sense of fear; strange sensations, such as numbness in the limbs; and motor phenomena, such as turning the head or eyes or spasm of a limb. The aura is part of the seizure. Knowledge of the aura can alert the dental team to the onset of a seizure, enabling them to initiate proper management quickly.

QUESTION. How long do your seizures last?

COMMENT. Seizures, except for status epilepticus, are self-limiting. The tonic-clonic phase of a grand mal seizure usually lasts not more than 2 to 5 minutes; the immediate recovery period lasts about 10 to 15 minutes, with complete return to normal preictal cerebral function in about 2 hours.[13] The duration of the convulsive phase of the seizure has important implications in clinical management. Once completed, seizures do not normally recur during the immediate postseizure period; however, recurrent seizures may occur, (as in status epilepticus).

QUESTION. Have you ever been hospitalized as a result of your seizures?

COMMENT. This question is asked to determine whether or not status epilepticus has ever occurred and whether or not serious injury to the patient has resulted from any previous seizures. In addition, most epileptics have probably been hospitalized on one or more occasions when emergency medical personnel were summoned by bystanders when a seizure occurred in a public area. Paramedical personnel follow strict treatment protocol and in instances when the postictal epileptic patient does not meet these criteria for recovery, a brief period of hospitalization will be required.

Physical Examination

There are no specific clinical signs or symptoms that can lead to a diagnosis of epilepsy if a patient is examined between seizures; however, over 50% of patients with recurring seizures demonstrate EEG abnormalities during the interictal period.

No specific treatment modification is indicated aside from possible psychosedation necessitated by obvious anxiety over the dental situation. Because most anticonvulsants are CNS depressants, such as the barbiturates (e.g., pentobarbital, secobarbital, and hexobarbital) and benzodiazepines (e.g., diazepam, oxazepam, midazolam), care must be observed whenever the use of psychosedative techniques is contemplated to avoid inadvertent oversedation (see discussion on treatment modifications.)

Psychologic Implications of Epilepsy

Folklore and myths have arisen connecting epilepsy to violent behavior.[54] Although there is very little evidence to link violence with epilepsy, many physicians and laypeople retain the belief that epileptics are dangerous, potentially violent people.[55] The incidence of epilepsy among prisoners in jails in the United States is approximately 1.8% compared to an incidence of between 0.5% and 1% in the general population.[56,57] Patients with psychomotor or grand mal seizures may exhibit signs of fright and may in fact struggle irrationally with anyone trying to help them during the seizure.

Most patients with recurrent seizures can and do adapt into the work force and social system despite occasional periods of disability caused by seizures and their immediate consequences. The most serious feature of epileptic disability is social ostracism. This ostracism is especially damaging to the school-aged child who is embarrassed by seizures and may be set apart from the other children because of fear and ignorance.[58] Many epileptics feel rejected and withdraw. This withdrawal, combined with the prejudice that may be experienced throughout childhood and adolescence, can lead to inadequate educational, matrimonial, and employ-ment opportunities. Because of low self-esteem, many epileptic persons may choose companions with emotional, physical, or mental handicaps of their own. Alcoholism and substance abuse may follow.

The overall risk of death among epileptics ranges from that of the general population to a rate 200% greater, and is significantly higher for the poorly controlled epileptic patient. Various factors contribute to the increased risk to life and health of the epileptic patient, including ictal brain injury, medication side effects, trauma during seizure episodes, and an increased rate of suicide.[59]

DENTAL THERAPY CONSIDERATIONS

The major consideration in dental care for the epileptic patient is to prepare to manage the patient if a seizure occurs. Specific modifications in dental treatment should be considered only if the situation warrants them. Psychologic stress and fatigue tend to increase the probability of a seizure developing. In the presence of dental-related fear, psychosedation during treatment should be considered.

Because of the greater degree of control maintained by the administrator over its actions, inhalation sedation with nitrous oxide and oxygen is a highly recommended route of sedation for the apprehensive epileptic patient. Nitrous oxide is not contraindicated for administration to the epileptic patient. Indeed, when administered with at least 20% oxygen, there are no medical contraindications to its administration.[60]

Oral medications may also be used effectively in the less apprehensive epileptic patient. The benzodiazepines (e.g., diazepam, oxazepam, triazolam, flurazepam) are highly recommended for adult patients, whereas chloral hydrate, promethazine, and hydroxyzine are suggested in children.

More profound levels of sedation (i.e., deep sedation) may be employed safely via intravenous or intramuscular routes of administration in the more fearful epileptic patient if the usual precautions associated with parenteral sedation techniques are applied. Hypoxia/anoxia will induce seizures in any patient, but are probably more likely to do so in patients with preexisting epilepsy. The use of supplemental oxygen during treatment, the pulse oximeter, and a pretracheal stethoscope are strongly suggested whenever deeper levels of sedation are employed.[60]

The use of alcohol is definitely contraindicated in epileptic patients because it may precipitate seizures.[61] It is therefore strongly suggested that epileptic patients not undergo dental treatment if it is obvious that they have recently ingested alcohol,

Table 21-3. Physical status classification of seizure disorders

	Physical status (ASA)	Considerations
History of seizures well controlled by medications (no acute seizures within past 3 months)	II	Usual ASA II considerations
History of seizure activity controlled by medications, yet seizures occurring more often than once a month	III	ASA III considerations, to include preparation for seizure management
History of status epilepticus	III-IV	Medical consultation before treatment
History of seizure activity poorly controlled by medications; frequency of acute seizures >1/week	IV	Medical consultation and better control of seizures before routine dental treatment

nor should the doctor consider the use of alcohol as a sedative agent in epileptic patients.

Table 21-3 lists the physical status classifications for epileptic patients. The typically well-controlled epileptic represents an ASA II risk, whereas less well-controlled patients may represent ASA III or ASA IV risks.

CLINICAL MANIFESTATIONS

The tonic-clonic seizure (grand mal, generalized seizure, major convulsion) will be described in depth following a description of other seizure types.

Partial Seizures

Partial seizures occur when an attack begins from a localized area of the brain and involves only one hemisphere. The seizure is called a simple partial seizure when consciousness is unaltered; for example, a focal motor seizure is a simple partial seizure in which the victim experiences jerking of a limb for several seconds while remaining fully alert and conscious.

If, however, the abnormal neuronal discharge spreads to the opposite hemisphere, consciousness is altered and the ability to respond is impaired. This is called a complex partial seizure and is associated with complex behavior patterns called automatisms. An example of a typical complex partial seizure is the sudden onset of a bad taste in the mouth (the aura), which is followed by a lack of responsiveness, fumbling of hands, and smacking of the lips. The patient slowly becomes reoriented in about 1 minute and is back to normal except for slight lethargy within 3 minutes.

The automatic behavior that occurs is associated with impaired consciousness and a loss of higher voluntary control. The nature of the automatic behavior is related to the degree and duration of the confusion and to the psychological and environmental conditions existing at the time of the attack.

Primitive, uncoordinated, purposeless activities, such as lip smacking, chewing movements, and sucking, occur in patients with moderate levels of impaired consciousness.

In patients with mild confusion on the other hand, the automatism may manifest itself as a mechanical continuation of activities initiated before the start of the seizure. The patient may continue to move a spoon toward the mouth in an eating movement, or may continue to pace around a room, if this was the activity at the onset of the seizure. The entire seizure lasts for a few minutes and there is only momentary postictal confusion and amnesia for ictal events.[62]

Focal status epilepticus is not common but is resistant to anticonvulsant drug therapy; characteristically, seizure activity lasts over a period of weeks despite vigorous treatment. Fortunately, this type of seizure is not life threatening. Both simple and complex partial seizures may progress to generalized tonic-clonic seizures.

Petit Mal (Absence Attacks)

Absence attacks occur primarily in children, with the onset between 3 and 15 years of age. The seizure has an abrupt onset, characterized by a complete suppression of all mental functions, manifested by sudden immobility and a blank stare. Simple automatisms and minor facial clonic movements may be noted. Intermittent blinking at a rate of 3 cycles per second and mouthing movements are examples. The absence attack may last for 5 to 30 seconds, whereas petit mal status may persist for hours or days. There is no prodromal or postictal period, the episode terminating as abruptly as it started. The blank stare is followed by the immediate resumption of normal activity. If the attacks occur during conversation, the patient may miss a few words or may break off in mid-sentence for a few seconds. The impairment of external awareness is so brief that the patient is unaware of it. Amnesia for ictal events is common and the patient may experience a subjective sense of lost time.[63]

It is not uncommon for an informal diagnosis of petit mal to occur when a young child first enters school. After a few weeks or months, the child's teacher may advise the parents that their child daydreams a lot or that he or she goes off into their own world for brief periods of time. Medical evaluation usually provides definitive evidence of petit mal epilepsy.

Generalized Tonic-Clonic Seizure

The generalized tonic-clonic seizure may be divided into three distinct clinical phases: a prodromal phase, including a preictal phase; a convulsive or ictal phase; and a postseizure or postictal phase.

Prodromal Phase

For a variable period of time (several minutes to several hours) before the occurrence of a generalized seizure, the epileptic patient exhibits subtle or obvious changes in emotional reactivity. The patient may exhibit an increase in either anxiety or depression. These changes are usually not evident to the staff of the dental office but might be detected by a close friend or relative of the patient. If such changes appear in an epileptic patient before a dental appointment, preparation for management of a seizure should be made and any planned dental treatment should be postponed until a later date.

The immediate onset of the seizure is marked by the appearance of an aura in most, but not all, patients. The aura is not truly a warning sign that a seizure is about to occur, but is an actual part of the seizure. The same aura usually recurs with each seizure in an epileptic patient. The duration of the aura is quite brief, usually only a few seconds. The clinical manifestations of the aura are related to the specific area of the brain from which the seizure originates. The aura itself may be considered a simple partial seizure that progresses to a generalized tonic-clonic seizure. It may be olfactory, visual, gustatory, or auditory in nature.

Unfortunately, many patients are unaware of their aura because they will later be amnesic of this period. Most persons with grand mal epilepsy remember nothing from the time immediately preceding the onset of the seizure until they fully recover, perhaps 15 or more minutes later. Patients will know their aura if a person who was near them when a seizure occurred relates it to them at a later time.

Preictal Phase

Soon after the appearance of the aura, the patient loses consciousness and, if standing, falls to the floor. It is at this time that most injuries are sustained. Simultaneously, a series of generalized bilateral, major myoclonic jerks occurs, usually in flexion, lasting for several seconds. The so-called "epileptic cry" occurs at this time. This is a sudden vocalization produced by air expelled through a partially closed glottis as the diaphragmatic muscles go into spasm. Autonomic changes are associated with this initial phase. These include an increase in the heart rate and blood pressure up to about twice baseline, markedly increased bladder pressure, cutaneous vascular congestion and piloerection, glandular hypersecretion, superior ocular deviation with mydriasis, and apnea.[50]

Ictal Phase: Tonic Component

A series of sustained generalized skeletal muscle contractions occur, first in flexion and then progressing to a tonic extensor rigidity of the extremities and the trunk (Fig. 21-1). During this phase of the seizure the muscles of respiration are also involved, and dyspnea and cyanosis may become evident, indicating inadequate ventilation. This tonic rigidity usually lasts from 10 to 20 seconds.

Ictal Phase: Clonic Component:

The tonic phase evolves into the clonic component. This is characterized by generalized clonic movements of the body accompanied by heavy, stertorous breathing. The clonic activity is manifested by alternating muscular relaxation and violent flexor contractions (Fig. 21-2). During this clonic phase, frothing at the mouth may be noted, because air and saliva are mixed. Blood may also appear in the mouth because the victim may injure intraoral soft tissues, biting the lateral side of the tongue and the cheek during the clonic portion of the seizure.[64] The usual duration of clonus is about 2 to 5 minutes. Clonic movements become less frequent, with the relaxation portions becoming prolonged as the seizure progresses, ending with a final flexor jerk. The ictal phase ends as respiratory movements return to normal and the tonic-clonic movements cease.

Postictal Phase

With the cessation of tonic-clonic movement and the return of normal respiration, the patient enters the postictal phase, during which consciousness gradually returns. The clinical manifestations of this phase largely depend on the severity of the ictal phase.

In the first several minutes of the immediate postictal phase there is a momentary period of muscular flaccidity during which urinary and/or fecal incontinence may occur, caused by sphincter relaxation. With the termination of normal seizure activity, the patient relaxes and sleeps deeply. If the seizure was more severe, the victim may initially be in a comatose or nonresponsive state. As consciousness gradually returns, a patient is initially quite disoriented and confused, unaware of where he or she is, what day of the week it is, and unable to count backward from 10 to 1 or do other simple mathematical calculations. With time an increasing level of alertness is observed. Patients sometimes then fall into a deep, but rousable, recuperative sleep and on awakening will complain of headache and muscle soreness.

Following most generalized seizures there is almost total amnesia of the ictal and postictal phases. Some persons do retain memory of the prodromal phase, however. Full recovery of preseizure cerebral functioning takes approximately 2 hours.[12]

Grand Mal Status (Status Epilepticus)

Status epilepticus is defined as a continuous seizure or the repetitive recurrence of any type of seizure without recovery between attacks.[22,23] In this discussion it is considered to be a direct continuation of the tonic-clonic seizure already described. As mentioned previously, grand mal status is a life-threatening situation. Patients in status epilepticus exhibit the same clinical signs and symptoms as those seen during the convulsive phase of a generalized seizure, the one major difference being their duration. Tonic-clonic seizures normally last from 2 to 5 minutes with variation noted on either extreme of time. Grand mal status may persist for hours or days and is the major cause of mortality directly related to seizure disorders. Mortality figures range from 3% to 23%, depending on the study cited.[65,66] The incidence of grand mal status has actually increased since the introduction of effective anticonvulsants. Most cases result from drug or alcohol withdrawal (barbiturate withdrawal is particularly severe), severe head injury, or metabolic derangements.[24,25,67]

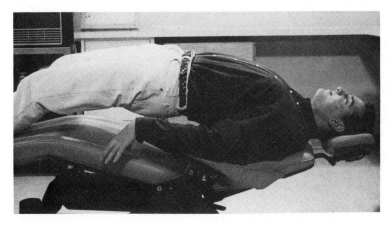

Fig. 21-1. Victim during tonic phase of generalized seizure (grand mal).

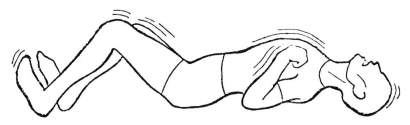

Fig. 21-2. Victim during clonic phase of generalized seizure (grand mal).

For the purposes of clinical management any continuous generalized (tonic-clonic) seizure lasting for 5 minutes or longer is classified as grand mal status.[23] The patient is nonresponsive (unconscious), cyanotic, perspires profusely, and demonstrates generalized clonic contractions with a very brief or entirely absent tonic phase. As grand mal status progresses, the patient becomes hyperthermic, with body temperature rising to 106° F or above. The cardiovascular system is greatly overworked; tachycardia and dysrhythmias occur, and the blood pressure is quite elevated—measurements of 300/150 mmHg are not uncommon. Unterminated grand mal status may progress to death resulting from cardiac arrest; irreversible neuronal damage from cerebral hypoxia, which occurs secondary to inadequate ventilation, the increased metabolic requirements of the entire body but of the central nervous system in particular; a decrease in cerebral blood flow in response to increased intracranial pressure; or a significant decrease in blood glucose levels as the brain utilizes large volumes for metabolism.

PATHOPHYSIOLOGY

Epilepsy is not a disease but a symptom. The symptom normally represents a primary form of brain dysfunction, although it is not possible to detect such a lesion in approximately 75% of patients with recurrent seizure disorders (idiopathic epilepsy). Epileptics should be viewed as people with brains that malfunction periodically.

Adult-onset epilepsy most often indicates the presence of a structural lesion of the brain, even though initial examination may fail to demonstrate it. Small tumors may take considerable time to enlarge to detectable size. Periodic medical examination every 4 to 6 months and annual EEGs are recommended. The use of the computed tomography (CAT) scan and magnetic resonance imaging (MRI) have greatly aided in detection of previously undetectable lesions. Experimental drug models of epilepsy presume that there are intrinsic intracellular and extracellular metabolic disturbances in neurons of epileptics that produce excessive and prolonged membrane depolarization. The common denominator is an increased permeability of the neuronal cell membrane with changes in sodium and potassium movement that effect the resting membrane potential and membrane excitability.[36,68] These hyperexcitable neurons are located in aggregates in an epileptogenic focus (the site of origin of the seizure) somewhere within the brain and tend toward recurrent, high-frequency bursts of action potentials.

Clinical seizure activity develops if the abnormal discharge is propagated along neural pathways or if local neuron recruitment occurs (if additional neighboring neurons are stimulated to discharge). Once a critical mass of neurons is recruited and a sustained excitation occurs, the seizure is propagated along conducting pathways to subcortical areas and thalamic centers. If this discharge remains localized within the focal area, a partial seizure develops with clinical signs and symptoms related to the specific focal area. If the discharge continues to spread through normal neuronal tissue and recruitment continues, generalized seizures occur. Clinical manifestations of the seizure depend on the focus of origin (e.g., partial seizures and aura of grand mal) and the region of the brain into which the discharge subsequently spreads.

That seizures can also arise in normal neurologic tissues is evidenced in clinical seizures caused by systemic metabolic and toxic disorders. Deficiencies in oxygen, as in hypoxia occurring during vasodepressor syncope, or glucose (e.g., hypoglycemia), or decreases in calcium ions (e.g., hypocalcemia) create a membrane instability that predispose otherwise normal neurons to paroxysmal discharge. Adequate electrical stimulation may also produce clinical seizures in normal neurologic tissues (e.g., electroconvulsive therapy [ECT]).

Significant alterations occur in both cerebral and systemic physiology during generalized motor seizures. Cerebral changes include marked increases in blood flow, oxygen and glucose utilization, and carbon dioxide production. These changes are associated with cerebral hypoxia and carbon dioxide retention, resulting in acidosis and lactic acid accumulation.[50,69] Following 20 minutes of continuous seizure activity, cerebral metabolic demands may exceed supply, potentially leading to neuronal destruction.[70]

Systemic effects of prolonged seizures are thought to be secondary to the massive autonomic discharge that produces tachycardia, hypertension, and hyperglycemia.[71] Other adverse systemic effects are produced secondary to massive skeletal muscle metabolism and disturbances in pulmonary ventilation, leading to lactic acidosis, hypoxia, hypoglycemia, and hyperpyrexia.[72,73]

MANAGEMENT

Management of a patient during the tonic-clonic phase of a generalized seizure is predicated on the prevention of injury and the assurance of adequate ventilation. In almost all cases there is no need to administer anticonvulsant medications, as most seizures are self-limiting. Should a seizure persist for an unusually long period of time (>5 minutes), anticonvulsant drug management should be considered. Following the convulsive phase of the seizure, patients will exhibit varying degrees of CNS, cardiovascular, and respiratory depression, which may require additional supportive management.

There will almost always be a prior knowledge of seizure activity in this patient, so it is highly unlikely that the dental office staff will be surprised when the seizure occurs.

Petit Mal and Partial Seizures

Management of petit mal and partial seizures is of a protective nature. The rescuer acts to prevent injury to the victim. In both of these seizure types there is little or no danger to the victim, so that even without assistance from staff members, morbidity seldom occurs. Indeed, many of these seizures will be of such short duration that the attending personnel will never even become aware of their occurrence. However, should these seizures persist for a significant length of time (average petit mal episode is 5 to 30 seconds; partial seizure lasts from 1 to 2 minutes), medical assistance may be summoned.

Diagnostic clues to the presence of petit mal and partial seizures include:

- Sudden onset of immobility and blank stare
- Simple automatic behavior
- Slow blinking of eyelids
- Short duration (seconds to minutes)
- Rapid recovery

Step 1: Terminate the dental procedure.

Step 2: Position the patient. In most cases of a petit mal or simple partial seizure there is neither the time nor the need to alter patient position before the seizure ends.

Step 3: Reassure the patient. Following the end of the seizure speak with the patient to determine their level of alertness. Seek to determine if there was any correlation between the dental treatment and the seizure. If this appears to be the case, appropriate procedures of the stress reduction protocol should be employed at future appointments. Medical consultation with the patient's primary care physician should be considered if there has been a recent increase in either the frequency of the seizures or of their severity. There is usually no need to seek outside medical assistance, nor is the administration of drugs necessary.

Step 4: Discharge of the patient and subsequent dental care. It is unlikely that the patient suffering from seizures is permitted to operate a motor vehicle. All states maintain requirements that prohibit epileptics from operating a motor vehicle until they

---

MANAGEMENT OF PETIT MAL AND PARTIAL SEIZURES

Terminate the dental procedure
↓
Position the patient
(leave alone during seizure)

Seizure stops / Reassure patient

Seizure continues (>5 minutes) / Summon medical assistance

↓
Allow patient to recover and discharge

↓
Basic life support, as indicated

---

can document control of their seizures for periods of time ranging from 1 year or longer.[74] The patient will therefore be discharged from the office in the care of an escort.

Subsequent dental care should take into consideration any dentally related factors that might have been involved in provoking the seizure. The accompanying box outlines the steps to follow to manage petit mal and partial seizures.

Generalized Tonic-Clonic Seizures (Grand mal)

Diagnostic clues to the presence of generalized tonic-clonic seizures include:[75]

- Presence of aura prior to loss of consciousness
- Loss of consciousness
- Tonic clonic muscle contraction
- Clenched teeth, tongue biting
- Incontinence

Preictal (Prodromal) Phase

Step 1: Terminate the dental procedure. When the patient with a prior history of grand mal epilepsy exhibits an aura, immediately terminate the dental procedure. A variable period of time will be available in order to remove as much dental equipment from the patient's mouth as is possible before he or she loses consciousness and progresses to the ictal phase of the event. Any removable dental appliances should also be removed from the patient's mouth at this time. There are reports of removable dental appliances having been aspirated during seizures.[76]

Step 2: Position the patient. When the seizure develops with the victim not in the dental chair, he or she should be placed on the floor in the supine position. When the seizure occurs in the dental chair, moving the patient will prove to be exceedingly difficult. In this situation the patient should be left in the dental chair, which should be placed in the supine position.

Step 3: Summon medical assistance. Although most generalized tonic-clonic seizures are of short duration, lasting not more than 5 minutes, it is the author's feeling that medical assistance should be sought at the very onset of the episode. This is done for two reasons: (1) Should the patient still be seizing upon arrival of medical assistance, obtaining a patent vein and the intravenous administration of anticonvulsant drug therapy may be more easily procured, and (2) in the more likely event that the patient has stopped seizing by the time medical assistance arrives at the dental office, their expertise can be utilized in evaluating the postical state of recovery of the patient, including the need for possible hospitalization or discharge home.

Step 4: Prevent injury. Prevention of injury to the convulsing patient is the next concern. If the victim is in bed or is on a well-padded, carpeted floor in an area devoid of hard objects that may cause injury, the rescuer can permit the patient to convulse with little chance of injury occurring. *Gently* restraining the victim's arms and legs from gross movements (allowing for minor movements) prevents injury from overextension or dislocation of joints. No attempt should be made to hold the convulsing patient's extremities in a fixed position as this may result in bony fractures.[23,50] If the floor is not padded, the head should be protected from traumatic injury by placing a thin, soft item, such as a blanket or jacket, beneath the head, making certain that the head is not flexed forward, thereby obstructing the airway.

With the victim in the dental chair, however, there is a possibility of injury from nearby dental equipment or falling from the chair. Fortunately, the typical dental chair is a good site in which to have a seizure. The headrest of most dental units is normally well padded so that no additional protection for the head is necessary. Any additional pillow or doughnut device that is placed atop the headrest should be removed, leaving the bare padded headrest. The doughnut or pillow will throw the patient's head forward and therefore increase the likelihood of partial or complete airway obstruction. Removing the headrest permits extension of the neck, lifting the tongue and creating greater airway patency (Fig. 21-3).

Our concern therefore must be to prevent the patient from impaling arms or legs on equipment, such as burs and hand instruments. One member of the office emergency team should move as much equipment as possible away from the victim while two other members stand by the patient to prevent injury from occurring. One member is positioned at the patient's chest and is responsible for the protection of the head and arms; the second member stands astride the victim's feet (Fig. 21-4).

NOTE. **Placement of any object in the oral cavity is usually *not* indicated during tonic-clonic seizures.**

Many dentists, physicians, and nurses have been trained to attempt to place objects into the mouth of the convulsing patient in an effort to prevent injury to the intraoral tissues and to prevent the patient from "swallowing the tongue". Soft items, such as handkerchiefs, towels, and gauze pads, have been recommended, as have ratchet-type and rubber mouth props, wooden tongue depressors wrapped in gauze, and even spoons. Airway maintenance is not improved by the forcible insertion of these objects into the victim's mouth. Indeed, the patient's muscles of mastication are in tetany during the seizure so that it is necessary to force the mouth open, greatly increasing the chances of injury to both the soft and hard tissues. Teeth have been fractured and aspirated during these attempts at helping the seizing patient.[77] The possibility of injury to the rescuer also exists when attempts are made to place protective objects into the convulsing patient's mouth. Under no circumstances should a rescuer's fingers be placed between the teeth of a convulsing patient.

In most grand mal seizures only minor degrees of bleeding develop, if bleeding occurs at all. Roberge and Maciera-Rodriguez[64] reported on the incidence of seizure-related intraoral lacerations in 100 patients. They found that 44% of seizing patients suffered intraoral lacerations, primarily on the lateral border of the tongue. Only two of these 44 patients subsequently required surgical repair of the lacerations. It has been the author's experience that there is usually no need to place any object into the mouth of a patient during the ictal phase of the seizure.

Tight, binding clothes should be loosened to prevent possible injury caused by the straining patient and to assist in breathing. This includes opening the collar and loosening a tie or belt.

Step 5: Basic life support, as indicated. During seizure activity, especially the tonic phase, respirations may not be adequate. Indeed, brief periods of apnea may occur with cyanosis evident. Secretions may also accumulate in the oral cavity and may, in large enough amounts, produce a degree of airway obstruction. Saliva and blood are the most common secretions. During the clonic phase respirations im-

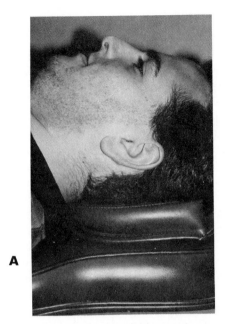 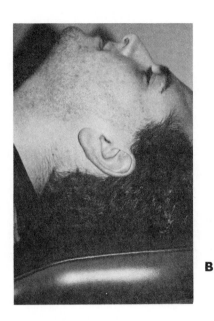

Fig. 21-3. A, Headrest of dental chair with doughnut or pillow. **B,** Bare headrest.

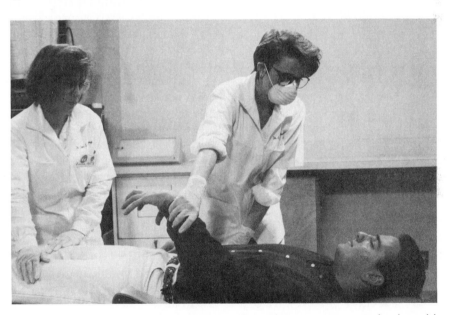

Fig. 21-4. To prevent injury from occurring to the patient, one team member is positioned at the patient's chest and the second member stands astride the victim's feet.

prove, but may still require assistance from rescuers in the form of airway maintenance (e.g., head tilt–chin lift). The heart rate and blood pressure will be significantly elevated above the patient's baseline values.

The victim's head should be extended (head tilt) to ensure airway patency, and if possible, the oral cavity should be suctioned carefully to remove secretions if they seem excessive. Suctioning is *not* usually required in the seizing patient. Soft rubber or plastic suction catheters are preferable to metallic ones, which can produce more soft and hard

tissue damage (e.g., bleeding, trauma). In either case the suction apparatus should be inserted between the buccal surface of the teeth and the cheek (Fig. 21-5). It should not be inserted between the teeth of the patient.

Step 6: Administer oxygen. If available, oxygen may be administered to any patient having a seizure.

Step 7: Monitor vital signs. Throughout the seizure the blood pressure, heart rate, and respiratory rate may be monitored, if possible. As mentioned previously, the blood pressure and heart rate will be markedly elevated and respiratory movements may

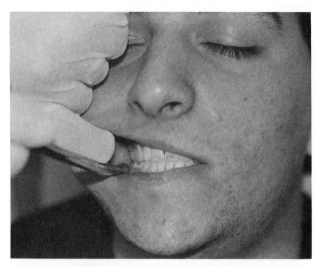

Fig. 21-5. The suction apparatus should be inserted between the buccal surface of the teeth and the cheek.

be absent during the tonic phase. During the subsequent clonic phase, heavy, stertorous breathing will be present.

Postictal Phase

Step 8: Basic life support, as indicated. With the cessation of seizures the patient enters the postictal phase, a phase of generalized depression (e.g., CNS, cardiovascular, and respiratory), with the degree of depression related to the degree of stimulation experienced during the preceding ictal phase. It is during the postictal phase that significant morbidity and even mortality may occur.

The ictal phase of a seizure is a highly dramatic and emotionally charged event for eyewitnesses, and attention is quickly focused on the patient. Once the convulsive phase ends, the patient relaxes and so, unfortunately, do the rescuers. This is quite premature because during the postictal period the patient may demonstrate significant CNS and respiratory depression to a degree that respiratory depression and/or airway obstruction may become evident.

Airway maintenance is almost always required and assisted or controlled artificial ventilation may, on rare occasion, be required. Oxygen may be administered by means of a full mask or nasal cannula, if indicated. Airway maintenance and adequacy of ventilation remain the primary considerations at this time.

Vital signs should be recorded at regular intervals (at least every 5 minutes). Blood pressure and respirations may be depressed in the immediate postictal period; however, they should gradually return toward the baseline level for that patient. The heart rate may be near baseline or only slightly depressed.

Step 9: Reassure patient and recovery. Recovery from the seizure will occur slowly, with the patient initially somnolent, but rousable, and gradually becoming increasingly alert. Return to normal preseizure cerebral functioning may require as long as 2 hours. There is also a significant degree of confusion and disorientation noted initially. The patient should be reassured that everything is alright. The author tells the patient, "This is Doctor Malamed. You are in the dental office. You had a seizure, and everything is alright." Many patients will respond more promptly when a familiar voice speaks to them. If a spouse, family member, relative, or friend accompanied the patient to the dental office, ask them to speak with the patient and reassure them at this time. Recovery includes a return of the vital signs to approximately the baseline level and recovery from the confusion and disorientation present during the early postictal period.

Step 10: Discharge from the office. For the author this is a very difficult step, and a primary reason to seek medical assistance early in the seizure. Following a seizure, should the patient be hospitalized, be sent to their private physician, or be sent home, and if so, how?

Paramedical personnel follow strict protocol for the management of emergency medical situations. In many jurisdictions criteria for hospitalization of a postseizure patient with a history of epilepsy include a lack of orientation to space (where are you?) and time (what day is it?). This decision is made simply, and if necessary, the patient is transported to the hospital for additional evaluation. In the event that the patient has recovered more completely and hospitalization is not warranted, the patient must be discharged from the dental office in the custody of a responsible adult. A relative or close friend should be called to the office, if not already present, to accompany the patient. The accompanying box outlines the steps to follow to manage generalized tonic-clonic seizures.

Grand Mal Status

In the event that generalized convulsive activity persists for unusually long periods (5 minutes or more), it may become necessary to terminate the seizure through the use of anticonvulsant drugs.

Step 1: Terminate the dental procedure.
Step 2: Position the patient.
Step 3: Summon medical assistance.
Step 4: Protect the patient from injury.
Step 5: Basic life support, as indicated.
Step 6: Administer oxygen.
Step 7: Monitor vital signs.

In the preceding seven steps we have managed a patient with generalized tonic-clonic seizures.

MANAGEMENT OF GENERALIZED TONIC-CLONIC SEIZURES (GRAND MAL)

Prodromal stage
    Terminate the dental procedure
        ↓

Ictal stage
    Position the patient
  (supine with legs elevated slightly)
        ↓
    Summon medical assistance
        ↓
  Protect the patient from injury
        ↓
  Basic life support, as indicated
        ↓
    Administer oxygen
        ↓
    Monitor vital signs
        ↓

Postictal stage
  Provide basic life support, as indicated
        ↓
  Reassure patient and allow to recover
        ↓
    Discharge patient
   ↙   ↓   ↘
To hospital To home To physician

Though most seizures stop spontaneously within 5 minutes, prolonged seizures are possible and are associated with a significantly increased risk of mortality and morbidity. Treatment options include (1) continuing basic life support and protecting the patient until medical assistance becomes available, or (2) providing definitive management of the seizure through the administration of anticonvulsant drugs. The first option is the most viable in many dental offices where drugs, equipment, and training for intravenous drug administration are not available, whereas the administration of anticonvulsant drugs should be considered only when the doctor and staff are well versed in the pharmacology of the agents and in artificial ventilation.

Step 8: Venipuncture and administration of anticonvulsant drug. Various anticonvulsant drugs may be used to terminate seizures. Ideally, the anticonvulsant should be of rapid onset and brief duration.[50] To be effective these agents must be administered intravenously; the intramuscular route is highly unpredictable and the oral route is contraindicated in an unconscious, convulsing patient. An intravenous infusion should be established, or the drugs may be injected directly into the vein of the patient. As the blood pressure is significantly elevated dur-

ing the seizure, superficial peripheral veins are usually quite evident, and with an assistant restraining the arm, an intravenous infusion can usually be established with little difficulty by a doctor trained in venipuncture. When proper equipment and adequately trained staff are not available, intravenous injections should not be attempted. In these instances it is advisable to continue with supportive therapy until more highly trained personnel arrive.

The anticonvulsant drug of choice for management of generalized tonic-clonic seizures is diazepam (Valium).[51,78] Diazepam is over 90% effective in instances of primary convulsive status.[79,80] A 10-mg dose is administered at a rate of 5 mg/min, and repeated every 10 minutes as necessary.[50] In children diazepam is administered in a dose of 0.3 mg/kg, and repeated every 10 minutes as necessary.[81]

If seizures persist, the injection may be repeated every 10 minutes. Potentially serious side effects of diazepam are related to excessively rapid injection and include transient hypotension, bradycardia, respiratory depression, and cardiac arrest.[82] These side effects are rarely observed if the agent is titrated slowly to effect. Generally, the total dose given should not exceed 0.5 mg/kg for acute therapy.[83]

Other benzodiazepines have been used to manage acute, generalized tonic-clonic seizures. Lorazepam may be as effective, but has a slower onset of action and a longer duration of action.[84] Midazolam, a water-soluble benzodiazepine, has also proved to be effective as an anticonvulsant following either intravenous or intramuscular administration.[85]

Until the introduction of the benzodiazepines in the 1960s, the barbiturates were used as the drugs of choice for seizure control. Pentobarbital (Nembutal), injected intravenously at a rate of 50 mg every 2 minutes, is an effective anticonvulsant. However, barbiturates have the disturbing ability to produce significant central nervous system and respiratory depression when employed in anticonvulsant doses, so the level of postictal depression may be intensified. Respiratory depression and apnea are not uncommon when barbiturates are employed as anticonvulsants. Effective airway maintenance and artificial ventilation must be provided until the patient has recovered.

Step 9: Administer 50% dextrose. The intravenous administration of 25 to 50 mL of 50% dextrose is recommended to rule out hypoglycemia as a possible cause of the seizure, as well as to maintain blood sugar levels because the brain is using large quantities of glucose in the ictal state.[50,51]

Step 10: Definitive management. All patients with grand mal status will require hospitalization follow-

---

MANAGEMENT OF GENERALIZED CONVULSIVE STATUS EPILEPTICUS

Prodromal stage
Terminate the dental procedure
↓

Ictal stage
Position the patient
(supine with legs elevated slightly)
↓
Summon medical assistance
↓
Protect patient from injury
↓
Basic life support, as indicated
↓
Administer oxygen
↓
Monitor vital signs
↓
(Seizure continues >5 minutes)
↙   ↘
Basic life support un-   Perform venipunc-
til assistance arrives   ture and administer
                            IV anticonvulsant
                            ↓
                            Administer 50%
                            dextrose IV
                            ↓
                            Definitive
                            management

---

ing the episode for neurologic evaluation and initiation of a treatment protocol to minimize further episodes. In the event that the seizure has not been terminated with the aforementioned drugs, other agents such as phenytoin (15 mg/kg)—for long-term seizure control; phenobarbital (10-15 mg/kg)—if seizures continue; and neuromuscular blockade (paralysis) with a nondepolarizing neuromuscular blocking agent such as pancuronium[86] may be required. The accompanying box outlines the steps to follow to manage generalized convulsive status epilepticus.

Drugs used in management: Yes: oxygen; anticonvulsant, if status epilepticus: diazepam, midazolam, pentobarbital
Medical assistance: Yes

DIFFERENTIAL DIAGNOSIS OF SEIZURES

The diagnosis of a seizure is not easily confused with other systemic medical conditions. There are, however, several systemic disorders that may have seizures as a part of their clinical signs (Table 21-4). The following discussion is presented to aid in diagnosing these possible causes of seizure activity.

Vasodepressor syncope is the most common cause of unconsciousness in the dental office. If hypoxia or anoxia persist, brief periods of seizure activity may occur. Differentiating factors indicating vasodepressor syncope include the presence of a definite precipitating factor, such as fear. Prodromal signs such as lightheadedness, nausea or vomiting, and profuse sweating are present before the loss of consciousness but are absent in epilepsy. The loss of consciousness in vasodepressor syncope is quite brief, recovery beginning once blood flow to the brain is increased. Muscles are flaccid, and there is no convulsive movement initially. The blood pressure and heart rate are depressed in vasodepressor syncope. Bladder and bowel incontinence rarely occur. Upon recovery of consciousness, the mental confusion and disorientation associated with epileptic convulsions are not present. The patient is alert and able to perform simple mental calculations. The primary cause of seizure activity in vasodepressor syncope is hypoxia/anoxia, which is treatable with airway management.

Cerebral vascular accident (CVA) may lead to the loss of consciousness with possible convulsions. Aids to differential diagnosis indicating CVA include the possible presence of an intense headache before the loss of consciousness and signs of neurologic dysfunction (e.g., muscle weakness or paralysis) before unconsciousness.

Hypoglycemia may also progress to the loss of consciousness and seizures. The patient's history, in addition to prior clinical signs and symptoms (see

Table 21-4. Possible causes of seizure disorders

Cause	Frequency	Where discussed in text
Epilepsy (grand mal)	Most common	Seizures (Section V)
Local anesthetic overdose reaction	Less common	Drug-related emergencies (Section VI)
Hyperventilation	Rare	Respiratory distress (Section III)
Cerebrovascular accident	Rare	Altered consciousness (Section IV)
Hypoglycemic reaction	Rare	Altered consciousness (Section IV)
Vasodepressor syncope	Rare	Unconsciousness (Section II)

Chapter 17), will provide evidence. Additional management in this situation requires the administration of intravenous dextrose.

REFERENCES

1. Taylor J, editor: Selected writings of John Hughlings Jackson, vol 1: On epilepsy and epileptiform convulsions, London 1931, Hodder and Stoughton (1958 reprint, New York: Basic Books).
2. Gastaut H: *Dictionary of Epilepsy*, Geneva, 1973, World Health Organization.
3. Sutherland JM, Eadie MJ: *The epilepsies: modern diagnosis and treatment*, ed 3, Edinburgh, 1980, Churchill Livingstone.
4. Commission on Classification and Terminology of the International League Against Epilepsy: Proposal for revised clinical and electroencephalographic classification of epileptic seizures, *Epilepsia* 22:489, 1981.
5. Delgado-Escueta AV, Treiman DM, Walsh GO: The treatable epilepsies: (2 parts), *N Engl J Med* 308:1508, 1983.
6. Hauser WA, Kurland LT: The epidemiology of epilepsy in Rochester, Minnesota, 1935 through 1967, *Epilepsia* 61:1, 1975.
7. Hauser WA: Epidemiology of epilepsy. In Schonberg BS, editor: *Advances in neurology*, vol 19, New York, 1978, Raven Press.
8. Camfield PR and others: Epilepsy after a first unprovoked seizure in childhood, *Neurology* 35:1657, 1985.
9. Shinnar S, and others: Discontinuing antiepileptic medication in children with epilepsy after two years without seizures: a prospective study, *N Engl J Med* 313:976, 1985.
10. Callaghan N, Garrett A, Goggin T: Withdrawal of anticonvulsant drugs in patients free of seizures for two years: a prospective study, *N Engl J Med* 318:942, 1988.
11. Epilepsy Foundation of America: *Basic statistics on the epilepsies*, Philadelphia, 1975, FA Davis.
12. Gastaut H, and others: *Generalized convulsive seizures without local onset*. In Vinken PJ, Bruyn GW, editors: *Handbook of clinical neurology*, vol 15, Amsterdam, 1974, Elsevier.
13. Gastaut H: *Epileptic seizures*, Springfield, Ill., 1972 Charles C Thomas.
14. Milichap J, Aymat F: Treatment and prognosis of petit mal epilepsy, *Pediatr Clin N Am* 14:905, 1967.
15. Livingston S, and others: Classification and clinical features of epileptic seizures, *Pediatr Ann* 8:176, 1979.
16. Gastaut H, and others: Generalized non-convulsive seizures without local onset. In Vinken PJ, Bruyn GW, editors: *Handbook of clinical neurology*, vol 15, Amsterdam, 1974, Elsevier.
17. Vick N: *Grinker's neurology*, ed 7, Springfield, Ill., 1976, Charles C Thomas.
18. Feindel W: Temporal lobe seizures. In Vinken PJ, Bruyn GW, editors: *Handbook of clinical neurology*, vol 15, Amsterdam, 1974, Elsevier.
19. Niedermeyer E: *Compendium of the epilepsies*, Springfield, Ill., 1974, Charles C Thomas.
20. Rasmussen T: Seizures with local onset and elementary symptomatology. In Vinken PJ, Bruyn GW, editors: *Handbook of clinical neurology*, vol 15, Amsterdam, 1974, Elsevier.
21. Gastaut H: Clinical and electroencephalographical classification of epileptic seizures, *Epilepsia* 11:114, 1970.
22. Hauser A: Status epilepticus: frequency, etiology and neurological sequelae. In Delgado-Escueta A, Wasterlain C, Treiman D, and others: editors: *Advances in neurology*, vol 34, New York, 1983, Raven Press.
23. *Emergency care and transportation for the sick and injured*, ed 4, Orco, IL, 1987, American Academy of Orthopedic Surgeons.
24. Celesia G, Messert B, Murphy M: Status epilepticus of late onset, *Neurology* 22:1047, 1972.
25. Aminoff MJ, Simon RP: Status epilepticus: Causes, clinical features and consequences in 98 patients, *Am J Med* 69:657, 1980.
26. Delgado-Escueta AV, Wasterlain C, Treiman DM, and others: Current concepts in neurology: management of status epilepticus, *N Engl J Med* 306:1337, 1982.
27. Oxbury J, Whitty C: Causes and consequences of status epilepticus in adults, *Brain* 94:733, 1971.
28. Treiman DM, Walton NY, Wickboldt C, and others: Predictable sequence of EEG changes during generalized convulsive status epilepticus in man and three experimental models of status epilepticus in the rat, *Neurology* 37(suppl 1):244, 1987.
29. Gumnit RJ, Sell MA, editors: Epilepsy: a handbook for physicians, ed 4, Minneapolis, 1981, University of Minnesota Comprehensive Epilepsy Program.
30. Janz D: Etiology of convulsive status epilepticus. In Delgado-Escueta A, Wasterlain C, Treiman D, and others, editors: *Advances in neurology*, vol 34, New York, 1983, Raven Press.
31. Andermann F, Robb J: Absence status: a reappraisal review of thirty-eight patients, *Epilepsia* 13:177, 1972.
32. Robb P, McNaughton F: Etiology of epilepsy: introduction. In Vinken PJ, Bruyn GW, editors: *Handbook of clinical neurology*, vol 15, Amsterdam, 1974, Elsevier.
33. Wilkinson DS, Prockop LD: Hypoglycemia: effects on the central nervous system. In Vinken PJ, Bruyn GW, editors: *Handbook of clinical neurology*, vol 15, Amsterdam, 1974, Elsevier.
34. Earnest MP, Yarnell PR: Seizure admissions to a city hospital: the role of alcohol, *Epilepsia* 17:387, 1976.
35. Newton R: Physostigmine salicylate in the treatment of tricyclic antidepressant overdosage, *JAMA* 231:941, 1975.
36. Tower DB: Neurochemistry of epilepsy. In Vinken PJ, Bruyn GW, editors: *Handbook of clinical neurology*, vol 15, Amsterdam, 1974, Elsevier.
37. Myers JA, Earnest MP: Generalized seizures and cocaine abuse, *Neurology* 34:675, 1984.
38. Jennett WB: *Epilepsy after non-missile head injuries*, Chicago, 1975, Mosby–Year Book.
39. Jennett WB: Posttraumatic epilepsy. In Thompson RA, Green JP, editors: *Advances in neurology*, vol 22, New York, 1979, Raven Press.
40. Friedlander WJ: Epilepsy, *Curr Med Diag Sept* 727, 1971.
41. Holmes GL: *Diagnosis and management of seizures in childhood*, Philadelphia, 1987, WB Saunders.
42. LeBlanc FE, Rasmussen T: Cerebral seizures and brain tumors. In Vinken PJ, Bruyn GW, editors: *Handbook of clinical neurology*, vol 15, Amsterdam, 1974, Elsevier.
43. Ketz E: Brain tumors and epilepsy. In Vinken PJ, Bruyn GW, editors: *Handbook of clinical neurology*, vol 16, Amsterdam, 1974, Elsevier.
44. Scheehan S: 1,000 cases of late onset epilepsy, *Irish J Med Sci* 6:261, 1958.
45. Schold C, Yarnell PR, Earnest MP: Origin of seizures in elderly patients, *JAMA* 238:1177, 1977.
46. Bauer G, Niedermeyer E: Acute convulsions, *Clin Electroenceph* 10:127, 1979.
47. Juul-Jensen P: Epilepsy: a clinical and social analysis of 1020 adult patients with epileptic seizures, *Acta Neurol Scand* 40(suppl 5):1, 1964.

48. Dahlquist NR, Mellinger JF, Klass DW: Hazard of video games in patients with light-sensitive epilepsy, *JAMA* 249:776, 1983.

49. Annegars J: Factors prognostic of unprovoked seizures after febrile convulsions, *N Engl J Med* 316:493, 1987:

50. Tomlanovich MC, Yee AS: Seizure. In Rosen P, editor: *Emergency medicine*, ed 2, St Louis 1988, Mosby—Year Book.

51. Aminoff MJ: Epilepsy. In Schroeder SA, Krupp MA, Tierney LM, and others, editors: *Current medical diagnosis and treatment 1990*, Norwalk, 1990, Appleton & Lange.

52. Porter RJ: How to use antiepileptic drugs. In Levy RH, Dreifuss EI, Mattson RH, and others; editors: *Antiepileptic drugs*, ed 3, New York, 1989, Raven Press.

53. Emerson R, D'Souza BJ, Vining EP, and others: Stopping medication in children with epilepsy: predictors of outcome, *N Engl J Med* 304:1125, 1981.

54. Vinson T: Towards demythologizing epilepsy, *Med J Aust* 2:663, 1975.

55. Lewis JA: Violence and epilepsy, *JAMA* 232:1165, 1975.

56. Gunn JC, Fenton G: Epilepsy in prisons: a diagnostic survey, *Br Med J* 4:326, 1969.

57. King LN, Young QD: Increased prevalence of seizure disorders among prisoners, *JAMA* 239:2674, 1978.

58. *New York Times*, Living with epilepsy, February 23, 1982.

59. Elwes R, Johnson A, Shorvan S, and others: The prognosis for seizure control in newly diagnosed epilepsy, *N Engl J Med* 311:944, 1984.

60. Malamed SF: *Sedation: a guide to patient management*, ed 2, St Louis, 1989, Mosby—Year Book.

61. Shaw G: Alcohol and the nervous system, *Clin Endocrinol Metab* 7:385, 1978.

62. Walter R: Clinical aspects of temporal lobe epilepsy, *Calif Med* 110:325, 1969.

63. Livingston S, and others: Medical treatment of epilepsy, *South Med J* 71:298, 1978.

64. Roberge RJ, Maciera-Rodriguez L: Seizure-related oral lacerations: incidence and distribution, *J Am Dent Assoc* 111:279, 1985.

65. Nicol CF: Status epilepticus, *JAMA* 234:419, 1975.

66. Maytal J: Low morbidity and mortality of status epilepticus in children, *Pediatrics* 83:323, 1989.

67. Rowan A, Scott D: Major status epilepticus, *Acta Neurol Scand* 46:573, 1970.

68. Reynolds EH: Water, electrolytes and epilepsy, *J Neurol Sci* 11:327, 1970.

69. Chapman AG, Meldrum BS, Siesjo BK: Cerebral metabolic changes during prolonged epileptic seizures in rats, *J Neurochem* 28:1025, 1977.

70. Kreisman NR, Rosenthal M, LaManna JC, and others: Cerebral oxygenation during recurrent seizures. In Delgado-Escueta A, Wasterlain C, Treiman D, and others, editors: *Advances in neurology*, vol 34, New York, 1983, Raven Press.

71. Laidlaw J, Richens A: *A textbook of epilepsy*, Edinburgh, 1976, Churchill-Livingstone.

72. Orringer CE, Eustace JC, Wunsch CD, and others: Natural history of lactic acidosis after grand mal seizures, *N Engl J Med* 297:796, 1977.

73. Meldrum BS, Vigouroux RA, Brierly JB: Systemic factors and epileptic brain damage: prolonged seizures in paralyzed artificially ventilated baboons, *Arch Neurol* 29:82, 1973.

74. Krumholz A, Fisher RS, Lesser RP, Hauser WA: Driving and epilepsy: a review and reappraisal, *JAMA* 265(5):622-626, 1991.

75. Pollakoff J, Pollakoff K: *EMT's guide to treatment*, 1991, Jeff Gould.

76. Giovannitti JA, Jr.: Aspiration of a partial denture during an epileptic seizure, *JADA* 103:895, 1981.

77. Scheuer ML, Pedley TA: The evaluation and treatment of seizures, *N Engl J Med* 323:1468, 1990.

78. Browne T: Drug therapy reviews: drug therapy of status epilepticus, *Am J Hosp Pharm* 35:915, 1978.

79. Browne T, Penry J: Benzodiazepines in the treatment of epilepsy, *Epilepsia* 14:277, 1973.

80. Tassinari C, Daniele O, Michelucci R, and others: Benzodiazepines: efficacy in status epilepticus. In Delgado-Escueta A, Wasterlain C, Treiman D, and others, editors: *Advances in neurology*, vol 34, New York, 1983, Raven Press.

81. Aicardi J, Chevrie JJ: Convulsive status epilepticus in infants and children: a study of 239 cases, *Epilepsia* 11:187, 1970.

82. *Physicians' Desk Reference*, 1991, ed 45, Oradell, N.J., 1991, Medical Economics Data.

83. Tintinalli J: Status epilepticus, *JACEP* 5:896, 1976.

84. Homan R, Walker J: Clinical studies of lorazepam in status epilepticus. In Delgado-Escueta A, Wasterlain C, Treiman D, and others, editors: *Advancess in neurology*, vol 34, New York, 1983, Raven Press.

85. Jaimovich DG, Shabino CL, Noorani PA, Bittle BK, Osborne JS: Intravenous midazolam suppression of pentylenetetrazol-induced epileptogenic activity in a porcine model, *Crit Care Med* 18(3):313-316, 1990.

86. Nugent S, Laravuso R, Rogers M: Pharmacology and use of muscle relaxants in infants and children, *J Pediatr* 94:481, 1979.

22 *Drug-Related Emergencies: General Considerations*

The administration of drugs has become commonplace within the practice of dentistry. The use of local anesthetics is considered an integral part of the dental treatment plan whenever potentially painful procedures are contemplated. Analgesic medications are prescribed for the relief of preexisting pain or for the alleviation of potential postoperative discomfort. Antibiotics are used whenever infection is present, and more commonly, antianxiety drugs are employed during all phases of the dental experience (pretreatment, during the appointment, and posttreatment). Other drugs are employed (Table 22-1), but the four categories mentioned constitute the overwhelming majority of all drugs used in the practice of dentistry.[1]

In all instances it is hoped that whenever a drug is administered or prescribed to a patient, a rational purpose exists for its administration. The indiscriminate administration of drugs has become one of the major causes of the great increase in the number of serious incidents of drug-related, life-threatening emergencies that are reported in the medical and dental literature.[2-5] Most drug-related emergencies are classified as one aspect of iatrogenic disease, a category that encompasses an entire spectrum of adverse effects produced unintentionally by physicians or dentists during the management of their patients.

The frequency of adverse drug reactions (ADRs) reported in the medical literature accounts for 3% to 20% of all hospital admissions.[5-7] An additional 5% to 40% of patients hospitalized for other reasons will experience an adverse drug reaction during their hospitalization. Furthermore, 10% to 18%

Table 22-1. Drug-prescribing habits in a U.S. dental school from 1983 to 1985

Drug category		Number of prescriptions
Analgesics		5730
Nonnarcotic	1139	
Combined with codeine	4570	
Plain narcotic	21	
Antibiotics		3931
Penicillin	2977	
Erythromycin	637	
Tetracycline	187	
Cephalosporin	130	
Minor tranquilizers		219
Sedative-hypnotics		65
Other categories		1500
TOTAL PRESCRIPTIONS FILLED		11,445

Data from Department of Pharmacology, University of Southern California School of Dentistry, Los Angeles.

of those patients admitted to the hospital because of an ADR have yet another drug reaction during their stay in the hospital, resulting in the length of hospitalization being doubled.[6] In most cases careful prescribing habits or care in the administration of drugs might have prevented the adverse drug reaction from occurring.

Some general principles of toxicology must be stated at this time so that the following material may be better understood (see accompanying box.) Toxicology is defined as the study of the harmful effects of chemicals (drugs) on biologic systems.

GENERAL PRINCIPLES OF TOXICOLOGY

1. No drug ever exerts a single action.
2. No clinically useful drug is entirely devoid of toxicity.
3. Potential toxicity of a drug rests in the hands of the user.

These harmful effects range from those that may prove inconsequential to the patient and are entirely reversible once the chemical is withdrawn, to those that prove uncomfortable but are not seriously harmful, to reactions that may seriously incapacitate the patient or cause death.[8]

Whenever a drug is administered, two types of drug actions may be observed: desirable drug actions—those that are clinically sought and are usually beneficial—and side effects, which are often undesirable drug actions.

An example of a desired drug action is the relief of anxiety achieved through the administration of diazepam to a fearful dental patient. A side effect of diazepam that is normally not desired but is not usually harmful to the patient is drowsiness. This effect of diazepam may even prove beneficial in certain circumstances; for example, a degree of drowsiness in an apprehensive dental patient can be desirable. However, the same degree of drowsiness while that patient is driving an automobile may prove to be hazardous. The side effect or undesired drug action may also prove to be harmful to a patient. Respiratory and cardiovascular depression although rarely observed with proper administration, have been reported after diazepam administration both parenterally (intramuscular and intravenous) and orally.[9]

A general principle of toxicology is: *No drug ever exerts a single action.* All chemicals exert many actions, some desirable, others undesirable. Ideally, the right drug in the right dose will be administered by the right route to the right patient at the right time for the right reason, and it will not produce any unwanted effects.[8] This clinical situation is rarely if ever attained, because no drug is so specific that it produces only the desired effects in all patients. *No clinically useful drug is entirely devoid of toxicity.* It must also be remembered that adverse drug reactions may occur when the wrong drug is administered to the wrong patient in the wrong dose by the wrong route at the wrong time and for the wrong reason.

PREVENTION

Although the preceding discussion may seem unduly pessimistic, it has not been presented with the intention of scaring dental practitioners away from the administration of drugs to their patients. Indeed, it is the author's firm conviction that drug use within the practice of dentistry is absolutely essential for the safe and proper management of many dental patients. For this reason it is extremely important for the doctor to become familiar with the pharmacologic properties of all the drugs that are used or prescribed by the doctor in his/her dental practice. Several excellent reference books are available that belong on the doctor's desk as readily available sources of information. These include *Facts and Comparisons* (revised monthly),[10] the *Physician's Desk Reference,*[11] and the American Medical Association's *AMA Drug Evaluations.*[12]

As Pallasch has stated[8]:

In most cases it is possible with sound clinical and pharmacological judgement to prevent serious toxicity from occurring. The aim of rational therapeutics is to maximize the therapeutic and minimize the toxic effects of a given drug.

No drug is "completely safe" or "completely harmful." All drugs are capable of producing harm if handled improperly, and conversely, any drug may be handled safely if proper precautions are observed. *The potential toxicity of a drug rests in the hands of the user.*

A second factor in the safe use of drugs is a consideration of the patient to whom the drug will be administered. Individuals may react in very different ways to the same stimulus; it should not be surprising then that patients will vary markedly in their reactions to drugs. Before administering any drug or prescribing any medication to a patient, the doctor must ask specific questions concerning the patient's past and present drug history.

Medical History Questionnaire

QUESTION 6. **Have you taken any medicine or drugs during the past 2 years?**

COMMENT. An accurate assessment of medications currently being taken or recently taken is essential if potential drug interactions, as well as side effects, are to be prevented.

QUESTION 7. **Are you allergic to (i.e., itching, rash, swelling of hands, feet, or eyes) or made sick by penicillin, aspirin, codeine, or any drugs or medications?**

COMMENT. Common signs and symptoms of allergy are presented in this question along with the names of three drugs commonly mentioned as producing ADRs. An alleged history of allergy to any drug must lead the doctor to an in-depth dialogue history of the patient concerning the incident or incidents (see Chapters 23 and 24).

QUESTION 9. Circle any of the following that you have had or have at present:
- Allergy or hives
- Chemotherapy (cancer, leukemia)
- Cortisone medicine

COMMENT. Affirmative responses must be followed by a thorough dialogue history to determine the drug(s) used, the reason for their administration, and the nature of any adverse reaction (if any) to the drug(s).

Dialogue History

Following a positive response to the question concerning allergy or adverse reaction (question 7), the doctor should obtain the following information from the patient concerning the incident:

What drug was used?

Was the patient taking any other medications at the time of the "allergy" or reaction?

Were vital signs recorded?

What was the time sequence of events during the reaction?

Where was the patient when the reaction occurred (home/medical-dental office)?

What were the clinical manifestations (signs and symptoms) of the reaction?

What acute treatment was given for the reaction?

Has the patient received the offending agent, or any chemical related to it, since the incident, and if so what reaction, if any, developed?

As will become evident in the chapters to follow, most patients will respond affirmatively to the question on allergy if they have ever experienced any adverse reaction to a drug in the past. In actuality the incidence of allergic phenomena is quite low; however, the reporting of allergy on dental and medical records is significantly higher. The reason for this variance lies in the fact that to the patient, any ADR is labeled an allergy. The layperson is often not familiar with the classification of drug reactions. For this reason, "allergy to Novocain" and "allergy to codeine" are commonly found as answers on dental history questionnaires. Although allergy to these agents is not impossible, the adverse reaction that did occur probably was not allergic. Careful questioning through the dialogue history by the doctor usually reveals that the "allergy to Novocain" was a psychogenic reaction such as hyperventilation or vasodepressor syncope, or an overdose (toxic) reaction to the agent; whereas the "allergy to codeine" most likely consisted of stom-

ach upset, or nausea or vomiting, which represent unwanted side effects of the drug but do not constitute an allergic reaction.

Questioning of the patient in order to determine the precise nature of the adverse drug reaction is vital. However, there are times when the patient's responses will be vague, thereby making it impossible to remove the doubt about the drug from the doctor's mind. In such cases the doctor should attempt to locate and speak to the person who observed or managed the so-called allergic reaction and attempt to determine more precisely the exact nature of the event.

Another factor to remember is that reactions that are often called adverse drug reactions may, in fact, be unrelated to the drug administered. In a fascinating paper entitled "Adverse Nondrug Reactions," Reidenberg and Lowenthal[13] demonstrated the occurrence of so-called drug side effects in persons who had not received any medications for a period of 2 weeks. Had they been receiving medications during this time, an ADR might well have been reported.

It is important to keep in mind that whenever doubt remains concerning the safety of any drug, it is prudent to initially assume that the patient is allergic to that agent and to avoid its use until the question can be answered definitively. This process may require referral of the patient to an allergist for further evaluation. In most instances, however, alternative agents can be used that possess the same beneficial clinical effects but do not have the allergic potential of the drug in question. These alternative agents should be used until the question of drug allergy can be conclusively decided.

Even in the absence of a positive history of ADR in the medical history questionnaire, it is still recommended that the patient be questioned directly concerning any drug that is being considered for use. Therefore, the doctor might ask the patient, "Have you ever taken Valium before?" and if the answer is yes, "What effect did it have?" Common, proprietary names (e.g., Valium) ought to be used because few patients are familiar with the generic names of drugs (e.g., diazepam).

In the absence of any prior adverse reaction to a medication, the doctor may feel more confident in administering the drug to the patient, always keeping in mind that adverse reactions can still arise despite prior administrations of the same agent without complication.

Care in Administration of Drugs

It is recognized that 85% of ADRs are related to the administration of an overdose of a particular agent.[6] Overdose of a drug may be an absolute overdose, (too many milligrams of a drug administered), or a relative overdose (a normal therapeutic dose for most patients that proves to be an overdose for an individual patient). Regardless of the type of overdose reaction encountered, most may be prevented through careful determination of the dosage (oral or intramuscular routes of administration) or through the careful administration of the drug to the patient (titration with the intravenous and inhalation routes). Most clinical responses to drugs will be related to the dose administered (i.e., they are dose-dependent); however, even minute quantities of a drug may precipitate a severe allergic reaction (anaphylaxis) in a previously sensitized individual.

The route of drug administration has an effect on the number and severity of ADRs. Two major routes of drug administration are considered: enteral and parenteral. Enteral routes of administration are those in which the drug is placed into the gastrointestinal tract, from which the drug is absorbed into the circulation. Enteral administration includes the oral and rectal routes. In parenteral administration the drug bypasses the gastrointestinal tract. Techniques of parenteral drug administration include intramuscular, submucosal, subcutaneous, intravenous, intraspinal, and intracapsular injections. Inhalation and topical application are other routes of administration that may be classified as parenteral.

In general, serious adverse drug reactions are observed more frequently following parenteral administration than following administration by enteral routes. Intravenous drug administration is the most effective route because it provides a rapid onset and high degree of reliability, but it also has a great potential for serious adverse drug reactions. However, when used properly, the intravenous route remains a very safe and very important route of drug administration in dentistry. Any ADRs seen following enteral drug administration are fewer in number and are usually of a less serious nature. However, the clinical effectiveness of drugs administered enterally is greatly diminished when compared to those administered parenterally.

When administering any drug to a patient, the choice of the proper route of administration must be carefully considered. Not all drugs can be administered by every route, and the degree of effectiveness may vary considerably when comparing one route to another with some agents. For example, 10 mg of diazepam administered intravenously usually provides a level of sedation adequate to permit a fearful dental patient to readily tolerate dental treatment; however, the level of sedation achieved when 10 mg of diazepam is administered orally will probably be inadequate to permit comfortable dental treatment for this same patient. On the other hand antibiotic prophylaxis for the patient with rheumatic heart disease may be achieved with either intramuscular injection or oral administration of penicillin 1 hour before therapy. In both instances of (intramuscular and oral) administration, the blood level of antibiotic achieved will prove adequate to prevent a transient bacteremia from producing a bacterial endocarditis. In this instance, however, the oral route is preferred over the parenteral route. As will be discussed later, penicillin has a high potential to cause allergy, and the route of drug administration may have significant bearing on the severity of any reaction that might occur.

A general rule in drug administration states that if a drug is clinically effective when administered enterally, this route is preferred over parenteral administration.

Most drug-related emergency situations are preventable. Carefully questioning the patient concerning any prior exposure and any reaction to a drug before administering it; carefully selecting the most appropriate route of administration to achieve the desired clinical effect; administering the drug using proper technique; and most importantly, being familiar with the pharmacology of all drugs prescribed to patients or used in the dental office will greatly reduce the incidence of adverse drug reactions.

CLASSIFICATION

Classifying adverse drug reactions has become a confusing task. In the past a variety of terms such as side effects, adverse experience, drug-induced disease, diseases of medical progress, secondary effects, and intolerance were used. The approach today is more simple, and most reactions are classified as adverse reactions.

The classification proposed by Pallasch,[8] shown in Table 22-2, represents a simplified approach to the problem of classifying adverse drug reactions. In this classification there are three major methods by which drugs may produce adverse reactions: (1) by a direct extension of a drug's pharmacologic actions, (2) by a deleterious effect on a chemically, genetically, metabolically, or morphologically altered recipient (the patient), and (3) by initiation of an immune (allergic) response.

Most adverse drug reactions are mere annoyances, but do not pose a threat to the patient's life. There are, however, several potential responses to

Table 22-2. Classification of adverse drug reactions

Toxicity resulting from direct extension of pharmacologic effects
Side effects
Abnormal dosage (overdosage)
Local toxic effects

Toxicity resulting from altered recipient (patient)
Presence of pathology
Emotional disturbances
Genetic aberrations (idiosyncrasy)
Teratogenicity
Drug-drug interactions

Toxicity resulting from drug allergy

From Pallasch TJ: *Pharmacology for dental students and practitioners*, Philadelphia, 1980, Lea & Febiger.

drugs that are life threatening, requiring immediate effective management if the patient is to fully recover to normal function. These include the overdose reaction (a direct extension of the pharmacologic activity of the drug) and the allergic response. Because of the critical nature of these responses and their importance in dentistry, they will be discussed in great depth in subsequent chapters.

In any discussion of drug-related or drug-induced emergencies there are normally three situations that are of immediate importance to the dental practitioner: overdose, allergy, and idiosyncrasy. Idiosyncrasy is discussed in this chapter; overdose and allergy are discussed more fully in later chapters but are also discussed briefly in this chapter. Approximately 85% of ADRs result from the pharmacologic effects of the drug, whereas 15% of ADRs result from immunologic reactions.[6]

Overdose Reaction

Overdose reaction (toxic reaction) may be defined as a condition that results from exposure to toxic amounts of a substance that does not cause adverse effects in smaller amounts.[14] It refers to the clinical signs and symptoms that are the result of an absolute or relative overadministration of a drug that produces elevated blood levels of that drug in various target organs and tissues. Clinical manifestations of overdose are related to a direct extension of the normal pharmacologic actions of the drug. In therapeutic doses, barbiturates, for example, produce a mild depression of the central nervous system, which results clinically in sedation or hypnosis (both desirable effects). Barbiturate overdose (higher blood levels of the barbiturate) produces more profound depression of the CNS with the real

possibility of respiratory and cardiovascular depression. Local anesthetics are also CNS depressants. When administered properly and in therapeutic doses, little or no evidence of CNS depression is evident; however, with increased blood levels, signs and symptoms of selective CNS depression are noted. Overdose reactions and their management are discussed in Chapter 23.

Allergy

Allergy may be defined as a hypersensitive response to an allergen to which an organism has previously been exposed and to which the organism has developed antibodies.[14] Clinically, there are a variety of ways in which allergy expresses itself. These include drug fever, angioedema, urticaria, dermatitis, depression of the blood-forming organs, photosensitivity, and anaphylaxis, the latter an acute systemic reaction possibly resulting in respiratory distress and cardiovascular collapse. Certain drugs and substances are much more likely to cause allergic reactions than are others (e.g., penicillin, aspirin, and bee stings). An allergic reaction is a possibility with any drug or chemical.

In marked contrast to the overdose reaction, in which clinical manifestations are related directly to the pharmacology of the drug administered, the observed clinical response in allergy is always a result of an exaggerated response of the body's immune system. The degree of response determines the acuteness and severity of the allergic reaction. Allergic responses to a barbiturate, a local anesthetic, and an antibiotic are produced by the same mechanism and may appear similar clinically. Indeed, allergic responses to bananas, shellfish, and bee stings are similar to each other and to those produced by drug allergy. All require the same basic management, whereas overdose reactions to these three agents are quite different clinically and require entirely different modes of treatment.

A third factor to consider when comparing overdose and allergy is the amount or dose of the drug administered. In overdose a dose of the drug or substance must be administered that is sufficient to produce a blood level high enough to produce adverse clinical actions. Overdose reactions are dose related. Allergy, in contrast, is not dose related. In the absence of allergy to penicillin, extremely large doses may be administered safely; yet in the presence of allergy, exposure to even a minute volume (<1mg) could result in the death of the patient. Consider the volume of venom injected into a person by a bee. In acutely allergic individuals clinical death (cardiopulmonary arrest) might be noted within seconds of exposure.

Idiosyncrasy

Idiosyncrasy, or idiosyncratic reactions, may be defined alternatively as "an individual's unique hypersensitivity to a particular drug, food, or other substance"[14]; those "adverse drug reactions that cannot be explained by any known pharmacologic or biochemical mechanism"; or as "any ADR that is neither an overdose nor an allergic reaction." An example of idiosyncratic reaction is CNS stimulation (e.g., excitation, agitation) produced following the administration of a known CNS-depressant agent, such as a barbiturate or antihistamine.

Idiosyncratic reactions cover an extremely wide range of clinical expression. Virtually any type of reaction may be seen; for example, reactions including depression following the administration of a stimulant, stimulation following administration of a depressant, and hyperpyrexia (markedly elevated body temperature) following the administration of a muscle relaxant, such as succinylcholine. It is difficult to predict which persons will experience idiosyncratic reactions or indeed the nature of the resulting reactions.

Management of Idiosyncrasy

Because of the unpredictability of the nature and of the occurrence of idiosyncratic reactions, their management is, of necessity, symptomatic. Of prime importance in the management of these situations are the essentials of basic life support: maintenance of the airway, adequate ventilation, and effective circulation.

If an idiosyncratic reaction presents as seizures, treatment consists of those procedures described in Chapter 21. Prevention of injury and airway management are the primary considerations. Knowledge of the basic steps in the management of the various categories of emergency situations presented in this text will better enable the doctor to successfully treat most idiosyncratic reactions.

It is currently thought that virtually all instances of idiosyncrasy have an underlying genetic mechanism. These genetic aberrations remain undetected until the individual receives a specific drug, such as succinylcholine, which then produces its bizarre (nonpharmacologic) clinical expression (e.g., malignant hyperthermia).

DRUG-RELATED EMERGENCIES

Before discussing the primary drugs used in dentistry and the major adverse reactions associated with each of them, it is important to discuss a factor responsible for more drug-related emergencies than any other. In the preceding discussion of ADRs all responses were related directly to the action of a drug on a biologic system. However, many drug reactions occur in association with the administration of a drug, but are not produced by the action of that drug on the body. Probably the major cause of drug-related emergency situations within the dental office is *the act* of administering local anesthetics. Although it is quite possible for true ADRs to occur in response to the local anesthetic drug, most reactions observed are related to the act of administering the local anesthetic. Psychogenic reactions, clinically vasodepressor syncope and hyperventilation, are the most common forms of drug-related emergency seen in dentistry. Both are often the result of extreme emotional stress produced by the act of giving the local anesthetic injection, not by the local anesthetic itself. Psychogenic reactions may also be observed with the parenteral administration of any drug. Whenever a needle and syringe are involved, the potential for a psychogenic reaction is increased. It is rare to observe a psychogenic reaction with an enterally administered drug.

DRUG USE IN DENTISTRY

Dentistry employs four major categories of drugs in the management of patients to the virtual exclusion of all others. Table 22-1 listed the drug-prescribing habits of faculty and students at the University of Southern California School of Dentistry over a 3-year period. The major categories of prescription drugs used in dentistry include analgesics, antibiotics, and antianxiety drugs. To these categories a fourth, local anesthetics, must be added. Local anesthetics are the most commonly employed drugs, routinely administered whenever a dental procedure appears capable of producing pain.

Examples of commonly prescribed or administered drugs and their potential for adverse drug reactions follow. It is recommended that the reader also consult a textbook on pharmacology when considering the use of any drug.

Local Anesthetics

Local anesthetics, the most widely used drugs in dentistry, have also proved to be among the safest agents available when properly administered. Table 22-3 lists the most commonly used local anesthetics in the United States, Canada, Europe, and Asia today. Lidocaine, mepivacaine, prilocaine, articaine, bupivacaine, and etidocaine are local anesthetics of the amide group, whereas benzocaine, propoxycaine, and procaine are agents of the ester group. Before lidocaine's introduction in the mid-

Table 22-3. Commonly used local anesthetics

Generic name	Proprietary name	Group
Articaine	Ultracaine	Amide
Benzocaine	—	Ester
Bupivacaine	Marcaine	Amide
Etidocaine	Duranest	Amide
Lidocaine	Octocaine, Xylocaine	Amide
Mepivacaine	Carbocaine, Isocaine, Polocaine, Scandanest	Amide
Prilocaine	Citanest	Amide
Procaine	Novocaine	Ester
Propoxycaine	Ravocaine	Ester

1940s, the esters were used exclusively. Although highly effective local anesthetics, the esters possess a significant allergy-producing potential.[15] This potential was one of the reasons for the development and introduction of the amide local anesthetics. Allergy to amide local anesthetics, although not impossible,[16,17] is extremely rare.[18] Reports occasionally appear in the medical and dental literature of allergy to an amide local anesthetic. However, with careful documentation most incidents prove to be psychogenic, overdose, or idiosyncratic reactions, or are the result of an allergy to some other component of the injected solution.[18] A more detailed discussion of local anesthetic allergy is presented in Chapter 24.

The most commonly observed ADRs to amide local anesthetics are those associated with the injection of the drugs; psychogenic responses, such as vasodepressor syncope and hyperventilation, comprise the greatest number of local anesthetic reactions observed today. The next most common cause (but a distant second) of adverse response to local anesthetics is the overdose reaction, which in many instances is produced by a relative overdose (i.e., caused by inadvertent intravascular injection) of the drug rather than by absolute overdose (i.e., caused by injection of too great a total dose).[19] True, documented, reproducible allergy is an extremely rare and unlikely cause of an adverse drug reaction to amide local anesthetics.

Topically applied local anesthetics are also capable of producing adverse reactions. Psychogenic responses are rare with these agents; indeed, topical anesthetics are usually employed to minimize the occurrence of psychogenic responses during the injection of local anesthetics. However, two adverse reactions to topical anesthetics are observed with a disturbing degree of frequency. The first adverse reaction, allergy, results because most topical anesthetics contain local anesthetics of the ester

type (e.g., benzocaine) in addition to a variety of other ingredients (e.g., methylparaben), which possess a relatively high degree of allergenicity. Allergic responses, such as erythema or angioedema of mucous membranes and lips, are not uncommon when these agents are employed. The second adverse reaction from topically applied local anesthetics is the overdose reaction. This reaction is related to the extremely rapid absorption of some of these agents through the mucous membranes of the oral cavity, with a consequent rapid elevation of local anesthetic blood level.[20]

The author strongly advocates the use of topical anesthetics prior to the administration of any local anesthetic by injection. The benefit to be gained by their use clearly outweighs any associated risk. Safer use of these agents may be achieved through the use of topical anesthetics of the amide type and the judicious administration of topical anesthetics to mucous membranes.

Antibiotics

Antibiotics are another frequently prescribed category of drugs in dentistry. They are properly employed in the treatment of an established active infection; they should not be prescribed prophylactically to prevent a possible infection from developing, except in special circumstances such as the prevention of bacterial endocarditis. Because of the potential for development of resistant bacterial strains and of allergy to these antibiotics, they should be used only when a therapeutic indication exists. As a group antibiotics possess a low incidence of adverse effects. This fact has probably been responsible for the current overadministration of these agents with the subsequent development of resistant bacterial strains (e.g., penicillin-resistant gonococcus). There is also increasing unease among medical personnel when administering parenteral antibiotics because of their high allergic potential.

Within the practice of dentistry there is little call for the parenteral administration of antibiotics. Most protocols for the prophylactic administration of antibiotics allow for enteral administration.[21] The blood levels of drugs and therapeutic efficacy should be much the same with both parenterally and orally administered antibiotics if proper attention is paid to dosage and to the sequence of administration. A major advantage of the oral route of administration is the decreased likelihood of adverse reactions. If these reactions should occur following oral administration, it is likely that they will be less acute than those following the parenteral administration of the same drug, although serious reactions can develop in either case.[22] If the parenteral administration of antibiotics, particularly penicillin, is required, the author strongly recommends that the medication *not* be administered in the dental office, but rather that the patient be referred to the emergency department of a nearby hospital where the drug can be administered parenterally and the patient kept under observation for approximately 1 hour. Table 22-4 lists commonly used antibiotics. The major ADR for which the doctor must be prepared when antibiotics are administered is allergy.

Table 22-4. Commonly prescribed antibiotics

Generic name	Proprietary name
Penicillin G	Pentids
	Pfizerpen
Penicillin V	Pen-vee K
	Deltapen-VK
	V-Cillin K
	Ledercillin-VK
	Uticillin-VK
	Betapen-VK
	Penapar-VK
	Robicillin-VK
Ampicillin	Amcill
	D-Amp
	Pfizerpen-A
	Principen
	Omnipen-N
	Polycillin-N
	Totacillin-N
Erythromycin	E-Mycin
	ERYC
	Ery-Tab
	Ilotycin
	Robimycin
	Ilosone
	Erythrocin
	Wyamycin
Clindamycin	Cleocin
	Dalacin-C
Cephalosporin	Keflin
	Seffin
	Keflex
	Novolexin
Amoxicillin	Augmentin
	Larotid
	Polymax
	Robamax
	Sumox
	Trimox
	Utimax
	Wymox

Analgesics

Drugs for the relief of pain comprise a significant portion of prescriptions written by dentists. Two major categories of analgesics are considered: mild analgesics (nonnarcotic) and strong analgesics (narcotics).

Nonsteroidal antiinflammatory drugs (NSAIDS), such as ibuprofen and naproxen, have become extremely popular and are relatively safe medications. Most adverse reactions are related to the gastrointestinal (GI) tract, including GI upset, nausea, and constipation. Also noted are headache, dizziness, and pruritis.[23]

Aspirin, acetaminophen, and codeine remain the most commonly prescribed analgesics in dentistry. The major adverse drug reactions associated with aspirin include a significant potential for allergy, with symptoms ranging from mild urticaria to bronchospasm to fatal anaphylaxis (see Chapter 24) and overdose (salicylism). Acetaminophen is most often associated with CNS depression or excitation, allergy, and overdose.[24]

Codeine is a narcotic agonist analgesic; however, it is a mild analgesic when compared to other opioids such as morphine and meperidine. Although allergy to codeine may occur, its incidence is quite low. The primary ADRs to codeine are nausea, vomiting, drowsiness, and constipation. These effects are more common in ambulatory than in nonambulatory patients.[24] With a 60-mg oral dose, approximately 22% of patients will become nauseated. A significantly lower incidence of nausea is found with smaller doses of codeine (30 mg). Codeine, given to excess or to sensitive patients, may produce the same clinical signs and symptoms of severe overdose as other, more potent narcotics (e.g., respiratory and cardiovascular depression). Thirty milligrams (orally) appears to be a highly effective analgesic dose of codeine and is associated with a minimal incidence of adverse reactions. The most likely ADR to be noted with codeine is GI upset, which is usually a dose-related phenomenon.

Meperidine (Demerol), hydromorphone (Dilaudid), and other narcotic agonists are occasionally employed in dentistry for the management of more intense pain. As with codeine the major ADRs observed are more often annoying than they are life threatening. Nausea and vomiting, dizziness, ataxia, sweating, and orthostatic hypotension are the most frequently noted side effects.[24] These ADRs are more likely to be noted in ambulatory patients, as are most dental patients, than in nonambulatory patients. Overdose may occur and, as with all narcotics, results in respiratory and cardio-

Table 22-5. Common analgesic drugs used in dentistry

Generic name	Proprietary name
Acetylsalicylic acid (aspirin)	Numerous
Acetaminophen	Anacin-3
	Datril
	Tempra
	Tylenol
Ibuprofen	Advil
	Medipren
	Motrin
	Nuprin
	Rufen
Mefenamic acid	Ponstel
Naproxen	Anaprox
	Naprosyn
Meclofenamate	Meclomen

Table 22-6. Common antianxiety/sedative-hypnotics

Generic name	Proprietary name
Barbiturates	
Hexobarbital	Presed
Pentobarbital	Nembutal
Secobarbital	Seconal
Benzodiazepines	
Diazepam	Valium
Oxazepam	Serax
Lorazepam	Ativan
Triazolam	Halcion
Flurazepam	Dalmane
Others	
Chloral hydrate	Cohidrate
	Noctec
Hydroxyzine	Atarax
	Durrax
	Orgatrax
	Vistaril
Promethazine	Ganphen
	Methazine
	Pentazine
	Phenergan
	Provigan
	Sigazine

vascular depression. Allergy, though possible, is rare. Table 22-5 lists commonly prescribed analgesic drugs.

Antianxiety Drugs

The use of drugs for the relief of anxiety during all phases of dental therapy has increased greatly in recent years. Although the enteral routes were almost the exclusive modes of administration in the past and are still very commonly employed today, the parenteral routes of drug administration (e.g., inhalation, intramuscular, and intravenous) have gained popularity. With this trend has come an increased potential for ADRs because of the much greater effectiveness of parenterally administered drugs. Although a wide variety of drugs are available for use for the management of anxiety in dental patients, the most frequently employed agents are barbiturates (administered orally and parenterally), nonbarbiturate antianxiety agents (administered orally and parenterally), and inhalation agents (primarily nitrous oxide and oxygen).

Barbiturates

Barbiturates are the oldest group of antianxiety drugs available, excluding alcohol. Examples of barbiturates prescribed in dentistry are given in Table 22-6. Effective orally and parenterally, the barbiturate sedative-hypnotics were the most frequently prescribed medications in dentistry for the management of fear and anxiety until the introduction of the benzodiazepines in the 1960s. Undesirable side effects are common following barbiturate administration. One of the most annoying side effects of barbiturate administration is the

"hangover" effect, consisting of lassitude, inebriation, and vertigo.[25] Allergy to barbiturates may also occur and represents an absolute contraindication to the use of any barbiturate. Probably the major factor behind the growing disenchantment with barbiturates, however, is their potential for overdose, both accidental and intentional.[26] Prior to the 1980s they were the leading drug cause of suicide. This trend has decreased as the barbiturates were reclassified as schedule II, III, and IV drugs, and as the benzodiazepines grew in popularity.[27] Overdose of barbiturates causes central nervous system depression to the point that respiratory function is depressed and eventually ceases.[28] Cardiovascular and central nervous system collapse follow, leading to death unless basic and advanced life support procedures are initiated immediately.

Nonbarbiturate Antianxiety Agents

Nonbarbiturate antianxiety agents were developed in the hope of managing anxiety effectively without the unpleasant and dangerous drug reactions associated with barbiturates. The major nonbarbiturate antianxiety and sedative-hypnotic agents are listed in Table 22-6.

Table 22-7. Common drugs and most likely adverse drug reactions (ADRs)

Drug	Allergy	Overdose	Side effects
Local anesthetics			
Esters	**Common,** especially with topical anesthetics; manifested as localized erythema and edema	**Unlikely with esters** unless genetic deficiency is present (e.g., atypical pseudocholinesterase)	**Rare;** sedation (drowsiness) most common
Amides	**Rare,** virtually nonexistent; most clinical reports prove alleged allergy to be overdose or allergy to other component of solution	**Most common ADR;** CNS depression; manifested as drowsiness, tremor, tonic-clonic seizures	**Rare;** sedation most common
Antibiotics	**Common;** high allergic potential to many antibiotics; manifested clinically over entire range of allergic phenomena	**Rare;** for penicillin, virtually nonexistent	**Rare;** gastrointestinal upset is most common
Analgesics			
Nonnarcotic	**Common;** high allergic potential (aspirin)	**Common;** salicylism	**Common**
Narcotic	**Uncommon**	**Common;** manifested as CNS depression (drowsiness), respiratory depression	**Most common ADR;** manifested clinically as nausea/vomiting, orthostatic hypotension
Antianxiety agents			
Barbiturates	**Uncommon**	**Most common ADR;** CNS depression; manifested as oversedation, loss of consciousness, respiratory and cardiovascular depression	**Common;** "barbiturate hangover"
Benzodiazepines	**Uncommon**	**Uncommon;** CNS depression; manifested as oversedation	Most common side effect is drowsiness
Nitrous oxide	**Rare,** never reported to date	**Common;** manifested as oversedation	**Most common ADR;** manifested as nausea/vomiting

The benzodiazepines represent a major advance in the management of anxiety; the first benzodiazepine, chlordiazepoxide (Librium), was introduced in 1960. Other benzodiazepines, diazepam (Valium), oxazepam (Serax), and clorazepate (Tranxene) are among the most prescribed drugs in the western world and are among the most effective and most widely used antianxiety agents in dentistry. Benzodiazepines may be administered orally and parenterally (e.g., diazepam, midazolam, lorazepam). Benzodiazepines are a decided improvement over barbiturates because of their remarkably lower incidence of side effects and overdose reactions. Benzodiazepines, probably because of their availability, are involved in more overdoses than any other class of drugs. However, there are extremely few well-documented reports of death solely from the ingestion of benzodiazepine.[29] Overdose to benzodiazepines, even when administered intravenously, usually consists of oversedation, drowsiness, and ataxia. Respiratory depression, although possible, is infrequent. Flurazepam

(Dalmane) and triazolam (Halcion) are benzodiazepines that are marketed as nonbarbiturate sedative-hypnotics. They are highly effective as substitutes for the barbiturates when used as "sleeping pills." Though the long-term administration of triazolam has been criticized, the use of either of these agents for specific indications in dentistry (e.g., for pretreatment sedation both the evening prior to, and the morning of, treatment) is recommended.[30]

Inhalation Sedation

Nitrous oxide and oxygen (N_2O-O_2) inhalation sedation is another method of anxiety control that has garnered increasing interest in the dental profession. Discovered in 1786 and first employed clinically in 1844, nitrous oxide is a highly effective antianxiety agent that, when employed properly, is remarkably free of unpleasant and potentially dangerous adverse reactions. Unwanted side effects from nitrous oxide and oxygen include nausea, vomiting, and oversedation. If inhalation sedation is administered with less than 20% oxygen, unconsciousness may ensue with cellular damage occurring from hypoxia but not from nitrous oxide. With the development of a new generation of inhalation sedation machines and an increasing awareness on the part of dental educators and manufacturers, safety features have been incorporated into current sedation units that make it extremely difficult to administer less than 20% oxygen to a patient receiving nitrous oxide and oxygen.[31]

Allergy to nitrous oxide has never been reported. Overdose consists of oversedation, which may manifest itself as a loss of consciousness. Management of this situation consists of decreasing the percentage of nitrous oxide and increasing the percentage of oxygen and employing the steps of basic life support until the patient regains consciousness.

The most commonly used drug categories in dentistry and their most likely adverse reactions are presented in Table 22-7. It must be remembered that all drugs are capable of producing virtually any of the three adverse reactions—allergy, overdose, and idiosyncrasy.

REFERENCES

1. Department of Pharmacology, University of Southern California School of Dentistry, Los Angeles, 1986.
2. Caranasos GJ, Stewart RB, Cluff LE: Drug-induced illness leading to hospitalization, *JAMA* 228:713, 1974.
3. Caranasos GJ, and others: Drug-associated deaths in hospital inpatients, *Arch Intern Med* 136:872, 1976.
4. Koch-Weser J: Fatal reactions to drug therapy, *N Engl J Med* 291:302, 1974.
5. McKeney JM, Harrison WL: Drug-related hospital admissions, *Am J Hosp Pharm* 33:792, 1976.
6. Caranasos GJ: Drug reactions. In Schwartz GR, Safar P, Stone JH, and others; editors: *Principles and practice of emergency medicine*, Philadelphia, 1978, WB Saunders.
7. Hallas J, Jensen KB, Grodum E, and others: Drug-related admissions to a department of medical gastroenterology: The role of self-medicated and prescribed drugs, *Scand J Gastroenterol* 26(2):174, 1991.
8. Pallasch TJ: *Pharmacology for dental students and practitioners*, Philadelphia, 1980, Lea & Febiger.
9. Forster A, Gardaz JP, Suter PM, and others: Respiratory depression by midazolam and diazepam, *Anesthesiology* 53:494, 1980.
10. Olin BR, editor-in-chief: Facts and Comparisons, St Louis, 1992, Facts and Comparisons.
11. *Physician's Desk Reference, 1991*, Oradell, N.J., 1991, Medical Economics Data.
12. American Medical Association: Drug evaluations annual (1992).
13. Reidenberg MM, Lowenthal DT: Adverse nondrug reactions, *N Engl J Med* 279:678, 1968.
14. *Mosby's Medical & Nursing Dictionary*, St Louis, 1983, Mosby–Year Book.
15. Criep LH, Castilho-Ribeiro C: Allergy to procaine hydrochloride with three fatalities, *JAMA* 151, 1185, 1955.
16. Brown DT, Beamish D, Wildsmith JA: Allergic reaction to an amide local anesthetic, *Br J Anaesth* 53:435, 1981.
17. Bateman PP: Multiple allergies to local anesthetics including prilocaine, *Med J Aust* 2:449, 1974.
18. Aldrete JA, Johnson DA: Allergy to local anesthetics, *JAMA* 207:356, 1969.
19. Adatia AK: Intravascular injection of local anesthetics, *Br Dent J* 138:328, 1975.
20. Adriani J: Reactions to local anesthetics, *JAMA* 196:405, 1955.
21. Dajani AS, Bisno AL, Chung KJ, and others: Prevention of bacterial endocarditis, *JAMA* 264(22):2919, 1990.
22. Gill CJ, Michaelides PL: Dental drugs and anaphylactic reactions: report of a case, *Oral Surg* 50:30, 1980.
23. Anaprox drug package insert, Syntex Puerto Rico, Inc., April 1990.
24. Tylenol with codeine drug package insert, McNeil Pharmaceutical Products, August 1990.
25. Harvey SC: Hypnotics and sedatives: the barbiturates. In Goodman IS and Gilman A, editors: *Pharmacological basis of therapeutics*, ed 6, New York, 1980 Macmillan.
26. Baltarowich LL: Sedative-hypnotics. In Rosen P, Baker FJ, Barkin RM, and others, editors: *Emergency medicine*, ed 2, St. Louis, 1988, Mosby–Year Book.
27. National Institute on Drug Abuse: Data from the Drug Abuse Warning Network, 1980 and 1984, Rockville, Md., U.S. Department of Health and Human Resources.
28. McCarron NM, Schulze BW, Walberg CB, and others: Short-acting barbiturate overdosage, *JAMA* 248:55, 1982.
29. Iserson KV: Tranquilizer overdose. In Rosen P, Baker FJ, Barkin RM, and others, editors: *Emergency medicine*, ed 2, St Louis, 1988, Mosby–Year Book.
30. The dark side of Halcion, *Time Magazine*, October 14, 1991.
31. Council on Dental Materials, Instruments, and Equipment: *Dentists' desk reference materials, instruments, and equipment*, Chicago, 1981, American Dental Association.

23 *Drug Overdose Reactions*

Drug overdose reactions have previously been defined as those clinical signs and symptoms that result from overly high blood levels of a drug in various target organs and tissues. Overdose reactions, also called toxic reactions, are the most common of all adverse drug reactions (ADRs), accounting for up to 85% in some estimates.[1] Overdose reactions represent a direct extension of the normal pharmacologic actions of the involved drug.

For an overdose to occur, the drug in question must gain access to the circulation in quantities sufficient to produce adverse effects on various tissues of the body. Under normal circumstances there is a constant absorption of a drug from its site of administration (e.g., gastrointestinal tract [oral], muscles [IM]) into the circulation, and a steady removal of the same drug from the blood as it undergoes redistribution (e.g., to skeletal muscle) and biotransformation (also known as metabolism and detoxification) in other parts of the body, primarily the liver. In this situation overly high blood levels of drugs seldom occur (Fig. 23-1). However, there are a number of ways in which this steady state may be altered, leading to either a rapid elevation in blood level—producing a sudden onset of signs and symptoms of an overdose reaction—or to a more gradual elevation of a drug's blood level—producing a slower onset of signs and symptoms. In either case an overdose reaction is caused by a blood (plasma) level of a drug sufficiently high to produce adverse effects in various organs and tissues of the body. The reaction will continue only as long as the blood level of the drug remains above the threshold for overdose.

In dentistry there are four commonly employed categories of drugs with significant overdose potential: local anesthetics, vasoconstrictors, such as epinephrine, sedative-hypnotics, and narcotic analgesics. Of these, the local anesthetics are by far the most frequently used drugs. A severe overdose reaction to a local anesthetic usually manifests itself as a generalized tonic-clonic seizure. The most commonly observed overdose reaction to the sedative-hypnotics and to narcotic analgesics is central nervous system and respiratory depression, whereas vasoconstrictor overdose causes an anxiety reaction along with a significant increase in the blood pressure and heart rate.

Because the usual route of administration of these drugs, the nature of the overdose reaction, and the management of the reaction differ so considerably in these groups, the following discussion on overdose will be divided into three sections: overdose reaction from (1) local anesthetics, (2) vasoconstricting drugs, and (3) sedative-hypnotic and narcotic analgesic drugs.

LOCAL ANESTHETIC OVERDOSE REACTION
General Considerations

Local anesthetics are the most commonly employed drugs in dentistry. The number of local anesthetic cartridges injected by dentists in the United States is conservatively estimated at 6 million cartridges per week, or in excess of 300 million per year. In actuality, the numbers probably greatly exceed this figure. In addition, local anesthetics are administered by many physicians and podiatrists. With the administration of this volume of local anesthetics per year, it is quite remarkable that more ADRs attributed to these agents are not reported. In all probability, however, a great many adverse reactions go unreported because they were transitory and innocuous enough to go unrecognized by the doctor, or were not deemed suitable to report. As discussed in Chapter 22, the most commonly observed and reported reactions to local anesthetics are normally labelled allergic reactions by

310

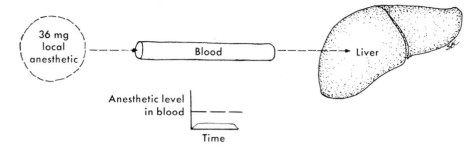

Fig. 23-1. Under normal conditions there is a constant absorption of local anesthetic from the site of deposition into the cardiovascular system and a constant removal of the agent from the blood by the liver. Local anesthetic levels in the blood remain low. (From Malamed SF: *Handbook of local anesthesia*, ed 3, St Louis, 1991, Mosby–Year Book.)

the patient and all too frequently by the doctor also; however, after careful scrutiny most of these are determined to have been either overdose reactions or, more likely, psychogenic responses.[2]

Predisposing Factors

An overdose reaction to a local anesthetic is related to the blood level of local anesthetic occurring in certain tissues and organs following its administration. There are several factors that can have a profound effect on the rate at which this blood level is elevated and the length of time for which it remains elevated. The presence of one or more of these factors predisposes the patient to the development of an overdose reaction. The first group of factors is related to the patient receiving the drug; the second group is related to the drug itself and the area into which it is administered.

Patient Factors

Predisposing patient factors are those that modify the response of an individual to the usual dose of a drug. This is commonly referred to as biologic or individual variation. The normal distribution curve demonstrates this variable response to drugs (Fig. 23-2). For a given dose of a drug, approximately 68% of patients will exhibit the appropriate response; 16% will be less responsive (hyporesponders), and 16% will be overresponsive (hyperresponders). Predisposing patient factors that influence drug responsiveness include age, body weight, the presence of pathology, genetics, mental attitude and environment, and sex.

Age. At either end of the age spectrum, individuals experience a higher incidence of ADRs. There are many reasons for this finding, several of which

are relevant to this discussion. The functions of absorption, metabolism, and excretion of drugs may be imperfectly developed, as in younger age groups, or these functions may be diminished, as in older age groups. Higher blood levels of drugs may occur because of the inability to transform the local anesthetic into an inactive substance, this in turn resulting from underdeveloped or decreased liver function. Or the individual may be unable to excrete the local anesthetic because of renal dysfunction. In patients aged 61 to 71 years, the half-life of lidocaine was increased by approximately 70% over a control group (ages 22 to 26 years).[3] As a general rule of thumb, drug dosages are decreased in patients under the age of 6 years and over the age of 65 years.

Body weight. In general, the greater the lean body weight of the individual (within limits), the greater the dose of a drug that can be tolerated before an overdose occurs. This is primarily related to the greater blood volume in larger, heavier, but nonobese individuals. This relationship does not apply to obese persons because the blood supply to fat is quite sparse compared to that supplying muscle. Therefore, a 200-pound obese patient usually cannot tolerate the same dose of local anesthetic as safely as a 200-pound muscular individual. Because most drugs are distributed evenly throughout the body, the larger the individual, the greater the blood volume, and the lower the blood level of the drug per milliliter of blood. For example, a dose of a local anesthetic administered to a 67.5 kg (150 pound) adult produces a lower blood level than the same dose administered to a 22.5 kg (50 pound) child. Drug doses are normally calculated on the basis of milligrams of drug per kilogram or pound of body weight. Such considera-

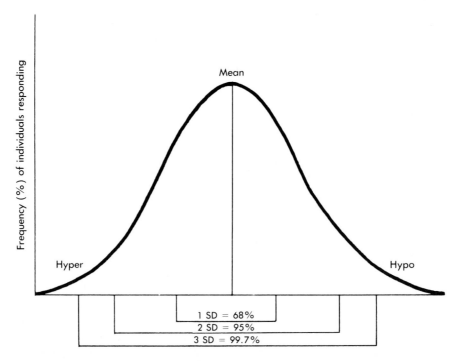

Fig. 23-2. Normal (bell-shaped) distribution curve. For any given drug, approximately 68% of patients experience desirable clinical effects with the usual adult dose; 95% exhibit desirable effects with a slightly lower or higher dose range. A small percentage of patients are hyporesponsive *(right side of curve)*, requiring doses in excess of "normal" before clinically desirable results appear. Of more importance, however, is the small group of hyperresponsive individuals *(left side of curve)*, who exhibit clinically desirable results at lower than normal dose levels. Drug overdose is more likely to develop in these patients. (From Pallasch TJ: *Pharmacology for dental students and practitioners*, Philadelphia, 1980, Lea & Febiger.)

tions are especially important in the pediatric and frail geriatric patient. One of the major factors involved in overdose reactions to local anesthetics in the past was a lack of consideration of this extremely important factor.

Drug dosages that are calculated in terms of milligrams per pound or per kilogram of body weight are based on the reaction of the normal responding patient, which is calculated from the responses of large numbers of patients. Individual patient responses to drug administration, however, may demonstrate significant variation. The normal distribution curve (see Fig. 23-2) illustrates this fact. The usual blood level of lidocaine required to induce seizure activity is 7.5 μg of lidocaine per milliliter of blood (μg/mL) in the brain. Hyporesponding patients may not demonstrate seizures until a significantly higher brain blood level is reached, whereas hyperresponders may exhibit seizures at a brain blood level of lidocaine considerably below 7.5 μg/m.L[4] It is therefore possible to see an overdose reaction to a drug occur even though the dose of drug administered was within the normal range for that patient.

Presence of pathology. The presence of preexisting disease may alter the ability of the body to biotransform a drug into a pharmacologically inactive substance. As is explained in a later section, most local anesthetics are biotransformed in the liver, with a small percentage of the drug excreted unchanged through the kidneys. Any disease state that reduces or increases hepatic blood flow is likely to alter various pharmacokinetic parameters of the amide local anesthetics.[5] However, renal dysfunction appears to have little effect on local anesthetic toxicity.

Patients with cardiovascular disease, especially congestive heart failure, demonstrate blood levels of local anesthetics almost twice those found in healthy patients receiving the same dose.[6,7] This is a result of several factors, including a reduced blood volume for drug distribution and a diminished hepatic blood flow secondary to low cardiac output.

Pulmonary disease states, especially those associated with carbon dioxide retention, lead to an increased risk of local anesthetic overdose. Carbon dioxide retention ($>PaCO_2$) leads to respiratory acidosis, which is accompanied by a decrease in the local anesthetic seizure threshold.[8,9] For lidocaine, an increase in PCO_2 from 25–40 torr to 65–81 torr lowered the convulsive threshold (CD_{100}) for lidocaine by 53%.[8]

Genetics. It has been reported with increasing frequency that certain individuals possess genetic deficiencies that alter their responses to certain drugs. A genetic deficiency in the enzyme serum cholinesterase is an important example. Produced in the liver, this enzyme circulates in the blood and is responsible for the biotransformation of two important drugs: succinylcholine[10] and the ester type of local anesthetics.[11,12]

Succinylcholine is a short-acting neuromuscular blocking agent that is frequently administered during the induction of general anesthesia for production of skeletal muscle relaxation and respiratory arrest during intubation. In normal individuals the action of succinylcholine is approximately 3 minutes, the drug being metabolized by serum cholinesterase. By contrast, in persons with deficient or atypical serum cholinesterase, succinylcholine is biotransformed at an extremely slow rate, with the ensuing period of apnea persisting for prolonged periods of time (up to several hours).[10] This same enzyme is responsible for the biotransformation of the ester local anesthetics (see Table 22-3). In the presence of atypical or deficient serum cholinesterase, the blood level of the ester local anesthetic continues to increase and remains elevated longer, greatly increasing the likelihood of an overdose reaction.[12]

Mental attitude and environment. The psychological attitude of a patient greatly influences the ultimate effect of a drug. This factor is of considerable importance with sedative-hypnotic and narcotic analgesic drugs; what a patient expects a drug to do greatly influences the clinical efficacy of that agent. This expectation of a drug's action is called the placebo response, and used properly, it is of great benefit to the doctor.

With regard to local anesthetics, it has been shown that the local anesthetic convulsive threshold is lowered in patients who are overly stressed (e.g., frightened). In addition, a patient's psychologic attitude will affect his or her response to stimulation. All dental personnel have encountered the apprehensive individual who overreacts to a stimulus, experiencing pain when gentle pressure is applied to tissues.

Sex. Differences between men and women regarding drug distribution, response, and metabolism have been described in animals but are not of major importance in humans. The only instance of sexual difference in the human species occurs in the pregnant woman. During pregnancy, renal function may be altered, leading to the impaired excretion of certain drugs and their accumulation in the blood, resulting in an increased risk of overdose. Although highly unlikely to prove clinically significant, this disturbance of renal function is a potential cause of local anesthetic overdose.

Drug Factors

The second group of predisposing factors in the development of overdose reactions relates to the drugs themselves and to their site of administration. Included are the vasoactivity of the drug, dose, route of administration, speed of administration, vascularity of the injection site, and the presence of vasoconstrictors.

Vasoactivity of drug. Several factors relating to the physicochemical properties of local anesthetics are important in determing whether or not the blood level of an agent following injection will be high or low. These include lipid solubility, protein binding, and vascular activity.

Local anesthetics that are more lipid soluble and more highly protein bound, such as etidocaine and bupivacaine, are retained in the fat and tissues at the site of injection and therefore exhibit a slower net systemic absorption rate compared to lidocaine and mepivacaine. This slower systemic absorption rate is associated with increased margins of safety for these agents. The rate of absorption of local anesthetics also depends on their direct actions on blood vessels at the injection site. All local anesthetics, with the notable exception of cocaine, have vasodilating properties.[13] Bupivacaine and etidocaine produce more vasodilation than do prilocaine, lidocaine, and mepivacaine. Vascular regulation of absorption appears to be a more important factor for the shorter-acting agents such as lidocaine, mepivacaine, and prilocaine, whereas tissue binding is of greater significance for the longer-acting agents, bupivacaine and etidocaine. Table 23-1 compares the lipid solubility, protein binding, and vasodilating properties of commonly used local anesthetics. The greater the degree of vasodilation produced by a local anesthetic, the more rapid its absorption into the circulation.

Dose of drug. For many years it was thought that the concentration of an injected solution was of major importance in determining overdose potential, even though the total milligram dosage re-

Table 23-1. Comparison of physicochemical properties of local anesthetics

	Lipid/ buffer partition coefficient	Protein binding (%)	Relative vasodilating values (lidocaine = 1.0)
Procaine	0.6	5.8	>2.5
Prilocaine	0.8	55	0.5
Mepivacaine	1.0	77	0.8
Lidocaine	2.9	64	1.0
Bupivacaine	28	95	2.5
Etidocaine	141	94	2.5

mained the same. This has been shown to be incorrect. Braid and Scott[14] demonstrated that 3% and 2% solutions of prilocaine yield the same blood level as an equivalent dose of a 1% solution, if the same number of milligrams are administered. Jebson[15] proved the same thing using 10% and 2% lidocaine.

Dosage, on the other hand, is a highly significant factor. Within the clinical dosage range for most local anesthetics, there is a linear relationship between dose and maximal blood concentration. Table 23-2 lists the concentrations of currently available local anesthetics. The larger the dose of local anesthetic injected, the higher the ultimate blood level of the drug will be.

Route of administration. Local anesthetics, when used for the control of pain, produce their clinical actions at the site of injection. Unlike most other drugs, it is not necessary for local anesthetics to enter into the circulation and to reach a certain minimal therapeutic blood level. The greater the length of time a local anesthetic remains in the area where pain control is required and the greater its

Table 23-2. Concentrations of commonly employed local anesthetics

Drug	Group	Available concentrations (%)
Propoxycaine	Ester	0.4 (Available with procaine)
Procaine	Ester	2 (Available with propoxycaine)
Lidocaine	Amide	2
Mepivacaine	Amide	2 (With vasoconstrictor)
		3 (Without vasoconstrictor)
Prilocaine	Amide	4
Bupivacaine	Amide	0.5
Etidocaine	Amide	1.5
Articaine	Amide	4

concentration at that site, the longer the duration of action. As the drug is absorbed into the circulation, it becomes less effective as a pain-controlling agent. When sufficient volume has been removed from the area, painful stimuli may again be felt. At the same time, the more rapidly the local anesthetic is removed from the site of injection, the more rapidly the blood level of the drug increases toward overdose levels.

A frequently noted factor in overdose reactions to local anesthetics is the inadvertent intravascular injection of these drugs. In this instance extremely high blood levels are produced in a brief period of time, producing acute overdose reactions; the peak anesthetic blood level is dependent upon the rate of intravascular administration. Absorption of topical anesthetics through the oral mucous membrane and the absorption of solutions from multiple injection sites are other ways in which overdose may develop. Some forms of topical anesthetic are absorbed quite rapidly through the oral mucous membrane.

Rate of injection. The rate of injection is a very important factor in the cause or prevention of overdose reactions to all drugs. The intravenous injection of a local anesthetic drug may or may not produce signs and symptoms of overdose. Indeed, lidocaine is frequently administered intravenously in doses of 75 mg to 100 mg in the management of several ventricular dysrhythmias. A major deciding factor in whether or not intravascular administration will prove clinically safe or hazardous is the rate at which the drug is administered. A 36-mg dose of lidocaine (one dental cartridge) administered intravenously in less than 15 seconds produces markedly elevated blood levels and the virtual guarantee of an overdose reaction. On the other hand 100 mg of lidocaine administered intravenously over several minutes as recommended in the management of cardiac dysrhythmias, produces a significantly lower blood level of lidocaine (greater distribution and biotransformation having occurred), with a decreased risk of developing an overdose. Fig. 23-3 shows representative blood levels after administration of 30 mg of tetracaine via various routes. The blood levels for the slow and the rapid intravenous administration of tetracaine are especially significant.[16] Many local anesthetic overdose reactions result from the combination of inadvertent intravascular injection and too rapid a rate of injection. Both of these causes are virtually 100% preventable.

Vascularity of injection site. The greater the vascularity of the site of injection, the more rapid is the absorption of a drug from that site into the

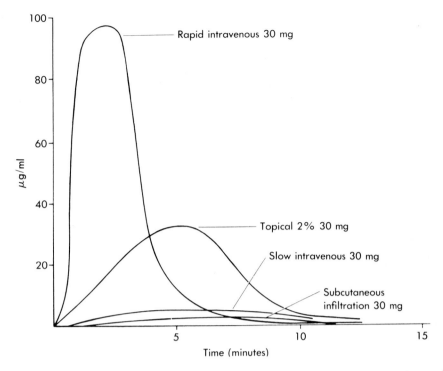

Fig. 23-3. Blood levels of local anesthetic (tetracaine) after administration by various routes. Note particularly the blood levels following rapid and slow intravenous administration. (From Adriani J, Campbell B: *JAMA* 162:1527, 1956.)

circulation. Although this is a desirable situation with most parenterally administered drugs when therapeutic blood levels are required, it is a decided disadvantage in the use of local anesthetics when used for pain control. Local anesthetics must remain in the area of injection in order to block nerve conduction. Unfortunately for the dental profession (at least as far as local anesthetic administration is concerned), the oral cavity is one of the more highly vascular areas of the entire body. A drug injected into the oral cavity can be expected to be absorbed into the blood more rapidly than the same drug injected elsewhere in the body. This factor, plus the inherent vasodilating properties of most local anesthetics, are the major reasons for the addition of vasoconstrictors to most local anesthetics.

Presence of vasoconstrictors. The addition of a vasoconstrictor into a local anesthetic solution results in a decrease in the rate of systemic absorption of the drug. The use of vasoconstrictors, along with proper injection technique, has greatly reduced the clinical toxicity of local anesthetics. The accompanying box summarizes risk factors for local anesthetic overdose.

OVERDOSE—PREDISPOSING FACTORS

Patient factors

Age (under the age of 6; over the age of 65)
Body weight (lower body weight increases risk)
Presence of pathology (e.g., liver disease, congestive heart failure, pulmonary disease)
Genetics (e.g., atypical plasma cholinesterase)
Mental attitude (anxiety decreases seizure threshold)
Sex (very slight increase in risk during pregnancy)

Drug factors

Vasoactivity of drug (vasodilation increases risk)
Dose of drug (higher dose increases risk)
Route of administration (intravascular route increases risk)
Rate of injection (rapid injection increases risk)
Vascularity of injection site (increased vascularity increases risk)
Presence of vasoconstrictor (decreases risk)

Prevention

Almost all overdose reactions to local anesthetics are preventable. Careful evaluation of the patient before the start of treatment and care in the technique of drug administration will minimize the risk of this potentially dangerous situation arising in all but a very few situations. Two sets of predisposing factors were presented in the previous section. The first set, patient factors, are those that cannot be eliminated but which, when present, may require specific modifications in dental care to prevent drug-related problems from developing. The second set of factors are related to the drugs themselves or to their administration. These factors are usually avoidable through proper drug selection and local anesthetic injection technique.

Medical History Questionnaire and Dialogue History

The only questions directly related to the use of local anesthetics are included in the general drug use questions (see Fig. 2-2). The doctor should carefully examine any adverse reaction to a local anesthetic and determine its precise nature. The detailed dialogue history for this type of questioning is presented in Chapter 24.

In the absence of a prior history of adverse reaction to local anesthetics, the patient should be questioned concerning past experiences with dental injections. Questions 2 and 3, relating to prior dental experiences in general, may provide some relevant information in this area. The information gathered from this response is useful in an evaluation of the psychologic status of this patient. A thorough medical history enables the doctor to eliminate two potential causes of local anesthetic overdose: unusually slow biotransformation of the local anesthetic and unusually slow elimination of the drug from the body.

Causes of Overdose Reactions

Before discussing the prevention of local anesthetic overdose, it is relevant to consider various ways in which high blood levels of local anesthetics may arise. Moore[17] has stated that high blood levels of local anesthetics may occur in one or more of the ways listed in the accompanying box. With these factors in mind, we can discuss the methods through which overdose reactions to local anesthetics may be avoided. As with the prevention of most other potentially life-threatening situations, the patient-completed medical history questionnaire is important.

CAUSES OF HIGH BLOOD LEVELS OF LOCAL ANESTHETICS

1. Biotransformation of the drug is unusually slow
2. Drug is slowly eliminated from the body through the kidneys
3. Total dose of local anesthetic administered is too large
4. Absorption of the local anesthetic from the site of injection is unusually rapid
5. Local anesthetic is inadvertently administered intravascularly

From Moore DC: *Complications of regional anesthesia,* Springfield, Ill., 1955, Charles C Thomas.

Biotransformation and elimination. Ester local anesthetics (see Table 22-3) undergo rapid biotransformation in the blood and liver.[18] The major portion of this biotransformation process occurs within the blood through hydrolysis to para-aminobenzoic acid by the enzyme pseudocholinesterase.[18] Patients with a familial history of atypical pseudocholinesterase are unable to detoxify ester-type agents at a normal rate, with the subsequent increased possibility that local anesthetic blood levels will reach overdose levels.[12] Atypical pseudocholinesterase is thought to occur in 1 out of 2820 individuals.[19] The patient with a questionable history should be referred to a physician for diagnostic tests, which may confirm or deny its existence. If atypical pseudocholinesterase is present, administration of ester local anesthetics is relatively contraindicated.

Amide local anesthetics may be administered without increased risk of overdose in these atypical plasma cholinesterase individuals. Amide local anesthetics are biotransformed in the liver by microsomal enzymes.[5] A history of liver disease (e.g., previous or present hepatitis or cirrhosis) does not absolutely contraindicate the use of these agents; however, prior liver disease is an indication that there may be some residual hepatic dysfunction and that the ability of the liver to biotransform amide local anesthetics may be altered to some degree. In an ambulatory patient with a history of liver disease, amide local anesthetics may still be used; however, they should be used judiciously (i.e., there is a relative contraindication to their administration). Minimal volumes should be employed for local anesthesia, bearing in mind that one cartridge may be capable of producing an overdose in this patient if liver function is compromised to a great enough degree. In the author's experience, however, such degrees of compromised liver function are more commonly observed in hospitalized patients than in ambulatory patients. Whenever doubt exists, medical consultation before injection of a local anesthetic is indicated. When a greater degree of liver dysfunction is present, the use of an ester local anesthetic is also relatively contraindicated because the hydrolytic enzyme cholinesterase is produced in the liver, and liver dysfunction may disturb their biotransformation as well.

A small percentage of a local anesthetic dose is eliminated from the blood in its active form through the kidneys. Values for urinary excretion have been cited as 3% for lidocaine,[20] <1% for prilocaine,[21] 1% for mepivacaine,[22] <1% for etidocaine,[23] and <1% for bupivacaine.[24] Renal dysfunction does not usually lead to excessive blood levels of local anesthetics. As with liver dysfunction, however, it may be prudent to limit the dose of anesthetic administered to the absolute minimum required for clinically effective pain control.

The patient requiring renal dialysis also represents a relative contraindication to the administration of large doses of local anesthetic. This patient is ambulatory between dialysis appointments and may come to the dental office for treatment. Undetoxified local anesthetic may accumulate in the blood of this patient, producing signs and symptoms (usually mild) of local anesthetic overdose.

The three remaining methods by which local anesthetic overdose may develop are (1) too large a total dose, (2) rapid absorption of the local anesthetic into the circulation, and (3) inadvertent intravascular injection. Prevention of these is best accomplished through adherence to proper technique of local anesthetic administration, which is reviewed following the discussion of each of these three factors.

Too large a total dose. If given in excess, all drugs are capable of producing signs and symptoms of overdose. The precise milligram dosage at which negative effects are first noted varies and is impossible to predict consistently for all people. The principle of biologic variability greatly influences the manner in which individuals respond to drugs. Most parenterally administered drugs are commonly administered in a dosage form that has been calculated after considering a number of factors, including the age and physical status of the patient. A third consideration in the determination of the maximum drug dosage is the weight of the patient receiving the drug. This factor is especially important in lighter weight patients. As mentioned previously, the larger the individual receiving the drug (within certain limits), the greater the drug distribution will be; therefore the resulting blood level of the drug will be lower and the milligram dosage that may safely be administered will be larger.*

The manufacturers of local anesthetic cartridges for dental use in the past did not indicate maximal dosages based on body weight. Instead, generations of dentists were taught, for example, that the maximal dosage of lidocaine was 300 mg (without epinephrine) or 500 mg (with epinephrine), for any adult patient.[25] Unfortunately, there have been cases in which these maximal dosages proved to be overly excessive for an individual patient's ability to tolerate, leading to morbidity or mortality. Such arbitrary doses for adult patients are meaningless when it is considered that one adult may weigh 200 pounds and another, 100 pounds. According to the old way of thinking, both of these persons were assumed to be capable of tolerating the same dosage of local anesthetic agent without adverse reaction. It becomes obvious that such thinking is erroneous. Distribution of the local anesthetic throughout the circulatory system of a muscular 200-pound adult results in a lower blood concentration than the same drug in a 100-pound adult. With all other potential factors being equal, the smaller adult has a greater risk of overdose than does the larger adult when both are exposed to the same drug dose. The overdose develops when the rate of absorption of the local anesthetic into the cardiovascular system exceeds the rate at which the liver is able to detoxify the agent.

Maximal dosages of local anesthetics should therefore be calculated on a milligram per weight basis (kilogram or pound).[26] Table 23-3 is a compilation of available information on maximal suggested dosages based on the patient's weight for several of the more commonly used dental local anesthetics.

It is highly unlikely that the dosages indicated in Table 23-3 will be reached. Rarely is there an indication for the administration of more than four or five cartridges during most conservative dental treatment. Indeed, it is possible to achieve full

---

*Although generally valid, there are always exceptions to this rule. Biologic variability and pathologic states can dramatically alter responsiveness to drugs; therefore, care must always be exhibited when administering any drug.

Table 23-3. Maximal recommended doses of commonly used local anesthetics*

Patient weight (lb)	Lidocaine 2%, with/without vasoconstrictor; 2.0 mg/lb up to 300 mg max		Mepivacaine 2% or 3%, 2.0 mg/lb up to 300 mg max			Prilocaine 4%, with/without vasoconstrictor; 2.7 mg/lb up to 400 mg max		Articaine (for adults) 4%, with vasoconstrictor; 3.2 mg/lb up to 500 mg max		Articaine (for children) 4%, with vasoconstrictor; 2.3 mg/lb up to 500 mg max	
	Mg	No. of cartridges	Mg	No. of cartridges		Mg	No. of cartridges	Mg	No. of cartridges	Mg	No. of cartridges
				2%	3%						
20	40	1.1	40	1.1	0.8	54	0.75	64	0.9	46	0.6
40	80	2.2	80	2.2	1.5	108	1.5	128	1.8	92	1.3
60	120	3.3	120	3.3	2.0	162	2.25	192	2.7	138	1.9
80	160	4.4	160	4.4	3.0	216	3.0	256	3.6	184	2.5
100	200	5.5†	200	5.5	3.5	270	3.75	320	4.4	230	3.0
120	240	6.5	240	6.5	4.0	324	4.5	384	5.33		
140	280	7.5	280	7.5	5.0	378	5.0	448	6.2		
160	300	8.0	300	8.0	5.5	400	5.5	500	7.0		
180	300	8.0	300	8.0	5.5	400	5.5	500	7.0		
200	300	8.0	300	8.0	5.5	400	5.5	500	7.0		

From Malamed SF: *Handbook of local anesthesia,* ed 3, St Louis, 1991, Mosby–Year Book.
*Doses indicated are for normal healthy patients. Drug doses should be decreased for debilitated or elderly patients.
†0.2 mg epinephrine dose is limiting factor for 1:50,000 epinephrine.

mouth anesthesia (palatal, maxillary, and mandibular) with fewer than six cartridges of local anesthetic. Exceptions to this exist in surgical procedures and in prolonged treatments.

It is suggested that the doctor begin to think in terms of milligrams of local anesthetic injected instead of number of cartridges. It is therefore necessary to review the relationship between percent solution and the number of milligrams contained in that solution.

A 1% solution of a local anesthetic contains 10 mg/mL of solution; a 2% solution contains 20 mg/mL, 3% is 30 mg/mL, 4% is 40 mg/mL, and so on. As a dental cartridge in the USA contains 1.8 mL of solution, the number of milligrams of anesthetic within a cartridge is determined by multiplying the volume of solution (1.8) by the number of milligrams per milliliter of the solution (e.g., 20, for a 2% solution). The result (1.8 × 20 = 36) is the number of milligrams in the dental cartridge. In some countries dental cartridges contain 2.2 mL of anesthetic. A cartridge of a 2% solution would therefore contain 44 mg of anesthetic drug. Table 23-4 summarizes the commonly used local anesthetic concentrations in dental practice and the number of milligrams found in the 1.8-mL dental cartridge.

Rapid absorption of drug into circulation. The addition of various vasoconstricting drugs to local anesthetics has proved to be of great benefit. Not

Table 23-4. Milligrams of local anesthetic per cartridge (1.8 mL) commonly used in dentistry

% concentration	= mg/mL	× 1.8 mL =	Total mg/cartridge
0.4	4		7.2
0.5	5		9
1	10		18
1.5	15		27
2	20		36
3	30		54
4	40		72

only do these agents increase the duration of action of local anesthetics by enabling them to remain at the site of injection for a greater length of time in adequate concentration to produce conduction blockade,[27] but vasoconstrictors also reduce the systemic toxicity of these drugs by retarding their absorption into the cardiovascular system (Table 23-5).[28] Vasoconstricting drugs should be considered an integral component of all local anesthetic solutions whenever depth and duration of anesthesia are important. There are but a few indications in dentistry for the use of a local anesthetic solution without a vasoconstrictor.

The addition of vasoconstrictors to local anesthetic solutions has brought with it another potential problem—overdose. Overdose of vasoconstricting agents has been reported.[29] Because in most

Table 23-5. Effect of vasoconstrictor (epinephrine 1:200,000) on peak local anesthetic level in blood

Local anesthetic	Dose (mg)	Peak level (µg/mL) Without vasoconstrictor	With vasoconstrictor
Mepivacaine	500	4.7	3.0
Lidocaine	400	4.3	3.0
Prilocaine	400	2.8	2.6
Etidocaine	300	1.4	1.3

From Malamed SF: *Handbook of local anesthesia*, ed 3, St Louis, 1991, Mosby–Year Book.

instances the vasoconstrictor in question is epinephrine, the potential reaction cannot be taken lightly. Overdose of vasoconstrictors is discussed more fully later in this chapter.

Clinical experience with vasoconstrictors has led to the use of more and more dilute solutions with equally effective clinical application. Early local anesthetics contained epinephrine concentrations of 1:50,000. Later combinations were produced with 1:80,000 and 1:100,000 concentrations. The most recent additions to the dental local anesthetic armamentarium: prilocaine, etidocaine, bupivacaine, and articaine all contain epinephrine in 1:200,000 concentrations. Mepivacaine is available in some countries in a 1:200,000 epinehrine concentration, and lidocaine with a 1:200,000 epinephrine concentration has recently become available in dental cartridges. Safety of a drug is increased with the use of the minimal effective concentration of both the local anesthetic and the vasoconstrictor.

Rapid uptake of local anesthetics may also arise following their topical application to the oral mucous membranes. As indicated in Fig. 23-3, absorption of some local anesthetics into the circulation following topical application is quite rapid, being exceeded only by direct intravenous injection.[16] Another important factor in increasing the overdose potential of topically applied local anesthetics is the need for them to be administered in a concentration that is greater than the injectable form of the same drug. This increased concentration is necessary in order to produce adequate anesthesia of the mucous membranes. For example, injectable lidocaine is effective as a 2% solution, whereas lidocaine for topical application is used in a 5% or 10% concentration. It is readily apparent that the injudicious use of topical anesthetics may readily produce signs and symptoms of local anesthetic overdose. Other local anesthetics commonly employed as topical anesthetics include benzocaine and tetracaine. Both of these agents are

esters and as such, are rapidly detoxified by plasma pseudocholinesterase. Tetracaine is rather rapidly absorbed from mucous membranes, whereas benzocaine is very poorly absorbed.[16] Overdose reactions to benzocaine are virtually unknown.[30] Tetracaine, on the other hand, has a significant toxicity potential and must therefore be employed judiciously. In addition, as esters, both of these agents are more likely to produce allergic reactions and localized tissue reaction (irritation) than are the amides.

Topical anesthetics are important components in the management of pain and anxiety. In spite of their low potential for adverse reactions, it is common practice to apply topical anesthetics to the site of needle penetration before any intraoral injection. When used in small localized areas, there is little chance of significant blood levels developing; however, it is not uncommon to find topical anesthetics applied over large areas (quadrants or whole arches) before soft tissue procedures such as scaling and curettage, when injections of local anesthetics are not planned. When used in this manner, significant blood levels are likely to be reached, with a greater likelihood of clinical overdose developing, particularly if this topical application is followed later by injection of local anesthetics.

The preceding comments must not be taken as a recommendation against the use of topical anesthetics. Indeed, it is the author's feeling that topical anesthetics form an extremely important part of every local anesthetic procedure. However, the dentist and dental hygienist must be aware of the potential complications so that they may be avoided. The following suggestions are offered for the use of topical anesthetics.

1. Amide type topical anesthetics should be employed whenever possible.

COMMENT. Although overdose potential exists for all local anesthetics, other adverse reactions (e.g., local tissue reaction and allergy) are more frequently observed with the ester-type topical anesthetics.

2. Area of application should be small.

COMMENT. There are only rare cases in which application of topical anesthetics to a full quadrant is indicated. Application of topical anesthetics to a full quadrant requires large quantities of the drug and results in an increase in the likelihood of overdose. It is the author's feeling that whenever larger areas (e.g., three or more teeth) require soft tissue anesthesia, injection of a local anesthetic should be considered.

3. Measured dosage forms of topical anesthetics should be used.

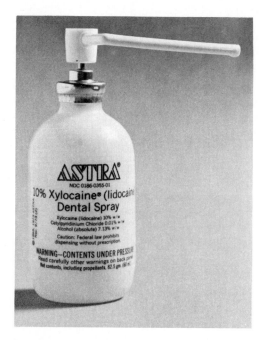

Fig. 23-4. Topical anesthetic spray with metered applicator. Depression of nozzle releases a 10-mg dosage of lidocaine.

COMMENT. Local anesthetics in the form of ointments and especially sprays are difficult to monitor as they are being applied. Overdose may be produced inadvertently with these devices. A spray form of an amide anesthetic (e.g., lidocaine 10%) is available that delivers a metered dose of 10 mg with each application (Fig. 23-4).[31]

Intravascular injection. Intravascular injection may occur with any intraoral injection but is much more likely to occur in certain anatomic areas. Table 23-6 lists the percentage of positive aspiration for various intraoral injections. Nerve block techniques usually possess the greatest potential for intravascular injection: 11% of aspiration tests in inferior alveolar nerve blocks, 5% of mental nerve

Table 23-6. Percentage of positive aspiration for various intraoral injections

Injection	*% positive aspiration*
Inferior alveolar block	11.7
Mental block	5.7
Posterior superior alveolar block	3.1
Anterior superior alveolar block	0.7
(Long) buccal block	0.5

From Barlett SZ: Clinical observations on the effects of injections of local anesthetics preceded by aspiration, *Oral Surg* 33:520, 1972.

blocks, and 3% posterior superior alveolar nerve blocks were positive, indicating that the needle bevel was lying within the lumen of a blood vessel (vein or artery).[32]

Both intravenous and intraarterial administration may produce overdose reactions. It had previously been thought that only intravenous injection of a local anesthetic was capable of producing an overdose reaction and that intraarterial injection would not lead to elevated blood levels, because arterial blood travels distally from the heart, not toward the heart as does venous blood. Aldrete[33,34] demonstrated that intraarterial administration of local anesthetics may produce an overdose as rapidly as, or more rapidly than, an intravenous injection. The mechanism of this reaction is a reversal of blood flow within the artery as the local anesthetic is injected rapidly. Such a mechanism during an inferior alveolar nerve block would entail the blood flowing in a retrograde fashion from the inferior alveolar artery to the internal maxillary artery, back to the external carotid, then to the common carotid, and finally to the internal carotid and the brain, a distance of only several inches.

Intravascular injection of local anesthetics in the practice of dentistry should almost never occur. With careful injection technique and a knowledge of the anatomy of the area to be anesthetized, the occurrence of overdose from an inadvertent intravascular injection will be minimal. Procedures necessary to prevent this complication include use of an aspirating syringe, use of a needle no smaller than 27 gauge, aspiration in at least two planes before injection, and the slow administration of the local anesthetic.

Recommending the use of an aspirating syringe for all injections would appear to be unnecessary because all dental schools teach its use to their students. However, in a survey on the injection techniques of practicing dentists, 21% of those surveyed stated that they employ nonaspirating syringes.[35] There is no justification for the use of such devices for any local anesthetic injection, because it is impossible to aspirate in order to determine the location of the needle bevel with these nonaspirating syringes.

Needle gauge is an important factor in determining whether or not a needle is within a vessel before injection. The needles most commonly available are 25, 27, and 30 gauge, with the 27 gauge being the most frequently used.[35] Needle gauge is of importance in several respects during local anesthetic injection. Accuracy in injection technique is one critical point. For a local anesthetic to control pain, it must be deposited near the nerve. As a

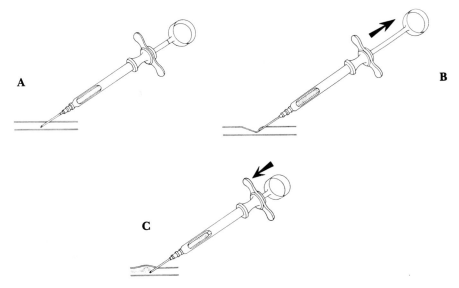

Fig. 23-5. Intravascular injection of local anesthetic. **A,** Needle is inserted in lumen of blood vessel. **B,** Aspiration test is performed. Negative pressure pulls vessel wall against bevel of needle; therefore no blood enters syringe (negative aspiration). **C,** Drug is injected. Positive pressure on plunger of syringe forces local anesthetic solution out through needle. Wall of vessel is forced away from bevel, and anesthetic solution is deposited directly into lumen of blood vessel.

needle is passed through tissue toward the target nerve, it is deflected to varying degrees. The extent of deflection has been tested and is related to the caliber or gauge of the needle. Needles with greater rigidity (i.e., larger gauge) were shown to deflect less when passed through tissues to the depth required for an inferior alveolar nerve block.[36] The second critical point relating to needle gauge concerns reliability of aspiration. In other words, if a needle is located within the lumen of a vessel, will aspiration tests always prove positive? Several studies have demonstrated that it is not possible to aspirate consistently with a needle gauge smaller than 25.[37-38] More recently, Trapp and Davies[39] reported that in vivo human blood may be aspirated through 23-, 25-, 27-, and 30-gauge needles without a clinically significant difference in resistance to flow. Small-gauge needles are occluded more readily with tissue plugs or with the wall of the vessel than are larger needles, leading to false-negative aspirations. For injection techniques that have a greater likelihood of positive aspiration, a 23- or 25-gauge needle should always be employed. These techniques include all block injections, especially the inferior alveolar nerve block. Unfortunately, the majority of practicing dentists surveyed use the 27-gauge needle for the inferior alveolar nerve block (64% use the 27-gauge needle; 34%, the 25-gauge needle).[35]

The method by which aspiration is carried out is yet another factor of importance in preventing intravascular injection. All local anesthetic needles have a bevel at the needle tip (Fig. 23-5, *A*). It is entirely possible for the bevel of the needle to be lying against the inner wall of a blood vessel. When negative pressure is created in the aspirating syringe (harpoon type or self-aspirating), the wall of the vessel may be sucked up against the bevel of the needle, preventing entry of blood into the needle and cartridge (Fig. 23-5, *B*). Clinically, the absence of blood return is interpreted as a negative aspiration and the injection of the anesthetic solution follows. Injection of the local anesthetic requires a positive pressure to be placed on the thumb ring in order to expel the local anesthetic from the cartridge through the needle and out into the tissues. However, in the case where the bevel of the needle is lying against the vessel wall, the positive pressure of the anesthetic solution pushes the vessel wall away from the needle bevel, and the local anesthetic solution is then deposited intravascularly (Fig. 23-5, *C*). A single aspiration test may therefore be inadequate to prevent intravascular injection. It is recommended that two or even three aspiration tests be made before and during injection of the drug. Each of these aspiration tests should be made with the bevel of the needle in a different position. To accomplish this, the hand holding the syringe must be turned approximately 45° to reorient the bevel of the needle relative to the wall of the vessel. Return of blood into the dental cartridge is considered a positive aspiration and mandates repositioning of the needle and reaspiration, with a negative result, before the administration of the local anesthetic. Only 60% of the dentists surveyed indicated they always aspirate before mandibular block, 25% said they rarely aspirate, and 15% said they never aspirate.[35]

The last factor related to prevention of overdose from intravascular injection concerns the rate of injection of the local anesthetic solution. Rapid intravascular injection of a dental cartridge (1.8 mL) of a 2% local anesthetic solution (36 mg) produces blood levels of anesthetic greatly in excess of those required for overdose. In addition, the elevation in blood level occurs rapidly so that the onset of signs and symptoms is immediate. Rapid injection may be defined as the administration of the contents of a dental cartridge in 30 seconds or less. The same quantity of solution injected intravascularly more slowly (60 seconds minimum) produces blood levels below the minimum for overdose (see slow intravenous, Fig 23-3).[16] In the event that the ensuing anesthetic blood level does exceed this minimal, the onset of the reaction is slower, with signs and symptoms less severe than those observed following rapid injection.

Slow injection of drugs is perhaps the most important factor in prevention of all adverse drug reactions. It is difficult to inject a drug too slowly, but it is quite easy to inject too rapidly. It is recommended that the administration of one full 1.8-mL cartridge of local anesthetic take a minimum of 60 seconds.[26] Such efforts significantly reduce the chance of an overdose reaction from intravascular injection. Of doctors surveyed, 46% administered a full cartridge of solution for the inferior alveolar nerve block in fewer than 30 seconds. Only 15% responded that they took 60 seconds or longer for the same injection.[35]

Technique of Local Anesthetic Administration

Overdose reactions, and indeed all ADRs related to local anesthesia, may be minimized through the proper administration of local anesthetics, described as follows:

1. Preliminary medical evaluation should be completed before local anesthetic administration.
2. Anxiety, fear, and apprehension should be managed before injecting a local anesthetic.
3. Dental injections should be administered whenever possible with the patient placed in

a supine or semisupine position. Patients should not receive local anesthetic injections while in an upright position unless absolutely necessary, as in severe cardiorespiratory disease.

4. Topical anesthetics should be applied to the site of needle penetration before all injections.
5. The weakest effective concentration of local anesthetic solution should be injected in the smallest volume compatible with successful anesthesia.
6. The anesthetic solution selected should be appropriate for the patient and for the planned dental treatment (e.g., duration of effect).
7. Vasoconstrictors should be included in all local anesthetics if not specifically contraindicated.
8. Aspirating syringes must always be employed for all injections.
9. Needles should be disposable, sharp, rigid, capable of reliable aspiration, and of adequate length for the contemplated injection techniques. Most block techniques require the use of long (1⅝-inch) 25-gauge needles. Short, 27-gauge needles may be used for other injection techniques.*
10. Aspiration should be carried out in at least two planes before injection.
11. Injection should be made slowly, with a minimum of 60 seconds being spent for each 1.8-mL dental cartridge.
12. The patient should remain under observation following all local anesthetic injections. A member of the dental office staff who is trained in the recognition of life-threatening situations should remain with the patient following the administration of the anesthetic. Not all local anesthetic overdose reactions occur immediately following the injection; many occur 5 or more minutes later. All too often, incidents are reported in which the doctor returns to the treatment room only to find the patient in the throes of a life-threatening adverse drug reaction. Continuous observation of the patient following drug administration permits prompt recognition and management of the situation with a greater probability of complete recovery.

---

*Variations may exist in needle selection for some regional nerve blocks. Textbooks on local anesthesia should be consulted for specific information.

Table 23-7. Comparison of forms of local anesthetic overdose

	Rapid intravascular	*Too large a total dose*	*Rapid absorption*	*Slow biotrans-formation*	*Slow elimination*
Likelihood of occurrence	Common	Most common	Likely with "high normal" dosages if no vasoconstrictors are used	Uncommon	Least common
Onset of signs and symptoms	Most rapid (seconds); intraarterial faster than intravenous	3-5 minutes	3-5 minutes	10-30 minutes	10 minutes to several hours
Intensity of signs and symptoms	Usually most intense	Gradual onset with increased intensity; may prove quite severe		Gradual onset with slow increase in intensity of symptoms	
Duration of signs and symptoms	2-3 minutes	Usually 5 to 30 minutes; depends on dose and ability to metabolize or excrete		Potentially longest duration because of inability to metabolize or excrete agents	
Primary prevention	Aspirate, slow injection	Administer minimal doses	Use vasoconstrictor; limit topical anesthetic use or use nonabsorbed type (base)	Adequate pretreatment physical evaluation of patient	
Drug groups	Amides and esters	Amides; esters only rarely	Amides; esters only rarely	Amides and esters	Amides and esters

Clinical Manifestations

Signs and symptoms of overdose will appear whenever the blood level of the local anesthetic in an organ, such as the brain, rises to the critical level at which adverse effects of the drug develop. The brain responds to the concentration of local anesthetic delivered to it by the circulatory system regardless of the manner in which the local anesthetic initially entered the blood. The blood or plasma level of local anesthetic dictates the degree of severity and the duration of the response. The rate of onset of signs and symptoms corresponds to the blood level. There is a considerable difference in the rate of onset noted among the various causes of local anesthetic overdose.

Onset, Intensity, and Duration

Rapid intravascular injection produces clinical signs and symptoms of overdose within seconds. The intensity of the reaction is normally greater following rapid intravascular injection, with unconsciousness and seizures appearing almost immediately. The duration of this form of overdose reaction, assuming adequate management, is usually more brief than other forms because of redistribution and continued biotransformation of the local anesthetic by the liver or serum cholinesterase while the reaction continues. This form of anesthetic overdose reaction is usually self-limiting and

may occur with all types of local anesthetics. Table 23-7 compares the different forms of local anesthetic overdose reaction.

Signs and symptoms of local anesthetic overdose from too large a total dose or from unusually rapid absorption of the agent into the cardiovascular system do not occur as rapidly as those from intravascular injection. In these two situations, signs and symptoms usually appear approximately 3 to 5 minutes after the administration of the drug and are initially of mild intensity. These may appear as a noticeable agitation of the patient, with an increase in intensity and progression of symptoms over the next few minutes or longer, if the blood level continues to rise. Clinically, the severity of these reactions may be as great as those witnessed in direct intravascular injection or they may not progress beyond a mild reaction. These reactions are also self-limiting because of the continued redistribution and biotransformation of the local anesthetic, but they tend to last significantly longer than the intravascular variety.

Unusually slow biotransformation or elimination of local anesthetics produces an even slower onset of clinical signs and symptoms. In two cases the author has witnessed, the patients obtained adequate mandibular anesthesia and were undergoing restorative procedures for a period of time (15 and 25 minutes, respectively) before any clinical manifestations were noted. These included mild tremor, which progressed slowly to a mild convulsion over the next half hour. Because of patient inability to rid the body of the local anesthetic, these forms of overdose have the potential to persist for long periods of time.

Signs and Symptoms

Local anesthetics produce depression of excitable membranes. The cardiovascular and, in particular, the central nervous systems are especially sensitive to these agents. The usual clinical expression of local anesthetic overdose is one of apparent stimulation followed by a period of depression.

Minimal to moderate blood levels. The initial signs of central nervous system overdose are usually excitatory. At low overdose blood levels the patient usually becomes confused, talkative, apprehensive, and excited; speech may be slurred. A generalized stuttering follows, which may lead to muscular twitching and tremor, commonly observed in the muscles of the face and in the distal parts of the extremities. Nystagmus may also be present. Blood pressure, heart rate, and respiratory rate are elevated.[40]

Symptoms of overdose may include headache. In addition, a generalized feeling of lightheadedness and dizziness is usually reported first (the lightheadedness described as being different from that produced by alcohol), leading to visual and auditory disturbances (e.g., difficulty in focusing, blurred vision, and ringing in the ears [tinnitus]). Numbness of the tongue and perioral tissues commonly develops, as does a feeling of either being flushed or chilled. As the reaction progresses and if the anesthetic blood level rises, drowsiness and disorientation occur, which may culminate in the loss of consciousness. The signs and symptoms of mild local anesthetic overdose may resemble psychomotor or temporal lobe epilepsy (see Chapter 21).

Moderate to high blood levels. As the local anesthetic blood level continues to rise, the clinical manifestations of the overdose reaction progress to a generalized convulsive state with tonic-clonic seizures. Following this phase of stimulation, there is an ensuing period of generalized central nervous system depression, characteristically of a degree of severity related to the degree of stimulation that preceded it. Therefore, it the patient underwent intensive tonic-clonic seizures, the postictal period of depression will be more profound, with probable unconsciousness, respiratory depression, and possible respiratory arrest. If the stimulatory phase was mild (e.g., talkativeness, agitation), the depressant phase will be milder, with perhaps a period of disorientation and lethargy as the only clinically observable signs. Blood pressure, heart rate, and respiratory rate are usually depressed during this phase of the local anesthetic overdose reaction, again to a degree proportionate to the degree of stimulation noted earlier. Table 23-8 summarizes clinical signs and symptoms.

Although the sequence just described is the usual sequence of clinical signs and symptoms of local anesthetic overdose, it is also possible for the excitatory phase of the reaction to be extremely brief or to not occur at all. This is true especially with lidocaine and mepivacaine, with which overdose

Table 23-8. Clinical manifestations of local anesthetic overdose

Signs	*Symptoms*
Low to moderate overdose levels	
Confusion	Headache
Talkativeness	Lightheadedness
Apprehension	Dizziness
Excitedness	Blurred vision, unable to focus
Slurred speech	Ringing in ears
Generalized stutter	Numbness of tongue and perioral tissues
Muscular twitching and tremor of face and extremities	Flushed or chilled feeling
Nystagmus	Drowsiness
Elevated blood pressure	Disorientation
Elevated heart rate	Loss of consciousness
Elevated respiratory rate	
Moderate to high blood levels	
Generalized tonic-clonic seizure, followed by:	
Generalized CNS depression	
Depressed blood pressure, heart rate, and respiratory rate	

may appear initially as drowsiness and nystagmus, leading directly to either unconsciousness or to generalized tonic-clonic seizure activity.[41] Etidocaine and bupivacaine do not cause drowsiness before seizures[42]; progression from the preseizure state of alertness to seizures is much more abrupt. The overdose reaction continues until the blood level of the local anesthetic falls below the minimal blood level for overdose or until the reaction is terminated through appropriate management, including possible drug therapy.

Pathophysiology

Local anesthetic overdose is produced by an overly high blood level of the drug in various organs and tissues. In instances in which the entry of the local anesthetic into the blood exceeds its rate of removal, overdose blood levels may be reached. The period of time required for clinical signs and symptoms to appear varies considerably with the cause of the elevated blood level.

Drugs do not merely affect a single organ or tissue, and all drugs have multiple actions. Local anesthetics are typical of all drugs in this regard. Though the primary pharmacological action of local anesthetics is the inhibition of the excitation conduction process in peripheral nerves, the ability of these drugs to stabilize membranes is not limited solely to peripheral nerves. Any excitable membranes, such as those that exist in the heart, brain, and neuromuscular junction, will be altered by local anesthetics if they achieve a sufficient tissue concentration.[43] In the following discussion both the desirable and the undesirable systemic actions of local anesthetics are discussed.

The term *blood* or *plasma level* refers to the amount of a drug that, following its administration, is absorbed into the circulation and transported in the blood plasma throughout the body. A sample of blood drawn from the patient may be analyzed to determine the amount of local anesthetic present per milliliter of blood. This is commonly referred to as the blood level or plasma level of a local anesthetic. Blood levels of drugs are measured in micrograms (μg) per milliliter (1000 μg = 1 mg).

An additional factor to consider when discussing blood levels of drugs is that, although ranges are mentioned for various systemic actions, patients will vary in their responses to drugs. Even though seizure activity may occur at a blood level of 7.5 μg/mL of lidocaine for most individuals, others may exhibit seizures at lower blood levels, whereas still others may tolerate blood levels that are greatly in excess of those listed without eliciting an adverse response. A second factor to consider is that different local anesthetics have different threshold

Table 23-9. Overdose thresholds

Agent	Usual threshold for CNS signs and symptoms
Bupivacaine, etidocaine	1-2 μg/mL
Prilocaine	4 μg/mL
Lidocaine, mepivacaine	5 μg/mL

levels at which the signs and symptoms of overdose usually appear (Table 23-9). It is not true that agents associated with higher plasma levels for overdose are less toxic, because these agents are usually less potent as local anesthetics and must therefore be injected at higher concentrations. For example, the ratio of CNS toxicity of bupivacaine, etidocaine, and lidocaine is approximately 4:2:1, which is similar to the relative potency of these drugs for the production of regional anesthesia in humans.[44]

Local Anesthetic Blood Levels

Following the intraoral injection of local anesthetics in the recommended manner, the drug slowly enters the blood. Circulating blood levels of lidocaine have been recorded following these injections and form the basis of the following discussion (Fig. 23-6). Blood levels of other anesthetic agents will differ from those reported for lidocaine. In studies published by Cannell and others,[45] it was demonstrated that following the administration of 40 to 160 mg of lidocaine by intraoral injection, the blood level rose to a maximum of approximately 1.0 μg/mL. No adverse reactions were reported at those levels.

As the blood level of lidocaine increases, systemic actions are noted, some of which have considerable therapeutic value. When a blood level of 4.5 to 7.0 μg/mL is reached, definite signs of CNS irritability are noted. With an increase to 7.5 μg/mL or greater, seizure activity is present, whereas above a level of 10 μg/mL, marked CNS depression is noted. Also noted at overdose levels are adverse actions on the cardiovascular system. Most adverse effects on the cardiovascular system do not develop until high overdose levels for the CNS have been reached. Fig. 23-3 shows the effect of the various routes of administration on the blood level of the anesthetic.

Systemic Activity of Local Anesthetics

Local anesthetic agents can inhibit the function of any excitable membrane. In the practice of dentistry these agents are normally applied to a very specific region of the body where they produce their primary function: reversible blockade or depression of peripheral nerve conduction. Other

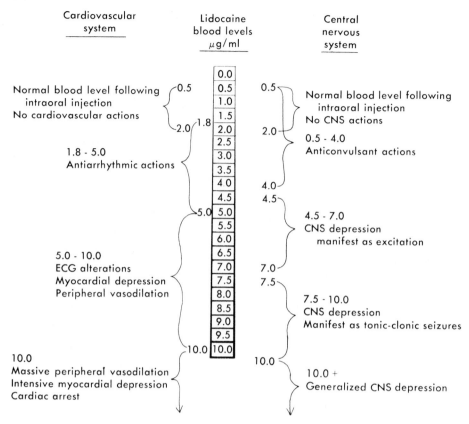

Fig. 23-6. Local anesthetic blood levels and actions on cardiovascular and central nervous systems.

actions of local anesthetics are related to the absorption of the drugs into the circulation and their systemic activities on various excitable membranes, including smooth muscle, the myocardium, and the central nervous system.

Although high blood levels of local anesthetics produce undesirable systemic responses, at non-overdose levels some desirable actions may be observed.

Cardiovascular action. Local anesthetics, particularly lidocaine, are frequently employed in the management of ventricular dysrhythmias, especially ventricular extrasystoles and ventricular tachycardia.[46] Considerable data are available today that illustrate the alterations occurring in the myocardium with increasing blood levels of lidocaine.[47,48]

It is generally considered that the minimal effective blood level of lidocaine for antidysrhythmic activity is 1.8 μg/mL.[46] In the range from approximately 2 to 5 μg/mL, the actions of lidocaine on the myocardium include electrophysiologic changes only. These include prolongation or abolition of the phase of slow depolarization during diastole in Purkinje fibers and a shortening of the

action potential duration and of the effective refractory period. At this therapeutic level no alterations in myocardial contractility, diastolic volume, intraventricular pressure, or cardiac output are observed.[43,49] The healthy as well as the diseased myocardium is well able to tolerate mildly elevated blood levels of local anesthetic without deleterious effect. When used to correct dysrhythmias, lidocaine is administered intravenously in a 50- to 100-mg bolus (1 mg/kg).[46] Overdose is a potential problem at this time, but the benefit-to-risk ratio allows for the judicious use of lidocaine. Increase of the lidocaine blood level to higher levels (5 to 10 μg/mL) produces a prolongation of conduction time through various portions of the heart, as well as an increase in diastolic threshold. This may be noted on the electrocardiogram (ECG) as an increased P-R interval and QRS duration, and sinus bradycardia. Along with this are noted decreased myocardial contractility, increased diastolic volume, decreased intraventricular pressure, and decreased cardiac output.[48,50] Peripheral vascular effects observed at this level include vasodilation, which produces a fall in the blood pressure. This occurs as a result of the direct relaxant effect of the agent on the peripheral vascular smooth muscle.[50]

Further increase in blood levels (>10 μg/mL of lidocaine) leads to an accentuation of the aforementioned electrophysiologic and hemodynamic effects, particularly a massive peripheral vasodilation, marked reduction in myocardial contractility, and a slowed heart rate, which may ultimately result in cardiac arrest.[48,50]

Central nervous system actions. The central nervous system is extremely sensitive to the actions of local anesthetics.[51] As cerebral blood levels of local anesthetics increase, clinical signs and symptoms are noted. Local anesthetics readily cross the blood-brain barrier, producing a depressant effect on central nervous system function.[43] At nonoverdose levels of lidocaine (<5 μg/mL) there are no clinical signs of adverse effects on the CNS; however, a CNS-depressant action that has certain therapeutic usefulness is observed. With blood levels between 0.5 and 4.0 μg/mL, lidocaine is able to terminate various forms of seizure.[52,53] Most clinically useful local anesthetic agents possess this anticonvulsant property (both procaine and lidocaine have been used to terminate or to decrease the duration of grand mal or petit mal seizures). The mechanism of this anticonvulsant action is thought to be a depression of hyperexcitable cortical neurons present in epileptic patients.

With an increase in the blood level above 4.5 μg/mL, initial signs and symptoms of CNS alteration appear. These are usually related to increased cortical irritability (e.g., agitation, talkativeness, and tremor). The symptom of numbness of the tongue and perioral tissues is thought to result from the rich blood supply to these tissues, allowing the drugs to produce blockade of the nerve endings.[49] With a further increase in the blood level to 7.5 μg/mL or greater of lidocaine, generalized tonic-clonic seizures occur. Following this period of CNS stimulation, a further increase in the blood level of the local anesthetic results in termination of seizure activity and an electroencephalographic pattern consistent with generalized CNS depression.[49] Respiratory depression and arrest are manifestations of this further depression.

It seems contradictory to state that local anesthetics are CNS depressants on the one hand, and then to claim that CNS stimulation is the first clinical manifestation of this CNS depression. This may be explained as follows: The stimulation and subsequent depression produced by high blood levels of local anesthetics result solely from depression of neuronal activity. The cerebral cortex receives both inhibitory and facilitory or stimulatory impulses. If it is considered that these two groups of neurons

are selectively depressed by different blood levels of local anesthetics, this seeming contradiction is explained. At anesthetic blood levels capable of producing seizures, the inhibitory pathways in the cerebral cortex are depressed, but the facilitory pathways are not. This depression of the inhibitory pathways permits the facilitory neurons to function unopposed, leading to an increased excitation of the CNS and ultimately to seizures.[54] With a further increase in the local anesthetic blood level, the facilitory neurons are depressed along with the inhibitory neurons, producing a state of generalized CNS depression. It must be noted here that the duration of the seizure, although primarily dependent on local anesthetic blood level, can be further modified by the acid-base status of the patient. The higher the arterial carbon dioxide tension ($Paco_2$), the lower the local anesthetic blood level required to precipitate generalized seizures. In contrast, the lower the $Paco_2$, the greater the drug blood level required to produce seizures.[8] Lowering a patient's $Paco_2$ through hyperventilation raises the cortical seizure threshold to local anesthetics and lessens the chance that a drug will cause seizures.

Drug-induced seizures, in and of themselves, are not necessarily fatal. However, the mortality rate in untreated animals is over 60%.[55] It appears that the duration of the seizure is a critical factor in determining the degree of morbidity. The convulsing brain requires greatly elevated oxygen and glucose levels to continue functioning. To a degree, the body's own mechanisms can compensate for this; however, respiratory and circulatory support can greatly enhance the chances of survival. As cardiovascular depression is produced by even more elevated blood levels of the local anesthetic and respirations are increasingly impaired by uncoordinated muscle spasm during the seizure, brain function will be affected even more through reduced cerebral blood flow and hypoxia.[56] Fig. 23-6 summarizes the clinical effects of local anesthetics seen with increasing blood levels.

Management

Management of a local anesthetic overdose is based on the severity of the reaction. In most cases the reaction will be mild and transitory, requiring little or no specific treatment. However, when the reaction is more severe and of longer duration, prompt management is necessary. Most local anesthetic overdoses are self-limiting. The blood level of the local anesthetic decreases as the reaction progresses because of the redistribution and biotransformation of the drug. It is a rare occasion indeed that drugs other than oxygen need to be administered to terminate a local anesthetic overdose. Overtreatment of local anesthetic overdose is a potential problem. In the rush of excitement that follows this unexpected reaction, emergency drugs, such as anticonvulsants, may be administered too freely. All anticonvulsants are CNS depressants and can delay recovery of consciousness.

The time for aggressive intravenous management of the local anesthetic overdose is when the simpler measures have failed to terminate the seizure. However, by ending the seizure, these agents may give the rescuer a false sense of accomplishment; none of these drugs is wholly innocuous.

Before discussing the management of the various types of local anesthetic overdose, it must be repeated that during and after administration of a local anesthetic, the patient should be observed continuously. Careful observation of any change in the patient's behavior following the administration of a local anesthetic will permit the reaction to be recognized and managed at an earlier stage, with less potential hazard for the patient.

Mild Overdose Reaction with Rapid Onset

An overdose reaction developing within 3 to 5 minutes of drug administration is considered rapid in onset. Possible causes of this reaction include intravascular injection, unusually rapid absorption, and administration of too large a total dose of the local anesthetic. If the clinical manifestations do not progress beyond a mild degree of CNS excitation with the retention of consciousness, no definitive therapy is necessary. The local anesthetic will undergo redistribution and biotransformation, and the blood level will fall below the overdose level in a short time.

Diagnostic clues to the presence of mild overdose to local anesthetic include:
- 3-5 minutes or longer onset after completion of the injection
- Talkativeness
- Increased anxiety
- Facial muscle twitching
- Increased heart rate, blood pressure, respirations

Step 1: Terminate the dental procedure.

Step 2: Position the patient. A comfortable position is recommended for a conscious patient.

Step 3: Reassure the patient.

Step 4: Administer oxygen. At this point, advantage may be taken of the fact that a lowered $Paco_2$ level will elevate the seizure threshold to local anesthetics. Instruct the patient to hyperventilate on room air or, if oxygen is readily available, use either a full face mask or nasal hood and ask the patient to

---

MANAGEMENT OF MILD LOCAL ANESTHETIC OVERDOSE WITH RAPID ONSET

Terminate the dental procedure
↓
Position the patient comfortably
↓
Reassure patient
↓
Administer oxygen
↓
Basic life support, as indicated
↓
Monitor vital signs
↓
Administer anticonvulsant drug, if needed
↓
Allow patient to recover and discharge

---

breathe deeply. This will usually suffice to prevent seizures from developing.

Step 5: Basic life support, as indicated. Assess airway, breathing, and circulation, and implement life support as needed. In a mild local anesthetic overdose reaction, basic life support will be quite adequate without any intervention required by the rescuer.

Step 6: Monitor vital signs. The stage of postexcitation depression is mild in this form of reaction, and little or no therapy is required in its management. Oxygen may be administered and the vital signs monitored and recorded.

Step 7: Administer anticonvulsant drug, if needed. The use of an anticonvulsant such as diazepam or midazolam is not usually indicated in the mild overdose described here. However, if the doctor is trained in venipuncture and has little difficulty in accessing a vein, diazepam or midazolam may be administered intravenously and titrated slowly until the clinical reaction abates. Intravenous agents should always be titrated to clinical effect (the cessation of muscular twitching in this situation). Small doses of intravenous diazepam or midazolam may prove effective.[57] Doses as low as 2.5 to 5 mg of diazepam have terminated seizures in humans. It must be reemphasized that for a mild reaction to a local anesthetic agent, as described, anticonvulsant drug therapy is normally not indicated.

Step 8: Recovery and discharge. The patient should be permitted to recover for as long as necessary. The scheduled dental treatment may or may not be continued following evaluation of the patient's physical and emotional status. Should the doctor have any doubt or concern about this patient's condition following this reaction, medical evaluation, preferably by an emergency room physician, should be seriously considered before discharging the patient. If any anticonvulsant drug was administered, the patient must not be permitted to leave unescorted and should receive medical evaluation prior to discharge. The accompanying box outlines the steps to follow to manage mild local anesthetic overdose with rapid onset.

Mild Overdose Reaction with Delayed Onset (>5 minutes)

If the patient exhibits signs and symptoms of an overdose after the local anesthetic has been administered in the recommended manner, if pain control has been achieved, and if dental treatment has begun, the most likely causes are abnormally slow biotransformation and excretion.

Step 1: Terminate the dental procedure.

Step 2: Position the patient in a comfortable position.

Step 3: Reassure the patient.

Step 4: Administer oxygen and instruct patient to hyperventilate.

Step 5: Basic life support, as indicated. With the patient conscious, implementing the steps of basic life support will not be necessary.

Step 6: Monitor vital signs.

Step 7: Administer anticonvulsant, if needed. Management of this situation entails terminating dental treatment, reassuring the patient, administering oxygen and controlled hyperventilation, and monitoring vital signs. Overdose reactions that result from either altered biotransformation or excretory dysfunction usually progress in intensity gradually and are of longer duration than those caused by other types of overdose. If venipuncture can be performed, an intravenous infusion may be established and an anticonvulsant (e.g., diazepam or midazolam) administered, titrating the drug until clinical signs and symptoms abate.

Step 8: Summon medical assistance (optional). When venipuncture is not practical, medical assistance should be sought as early as possible. Postexcitement depression is relatively mild following a mild excitement phase. The use of an anticonvulsant to help end the reaction may increase the level of postexcitation depression but only to a minor degree. Monitoring the patient and adhering to the steps of basic life support are normally entirely adequate to manage this situation. Oxygen should be administered to the patient. When an anticonvulsant drug has been administered to the patient, medical assistance should be sought.

Step 9: Medical consultation. Following successful treatment of a mild overdose with slow onset, the

---

> **MANAGEMENT OF MILD LOCAL ANESTHETIC OVERDOSE WITH DELAYED ONSET**
>
> Terminate the dental procedure
> ↓
> Position the patient comfortably
> ↓
> Reassure patient
> ↓
> Administer oxygen
> ↓
> Basic life support, as indicated
> ↓
> Monitor vital signs
> ↓
> Administer anticonvulsant drug, if needed
> ↓
> Summon medical assistance, if needed
> ↓
> Recovery and discharge

---

patient should undergo evaluation by a physician to determine the possible causes of the reaction. This examination might include blood tests and renal and liver function tests to determine the ability of the patient to adequately metabolize and excrete these drugs. The doctor should make the initial consultation with the physician while the patient is still present in the office.

Step 10: Recovery and discharge. Allow the patient to recover for as long as is necessary, and then arrange for the patient to be escorted by an adult companion (e.g., spouse, relative, friend) to a local hospital or the physician's office. Before further dental treatment requiring local anesthetics is scheduled, a complete evaluation of the patient to help determine the cause of the overdose reaction should be completed. The accompanying box outlines the steps to follow to manage mild local anesthetic overdose with delayed onset.

Severe Overdose Reaction with Rapid Onset

If the signs and symptoms of overdose appear almost immediately (e.g., with the anesthetic syringe still in the patient's mouth or within a few seconds of the injection having been completed), intravascular injection, either intravenous or intra-arterial, is the most likely cause of the reaction. Because of the extremely rapid elevation of the anesthetic blood level, clinical manifestations are likely to be severe. Unconsciousness with or without seizures may be the initial clinical sign of the reaction.

Diagnostic clues to the presence of severe overdose to local anesthetic with a rapid onset include:

- Signs and symptoms appear either during injection, or within seconds of its completion
- Generalized tonic-clonic seizure
- Loss of consciousness

Step 1: Position the patient. Remove the syringe, if still present, from the patient's mouth and place the patient into the supine position with the feet elevated slightly. Subsequent management is based on the presence or absence of seizures.

Step 2: Summon medical assistance. When a seizure develops either during or following an injection of a local anesthetic, the immediate activation of the emergency medical system (EMS) is indicated.

When the loss of consciousness is the sole clinical sign present, position the patient (step 1) and manage the patient as described in Chapter 5. If the return of consciousness is rapid, the likely cause of the unconsciousness was vasodepressor syncope and medical assistance is not usually required. Should the patient not respond rapidly then prompt activation of EMS is urged.

Step 3: Protect the patient. Should seizures occur, which is common, management follows that described in Chapter 21 for all seizures. Recommended management includes the prevention of injury to the patient by protecting the arms, legs, and head. If possible (and only if easily possible), a soft object such as a handkerchief or cloth towel should be placed between the teeth of the patient to prevent possible injury to the tongue and lips. Extreme care must be exercised by the rescuer in this effort. Never place fingers between the teeth of a convulsing individual. As mentioned in Chapter 21, this is highly unlikely to be completed easily, so that in most instances of seizures, nothing will be placed into the patient's mouth. Tight, binding articles of clothing such as ties, collars, and belts should be loosened. Prevention of injury is the primary aim of management during the seizure.

Step 4: Basic life support, as indicated. Basic life support procedures are instituted as needed and oxygen is administered. Maintenance of adequate ventilation—the removal of carbon dioxide and the administration of oxygen—will minimize or prevent hypercarbia and hypoxia from developing and aid in maintaining the seizure threshold of the anesthetic drug (the local anesthetic seizure threshold is lowered as the patient becomes acidotic). In most instances of local anesthetic-induced seizures, airway maintenance and assisted ventilation will be necessary, but the heart should remain functional (e.g., adequate blood pressure and heart rate).

Step 5: Administer oxygen. Adequate oxygenation and ventilation of the patient during local anesthetic-induced seizures is extremely important in the termination of seizures and minimizing morbidity associated with the episode.

Step 6: Monitor vital signs. The blood level of the local anesthetic will continue to decrease as it undergoes redistribution and biotransformation. Within several minutes the anesthetic blood level will fall below the seizure threshold and the seizure will cease *unless* the patient has become acidotic during the seizure. In most cases of local anesthetic-induced seizures, definitive drug therapy to terminate the seizure is unnecessary.

Step 7: Venipuncture and IV anticonvulsant. The intravenous administration of an anticonvulsant should not be considered unless the doctor is well trained in venipuncture, has the appropriate drug(s) available, and is able to manage an apneic patient during the postseizure period. If possible, diazepam or midazolam should be titrated slowly until the seizure ends. In some cases, however, it may prove difficult to secure a vein on a convulsing patient. In these situations basic life support should be continued until the arrival of medical assistance.

Step 8: Postictal management. Following the seizure, there is a period of generalized CNS depression that is usually equal in intensity to the stimulatory phase. During this period the patient may be drowsy or may be unconscious, breathing may be shallow or absent, the airway may be partially or totally obstructed, and the blood pressure and heart rate may be depressed or even absent. Management of the patient will be predicated upon which signs and symptoms are present.

The use of anticonvulsants to terminate a seizure only adds to this postictal state of depression. Barbiturates have a greater depressant effect than the benzodiazepines, diazepam and midazolam, although all are equally effective as anticonvulsants, thus the choice of a benzodiazepine for management of seizures.

Management of the postictal period requires adherence to the steps of basic life support. A patent airway must be maintained and oxygen or artificial ventilation administered, as indicated. Vital signs must continue to be monitored and recorded. If the blood pressure or heart beat is lost, CPR is begun (see Chapter 30). Most commonly, the blood pressure and heart rate in the postictal period are low, with a gradual return toward baseline levels as the patient recovers.

Step 9: Additional management considerations. Should the blood pressure remain depressed for extended periods (>30 minutes) and medical assistance is not available, the administration of a drug to elevate the blood pressure should be considered. Once again, this step should only be considered when the doctor is well trained in the administration of these drugs and in the management of any complications associated with their administration. A vasopressor such as 20 mg of methoxamine intramuscularly should be considered. Methoxamine administered intramuscularly produces a mild elevation in blood pressure; the effect lasts for 1 hour or longer. Another means of elevating blood pressure is the administration of 1000 mL of either normal saline or 5% dextrose and water via intravenous infusion.

Step 10: Recovery and discharge. The condition of the patient will be stabilized by the emergency medical personnel, who will then transfer the patient via ambulance to the emergency department of a local hospital for definitive management, observation, and recovery.

It was mentioned earlier in this chapter that with the rapid rise in local anesthetic blood level following inadvertent intravascular administration, the first clinical sign may be unconsciousness. When this occurs, management should follow that outlined in Chapter 5. Follow-up therapy is identical to that suggested for the postseizure patient.

Severe Overdose Reaction with Slow Onset

Local anesthetic overdose reactions that evolve slowly over a period of 15 to 30 minutes are unlikely to progress to severe clinical signs and symptoms if the patient is continuously observed and management is initiated promptly. Clinical signs and symptoms most often progress from those of a mild nature to tonic-clonic seizures over a relatively short period of time (5 minutes), or the progression may be much less pronounced. In either case dental treatment must be stopped as soon as signs and symptoms are observed.

Step 1: Terminate the dental treatment. It is likely that dental treatment has started before signs and symptoms of the overdose become obvious. Immediately cease the dental procedure and initiate emergency care.

Step 2: Position the patient. Positioning will depend upon the status of the patient. If conscious, positioning is initially based upon comfort; if unconscious, the supine position with legs elevated slightly is recommended.

Step 3: Summon medical assistance.
Step 4: Protect the patient.
Step 5: Basic life support, as indicated.
Step 6: Administer oxygen.
Step 7: Monitor vital signs.
Step 8: Venipuncture and administer IV anticonvul-

sant. If symptoms are mild at the onset but progress in severity, definitive drug therapy with an anticonvulsant is indicated if available. Titration of a suitable anticonvulsant is indicated.

Step 9: Postictal management. The postictal state of depression requires strict adherence to the steps of basic life support to minimize any potential morbidity and mortality. A mild vasopressor (e.g., methoxamine) or infusion of intravenous fluids may be necessary if the blood pressure remains depressed for prolonged periods of time.

Step 10: Recovery and discharge. Patients will be stabilized at the scene and then transported by emergency medical personnel to a local emergency department of a hospital for definitive management, recovery, and discharge. The accompanying box outlines the steps to follow to manage severe local anesthetic overdose with slow or rapid onset.

Local anesthetic-induced seizures need not lead to significant morbidity or to death if the patient is properly prepared for the injection; if the person administering the local anesthetic is well trained in the management of complications, including seizures; and if appropriate resuscitation equipment is available. The administration of local anesthetics should not be carried out in any situation without these precautions.

MANAGEMENT OF A SEVERE LOCAL ANESTHETIC OVERDOSE WITH SLOW OR RAPID ONSET

Position the patient
(supine with legs elevated)
↓
Summon medical assistance
↓
Protect the patient
↓
Basic life support, as indicated
↓
Administer oxygen
↓
Monitor vital signs
↓
Venipuncture and administer IV anticonvulsant
(for prolonged seizure)
↓
Postictal management
↓
Consider additional management
↓
Recovery and discharge

Drugs used in management: Oxygen; anticonvulsant (e.g., diazepam, midazolam)

Medical assistance: If mild, no; if severe or if anticonvulsant is administered, yes

EPINEPHRINE (VASOCONSTRICTOR) OVERDOSE REACTION
Precipitating Factors and Prevention

With the increasing use of vasoconstrictors in local anesthetic solutions, a potentially new ADR has been introduced—overdose from the vasoconstrictor. Although a variety of vasoconstrictors is currently used in dentistry (Table 23-10), the most effective and the most widely employed is epinephrine. Overdose reactions are uncommon when agents other than epinephrine are employed because of the decreased potency of these agents. These reactions are also more likely to occur when greater concentrations of epinephrine are used. Table 23-11 outlines the concentrations (mg/mL) of the various epinephrine dilutions currently in use.

The optimal concentration of epinephrine for the prolongation of anesthesia with lidocaine is a 1:250,000 dilution.[58] There is no apparent reason for the use of the 1:50,000 dilution so frequently employed today for pain control. It contains twice the epinephrine per milliliter as a 1:100,000 dilution and four times that contained in a 1:200,000 dilution, while not adding any positive attributes to the anesthetic. The only benefit of the 1:50,000 concentration of epinephrine over other concentrations appears to be the control of bleeding (hemostasis). However, when used as a hemostatic agent, epinephrine must be applied directly to the area where the bleeding is occurring or will occur. Only small quantities of the solution are necessary, and in many surgical areas only small quantities are feasible, because larger volumes actually interfere with the surgical procedure. Overdose reactions from this use of 1:50,000 epinephrine are rare.

There is yet another form in which epinephrine is used in dentistry that is even more likely to produce an overdose reaction or precipitate other life-threatening situations. This is the racemic epinephrine gingival retraction cord that is commonly used prior to impression taking in crown and bridge procedures. The currently available epinephrine-impregnated cord contains from 310 to 1000 μg of racemic epinephrine per inch of cord.[59] Racemic epinephrine is a combination of the levorotatory and dextrorotatory forms of epineph-

Table 23-10. Vasoconstrictors commonly employed in dentistry

Agent	Available concentrations	Maximal dose	Local anesthetic agents used with
Epinephrine	1:50,000	Healthy adult: 0.2 mg	Lidocaine 2%
	1:100,000	Cardiac patient: 0.04 mg	Articaine 4%
			Lidocaine 2%
	1:200,000		Articaine 4%
			Lidocaine 2%*
			Prilocaine 4%
Levonordefrin (Neo-Cobefrin)	1:20,000	Healthy adult: 1.00 mg	Mepivacaine 2%
		Cardiac patient: 0.2 mg	Procaine 2% with propoxycaine 0.4%
Levarterenol (Levophed)	1:30,000	Healthy adult: 0.34 mg	Procaine 2% with propoxycaine 0.4%
		Cardiac patient: 0.14 mg	

*Available in Europe (7/92)

Table 23-11. Dilutions of vasoconstrictors used in dentistry

Dilution	Drug available	Mg/mL	Mg per cartridge (1.8 mL)	Maximum no. of cartridges used for healthy patient (H) and cardiac patient (C)
1:1000	Epinephrine (emergency kit)	1.0	Not applicable	Not available in local anesthetic cartridge
1:10,000	Epinephrine (emergency kit)	0.1	Not applicable	Not available in local anesthetic cartridge
1:20,000	Levonordefrin	0.5	0.09	10 (H), 2 (C)
1:30,000	Levarterenol	0.034	0.06	5 (H), 2 (C)
1:50,000	Epinephrine	0.02	0.036	5 (H), 1 (C)
1:100,000	Epinephrine	0.01	0.018	10 (H), 2 (C)
1:200,000	Epinephrine	0.005	0.009	20 (H), 4 (C)

rine; the dextro form is about one-twelfth to one-eighteenth as potent as the levo form. However, because of the high concentration of epinephrine in this preparation, these retraction cords are a potential source of danger to all patients, especially cardiac-risk patients. Epinephrine in an epinephrine-impregnated cord is absorbed rapidly through gingival epithelium that has been disturbed (i.e., abraded) by dental procedures, such as cavity preparation, whereas little absorption into the systemic circulation occurs through intact oral epithelium. Studies have demonstrated that from 24% to 92% of the applied epinephrine is absorbed into the circulation;[59] the extreme variability is thought to result from the degree of vascular exposure (bleeding) and the length of time of the exposure.

When gingival retraction is necessary, it is recommended that other nonvasoactive retraction materials be used. Effective agents that do not possess the adverse systemic actions of epinephrine are available and should be used in its place. Commercial preparations of hemostatics that do not contain vasoactive substances include: Hemodent: (containing aluminum chloride, hydroxyquinoline sulfate, phenocainium chloride, and ethyl aminobenzoate), and alum (a saturated alum solution).

The American Dental Association[59] states that "since effective agents which are devoid of systemic effects are available, it is not advisable to use epinephrine for gingival retraction, and its use is contraindicated in individuals with a history of cardiovascular disease."

Clinical Manifestations and Pathophysiology

The clinical manifestations of epinephrine (vasoconstrictor) overdose appear in many ways to be similar to an acute anxiety response. Indeed, in the acute anxiety response most of the signs and symptoms are produced by the large increase in endogenous catecholamine release (e.g., epinephrine and norepinephrine) by the adrenal medulla. As with all drug overdose reactions, clinical signs and symptoms relate to the normal pharmacology of the drug administered. Symptoms of an epinephrine overdose are listed in Table 23-12. The patient may make complaints such as "My heart is pounding" or "I feel nervous."

Signs of epinephrine overdose include a sharp rise in both the blood pressure, especially systolic, and heart rate. The rise in blood pressure is potentially hazardous, especially following inadvertent intravascular injection. Cerebral hemorrhage and cardiac dysrhythmias may be produced by an overdose of epinephrine. Subarachnoid hemorrhage has been recorded following the subcutaneous administration of 0.5 mg of epinephrine.

Table 23-12. Clinical manifestations of epinephrine overdose

Symptoms	Signs
Fear	Elevated blood pressure
Anxiety	Elevated heart rate
Tenseness	
Restlessness	
Throbbing headache	
Tremor	
Perspiration	
Weakness	
Dizziness	
Pallor	
Respiratory difficulty	
Palpitation	

Blood pressures in excess of 400/300 torr have been recorded for a short time following this occurrence.[60] In addition, epinephrine, a powerful cardiac stimulant, may predispose a patient toward ventricular dysrhythmias. The heart rate increases (>140 to 160 beats per minute is common), and the rhythm may be altered. Ventricular premature contractions occur first, followed by ventricular tachycardia. Ventricular fibrillation may follow and is usually fatal unless immediately recognized and managed (see Chapter 30).

Patients with preexisting cardiovascular disease are at greater risk of these adverse actions of epinephrine. Increased workload on an already impaired cardiovascular system is likely to precipitate an acute exacerbation of a preexisting problem such as anginal pain, myocardial infarction, heart failure, or cerebrovascular accident.[61,62]

Overdose reaction from epinephrine is transitory, the acute phase rarely lasting for more than a few minutes; however, the patient may feel tired and depressed ("washed out") for a prolonged period following the episode. The normally short duration of the epinephrine overdose reaction is related to the rapid biotransformation of epinephrine in the body. The liver produces the enzymes monoamine oxidase (MAO) and catecholamine O-methyltransferase (COMT), necessary for the biotransformation of epinephrine. Patients receiving monoamine oxidase inhibitors (MAO-I) in the management of depression are unable to eliminate epinephrine at the normal rate and are therefore more susceptible to overdose from epinephrine.

Management

Most instances of epinephrine overdose are of such short duration that little or no formal management is necessary. On occasion, however, the reaction may appear prolonged, and some management will be desired. Management will parallel that of a cerebrovascular accident associated with markedly elevated blood pressure (see Chapter 19).

Diagnostic clues to the presence of an overdose of vasoconstrictor include:

- Increased anxiety after injection
- Tremor of limbs
- Diaphoresis (sweating)
- Headache
- Florid appearance
- Palpitation (tachycardia)
- Elevated blood pressure

Step 1: Terminate the dental procedure. As soon as the clinical manifestations of the overdose reaction appear, terminate the dental procedure and, if possible, remove the source of epinephrine from the patient. This is obviously impossible following administration of a local anesthetic, however, gingival retraction cord should be removed immediately.

Step 2: Position the patient. The conscious patient should be placed in a comfortable position (patient may determine position). The supine position is not recommended because it accentuates the cardiovascular effects, particularly the increased cerebrovascular blood flow, noted in that position. The semisitting or erect position minimizes this elevation in cerebral blood pressure to a slight degree.

Step 3: Reassure the patient. Increased anxiety and restlessness are usually noted in this reaction, along with other signs and symptoms such as palpitation and respiratory distress. These further increase the patient's apprehension and lead to an accentuation of the clinical problem. The doctor should reassure the patient.

Step 4: Basic life support, as indicated. Assess airway, breathing, and circulation and implement basic life support as needed. Rapid assessment in this situation will confirm the adequacy of basic life support.

Step 5: Monitor vital signs. Blood pressure and heart rate should be monitored and recorded every 5 minutes during the episode. Rather striking elevations may be noted in both of these parameters, which should gradually decline toward baseline over a period of time. This is especially true when epinephrine-impregnated retraction cord was applied and then removed from the gingival tissues.

Step 6: Summon medical assistance. With a markedly elevated blood pressure and heart rate and signs and symptoms associated with cerebrovascular problems (e.g., headache, flushing), medical assistance should be sought immediately.

Step 7: Administer oxygen. Oxygen may be administered to the patient if necessary. If the patient complains of difficulty in breathing, oxygen should be administered by means of a nasal cannula, nasal hood, or full face mask.

Step 8: Recovery. Vital signs will gradually return toward baseline levels. Continue to monitor and record the blood pressure and heart rate during this time (every 5 minutes). Permit the patient to remain seated in the dental chair for as long as necessary following the episode. Patients invariably feel fatigued and depressed for considerable lengths of time following this epinephrine overdose.

Step 9: Discharge. With arrival of emergency medical assistance, the patient's cardiovascular status will be more completely evaluated (e.g., through ECG). A decision on the patient's disposition will be made in consultation with the emergency medical team, dentist, and emergency room physicians.

In most situations in which the severity of cardiovascular symptoms and signs was not great, the patient will not require hospitalization. However, when signs and symptoms of cardiovascular stimulation persist, a period of hospitalization for evaluation will be suggested. The accompanying box outlines steps to follow to manage an epinephrine overdose.

Drugs used in management: Oxygen
Medical assistance: If minor, no; if severe, yes

MANAGEMENT OF AN EPINEPHRINE (VASOCONSTRICTOR) OVERDOSE

Terminate the dental procedure
(remove gingival retraction cord)
↓
Position the patient in upright position
↓
Reassure the patient
↓
Basic life support, as indicated
↓
Monitor vital signs
↓
Summon medical assistance
↓
Administer oxygen
↓
Recovery
↓
Discharge

CENTRAL NERVOUS SYSTEM DEPRESSANT OVERDOSE REACTIONS

Whenever CNS depressant drugs are administered to a patient, there is always the possibility that an exaggerated degree of CNS depression may develop. Clinically, this might simply be noted as slight oversedation, or it might result in an unconscious patient who has ceased breathing.

In the opinion of many, the drugs most likely to produce an overdose are the barbiturates.[63] The barbiturates represented the first major breakthrough in the pharmacologic management of anxiety and because of this, adverse drug reactions such as allergy, addiction, and overdose, which are associated with barbiturate use, were tolerated. However, with the introduction of newer antianxiety drugs (e.g., the benzodiazepines) that do not possess the same potential for abuse and overdose, the use of barbiturates has declined.[63] The barbiturates still remain a very useful therapeutic group in the dentist's and physician's armamentarium for management of anxiety.

Although the barbiturates present the greatest potential for adverse reaction, the narcotic agonist analgesics are responsible for a greater number of clinically significant episodes of overdose and respiratory depression in dentistry. This is simply because the narcotics are used today to a much greater degree than the barbiturates. The administration of narcotics is popular in the management of uncooperative pediatric patients.[64] In addition, narcotics are often employed intravenously in conjunction with other sedative drugs to aid in achieving sedation and pain control in fearful patients. Goodson and Moore[65] reported on 14 cases in pediatric dentistry in which the administration of narcotics and other drugs led to seven deaths and three cases of brain damage. Several narcotics were implicated in these reactions: alphaprodine (seven cases), meperidine (six cases), and pentazocine (one case).

Predisposing Factors and Prevention

Because barbiturates and narcotics are commonly used for the preoperative management of anxiety, they are most often administered orally or intramuscularly. The clinical efficacy of a drug depends in large part on its absorption into the cardiovascular system and its subsequent blood level in different organs of the body. Only the inhalation and intravenous routes of drug administration, with rapid onsets of action, permit titration.[66] With oral and intramuscular administration, drug absorption is erratic, as demonstrated by the wide range of variability in clinical effectiveness. The normal distribution curve becomes important when drugs are administered by those routes in which titration is not possible. Average drug doses are based on this curve; therefore, 100 mg of secobarbital, or 5 mg diazepam orally produce a desired effect (drowsiness for secobarbital; anxiolysis for diazepam) in the majority of patients who receive them. For some patients, however, these doses are ineffective, and these persons will require a larger dose to attain the same clinical level of sedation. These persons, called hyporesponders, do not risk potential overdose when administered an average dose, because a lack of adequate sedation is the clinical result.

The potential danger in the use of drugs lies with patients for whom an average dose of secobarbital or diazepam is too great. These are persons who are quite sensitive (do not mistake this term for allergy; for they are quite different) to the drug and require smaller than usual doses to obtain clinically effective sedation. These persons are called hyperresponders. Normally it is not possible to predict in advance which patients will react in this manner. Only a previous history of an ADR can provide a clue to this occurrence. The medical history questionnaire should be carefully examined in relation to all drug reactions. When a history of drug sensitivity is obtained, great care must be exercised whenever considering the administration of either barbiturates or narcotics. Lower than usual doses should be considered for use or different drug categories substituted. Nonbarbiturate sedative-hypnotic drugs, the benzodiazepines, and the narcotic agonist/antagonists may be effectively substituted for these drugs.

Although the nature of the overdose cannot be easily predicted in advance, there is another way in which these drugs can produce an overdose reaction, a way that is usually preventable. It relates to the clinical goal sought by the doctor when these drugs are administered. Some clinicians use barbiturates or narcotics to achieve deeper levels of sedation in fearful patients. When used in this manner via the oral or intramuscular routes of drug administration, the potential for overdose is greatly increased. Most doctors who employ barbiturates for sedation in their practices have encountered patients who became uncooperative (e.g., less inhibited) after receiving these drugs. The planned dental treatment could not be completed because of the difficulty in managing the individual who received a small overdose of the barbiturate and became less inhibited. Larger doses of this drug given to an anxious patient in an attempt to produce deeper levels of sedation will produce even

Table 23-13. Summary of routes of drug administration

Route of administration	Control		Recommended safe sedative levels
	Titrate	*Rapid reversal*	
Oral	No	No	Light only
Rectal	No	No	Light only
Intramuscular	No	No	Adults: light, moderate
			Children: light, moderate, profound
Intravenous	Yes	No (most drugs);	Adults and children*: light, moderate,
		yes (narcotics)	profound
Inhalation	Yes	Yes	Any sedation level

*There is usually little need for intravenous sedation in normal healthy children. Most children who will permit a venipuncture will also permit a local anesthetic to be administered intraorally. Intravenous sedation is of great benefit in managing handicapped children and adults.

greater degrees of CNS depression, with respiratory depression and the possible loss of consciousness.

Employing any CNS depressant drug to obtain deeper levels of sedation by routes of administration in which titration is not possible is, therefore, not advised and is an invitation to overdose. It cannot be recommended unless no alternative method of treatment exists. Only those techniques that permit titration can be safely employed to achieve deeper levels of sedation, and then only in cases in which the doctor is thoroughly familiar with both the technique of administration and with the drugs to be administered, and is able to manage all possible complications associated with the procedure.

The inhalation and intravenous routes are the only ones that permit titration of drugs. A factor that must be considered regarding inhalation and intravenous sedation is that absorption of the drug(s) into the systemic circulation occurs rapidly so that drug responses, both therapeutic and adverse, may occur quite suddenly. Titration must always be employed when these techniques are used. Titration remains the greatest safety feature that these techniques possess. Table 23-13 summarizes recommendations for the various routes of drug administration.

Clinical Manifestations
Barbiturate and Nonbarbiturate Sedative Hypnotics

Barbiturates produce depression of a number of physiologic properties, including nerve tissue; respiration; and skeletal, smooth, and cardiac muscle. The mechanism of action (sedation and hypnosis) is depression at the level of the hypothalamus and the ascending reticular activating system, which produces a decrease in the transmission of impulses to the cerebral cortex. Further increases in the blood level of barbiturates produce depression at other levels of the central nervous system, such as profound cortical depression, depression of motor function, and finally, depression of the medulla.[67] This may be represented as follows:

Sedation (calming) → hypnosis (sleep) → general anesthesia (unconsciousness with progressive respiratory and cardiovascular depression) → respiratory arrest

Sedation and oversedation. At low (therapeutic) blood levels, the patient will appear calm and cooperative (sedated). As the barbiturate blood level increases, the patient begins to fall into a rousable sleep (hypnosis). The doctor will notice the patient's inability to keep the mouth open in spite of constant reminders to do so. In addition, patients at this level of barbiturate-induced CNS depression have a tendency to overrespond to stimulation, especially that of a noxious nature. The unsedated adult patient may grimace in response to pain; but the oversedated (with barbiturates) adult has an exaggerated response—perhaps yelling or jumping. This reflects the loss of self-control over emotion that is produced by the generalized CNS-depressant action of the barbiturate.[67]

Hypnosis. With continued elevation of the barbiturate blood level, hypnosis (sleep) ensues, with a minor degree of depression of respiratory function (decreased depth and increased rate of ventilation). At this barbiturate blood level there is virtually no adverse action on the cardiovascular system, only a slight decrease in blood pressure and heart rate similar to that occurring in normal sleep. Dental treatment cannot be continued at this level of CNS depression because the patient is unable to cooperate with the doctor by keeping the mouth open and may well require assistance in maintenance of a patent airway (e.g., head tilt). The patient will still respond to noxious stimulation but in a sluggish, still exaggerated manner.

General anesthesia. With a further increase in the barbiturate blood level, the degree of CNS depression broadens so that the patient now loses consciousness (i.e., incapable of response to sensory stimulation, loss of protective reflexes, with attendant inability to maintain a patent airway). Respiratory movements are still present; however, with a further increase in barbiturate blood levels, medullary depression occurs and is clinically evident as respiratory and cardiovascular depression. Respiratory depression is seen as shallow breathing movements at a slow or, more commonly, rapid rate. Expansive movements of the chest do not indicate that air is entering or leaving the lungs, but only that the body is attempting to bring air into the lungs. Airway obstruction may be present as the muscular tongue relaxes. Cardiovascular depression is noted by a continued decrease in blood pressure, caused by medullary depression and a direct depression of the myocardium and vascular smooth muscle, and an increased heart rate. The patient develops a shocklike appearance, with a weak and rapid pulse and cold, moist skin.

Respiratory arrest. As the barbiturate blood level continues to increase or if the patient does not receive adequate treatment in the previous stage, respiratory arrest may occur. Respiratory arrest is readily diagnosed and managed by assessing the airway and breathing. If not managed rapidly and adequately, it will soon progress to cardiac arrest.

Other nonbarbiturate sedative-hypnotic drugs, such as hydroxyzine, chloral hydrate, and promethazine, also possess the potential to produce overdose, although this is not as likely to occur as with the barbiturates.[68,69] The potential for overdose varies significantly from drug to drug, but all sedative-hypnotic drugs have this potential to some degree.

Narcotic Agonists

Meperidine, morphine, and fentanyl are the most frequently used parenteral narcotics, with meperidine and fentanyl the most popular in dentistry.

For many years alphaprodine (Nisentil), because of its rapid onset and short duration of action, was extremely popular as a sedative in pediatric dentistry. Alphaprodine is no longer marketed in the United States. It was withdrawn in 1986 following several reports of fatalities associated with its administration in dental situations.[65,70-72]

Meperidine, like most narcotic agonists, exerts its primary pharmacologic actions on the central nervous system. Therapeutic doses of meperidine produce analgesia, sedation, euphoria, and a degree of respiratory depression. Of principle concern, of course, is the respiratory depressant action of the narcotic agonists. They are direct depressants of the medullary respiratory center. In human subjects respiratory depression from narcotic agonists is evident even at doses that do not disturb the level of consciousness. The degree of respiratory depression produced by narcotics is dose-dependent: the greater the dose of the drug, the more significant the level of depression of respiration.[66] The newer narcotic agonists/antagonists, nalbuphine and butorphanol, offer the prospect of analgesia and sedation with minimal respiratory depression.[73,74]

Death from narcotic overdose almost always is the result of respiratory arrest.[75] All phases of respiration are depressed—rate, minute volume, and tidal volume.[76] The respiratory rate may fall below 10 per minute. Rates of 5 to 6 per minute are not uncommon. The cause of the decreased respiratory activity is a reduction in responsiveness of the medullary respiratory centers to increases in carbon dioxide tension (PCO_2) and also a depression of the pontine and medullary centers that are responsible for respiratory rhythm.[75]

The cardiovascular effects of meperidine are not clinically significant when the drug is administered within the usual therapeutic dose range. Following the intravenous administration of meperidine, however, there is normally an increase in the heart rate, produced by atropine-like vagolytic properties of meperidine. At overdose levels the blood pressure remains quite stable until late in the course of the reaction, when it falls primarily as a result of hypoxia. The administration of oxygen at this time will produce an increase in blood pressure despite continued medullary depression. Overly high blood levels of narcotic agonists can lead to the loss of consciousness.

Overdose reactions to both the sedative-hypnotic drugs and narcotic agonists are produced by a progressive depression of the central nervous system that is manifested by alterations in the level of consciousness and as respiratory depression that ultimately results in respiratory arrest. The loss of consciousness produced by barbiturates or narcotic agonists is not always due to overdose; in other words, loss of consciousness is sometimes desirable. For example, these drugs are very commonly administered as the primary agents in general anesthesia. However, when sedation is the goal, the loss of consciousness and respiratory depression must be considered to be serious, though not always preventable, complications of drug administration.

The duration and the degree of this clinical reaction will vary according to the route of administration, the dose of the drug administered, and the patient's individual sensitivity to the drug. In most situations oral and rectal administration result in less CNS depression but with a longer duration; intramuscular and submucosal administration result in a more profound level of depression that is relatively long lasting, whereas intravenous administration produces a rapid onset of a profound level of depression that is of a shorter duration than that seen with the other techniques. The onset of respiratory depression following intravenous administration may be quite rapid; that following oral or rectal administration is considerably slower. Onset is intermediate in intramuscular and subcutaneous administration.

Management
Sedative-Hypnotic Drugs

Management of an overdose to sedative-hypnotic drug administration is concerned with correction of the clinical effects of CNS depression. Of primary importance is the management of respiratory depression through the administration of BLS (basic life support). Unfortunately, there is no effective antagonist that can reverse the CNS-depressant properties of the barbiturate sedative-hypnotics.

Diagnostic clues to the presence of an overdose of a sedative-hypnotic drug include:[77]

- Recent administration of sedative-hypnotic drug
- Decreased level of consciousness
- Respiratory depression (rapid rate, shallow depth)
- Loss of motor coordination (ataxia)
- Slurred speech

Step 1: Terminate the dental treatment. The rate at which clinical signs and symptoms of overdose develop will vary with routes of administration. Onset following intravenous administration will occur within minutes; within 10 to 30 minutes following intramuscular administration; and within 45 minutes to an hour following oral administration.

Step 2: Position the patient. The patient, who is either semiconscious or unconscious, is placed in the supine position with the legs elevated slightly (Fig. 23-7). The goal in this situation, regardless of the level of consciousness of the patient, is to maintain an adequate cerebral blood flow.

Step 3: Basic life support, as indicated. A patent airway must be ensured and the adequacy of breathing assessed. Head tilt or head tilt–chin lift techniques may be necessary at this time (Fig. 23-8). The presence or adequacy of the patient's spontaneous ventilatory efforts is next assessed by the rescuer, who places his or her ear 1 inch from the patient's mouth and nose and listens and feels for exhaled air while looking at the patient's chest to see if the patient is attempting to breathe spontaneously.

Maintenance of a patent airway is the most important step in management of this patient. Step

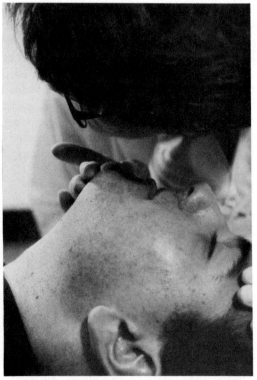

Fig. 23-8. Head tilt–chin lift.

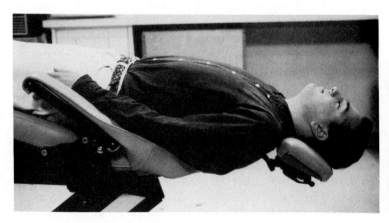

Fig. 23-7. Unconscious patient is placed in supine position with feet elevated slightly.

5, providing adequate oxygenation, is contingent on successfully maintaining a patent airway.

Step 4: Summon medical assistance, if needed. In a situation in which the patient loses consciousness following barbiturate administration, it might be prudent to seek medical assistance immediately. The need for medical assistance will vary depending upon the doctor's training in airway management and anesthesiology. When the patient remains conscious, but is overly sedated, seeking medical assistance is more of a judgment call by the doctor. When in doubt, seek assistance sooner rather than later.

Step 5: Administer oxygen. The patient may exhibit different degrees of breathing. He or she may be conscious but overly sedated—responding slowly to painful stimulation. In this situation the patient will probably be able to maintain his or her own airway and will be breathing spontaneously and somewhat effectively. The rescuer need only monitor the patient, assist in airway maintenance (e.g., head tilt—chin lift) and, if desired, administer oxygen through a demand valve or nasal cannula.

The patient may also be more deeply sedated and barely responsive to stimulation, with the airway partially or totally obstructed. In this situation airway maintenance is essential in addition to assisted ventilation. With patency of the airway ensured, the patient should receive oxygen through a full face mask. If spontaneous breathing is present but shallow, assisted positive-pressure ventilation is indicated. This is accomplished by activating the positive-pressure mask as the patient begins each breathing movement. Use of the positive-pressure mask is accomplished by depressing the button on top of the mask until the patient's chest rises and then releasing the button (Fig. 23-9). With the self-inflating bag-valve-mask device, the bellows bag is squeezed at the start of each inhalation. An air-tight seal and head tilt must be maintained at all times.

If respiratory arrest has occurred, controlled artificial ventilation must be started immediately. The recommended rate for the adult is one breath every 5 seconds (12 per minute), one breath every 4 seconds for the child aged 1 through 8 years (15 per minute), and one breath every 3 seconds for the infant under 1 year of age (20 per minute).[78] Successful ventilation is indicated by expansion of the patient's chest. Overinflation is to be avoided because this leads to abdominal distention and may result in inadequate ventilation and regurgitation.

Step 6: Monitor vital signs. The patient's vital signs must be monitored throughout the episode. Blood

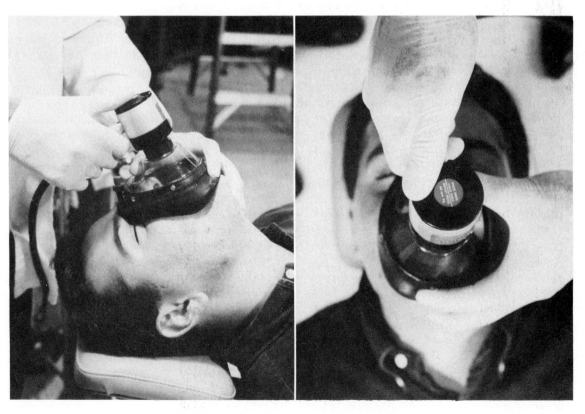

Fig. 23-9. Use of positive pressure mask.

pressure, heart rate and rhythm, and respiratory rate should be recorded every 5 minutes, and a written record maintained. A member of the emergency team is responsible for this task. If the blood level of the sedative-hypnotic drug increases significantly, the blood pressure will decrease while the heart rate increases.[79] Should blood pressure and the pulse disappear, cardiopulmonary resuscitation must be instituted immediately.

In most cases of barbiturate or nonbarbiturate sedative-hypnotic drug overdose, the patient will be maintained in this manner until the blood level of the drug decreases and the patient clinically recovers, or medical assistance arrives. In most cases recovery is the result of a redistribution of the drug within compartments in the body, not of biotransformation. However, the patient will appear to be more alert and responsive, breathing will improve (become deeper), and if previously depressed, the blood pressure will return to approximately baseline levels. The length of time for this process to occur depends on the drug administered (short versus long acting) and its route of administration.

Step 7: Establish an intravenous line, if possible. If an intravenous infusion has not previously been established, it is prudent to establish one at this time, if the presence of training and equipment permit. Although there are no effective antidotal drugs for sedative-hypnotic drug overdosage, hypotension may be treated most effectively through intravenously administered solutions or medications. As the blood pressure decreases, however, veins will become progressively more difficult to locate and cannulate. Establishing an intravenous line at the earliest possible time may prove invaluable later.

Venipuncture should be attempted only if the doctor is trained in this technique, has the necessary equipment available, and if the patient continues to receive adequate care (BLS) from other personnel. *A patent airway is more important than a patent vein.*

Step 8: Definitive management. Definitive management of a sedative-hypnotic overdose is based primarily on the maintenance of an adequate airway and ventilation until the patient recovers. Signs and symptoms of hypotension are checked by monitoring vital signs and determining the adequacy of tissue perfusion.*

---

*Adequacy of tissue perfusion may be determined by pressing on a nailbed or skin and releasing pressure. Adequate perfusion is present if color returns in not more than 3 seconds. If 4 or more seconds are required, tissue perfusion is inadequate and consideration must be given to the immediate infusion of intravenous fluids.

> **MANAGEMENT OF SEDATIVE-HYPNOTIC OVERDOSE**
>
> Terminate dental treatment
> ↓
> Position the patient
> (supine with legs elevated)
> ↓
> Basic life support, as indicated
> ↓
> Summon medical assistance, if necessary
> ↓
> Administer oxygen
> ↓
> Monitor vital signs
> ↓
> Establish IV infusion, if possible
> ↓
> Definitive management
> ↓
> Recovery and discharge

Step 9: Recovery and discharge. In the event that the overdose is profound and requires the assistance of outside medical personnel, the patient may require stabilization and transportation to a hospital for observation and full recovery. Should this be necessary, the doctor should always accompany the patient to the hospital. The accompanying box outlines the steps to follow to manage sedative-hypnotic overdose.

In most cases, however, the sedative-hypnotic overdose is significantly less severe, with diminished responsiveness and slight respiratory depression noted clinically. Management consists of positioning, airway maintenance, and assisted ventilation until recovery. Medical assistance is not usually required. Prior to discharge in the custody of a responsible adult, the patient must be capable of standing and walking without assistance. Under no circumstances should the patient be discharged alone or if not adequately recovered.

Drugs used in management: Oxygen

Medical assistance: Altered consciousness: varies by training and experience of doctor; unconscious: yes

Narcotic Analgesics

Oversedation and respiratory depression are the primary clinical manifestations of narcotic overdose. Cardiovascular depression normally does not develop until quite late in the overdose reaction, especially in supine patients. Management of the patient who has received an absolute or relative overdose of a narcotic is the same as that described for the sedative-hypnotic drugs with one major addition: specific antagonist drugs are available that reverse the clinical actions of the narcotic agonists. Steps in the management of this patient follow. The clinical picture may vary from slightly altered levels of consciousness with minimal respiratory depression, to the unconscious, apneic patient.

Diagnostic clues to the presence of an overdose of a narcotic include:[77]

- Altered level of consciousness
- Respiratory depression (slow rate, normal to deep depth)
- Miosis (contraction of pupils of the eyes)

Step 1: Terminate the dental treatment.

Step 2: Position the patient. The patient is placed in the supine position with the legs elevated slightly.

Step 3: Basic life support, as indicated. The presence of a patent airway is ensured, and breathing is monitored. Narcotics produce a decreased rate of respiration with little change in the tidal volume. Therefore the depth of ventilation is increased.[76]

In most cases of narcotic overdose the patient remains conscious though not fully alert or responsive. Assistance in maintenance of the airway may be desirable (e.g., head tilt–chin lift). When more profound depression is present, unconsciousness and respiratory arrest may occur, necessitating assessment of airway and breathing. As the cardiovascular system is relatively unaffected in narcotic overdose (if the airway and breathing are maintained), especially in the supine patient, the blood pressure and heart rate will be near baseline.[80]

Step 4: Summon medical assistance, if necessary. Depending upon the level of consciousness, the degree of respiratory depression, the training of the doctor in anesthesiology, and the availability of equipment and drugs, it might be prudent to summon medical assistance at this time.

When unconsciousness and respiratory arrest are present, medical assistance should be summoned immediately if the doctor is not well trained in anesthesiology. In the hands of a doctor well-trained in anesthesiology (e.g., general anesthesia), management of this patient may continue to include the administration of antidotal drugs (see text that follows).

Step 5: Administer oxygen. Oxygen and/or artificial ventilation is administered, if necessary. The administration of oxygen is especially important in the early management of a narcotic overdose. Little cardiovascular depression is normally observed, and when present, it occurs as a result of hypoxia secondary to respiratory depression. The administration of oxygen to a patient with a patent airway prevents or reverses any cardiovascular depression, including dysrhythmias, that are evident.[81]

Step 6: Monitor vital signs. Vital signs are monitored every 5 minutes and entered on a record sheet. Should pulse and blood pressure be absent, cardiopulmonary resuscitation is initiated immediately.

Step 7: Establish an intravenous line, if possible. With the cardiovascular system minimally effected by narcotic overdose in the supine position, it will be possible to establish an intravenous infusion in most patients. The availability of an intravenous access will expedite definitive therapy.

Step 8: Definitive management. Definitive management is available in cases in which a narcotic is the likely cause of the overdose reaction. Even when what could normally be considered to be a small dose of a narcotic has been given, a narcotic antagonist should be administered to the patient if excessive respiratory depression has developed.

No drug will be administered to the patient until a patent airway and adequacy of ventilation have been ensured and the vital signs are monitored. At this time a narcotic antagonist will be administered. The agent of choice, naloxone, should be administered intravenously, if possible, to take advantage of the more rapid onset of action with this route. If the intravenous route is unavailable, intramuscular administration is acceptable. The onset of action is slower after intramuscular administration, but naloxone will prove to be effective if a narcotic has produced the respiratory depression. Regardless of the route by which naloxone is administered, the emergency team must continue to provide basic life support as indicated from the time of naloxone administration until its onset of action, which is determined by increased patient responsiveness and more adequate and rapid ventilatory efforts. Following intravenous administration, naloxone will demonstrate its actions within 1 to 2 minutes, and within 10 minutes following intramuscular administration.

Naloxone is available in a 1-mL ampule containing 0.4 mg (adult dosage form) and 0.02 mg (pediatric dosage form). The drug is loaded into a plastic disposable syringe, and if the intravenous route is available, 3 mL of diluent (any intravenous fluid) is added to the syringe, producing a final concentration of 0.1 mg/mL of naloxone (adult) or 0.005 mg/mL (pediatric). The drug is then administered intravenously to the adult patient at a rate of 1 mL per minute until the patient's ventilatory rate increases and there is increased alertness. In children the intravenous dose is 0.01 mg/kg.[82] If administered intramuscularly, a dose of 0.4 mg (adult) or 0.01 mg/kg (pediatric) is administered into a suitable muscle mass, such as the mid-deltoid or vastus lateralis, or sublingually (if the patient is unconscious).

A potential problem with naloxone is the fact that its duration of clinical activity may be shorter than that of the narcotic it is being used to reverse. This is especially true in cases in which longer-acting narcotic agonists such as morphine are administered; it is less likely to occur with meperidine and still less likely with fentanyl and its anologues alfentanil[83] and sufentanil.[84] When the narcotic action is of greater duration than the intravenously administered naloxone, the doctor and staff would notice an improvement in the patient's clinical picture as the naloxone began to act, and then see a recurrence of CNS depression approximately 10 or more minutes later, (following intravenous administration of naloxone). Because the narcotic producing the overdose continues to undergo redistribution and biotransformation during this time, in the event that such a rebound effect does occur, it would quite likely be of a much milder nature than the initial response. In cases in which longer-acting narcotics have been administered intramuscularly or submucosally, it is recommended that the initial intravenous dose of naloxone be followed with an intramuscular dose (0.4 mg [adult] or 0.01 mg/kg [pediatric]). In this manner, as the effect of the original naloxone dose is diminishing, the level of naloxone from the intramuscular dose will be reaching a peak, thus minimizing the risk of a relapse. The availability in the near future of naltrexone, a longer-acting narcotic antagonist, will minimize this risk. The administration of naloxone in cases of narcotic overdose is important but not the most critical step in overall patient management (see text that follows).

Step 9: Permit recovery. The patient is observed and monitored following the administration of naloxone and apparent clinical recovery. The patient may be transported to a recovery area within the dental office, but should remain there under constant supervision for at least 1 hour; on the other hand, if the doctor considers it prudent, the planned dental treatment may continue. Once again, whether or not to treat the patient at this visit is a judgment call to be made by the doctor after taking into consideration the status of the patient and the level of expertise of the doctor and staff in recognizing and managing this problem. When any doubt exists, do not continue with dental

---

MANAGEMENT OF NARCOTIC OVERDOSE

Terminate dental treatment
↓
Position the patient
(supine with legs elevated)
↓
Basic life support, as indicated
↓
Summon medical assistance, if necessary
↓
Administer oxygen
↓
Monitor vital signs
↓
Establish IV infusion, if possible
↓
Definitive management
(naloxone IV or IM)
↓
Recovery and discharge

---

care. Vital signs should be recorded every 5 minutes during the recovery period, oxygen and suction must be available, and trained personnel must be present.

Step 10: Discharge. Patient discharge may require the transport of the patient to a hospital facility for observation or follow-up care.

In most cases hospitalization will not be necessary. Following a period of recovery in the dental or medical office, the patient can be discharged in the custody of a responsible adult companion, using the same recovery criteria established for parenteral sedation and general anesthesia.[66] The accompanying box outlines the steps to follow to manage narcotic overdose.

Drugs used in management: Oxygen, naloxone
Medical assistance: If altered consciousness: varies by doctor's training and experience; if unconscious: varies by doctor's training and experience

SUMMARY

The previous discussions dealt with overdose reactions of varying levels of severity that occur following the administration of a single drug. Although single-drug overdose can and does occur, especially following intramuscular or submucosal administration (e.g., inability to titrate to effect), most overdose reactions that are reported involve the administration of more than one medication. In many of these cases, drugs such as an antianxiety drug are combined with a narcotic to provide a level

Table 23-14. Dose administered relative to recommended maximum dose

Case	Narcotic analgesics (percentage)*	Antiemetic sedatives (percentage)*	Local anesthetics		
			Percentage*	N₂O-O₂	Result
1	216	36	172	—	Fatality
2	173	145	237	—	Fatality
3	336	0	342	—	Fatality
4	127	27	267	+	Fatality
5	309	372	230	+	Brain damage
6	436	?	?	—	Fatality
7	100	136	107	—	Fatality
8	167	300	219	+	Brain damage
9	66	0	60	—	Recovery
10	66	92	?	+	Recovery
11	183	0	?	—	Recovery
12	200	558	0	—	Recovery
13	250	136	127	—	Brain damage
14	50	0	370	+	Fatality

From Goodson JM, Moore PA: *J Am Dent Assoc* 107:239, 1983. Copyright by the American Dental Association. Reprinted by permission.
*Expressed as percentage of maximal recommended dose for that patient.

of sedation and some analgesia. To these a local anesthetic will usually be added for the control of operative pain. All three drug categories are CNS depressants. Added to this, in many cases, will be nitrous oxide and oxygen, adding yet another degree of CNS depression.

Whenever more than one CNS-depressant drug is administered to a patient, the dosages of both agents must be reduced from their usual dosage to prevent exaggerated, undesirable clinical responses. As is demonstrated in Table 23-14, in most of the cases reported by Goodson and Moore,[65] this step was not taken, with disastrous results occurring in many cases.

Another factor must be considered, one that most health professionals do not, as a rule, give much thought when using sedative techniques. That is the fact that local anesthetics themselves are CNS depressants and can produce additive actions when administered in conjunction with the drugs commonly employed for sedation. The maximal dosage of local anesthetic to be administered to any patient, but especially to a child or lighter-weight adult, should be based on the patient's body weight in kilograms or pounds. When no other CNS depressants are being administered, this maximal dose could be reached without adverse effects if the patient is an ASA I and falls within the normal range on the bell-shaped curve. Maximal recommended doses of the most commonly used local anesthetics are presented in Table 23-15. When used in conjunction with other CNS depressants, the dosage of the local anesthetic should be minimized.

Table 23-15. Maximal recommended local anesthetic doses

Drug	Dose		Absolute maximal dose
	mg/kg	mg/lb	
Lidocaine	4.4	2.0	300
Mepivacaine	4.4	2.0	300
Prilocaine	6.0	2.7	400
Bupivacaine	2.0	0.9	90

A primary goal of sedation is to produce a cooperative patient who still maintains protective reflexes (e.g., swallowing, coughing, maintenance of the airway). When possible, this goal should be achieved using the simplest technique available, as well as the fewest number of drugs possible. Polypharmacy, the combination of several drugs, is necessary in many patients in order to achieve the desired level of sedation; however, if it is possible to reach this same desired effect with one drug, the combination ought not be employed. The use of drug combinations simply increases the opportunity for ADRs, as well as making it less obvious which drug may have produced the problem, thereby making management of the situation more difficult.

Within the individual techniques of sedation, it is suggested that single-drug regimens are preferable to combinations of drugs. Rational drug combinations are available for use in cases in which they are specifically indicated. With intravenous drug administration, the problem of severe ADRs should not occur if the titration technique is adhered to at all times. With intramuscular and oral drug administration, however, titration is not available. The doctor must modify individual drug dosages prior to their administration. Serious ADRs are more likely to occur with techniques in which titration is not possible.

Consideration must also be given to the use of multiple techniques of sedation, as opposed to multiple drugs by one technique of administration, in a patient. It is not be uncommon for a patient who represents a significant management problem to receive an oral antianxiety drug prior to arrival in the office, followed by either intramuscular, submucosal, or intravenous sedation, as well as inhalation sedation and local anesthesia during the course of the appointment. Whenever oral sedation with CNS depressants has been used, the dosages of all subsequent CNS depressants should be carefully evaluated prior to their administration. This is critical when either the intramuscular or submucosal routes are used, because they do not permit titration of the drug(s). With inhalation and intravenous sedation, careful titration of CNS-depressant drugs to the previously orally premedicated patient will usually produce the desired level of clinical sedation with a minimal risk of adverse response by the patient.

How, then, may overdose reactions best be prevented? Goodson and Moore made the following recommendations concerning the use of sedative techniques in which narcotics are being administered:[65]

1. Be prepared for emergencies: Continuous monitoring of the cardiovascular and respiratory systems should be employed. An emergency kit containing drugs such as adrenaline, oxygen, and naloxone should be readily available, in addition to equipment and trained personnel. In their article Goodson and Moore state that "because multiple sedative drug techniques can easily induce unconsciousness, respiratory arrest, and convulsions, practitioners should be prepared and trained to recognize and control these occurrences."

2. Individualize the drug dosage: When drugs are used in combination, the dosage of each drug must be carefully selected. The toxic effects of drug combinations appear to be additive. Drug selection must be based on the patient's general health history. The presence of systemic disease usually indicates the need for a reduction of dosage. Because most sedative drugs are available in quite concentrated form, and because children will require very small dosages, extreme care must be taken when these drugs are being prepared for administration.

Fixed-dose administration of drugs based on a range of ages (e.g., 4 to 6 years: 50 mg) should *not* be employed. Dosages based on body weight or surface area of the patient, or titration are preferred, if possible.[85]

Should the selected drug dosage prove to be inadequate to produce the desired effect in the patient, it is prudent to consider a change in the sedation technique or in the drugs being used (at a subsequent appointment), rather than increasing the drug dosage to a higher and potentially more dangerous level at the same visit.

3. Recognize and expect adverse drug effects: When combinations of CNS-depressant drugs have been administered, the potential for excessive CNS and respiration depression is increased and should be expected.

The Dentists Insurance Company (TDIC), in a retrospective study of deaths and morbidity in dental practices over a 3-year period, concluded that in most of those incidents related to the administration of drugs, there were three common factors.[86]

1. Improper preoperative evaluation of the patient
2. Lack of knowledge of drug pharmacology by the doctor
3. Lack of adequate monitoring during the procedure

These three factors greatly increased the risk of serious ADRs developing, with a negative outcome the usual result.

An overdose reaction to the administration of CNS-depressant drugs may not always be a preventable complication; however, with care taken on the part of the doctor, the incidence of these events should be extremely low, and a successful outcome should be the result virtually every time. With techniques such as intravenous and inhalation sedation, in which titration is possible, overdosage should be rare. With oral, intramuscular, and submucosal drug administration, in which the doctor has little control over the drug's ultimate effect because of the inability to titrate, greater care must be expended by the doctor in the preoperative evaluation of the patient, the determination of the appropriate drug dosage, and in monitoring throughout the procedure so that excessive CNS or respiratory depression may be observed and treated immediately. When the oral, submucosal, and intramuscular routes of administration are employed, the onset of adverse reactions may be delayed. The adverse reaction may not develop until after the rubber dam is in place and the dental procedure is started. Monitoring of the patient throughout the procedure therefore becomes extremely important to patient safety. The author's preferences, as of August 1992, in monitoring during parenteral sedation are as follows:[66]

1. Central nervous system
   Direct verbal contact with patient
2. Respiratory system
   Pretracheal stethoscope
   Pulse oximetry
3. Cardiovascular system
   Continuous monitoring of vital signs
   ECG

REFERENCES

1. Caranasos GJ: Drug reactions. In Schwartz GR, Safar P, Stone JH, and others, editors: *Principles and practice of emergency medicine*, Philadelphia, 1978, WB Saunders.
2. Aldrete JA, Johnson DA: Evaluation of intracutaneous testing for investigation of allergy to local anesthetic agents, *Anesth Analg* 49:173, 1970.
3. Nation RL, Triggs EJ, Selig M: Lignocaine kinetics in cardiac patients and aged subjects, *Br J Clin Pharmacol* 4:439, 1977.
4. Demetrescu M, Julien RM: Local anesthesia and experimental epilepsy, *Epilepsia* 15:235, 1974.
5. Arthur GR: Pharmacokinetics of local anesthetics. In Strichartz GR, editor: *Local anesthetics, handbook of experimental pharmacology*, vol 81, Berlin, 1987, Springer-Verlag.
6. Bax ND, Tucker GT, Woods HF: Lignocaine and indocyanine green kinetics in patients following myocardial infarction, *Br J Clin Pharmacol* 10:353, 1980.
7. Sawyer DR, Ludden TM, Crawford MH: Continuous infusion of lidocaine in patients with cardiac arrhythmias: unpredictability of plasma concentrations, *Arch Intern Med* 141:34, 1981.
8. Englesson S: The influence of acid-base changes on central nervous system toxicity of local anaesthetic agents. I. an experimental study in cats, *Acta Anaesthesiol Scand* 18:79, 1974.
9. DeJong RH, Wagman IH, Prince DA: Effect of carbon dioxide on the cortical seizure threshold to lidocaine, *Exp Neurol* 17:221, 1982.
10. Lear E, and others: Atypical pseudocholinesterase: a clinical report, *Anesth Analg* 55:243, 1976.
11. Lanks KW, Sklar GS: Pseudocholinsterase levels and rates of chloroprocaine hydrolysis in patients receiving adequate doses of phospholine iodide, *Anesthesiology* 52:434, 1980.
12. Zsigmond EK, Eilderton TE: Survey of local anesthetic toxicity in the families of patients with atypical plasma cholinesterase, –J Oral Surg 33:833, 1975.
13. Lindorf HH, Ganssen A, Mayer P: Thermographic representation of the vascular effects of local anesthetics, *Electromedica* 4:106, 1974.
14. Braid DP, Scott DB: The systemic absorption of local analgesic drugs, *Br J Anaesth* 37:394, 1965.
15. Jebson PR: Intramuscular lignocaine 2% and 10%, *Br Med J* 3:566, 1971.
16. Adriani J, Campbell B: Fatalities following topical application of local anesthetics to mucous membranes, *JAMA* 162:1527, 1956.
17. Moore DC: *Complications of regional anesthesia*, Springfield, Ill., 1955, Charles C Thomas.
18. DuSouich P, Erill P: Altered metabolism of procainamide and procaine in patients with pulmonary and cardiac disease, *Clin Pharmacol Ther* 21:101, 1977.
19. Downs JR: Atypical cholinesterase activity: its importance in dentistry, *J Oral Surg* 24:256, 1966.
20. Keenaghan JB, Boyes RN: The tissue distribution, metabolism and excretion of lidocaine in rats, guinea pigs, dogs and man, *J Pharmacol Exp Ther* 180:454, 1972.
21. Mather LE, Tucker GT: Pharmacokinetics and biotransformation of local anesthetics, *Anesthesiol Clin* 16:23, 1978.
22. Meffin P, Robertson RAV, Thomas J, and others: Neutral metabolites of mepivacaine in humans, *Xenobiotica* 3:191, 1973.
23. Thomas J, Morgan D, Vine J: Metabolism of etidocaine in man, *Xenobiotica* 6:39, 1976.
24. Friedman GA, Rowlingson JC, Difazio CA, and others: Evaluation of the analgesic effect and urinary excretion of systemic bupivacaine in man, *Anesth Analg* 61:23, 1982.
25. Monheim LM: *Local anesthesia and pain control in dental practice*, St Louis, 1957, Mosby–Year Book.
26. Malamed SF: *Handbook of local anesthesia*, ed 3, St Louis, 1991, Mosby–Year Book.
27. Bieter RN: Applied pharmacology of local anesthetics, *Am J Surg* 34:500, 1936.
28. Vandam LD: Some aspects of the history of local anesthesia. In Strichartz GR, editor: *Local anesthetics, handbook of experimental pharmacology*, vol 81, Berlin, 1987, Springer-Verlag.
29. Larsen LS, Larsen A: Labetalol in the treatment of epinephrine overdose, *Ann Emerg Med* 19(6):680-682, 1990.
30. Marcovitz PA, Williamson BD, Armstrong WF: Toxic methemoglobinemia caused by topical anesthetic given before transesophageal echocardiography, *J Amer Soc Echocardiog* 4(6):615-618, 1991.
31. Xylocaine 10% oral spray, Drug package insert, Astra Pharmaceutical Products, Westboro, Mass., March 1989.
32. Bartlett SZ: Clinical observations on the effects of injections of local anesthetics preceded by aspiration, *Oral Surg* 33:520, 1972.
33. Aldrete JA, Narang R, Sada T: Untoward reactions to local anesthetics via reverse intracarotid flow, *J Dent Res* 54:145, 1975.
34. Aldrete JA, others: Reverse carotid blood flow—a possible explanation for some reactions to local anesthetics, *J Am Dent Assoc* 94:142, 1977.
35. Malamed SF: Local anesthetic survey, unpublished data, 1980.
36. Jeske AH, Boshart BF: Deflection of conventional versus non-deflecting dental needles in vitro, *Anesth Prog* 32:62, 1985.
37. Foldes FF, McNall PG: Toxicity of local anesthetics in man, *Dent Clin N Am*, July: 257, 1961.
38. Kramer H, Mitton V: Dental emergencies, *Dent Clin N Amer* 17:443, 1973.
39. Trapp LD, Davies RO: Aspiration as a function of hypodermic needle internal diameter in the in-vivo human upper limb, *Anesth Prog* 27:49, 1980.
40. Covino BG, Vassallo HG: *Local anesthetics: mechanisms of action and clinical use*, New York, 1976, Grune & Stratton.
41. Scott DB, Cousins MJ: Clinical pharmacology of local anesthetic agents. In Cousins MJ, Bridenbaugh PO editors: *Neural blockade*, Philadelphia, 1980, JB Lippincott.
42. Munson ES, Tucker WK, Ausinsch B, Malagodi H: Etidocaine, bupivacaine, and lidocaine seizure thresholds in monkeys, *Anesthesiology* 42:471-478, 1975.

43. Covino BG: Toxic and systemic effects of local anesthetic agents. In Strichartz GR, editor: *Local anesthetics, handbook of experimental pharmacology*, vol 81, Berlin, 1987, Springer-Verlag.

44. Liu PL, Feldman HS, Giasi R, and others: Comparative CNS toxicity of lidocaine, etidocaine, bupivcaine, and tetracaine in awake dogs following rapid IV administration, *Anesth Analg* 62:375, 1983.

45. Cannell H, and others: Circulating levels of lignocaine after peri-oral injections, *Br Dent J* 138:87, 1975.

46. Harrison DC, Alderman FL: Relation of blood levels to clinical effectiveness of lidocaine. In Scott DB, Julian DC, editors: *Lidocaine in the treatment of ventricular arrhythmias*, Edinburgh, 1971, E & S Livingstone.

47. Block A, Covino BG: Effects of local anesthetic agents on cardiac conduction and contractility, *Reg Anaesth* 6:55, 1982.

48. Liu PL, Feldman HS, Covino BM, and others: Acute cardiovascular toxicity of intravenous amide anesthetics in anesthetized ventilated dogs, *Anesth Analg* 61:317, 1982.

49. Strichartz GR, Covino BG: Local anesthetics. In Miller RD editor: *Anesthesia*, ed 2, New York, 1990, Churchill-Livingstone.

50. Liu PL, Feldman HS, Covino BM, and others: Acute cardiovascular toxicity of procaine, chloroprocaine, and tetracaine in anesthetized ventilated dogs, *Reg Anaesth* 7:14, 19, 1982.

51. Scott DB: Toxicity caused by local anaesthetic drugs, *Br J Anaesth* 53:553–554, 1981.

52. Julien RM: Lidocaine in experimental epilepsy: correlation of anticonvulsant effect with blood concentration, *Electroencephalogr Clin Neurophysiol* 34:639, 1973.

53. Julien RM, Demetrescu M: A neutral local anesthetic for research in experimental epilepsy, *J Life Sci* 4:27, 1974.

54. Wagman IH, DeJong RH, Prince DA: Effects of lidocaine on the central nervous system, *Anesthesiology* 28:155, 1967.

55. Adatia AK: Intravascular injection of local anesthetics, *Br Dent J* 138:328, 1975.

56. Ingvar M, Siesjo BK: Local blood flow and glucose consumption in the rat brain during sustained bicuculline-induced seizures, *Acta Neurol Scand* 68:129, 1983.

57. Jaimovich DG, Shabino CL, Noorani PA, and others: Intravenous midazolam suppression of pentylene tetrazol-induced epileptogenic activity in a porcine model, *Crit Care Med* 18(3):313, 1990.

58. Jakob W: Local anaesthesia and vasoconstrictive additional components, *Newslett Int Fed Dent Anesthesiol Soc* 2(1):3, 1989.

59. American Dental Association: *Accepted dental therapeutics*, ed 40, Chicago, 1984, American Dental Association.

60. Verrill PJ: Adverse reactions to local anesthetics and vasoconstrictor drugs, *Practitioner* 214:380, 1975.

61. Alexander RE: Epinephrine is safe for heart patients, *Med Times* 99:132, 1971.

62. Campbell RL: Cardiovascular effects of epinephrine overdose: case report, *Anesth Prog* 24:190, 1977.

63. Baltarowich LL: Sedative-hypnotics. In Rosen P, editor: *Emergency medicine*, ed 2, St Louis, 1988, Mosby–Year Book.

64. Braham RL: *Textbook of pediatric dentistry*, Baltimore, 1985, Williams & Wilkins.

65. Goodson JM, Moore PA: Life-threatening reactions after pedodontic sedation: an assessment of narcotic, local anesthetic, and antiemetic drug interaction, *J Am Dent Assoc* 107:239, 1983.

66. Malamed SF: *Sedation: a guide to patient management*, ed 2, St Louis, 1989, Mosby–Year Book.

67. Harvey SC: Hypnotics and sedatives: the barbiturates. In Goodman IS, Gilman A, editors: *Pharmacological basis of therapeutics*, ed 6, New York, 1980, Macmillan.

68. Zendell E: Chloral hydrate overdose: a case report, *Anesth Prog* 19:6, 1972.

69. Benusis KP, Kapuan D, Furnam LJ: Respiratory depression in a child following meperidine, promethazine and chlorpromazine premedication: report of a case, *J Dent Child* 46:50, 1979.

70. Del Vecchio PJ Jr: 20/20 (letter), *Am Dent Assoc News* 14:4, 1983.

71. Hine CH, Pasi A: Fatality after use of alphaprodine in analgesia for dental surgery: report of a case, *J Am Dent Assoc* 84:858, 1972.

72. Okuji DM: Hypoxic encephalopathy after the administration of alphaprodine hydrochloride, *J Am Dent Assoc* 103:50, 1981.

73. Gal TJ, DiFazio CA, Moscicki J: Analgesic and respiratory depressant activity of nalbuphine: a comparison with morphine, *Anesthesiology* 57:367, 1982.

74. Heel RC, Brogden RN, Speight TM, and others: Butorphanol: a review of its pharmacological properties and therapeutic efficacy, *Drugs* 16:473, 1978.

75. Jaffe JH, Martin WR: Opioid analgesics and antagonists. In Goodman L, Gilman A, editors: *The pharmacological basis of therapeutics*, ed 6, New York, 1980, Macmillan.

76. Allen T: Narcotics. In Rosen P, editor: *Emergency medicine*, ed 2, St Louis, 1988, Mosby–Year Book.

77. Pollakoff J, Pollakoff K: *EMT's guide to signs and symptoms*, 1991.

78. American Heart Association and National Academy of Sciences: National Research Council: Standards for cardiopulmonary resuscitation (CPR) and emergency cardiac care (ECC), *JAMA* 255:2905, 1986.

79. Matthew H: Barbiturates, *Clin Toxicol* 8:495, 1975.

80. Lowenstein E: Morphine anesthesia in perspective, *Anesthesiology* 35:563, 1971.

81. Duberstein JL, Kaufman DM: A clinical study of an epidemic of heroin-induced pulmonary edema, *Am J Med* 51:704, 1971.

82. Narcan drug package insert, DuPont Pharmaceuticals, July 1988.

83. Janssens F, Torremans J, Janssen PA: Synthetic 1,4-disubstituted-1,4-dihydro-5H-tetrazol-5-one derivatives of fentanil: alfentanil (R 39209), a potent, extremely short-acting narcotic analgesic, *J Med Chem* 29:2290, 1986.

84. Clotz MA, Nahata MC: Clinical uses of fentanyl, sufentanil, and alfentanil, *Clin Pharamcy* 10(8):581-593, 1991.

85. Done AK: In Modell W, editor *Drugs of choice 1972-1973*, St Louis, 1972, Mosby–Year Book.

86. deJulien LE: Causes of severe morbidity/mortality cases, *J Cal Dent Assoc* 11:45, 1983.

24 *Allergy*

Allergy has previously been defined as a hypersensitive state acquired through exposure to a particular allergen, reexposure to which produces a heightened capacity to react.[1] Allergic reactions cover a broad range of clinical manifestations, from mild, delayed reactions that develop as long as 48 hours after exposure to the antigen, to immediate and life-threatening reactions that develop within seconds of exposure. A classification of allergic reactions is presented in Table 24-1.[2] Although all allergic phenomena are important, two forms of allergy are of particular consequence in the practice of dentistry. The type I, or anaphylactic (immediate), reaction may present the dental office staff with the most acute life-threatening emergency situation of any discussed in this textbook. The type IV, or delayed, allergic reaction, seen clinically as contact dermatitis, is particularly relevant because of the significant number of dental personnel who develop this form of allergy. Allergic reactions in health workers to latex gloves are being reported with increasing frequency[3] as are reports of allergy in patients to the latex gloves worn by their doctors.[4]

Immediate allergic reactions are of primary concern and will receive major emphasis in the following discussion. The type I reaction may be subdivided into several forms of response, including generalized and localized anaphylaxis.[2] A list of type I allergic reactions follows:

Type I immediate hypersensitivity:
Generalized (systemic) anaphylaxis
Localized anaphylaxis
   Urticaria (in the skin)
   Bronchial asthma (in the respiratory tract)
   Food allergy (in the gastrointestinal tract and other organs)

The major forms of type I reaction are discussed following a presentation of several terms relevant to this chapter.

Allergen. An antigen that can elicit allergic symptoms

Anaphylactic. From the Greek *ana* = against or backward; *phylax* = guard or protect, meaning "without protection" to be distinguished from prophylaxis, as in "for protection"[5]

Anaphylactoid. Anaphylactoid reactions, which mimic true IgE-mediated anaphylaxis, are idiosyncratic reactions that occur generally when the patient is first exposed to a particular drug or agent. Although not immunologically mediated, their emergency management is the same as that of immunologically mediated reactions.

Angioedema (angioneurotic edema). Noninflammatory edema involving the skin, subcutaneous tissue, underlying muscle, and mucous membranes, especially those of the gastrointestinal and upper respiratory tracts; occurs in response to exposure to an allergen; the most critical area of involvement is the larynx (laryngeal edema)

Antibody. Those substances found in the blood or tissues that respond to the administration of, or react with, an antigen; they differ in structure (e.g., IgE and IgG) and are capable of eliciting distinctly different responses (e.g., anaphylaxis or serum sickness)

Antigen. Any substance foreign to the host that is capable of activating an immune (e.g., allergic) response by stimulating the development of a specific antibody

Atopy. A "strange disease"; a clinical hypersensitivity state subject to hereditary influences; examples include asthma, hay fever, and eczema

Pruritus. Itching

Urticaria. A vascular reaction of the skin marked by the transient appearance of smooth, slightly elevated patches, which are redder or paler than the surrounding skin and are often accompanied by severe itching

All allergic reactions are mediated through immunologic mechanisms that are similar, regardless of the specific antigen that is responsible for initiating the reaction. Therefore, it is possible, and likely, that an allergic reaction to the venom of a

348   *Drug-related emergencies*

Table 24-1. Classification of allergic diseases (after Gell and Coombs)

Type	Mechanism	Principal antibody or cell	Time of reactions	Clinical examples
I	Anaphylactic (immediate, homocytotropic, antigen-induced, antibody-mediated)	IgE	Seconds to minutes	Anaphylaxis (drugs, insect venom, antisera) Atopic bronchial asthma Allergic rhinitis Urticaria Angioedema Hay fever
II	Cytotoxic (antimembrane)	IgG IgM (activate complement)	—	Transfusion reactions Goodpasture's syndrome Autoimmune hemolysis Hemolytic anemia Certain drug reactions Membranous glomerulonephrosis
III	Immune complex (serum sickness-like)	IgG (form complexes with complement)	6-8 hours	Serum sickness Lupus nephritis Occupational allergic alveolitis Acute viral hepatitis
IV	Cell-mediated (delayed) or tuberculin-type response	—	48 hours	Allergic contact dermatitis Infectious granulomas (tuberculosis, mycoses) Tissue graft rejection Chronic hepatitis

Adapted from Krupp MA, Chatton MJ: *Current medical diagnosis and treatment,* Los Altos, Calif., 1984, Lange Medical.

stinging insect, such as a wasp, may be identical to the reaction to eating a strawberry, or after aspirin or penicillin administration to a previously sensitized individual. This must be differentiated from an overdose or toxic drug reaction that represents a direct extension of the normal pharmacologic actions of the drug involved. Overdose reactions are much more frequently encountered than are allergic drug reactions (85% of adverse drug reactions [ADRs] result from the pharmacologic actions of the drug; 15% are immunologic reactions[6]), even though to the non-medical individual any adverse drug reaction is usually considered an allergy. It is hoped that following the discussions in this section, the reader will be able to fully evaluate any history of supposed allergy to determine what really occurred, and will be able to differentiate between these two important ADRs, allergy and overdose. Chapter 25 presents a differential diagnosis of the several ADRs and other clinically similar reactions.

Allergy is a frightening word to those health professionals who are responsible for the primary care of patients. In the dental profession many drugs that have a significant potential for producing allergy are regularly administered or prescribed to patients. Although the concept of prevention has been emphasized repeatedly through-

out this book, in no other situation is the concept of prevention of greater importance than in allergy. Although allergy is not the most common adverse drug reaction, it is frequently involved with the most serious of these reactions. Emphasis will be placed on the more immediate allergic reaction and on those specific drugs and chemicals in common use in dental practice.

PREDISPOSING FACTORS

The number of persons with significant allergy is not small. Of the population in the United States, 15% have allergic conditions that are severe enough to require medical management. Thirty-three percent of all chronic disease in children is allergic in nature.[7,8] Individuals with allergy problems represent a potentially serious risk when receiving dental treatment. Although never without risk, the administration of drugs is normally accomplished without any significant frequency of adverse reactions (indeed, if ADRs occurred with greater frequency, dentists would avoid using many drugs in dental practice). However, in an individual with a genetic predisposition to allergy (e.g., the atopic patient), great care must be taken when considering the use of any drug. The patient with multiple allergies (e.g., hay fever, asthma, or allergy to numerous foods) is much more likely to elicit an allergic response to the drugs used in dentistry than is a patient with no prior history of allergy.

Although the patient's prior history is the major factor in determining the risk of allergy, the specific drug to be employed is also of extreme importance. In allergy, as opposed to overdose, prior contact (the sensitizing dose) is almost always necessary for the reaction to develop. Such is not the case in anaphylactoid reactions, however. Signs and symptoms of allergy appear only after a subsequent (challenge) dose is administered to the patient. Without the sensitizing and challenge doses, allergy will not occur.

Various drug groups are more highly allergenic than are others. In one survey barbiturates, penicillins, meprobamate, codeine, and thiazide diuretics were responsible for over 70% of the allergic reactions encountered.[9] Laryngeal edema, acute bronchospasm with respiratory failure, and circulatory collapse, occurring alone or in combination, are responsible for 400 to 800 anaphylactic deaths annually in the United States.[10] Leading causes of death from anaphylaxis are parenterally administered penicillin (100 to 500 deaths per year) and Hymenoptera stings (40 to 100 deaths per year).[11,12] Medications frequently involved in anaphylactoid deaths include radiopaque contrast media reactions (up to 500 deaths per year),[13] and the iatrogenic administration of common medications such as aspirin and other nonsteroidal antiinflammatory drugs.[14,15]

Listed below are the more commonly used drugs in dental practice that possess a significant potential for allergy.

Antibiotics
  Penicillins
  Cephalosporins
  Tetracyclines
  Sulfonamides
Analgesics
  Acetylsalicylic acid (ASA—aspirin)
  Nonsteroidal antiinflammatory drugs
    (NSAIDs)
Narcotics
  Morphine
  Meperidine
  Codeine
Antianxiety drugs
  Barbiturates
Local anesthetics
  Esters
    Procaine
    Propoxycaine
      Benzocaine
      Tetracaine
    Methylparaben preservative
Preservatives
  Parabens—methylparaben
  Bisulfites
  Metasulfites
Other agents
  Acrylic monomer (methyl methacrylate)

Antibiotics

Probably the most significant ADR associated with antibiotics is the ability of many of these agents to produce allergic reactions. Some antibiotics, such as erythromycin, are associated with a very low incidence of allergy; whereas others, particularly the sulfonamides and penicillins, frequently produce allergic responses. In virtually all cases the allergic reactions associated with antibiotic therapy are not life threatening. The penicillins, the most commonly used antibiotics in dentistry, are the major exceptions. The first anaphylactic-induced fatality caused by penicillin was reported in 1949.[16] Penicillin has remained the leading cause of fatal anaphylaxis since that time.[17,18]

It has been estimated that the incidence of allergy to penicillin ranges anywhere from 0.7% to 10% of those receiving the drug.[11] Approximately 2.5 million persons in the United States are allergic to penicillin. Of patients receiving penicillin, 0.015% to 0.04% will develop anaphylaxis, with a fatality rate of 0.0015% to 0.002%.[11] This accounts for 100 to 500 deaths per year.

In a survey on the nature and extent of penicillin side reactions, 150 cases of anaphylaxis were studied. Of the patients observed, 14% had a history of other allergies, 70% had previously received penicillin, and over 33% had experienced a prior immediate allergic reaction to the drug. When death occurred, it normally occurred within 15 minutes.[19]

Allergy to penicillin may be induced by any mode of administration. The topical route is probably the most likely to sensitize (5% to 12% sensitized), the oral route the least likely (0.1% sensitized). However, it is also possible to be sensitized to penicillin without knowledge of prior exposure, because penicillin is a natural contaminant of our environment. The penicillin mold is airborne and may be found in bread, cheese, milk, and fruit. Parenterally administered penicillin is responsible for the vast majority of severe anaphylactic reactions, with only six fatalities reported from oral penicillin.[9] Cephalosporins, structurally similar to penicillin, have been reported to be cross-allergenic in 5% to 16% of patients.[20]

Analgesics

Allergy may develop to any of the pain-relieving drugs commonly used in dentistry. This is somewhat true regarding the narcotic agonist analgesics, such as codeine and meperidine, but the incidence of true allergy to these agents is quite low, even though "allergic to codeine" is listed frequently on medical history questionnaires. A thorough dialogue history is required to determine the exact nature of the ADR that occurred. In most instances the allergy to codeine turns out to be merely annoying side effects such as nausea, vomiting, drowsiness, dysphoria (restlessness), or constipation.

The incidence of allergy to aspirin is relatively high (estimated to be from 0.2% to 0.9%), with symptoms ranging from mild urticaria to anaphylaxis.[21,22] Previous ingestion of aspirin without ill effect is no guarantee against a subsequent allergic reaction to the drug. Allergic reactions to aspirin also take the form of angioedema and asthma (bronchospasm). Asthma is the chief allergic manifestation in most persons sensitive to aspirin, but especially in the middle-aged female who also has nasal polyps, pansinusitis and rhinitis.[23,24] Anaphylaxis may also occur.[25] Other nonsteroidal antiinflammatory drugs also carry risk for allergy.[14,15,26]

Antianxiety Drugs

Of the many drugs commonly used for the management of anxiety in dentistry, the barbiturates probably possess the greatest potential for sensitization of patients. Although not as common as allergy to penicillin or aspirin, allergy to barbiturates usually manifests itself in the form of skin lesions such as hives and urticaria or, less frequently, in the form of blood dyscrasias such as agranulocytosis or thrombocytopenia.[27] Allergy to barbiturates occurs much more frequently in persons with a history of asthma, urticaria, and angioedema. A history of allergy to any of the barbiturates is an absolute contraindication to the use of any of these agents.

Local Anesthetics

Local anesthetics are the most commonly used drugs in dentistry and probably the most important. Without their availability dentistry would revert back to the days when all dental procedures were associated with pain. Adverse drug reactions, though uncommon, are seen with the use of local anesthetics. The overwhelming majority of these reactions are not allergic in nature, but are related to a direct effect of the drug.[28,29] Allergy to local anesthetics does occur; however, the incidence of such reactions has dramatically decreased since the introduction of amide-type local anesthetics in the 1940s. Allergic manifestations of local anesthetics may range from an allergic dermatitis (commonly occurring among dental office personnel) to a typical asthmatic attack to fatal systemic anaphylaxis.

Hypersensitivity to local anesthetics occurs much more frequently in response to the ester local anesthetics such as procaine, propoxycaine, benzocaine, tetracaine, and compounds related to them, such as procaine penicillin G, and procainamide (an antidysrhythmic drug).[28,30] Local anesthetics of the amide type are essentially free of this problem, yet the frequency of reports of allergy to amide local anesthetics in the dental and medical literature and on medical history questionnaires seems to be increasing. This apparent contradiction may be cleared up with careful evaluation of these alleged local anesthetic allergies. Several investigators, most notably Aldrete and Johnson,[31] have investigated these reports and performed extensive evaluations of each case, seeking to determine the nature of the reaction. In most cases the reaction was the result of either psychogenic factors or drug overdose (see Chapter 23); in other cases, the reactions demonstrated were of an allergic nature. When an ester local anesthetic is employed, a true allergic reaction is frequently elicited; however, with use of the amide local anesthetics, a purported allergic reaction is frequently shown to be another type of response (e.g., overdose, idiosyncrasy, or psychogenic). Malamed[32] examined 188 patients referred for evaluation of "local anesthetic allergy." Careful dialogue history and intracutaneous testing found no patient to be allergic to an amide local anesthetic and four patients with allergy to the paraben preservative. Esters were not evaluated in these patients.

Although true allergy to amide local anesthetics is rare, patients have more frequently demonstrated true allergic reactions to components of the dental cartridge. The dental cartridge contains a number of components besides the local anesthetic solution (Table 24-2). Of special interest with respect to allergy are two items: methylparaben and sodium metabisulfite.

The parabens—methyl, ethyl, and propyl—are bacteriostatic agents and are added to many drugs, foods, and cosmetics that are meant for multiple use. The parabens are structurally related to the ester local anesthetics, thus their increased allergenicity. It is difficult if not impossible to avoid contact with the parabens. Because of their increas-

Table 24-2. Contents of local anesthetic cartridge

Ingredient	Function
Local anesthetic agent	Conduction blockade
Vasoconstrictor	Decrease absorption of local anesthetic into blood, thus increasing duration of anesthesia and decreasing toxicity of anesthetic
Sodium metabisulfite	Antioxidant for vasoconstrictor
Methylparaben*	Preservative to increase shelf life; bacteriostatic
Sodium chloride	Isotonicity of solution
Sterile water	Diluent

*Methylparaben has been excluded from all local anesthetic cartridges manufactured in the United States since January, 1984. It is still found in multiple-dose vials of medications and in some local anesthetic solutions manufactured in other countries.

ing use, the frequency of sensitization to the parabens has greatly increased. Parabens are used increasingly in nondrug items such as skin creams, hair lotions, suntan preparations, face powder, soaps, lipsticks, toothpastes, syrups, soft drinks, and candies. In response to the increasing incidence of allergic reactions to these products, certain products have been marked as "hypoallergenic" and do not contain any parabens. Though anaphylaxis has been reported, paraben allergy is rarely systemic, most commonly appearing as a localized skin eruption or as localized edema.

Patients with a history of allergy to an amide local anesthetic were tested, using the anesthetic without methylparaben and with the preservative alone.[31,32] In every instance the patient reacted to the preservative but did not react to the same anesthetic without the preservative. Paraben allergy is almost exclusively limited to a dermatologic type response. In 1984 the Food and Drug Administration (FDA) ordered the removal of paraben preservatives from all single-use local anesthetic cartridges manufactured in the United States. Methylparaben is still included in dental cartridges of local anesthetics in some countries, and is found in all multiple-dose containers of injectable drugs.

Allergy to sodium bisulfite or metabisulfite is being reported with increasing frequency.[33-35] Bisulfites are antioxidants and are commonly used in restaurants where they are sprayed on fruits and vegetables as a preservative and to prevent discoloration. For example, sliced apples sprayed with bisulfite do not turn brown (i.e., become oxidized). Bisulfites are also used to prevent bacterial contamination of wines, beers, and distilled beverages.[36] Persons with bisulfite allergy frequently respond to contact with bisulfite with severe respiratory allergy, such as bronchospasm. Within the asthmatic population reports demonstrate that up to 10% are allergic to bisulfites.[33,37] It is not known if bisulfites are triggers of anaphylaxis.[33,37] A history of bisulfite allergy should alert the doctor to the possibility of this same type of response if sodium bisulfite or metabisulfite are included in the anesthetic cartridge. Bisulfites are present in all cartridges of local anesthetic that contain a vasoconstrictor. Local anesthetic solutions that do not contain vasoconstrictor additives do not contain bisulfites.

Topical anesthetics are also potential allergens. Most topical anesthetics are esters, with benzocaine and tetracaine the most commonly employed. Many topical anesthetics, even the amides (e.g., lidocaine), contain preservatives such as the parabens (methyl, ethyl, propyl), so that allergy must always be considered when these agents are used.

Clinical manifestations of allergy related to topical anesthetic application may span the entire spectrum of allergic responses; however, the most common response is allergic contact stomatitis, which may include mild erythema, edema, and ulcerations. If widespread and severe, the edema may lead to difficulty in swallowing and breathing.

Other Agents

"Denture sore mouth" is the name commonly given to inflammatory changes of the mucous membranes developing beneath dentures. Most frequently the oral mucosa of the palate and maxillary ridges are involved, with the tissue appearing bright red and edematous and the patient complaining of soreness, rawness, dryness, and burning.

The acrylic resins used in most dentures today are capable of producing allergy. This is much more likely to occur when self-cured acrylics are used instead of heat-cured acrylics. In addition, dental personnel and laboratory technicians may develop contact dermatitis to these materials. These reactions occur most frequently on the fingers and hands and are almost always caused by the acrylic monomer (the liquid), methyl methacrylate.

Heat-cured acrylics are less frequently associated with allergy because the monomer is more completely utilized in the polymerization process. In cold-cured or self-cured acrylics, it is likely that small amounts of monomer will remain unpolymerized, and it is this that produces the allergic response in previously sensitized individuals. Cold-

352   *Drug-related emergencies*

curing or self-curing acrylics are employed in denture repair and relining procedures, as well as in the fabrication of temporary crowns, bridges, and splints.

PREVENTION
Medical History Questionnaire

The medical history questionnaire contains several questions relating to allergy.

QUESTION 7. Are you allergic to (i.e., experience itching, rash, swelling of hands, feet, or eyes) or made sick by penicillin, aspirin, codeine, or any drugs or medications?

QUESTION 9. Circle any of the following that you have had or have at present:
• Asthma
• Hay fever
• Sinus trouble
• Allergies or hives

COMMENT. These questions seek to determine if ADRs have occurred. Adverse drug reactions are not uncommon; those most frequently reported are usually labeled "allergy." Any positive response to these questions must be thoroughly evaluated by means of the dialogue history.

In all instances in which the possibility of allergy does exist, it is prudent for the doctor to assume that the claim of allergy is valid and to continue to do so until the exact nature of the reaction can be determined. The dialogue history is a vital part of this determination process, as is possible medical consultation in the event that any doubt remains concerning the allergy following the dentist's evaluation of the patient. The drug or drugs in question, as well as any closely related drugs, should not be used until the alleged allergy has been thoroughly evaluated.

Fortunately, substitute drugs exist and may be employed in place of most of those that commonly cause allergy. These substitute drugs possess most of the same desirable clinical actions as the primary drugs, but are not as allergenic. The only group in which the substitute drugs are not as effective clinically as the primary agents is the local anesthetics. Because these are also the most important drugs employed in dental practice, much of the following discussion is related to the problem of local anesthetic allergy.

Dialogue History

Following an affirmative response to the question about a previous adverse drug reaction, the doctor should seek as much information as possible from the patient directly. The following questions should be asked, with slight modification where appropriate, in the evaluation of an alleged drug allergy.

QUESTION. What drug was used?

COMMENT. A patient who is truly allergic to a drug should be told the exact generic name of the substance. Many persons with documented allergic histories wear a Medic Alert tag (Fig. 24-1), which lists the items to which they are sensitive as well as other medical conditions. However, the most common responses to this question are, "I'm allergic to local anesthetics," "I'm allergic to Novocain," or "I'm allergic to all '-caine' drugs." Novocaine (procaine), an ester, is rarely used today as a local anesthetic in dentistry, the amides having virtually replaced the esters. Yet patients routinely refer to the local anesthetics they receive as "shots of Novocain." There are two reasons for this: first, the name Novocain has become virtually synonymous with dental injections. Second, in spite of the fact that most doctors do not use procaine or procaine-propoxycaine, many doctors themselves still refer to local anesthetics as Novocain, although they use amide local anesthetics almost exclusively. Therefore, the usual response to the question remains, "I'm allergic to Novocain." This response, if received from a patient who has truly been managed properly (see text that follows) in the past following an adverse reaction to a local anesthetic, indicates that the patient was sensitive to an ester local anesthetic but not to the amide local anesthetic. However, the answers received are usually too general and too vague to permit any conclusions to be drawn without further questioning.

QUESTION. What amount of drug was administered?

COMMENT. This question seeks to determine whether or not there was a definite dose-response relationship, as might be seen in an overdose reaction. The problem is that the patient rarely knows these clinical details and can provide little or no assistance.

QUESTION. Did the solution contain vasoconstrictors or preservatives?

COMMENT. The reaction may have been an overdose to the vasoconstrictors in the solution. If an allergic reaction did occur, perhaps it was related to the preservative and not to the local anesthetic. Unfortunately, however, most patients are unable to furnish this information.

QUESTION. Were you taking any other medication at the time?

COMMENT. This question seeks to determine the possibility that drug interaction or another drug was responsible for the reported adverse reaction.

QUESTION. What was the time sequence of events?

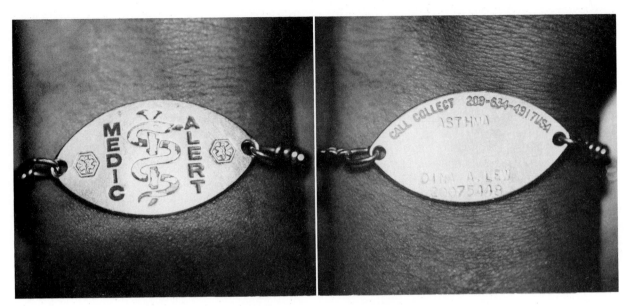

Fig. 24-1. Medical alert bracelet.

COMMENT. When, in relation to the administration of the drug, did the reaction occur? Most ADRs associated with local anesthetic administration occur during or immediately following their injection. Syncope, hyperventilation, overdose, and anaphylaxis are most likely to develop at the time of injection, although any of these reactions may also occur later during dental therapy. Try to determine how long the episode lasted. How long was it until the patient was discharged from the office? Was dental treatment continued followed the episode? Dental treatment that continued following the episode indicates that the reaction was probably not an allergic response.

QUESTION. What position were you in when the reaction took place?

COMMENT. Injection of local anesthetics with the patient in an upright position is most likely to produce a psychogenic reaction (e.g., vasodepressor syncope). This does not exclude the possibility of other reactions having occurred; however, if the patient was in a supine position during injection, vasodepressor syncope seems less likely to be the cause of the reaction, even though loss of consciousness may occur on rare occasion in these circumstances.

QUESTION. How did the reaction manifest itself? What happened?

COMMENT. This is a very important question because it asks the patient to describe what actually occurred. The allergy in many instances is explained by the answer to this question. The signs and symptoms the patient describes should be recorded and evaluated to make a tentative diagnosis of the ADR. See the chapters on overdose reaction (Chapter 23), vasodepressor syncope (Chapter 6), and the differential diagnosis of drug reactions (Chapter 25), as well as this chapter for complete listings of clinical signs and symptoms of each of these responses. Did the patient lose consciousness? Did seizures occur? Was there a skin reaction or respiratory distress?

Allergic reactions normally involve one or more of the following systems: the skin (e.g., itching, swelling, rash), the gastrointestinal system (e.g., diarrhea, nausea and vomiting, cramping), the exocrine glands (e.g., running nose, watery eyes), the respiratory system (e.g., wheezing, laryngeal edema), and the cardiovascular (e.g., hypotension, tachycardia) and/or genitourinary system.

Most often, patients describe their allergic reaction as one in which they suffered palpitations, severe headache, sweating, and mild shaking (tremor). Such reactions are usually of psychogenic origin or are related to the administration of large doses of vasoconstrictors and are not allergic in nature. Hyperventilation, an anxiety-induced reaction in which the patient loses control of his or her breathing—breathing rapidly and deeply—leads to signs and symptoms of dizziness, lightheadedness, and peripheral (e.g., fingers, toes, lips) paresthesias.

QUESTION. **What treatment was given?**

COMMENT. When the patient is able to describe the management of the reaction, the doctor can usually determine its cause. Were drugs administered? If so, what drugs? Epinephrine, anticonvulsants, aromatic ammonia? Knowledge of the definitive management of each of these situations can lead to an accurate diagnosis.

Drugs employed in the management of allergy include three drug types or categories: epinephrine (Adrenalin); antihistamines, including diphenhydramine (Benadryl) or chlorpheniramine (Chlor-Trimeton); and corticosteroids, including hydrocortisone sodium succinate (SoluCortef). The use of one or more of these drugs greatly increases the possibility that an allergic reaction did occur.

Anticonvulsants such as diazepam (Valium), midazolam (Versed, Hypnovel, Dormicum), and the injectable barbiturates, including pentobarbital (Nembutal), are administered to manage seizures, either generalized tonic-clonic or those induced by local anesthetics. Aromatic ammonia is frequently used in the treatment of syncopal episodes. Oxygen may be administered in any or all of these reactions.

QUESTION. **Were the services of a physician or paramedical personnel required? Were you hospitalized?**

COMMENT. A positive response indicates that a more serious reaction occurred. Most psychogenic responses can be ruled out in this instance.

QUESTION. **What is the name and address of the doctor (dentist, physician, or hospital) who was treating you at the time the adverse reaction took place?**

COMMENT. If possible, it is usually valuable to speak to the doctor who managed the previous episode. He or she is, in most instances, able to locate the records and to describe in detail what actually occurred. Direct discussion with the dentist or physician normally provides a wealth of information with which the knowledgeable practitioner can determine the precise nature of the previous reaction. It is quite unlikely that a health professional will ever forget a case of anaphylaxis that occurred during the management of a patient. It is much more likely that details of a syncopal episode will be forgotten with time.

Medical Consultation

If doubt remains in the doctor's mind following completion of the dialogue history, allergy must still be assumed, and the drugs in question should not be used. At this point, referral of the patient should be considered, to a doctor who will be able to more fully evaluate the nature of the previous reaction. Physicians, primarily allergists and anesthesiologists, and some dentists (dentist anesthesiologists) are likely to be willing and able to completely evaluate this patient. This doctor will also be able to perform certain tests that will prove more reliable in assessing the patient's local anesthetic allergy. Among the more commonly used tests are skin testing, passive transfer methods, and blood tests, such as the basophil degranulation test.[38]

Skin testing is still the primary mode of testing for local anesthetic allergy. Although several varieties of skin tests are used, the intracutaneous test is considered to be among the most reliable.[31] Intracutaneous testing involves the injection of 0.1 mL of the test solution and is thought to be 100 times more sensitive than the cutaneous test. It is, however, more unpleasant because it requires multiple needle punctures. Other problems associated with its use involve false-positives produced by the local release of histamine in response to skin puncture by the needle. However, intracutaneous testing is clinically useful, since a negative response probably means that the patient can safely receive the local anesthetic tested. No instance of an immediate allergic reaction has ever been reported in a patient with a previously negative intracutaneous response for a given agent.[31,32]

In all instances in which skin testing is employed, the anesthetic solutions should not contain any preservatives. Tests for allergy to methylparaben should be done separately. If a positive response to paraben occurs, local anesthetics to which the patient is not allergic should be used during the patient's dental treatment provided they do not contain any preservative. All dental cartridges manufactured in the United States since January, 1984, do not contain methylparaben.

The protocol for intracutaneous testing for allergy to local anesthetics currently in use at the University of Southern California School of Dentistry is summarized as follows: After an extensive dialogue history, review of the patient's medical history, informed consent, and establishment of an intravenous line, 0.1 mL of each of the following is deposited intracutaneously: 0.9% normal saline, 1% or 2% lidocaine, 3% mepivacaine, and 4% prilocaine, all without methylparaben, followed by 0.1 mL of bacteriostatic water and/or one or more local anesthetics containing methylparaben. The patient's vital signs are monitored every 5 minutes throughout the testing procedure. Following successful completion of this phase of the testing (60 minutes), 1 mL of one of the preceding local anesthetic solutions that tested negative is administered intraorally by means of supraperiosteal (infiltration) injection, atraumatically, but without use of topical anesthetic, above a maxillary anterior tooth. This is called a challenge test, and it frequently provokes the so-called allergic reaction, that is, signs and symptoms of a psychogenic response.[32]

After having completed more than 188 local anesthetic allergy test procedures, the author has encountered four allergic responses to the paraben preservative and none to the local anesthetic itself. Numerous psychogenic responses have developed during either the intracutaneous or intraoral testing procedures.

Skin testing is not without risk. Severe, immediate allergic reactions may be precipitated by the administration of as little as 0.1 mL of a drug to a sensitized patient. Emergency drugs, equipment, and personnel for resuscitation must always be readily available when allergy testing is contemplated.

Allergy Testing in the Dental Office

It is occasionally suggested that in an emergency situation (such as a toothache or infection) the doctor should carry out the aforementioned testing procedure in the dental office. It is the author's firm conviction that dental office allergy testing not be considered for the following reasons. First, skin testing, although potentially valuable, is not foolproof. Localized histamine release (false-positives) may result from the trauma of the needle insertion. A negative reaction, although commonly taken to indicate that a drug may safely be injected, may also prove unreliable. In some cases the drug itself is not the agent to which the patient is sensitive. Instead, a metabolite resulting from biotransformation of the drug may be the causative agent. The skin test would be negative or a positive response would be delayed for many hours under these circumstances. A second and even more compelling factor for not using skin testing in the dental office is the possibility that even the minute quantity of drug being employed (0.1 mL) might precipitate an immediate and acute systemic anaphylactic response in a truly allergic patient. Drugs, equipment, and personnel needed for the management of anaphylaxis and cardiopulmonary arrest must always be available when allergy tests are undertaken.

Dental Therapy Modifications
Allergy to Drugs Other Than Local Anesthetics

When a patient is proved to be truly allergic to a drug, precautions must be taken to prevent the

patient from receiving that substance. The outside of the dental chart should be marked with a medical alert sign that is easily visible, alerting the dental office staff to look at the medical history carefully. Inside the chart it should be noted that the patient "is allergic to _____."* For all of the more highly allergenic drugs prescribed in dentistry, substitute drugs are available that are usually equipotent in therapeutic effect but that pose less of a risk of allergy.

Penicillin allergy may be circumvented through the use of erythromycin; it is a drug possessing virtually the same clinical spectrum of effectiveness as penciillin G, but with a lower incidence of allergy. Sensitization reactions to erythromycin, including skin lesions, fever, and anaphylaxis, have been reported but are much less frequent than penicillin allergy.[39] Erythromycin remains the classic substitute drug for penicillin G.

Acetaminophen is the drug employed in cases of allergy to aspirin. Although as effective an analgesic as aspirin, acetaminophen is not as effective as an antipyretic. However, it is not cross-allergenic with aspirin and may be administered to the salicylate-sensitive patient.

Allergy to the narcotic analgesics is rare, with the unpleasant side effects of nausea and vomiting the most commonly encountered reactions. However, in the presence of a true narcotic allergy, no narcotic may be used because they are cross-allergenic. Nonnarcotic analgesics may be of some value in this situation.

Barbiturate allergy is an absolute contraindication to the use of any barbiturate, because cross-allergenicity exists among all group members. However, the chemical structures of the nonbarbiturate sedative-hypnotics are sufficiently different so that cross-allergenicity does not occur. These drugs may safely be employed in patients with barbiturate allergy. Included in this group of drugs are flurazepam, diazepam, midazolam, oxazepam, triazolam, chloral hydrate, and hydroxyzine.

Allergy to methyl methacrylate monomer is most readily avoided by not employing acrylic resins. If, however, acrylic resins must be used, heat-cured acrylic is much less allergenic than cold-cured or self-cured acrylic.

Table 24-3 summarizes the substitute drugs discussed here. In all cases it is possible for a patient to be allergic to one of the substitute drugs. There-

*Patient confidentiality laws preclude writing a patient's medical information on the outside of the chart where it may be seen by other persons. A general notice on the outside, "Medical Alert," is adequate to alert the staff to check the patient's medical history prior to the start of treatment.

Table 24-3. Allergenic drugs and possible substitutes

Category	Drug	Usual substitute	
		Generic	*Proprietary*
Antibiotics	Penicillin	Erythromycin	Ilosone
			Erythrocin
Analgesics	Acetylsalicylic acid (aspirin)	Acetaminophen	Tylenol
			Tempra
			Datril
	Narcotic	No equally effective substitute presently available	
Sedative-hypnotics	Barbiturates	Flurazepam	Dalmane
		Diazepam	Valium
		Triazolam	Halcion
		Chloral hydrate	Noctec
		Hydroxyzine	Atarax, Vistaril
Acrylic	Methyl methacrylate	Avoid use if possible, otherwise, use heat-cured acrylic	

fore, the doctor must specifically question the patient about any drug before it is administered.

When considering the use of these or any other drugs, several additional factors must be considered. The likelihood of an allergic reaction to a drug increases with the duration and the number of courses of therapy. One remarkable example is a patient who had received 16 courses of penicillin therapy without adverse reaction over many years but developed anaphylactic shock with the seventeenth. Although long-term drug therapy is rarely necessary in dentistry, one must remember that acute allergic reactions may occur even in the absence of a previous history of allergy.

The route of drug administration is also of importance. It must be understood that allergic symptoms can arise following any route of administration. The site of administration is frequently the main target area for the allergic symptoms, especially following topical application of drugs. Of significance, however, is the finding that anaphylactic reactions occur much less commonly following enteral rather than parenteral administration of drugs. The frequency of other types of allergic drug reaction may also be decreased by using the oral route. It is important therefore to consider the method of administration of a drug and, when it is possible, to administer the drug orally rather than parenterally. Penicillin is an example of a highly allergenic drug. There are extremely few indications for the parenteral administration of this agent in the dental office, because oral administration has been shown to result in adequate blood levels of penicillin in a relatively short time.[40] However, anaphylaxis has been reported following the oral administration of penicillin.[9,41] Antianxiety agents may require parenteral administration when used in a fearful patient. The risk of allergy to the drug must be weighed against the potential benefit to be gained from its use by this route. Local anesthetics, however, are a drug group that must be administered parenterally to be effective. Allergic reactions observed following parenteral drug administration tend to be more severe.

Management
Alleged Allergy to Local Anesthetics

Elective dental care: With a doubtful history of allergy to local anesthesia, these drugs should not be administered to the patient. Elective dental care that requires local anesthesia (e.g., topical or injectable) may need to be postponed until a thorough evaluation of the patient is completed by a competent person. Dental care not requiring local or topical anesthesia may be carried out during this period.

Emergency dental care: The patient in pain or with an oral infection presents a more difficult situation. In many cases the patient is new to the office, has a tooth requiring extraction or pulpal extirpation, and has a normal medical history except for an alleged allergy to Novocain. Following questioning of this patient, the allergy seems most likely to have been of psychogenic origin (e.g., vasodepressor syncope), but some doubt remains. How might this patient be managed?

Option 1: The most practical approach to this patient is an immediate consultation with a person who is able to test the patient for response to local anesthetics. Dental treatment should be postponed if possible. If pain is present it may be managed orally with various analgesics; infection can be controlled with antibiotics. These are temporary measures only. Following evaluation of the patient's claim of allergy, definitive dental care may be carried out.

Option 2: A second approach might be to use general anesthesia in place of a local anesthetic for the management of the dental emergency. Although a highly useful and relatively safe technique when properly performed, there are complications and problems associated with the use of general anesthesia, not the least of which is the fact that it is unavailable in most dental offices. However, general anesthesia remains a viable alternative to local anesthesia in the management of the allergic patient, provided adequate facilities and well-trained personnel are available.

Option 3: A third option to consider when emergency treatment is necessary and general anesthesia is not available is to use an antihistamine, such as diphenhydramine, as a local anesthetic for the management of pain during treatment. Most injectable antihistamines possess local anesthetic properties. Several are more potent local anesthetics than procaine. Diphenhydramine (Benadryl) has been the most commonly used antihistamine in this regard. Used as a 1% solution with 1:100,000 epinephrine, diphenhydramine has produced pulpal anesthesia of up to 30 minutes' duration.[42]

An unwanted side effect frequently noted during the intraoral administration of diphenhydramine is a burning or stinging sensation. The use of nitrous oxide and oxygen along with this agent minimizes discomfort. Another possible unwanted result of the use of antihistamine as a local anesthetic is postoperative tissue swelling and soreness. These unpleasant actions must be considered before the use of these agents. For these reasons the use of diphenhydramine as a local anesthetic is usually limited to those instances in which there is a questionable history of local anesthetic allergy, the patient has a dental emergency requiring immediate physical intervention, and general anesthesia is not a reasonable alternative. It must again be kept in mind that allergy may develop to any drug, including the antihistamines.[43] The patient should be questioned concerning prior exposure to antihistamines or other drugs before they are used.

It is important to remember that there are almost no dental emergency situations in which physical intervention is absolutely required. Appropriate drug therapy with immediate medical consultation (option 1) probably remains the most reasonable mode of action in these cases of alleged local anesthetic allergy coupled with a dental emergency.

Confirmed Allergy to Local Anesthetics

Management of the patient with a true, documented, and reproducible allergy to local anesthetics varies according to the nature of the allergy. If the local anesthetic allergy is limited to the ester drugs (e.g., procaine, propoxycaine, benzocaine, or tetracaine), the amides (e.g., lidocaine, mepivacaine, or prilocaine) may be used as cross-allergenicity, though possible, is rare. If the local anesthetic allergy was actually an allergy to the paraben preservative, an amide local anesthetic may be injected if it does not contain any preservative. Dental cartridges in the United States have not contained parabens since 1984; however, if the local anesthetic was administered by a nondental health professional, it is possible that the drug contained paraben because multiple-dose containers of local anesthetics (all of which contain paraben) are frequently used by medical personnel other than dentists. On occasion, however, it is reported that a patient is allergic to all "-caine" drugs. The author recommends that this report undergo careful scrutiny and that the method by which this conclusion was reached be reexamined (What tests were carried out? By whom? Were pure solutions used? Or were preservatives present?). All too often patients are labeled allergic to all local anesthetics when in reality they are not. These patients often have their dental treatment carried out in a hospital setting under general anesthesia, when a proper evaluation might have prevented this, saving the patient much time and money in addition to decreasing the operative and anesthetic risk.

The following statement on local anesthetic allergy by Aldrete and Johnson[31] concludes this important section on the prevention of allergy.

"A strong plea is made for a thorough evaluation of the circumstances surrounding an adverse reaction to a local anesthetic before the label of "allergic to procaine," "allergic to lidocaine," or "allergic to all 'caine' drugs" is entered on the front of the patient's chart. We believe that untoward reactions observed during the use of local anesthetic agents are quite frequently the result of overdosage. . . . The benefits obtained from the use of local anesthetic agents should not be denied to a patient just because of an untoward response during a previous exposure to one of them. Instead, details of the circumstances surrounding the incident, such as sequence of events, other drugs administered, and the type of procedure, must be evaluated."

CLINICAL MANIFESTATIONS

The various forms that allergic reactions may take are listed in Table 24-1. In addition to these classifications, it is also possible to list reactions according to the length of time that elapses between contact with the antigen and the appearance of clinical signs and symptoms. The two categories in this grouping are immediate and delayed reactions. Immediate allergic reactions are those that occur within seconds to hours of exposure and include types I, II, and III of the Gell and Coombs classification system (Table 24-1). Delayed allergic reactions occur hours to days following antigenic exposure. The type IV reaction is an example of delayed response.

Of greatest significance to the dentist are the immediate reactions, in particular the type I, or anaphylactic, reaction. Most allergic drug reactions are immediate. A number of organs and tissues are affected during immediate allergic reactions, particularly the skin, cardiovascular system, respiratory system, the eyes, and gastrointestinal tract. Generalized (systemic) anaphylaxis by definition affects all of the aforementioned systems. When hypotension occurs as a part of the reaction, resulting in the loss of consciousness, the term *anaphylactic shock* may be employed.

Immediate allergic reactions may also manifest themselves through any number of combinations involving these systems. Reactions involving one organ system are referred to as localized anaphylaxis. Examples include bronchial asthma, in which the respiratory system is the target, and urticaria, in which the skin is the target organ. The skin and respiratory reactions are discussed individually, followed by a description of generalized anaphylaxis.

Onset

The period elapsing between the exposure of the patient to the antigen and the development of clinical symptoms is of great importance. In general, the more rapidly signs and symptoms of allergy occur following exposure, the more intense the ultimate reaction.[44] Conversely, the greater the time elapsing between exposure and onset, the less intense the reaction. However, rare cases have been reported of systemic anaphylaxis developing up to several hours following antigenic exposure.[45] Of importance too is the rate at which signs and symptoms progress once they appear. If they appear and rapidly increase in intensity, the reaction is more likely to be life threatening than is one that progresses slowly or not at all once initial signs and symptoms appear. These time factors have a bearing on the management of allergic reactions.

NOTE. **The more rapidly signs and symptoms of allergy occur following exposure, the more intense the ultimate reaction.**

Skin Reaction

Allergic skin reactions are the most common sensitization reaction to drug administration. Many types of allergic skin reactions may occur; the three most important types are localized anaphylaxis, contact dermatitis, and drug eruption. Drug eruption constitutes the most common group of skin manifestations of drug allergy. Included in this category are urticaria (itching, hives), erythema (rash), and angioedema (localized swelling measuring several centimeters in diameter).

Urticaria is associated with wheals (smooth, slightly elevated patches of skin) and frequently with intense itching (pruritis). Angioedema is a process in which localized swelling occurs in response to an allergen. Several forms of angioedema exist, but they are clinically similar.[46,47] The skin is usually of normal temperature and color, unless accompanied by urticaria and/or erythema, and pain and itching are uncommon. The areas most frequently involved include the periorbital, perioral, and intraoral regions of the face, as well as the extremities. Of special interest in dentistry is the potential involvement of the lips, tongue, pharynx, and larynx, which can lead to obstruction of the airway. The preceding group of signs and symptoms are most often noted in heritary angioneurotic edema. Angioedema is observed most frequently following administration of topical anesthetics (e.g., ester local anesthetics or methylparaben) to the oral mucosa. Within 30 to 60 minutes, the tissue in contact with the allergen appears quite swollen and erythematous.

Allergic skin reactions, if they are the sole manifestation of an allergic response, are normally not considered to be life threatening. Yet a skin reaction that develops rapidly following drug administration may be only the first indication of a more generalized reaction to follow.

Contact dermatitis is an allergic reaction that is most often observed in members of the dental profession. The sensitization process may require years of constant exposure before clinical symptoms occur. These include erythema, induration (hardness), edema, and vesicle formation. Chronic reexposure to the specific antigen results in dry, scaly lesions resembling eczema. Signs and symptoms related to allergic skin reactions are presented in Table 24-4.

Respiratory Reactions

Clinical signs and symptoms of allergy may be related entirely to the respiratory tract, or signs and symptoms of respiratory tract involvement may occur along with other systemic responses. In a slowly

Table 24-4. Clinical manifestations of allergic skin reactions

Reaction	Symptoms	Signs	Pathophysiology
Urticaria	Pruritis, tingling and warmth, flushing, hives	Urticaria, diffuse erythema	Increased vascular permeability, vasodilation
Angioedema	Nonpruritic extremity, periorbital and perioral swelling	Nonpitting edema, frequently asymmetrical	Increased vascular permeability, vasodilation

From Lindzon RD, Silvers WS: Anaphylaxis. In Rosen P, Baker FJ, Barkin RM, and others, editors. *Emergency medicine*, ed 2, St Louis, 1988, Mosby–Year Book.

Table 24-5. Clinical manifestations of respiratory allergic reactions

Reaction	Symptoms	Signs	Pathophysiology
Rhinitis	Nasal congestion, nasal itching, sneezing	Nasal mucosal edema, rhinorrhea	Increased vascular permeability, vasodilation, stimulation of nerve endings
Laryngeal edema	Dyspnea, hoarseness, throat tightness, hypersalivation	Laryngeal stridor, supraglottic and glottic edema	As above, plus increased exocrine gland secretions
Bronchospasm	Cough, wheezing, retrosternal tightness, dyspnea	Cough, wheeze (bronchi), tachypnea, respiratory distress, cyanosis	As above, plus bronchiole smooth muscle contraction

From Lindzon RD, Silvers WS: Anaphylaxis. In Rosen P, Baker FJ, Barkin RM, and others, editors: *Emergency medicine*, ed 2, St Louis, 1988, Mosby–Year Book.

evolving generalized allergic reaction, respiratory reactions normally follow the skin, exocrine, and gastrointestinal responses, but precede cardiovascular signs and symptoms. Bronchospasm is the classic respiratory manifestation of allergy. It represents the clinical result of constriction of bronchial smooth muscle. Signs and symptoms of an acute episode of allergic asthma are identical to nonallergic asthma. They include respiratory distress, dyspnea, wheezing, flushing, possible cyanosis, perspiration, tachycardia, greatly increased anxiety, and the use of the accessory muscles of respiration. Asthma is described fully in Chapter 13.

A second respiratory manifestation of allergy may be the extension of angioedema to the larynx, which produces swelling of the vocal apparatus with subsequent obstruction of the airway. Clinical signs and symptoms of this acutely life-threatening situation include little or no exchange of air from the lungs (look to see if the chest is moving; feel that there is little or no air; listen for wheezing, indicative of a partial airway obstruction, or no sound, indicating total obstruction of the airway). The occurrence of significant angioedema represents one of the most ominous clinical signs. Acute airway obstruction leads rapidly to death unless immediately corrected.

Laryngeal edema represents the effects of allergy on the upper airway. Asthma represents the actions of allergy on the lower airway. Table 24-5 summarizes the clinical signs and symptoms of allergy on the respiratory system.

Generalized Anaphylaxis

Generalized anaphylaxis is a most dramatic and acutely life-threatening allergic reaction and may cause death within a few minutes. Most fatalities from anaphylaxis occur within the first 30 minutes postantigenic exposure, although many will succumb up to 120 minutes after the onset of the anaphylactic reaction.[48] It may develop following the administration of an antigen by any route, but is most likely to occur following parenteral administration. The time from antigenic challenge to the onset of signs and symptoms is quite variable, but typically the reaction develops rapidly, reaching a maximal intensity within 5 to 30 minutes. Delayed responses of an hour or more have also been reported. It is thought that this is a result of the rate at which the antigen enters the circulatory system.

The signs and symptoms of generalized anaphylaxis are highly variable.[10] Four major clinical syndromes are recognized: skin reactions, smooth muscle spasm (gastrointestinal and genitourinary tracts and respiratory smooth muscle), respiratory distress, and cardiovascular collapse. In typical generalized anaphylaxis, the symptoms progressively evolve through these four areas; however, in cases of fatal anaphylaxis, respiratory and cardiovascular

Table 24-6. Clinical manifestations of allergic cardiovascular reactions

Reaction	Symptoms	Signs	Pathophysiology
Circulatory collapse	Light-headedness, generalized weakness, syncope, ischemic chest pain	Tachycardia, hypotension, shock	Increased vascular permeability, vasodilation a. Loss of vasomotor tone b. Increased venous capacitance
Dysrhythmias	As above, plus palpitations	ECG changes: tachycardia, nonspecific and ischemic ST-T wave changes, premature atrial and ventricular contractions, nodal rhythm, atrial fibrillation	Decreased cardiac output a. Direct mediator-induced myocardial suppression b. Decreased effective plasma volume c. Decreased preload d. Decreased afterload e. Hypoxia and ischemia f. Dysrhythmias g. Iatrogenic effects of drugs used in treatment h. Preexisting heart disease
Cardiac arrest		Pulselessness; ECG changes: ventricular fibrillation, asystole	

From Lindzon RD, Silvers WS: Anaphylaxis. In Rosen P, Baker FJ, Barkin RM, and others, editors: *Emergency medicine*, ed 2, St Louis, 1988, Mosby–Year Book.

disturbances predominate and are evident early in the reaction.

In a typical generalized anaphylactic reaction, the first involvement is with the skin. The patient experiences a generalized warmth and tingling of the face, mouth, upper chest, palms, soles, or the site of antigenic exposure. Pruritis is a universal feature, and may be accompanied by generalized flushing and urticaria, while nonpruritic angioedema may also be evident initially. Other reactions that are noted during the early phase of the reaction include conjunctivitis, vasomotor rhinitis (inflammation of the mucous membranes of the nose, marked by increased mucous secretion), and pilomotor erection (the feeling of "hair standing on end"). Cramping abdominal pain with nausea, vomiting, diarrhea, and tenesmus (persistent, ineffectual spasms of the rectum or bladder, accompanied by the desire to empty the bowel or bladder), incontinence, pelvic pain, headache, a sense of impending doom, or a decrease in the level of consciousness.

These manifestations may soon be followed by mild to severe respiratory distress. The patient may describe a cough, a sense of pressure on the chest, dyspnea, and wheeze from bronchospasm, or throat tightness, odynophagia (a severe sensation of burning, squeezing pain while swallowing), or hoarseness associated with laryngeal edema or oropharyngeal angioedema. In a rapidly developing

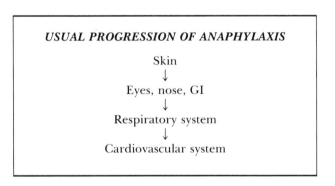

reaction, all symptoms may occur within a very short time with considerable overlap. In particularly severe reactions, respiratory and cardiovascular symptoms may be the only signs present.

Signs and symptoms of cardiovascular disturbance occur next and include pallor, lightheadedness, palpitation, tachycardia, hypotension, and cardiac dysrhythmias, followed by the loss of consciousness and cardiac arrest. With the loss of consciousness the anaphylactic reaction may more properly be called anaphylactic shock.

Cardiovascular signs and symptoms of allergy are summarized in Table 24-6. Any of these patterns may occur singly or in combination.[10]

The duration of the anaphylactic reaction or any part of it may vary from minutes to a day or more. With prompt and appropriate therapy the entire reaction may be terminated rapidly; however, the two most serious sequelae, hypotension and laryngeal edema, may persist for hours or days in spite of therapy. Death may occur at any time, the usual cause (from autopsy reports) being upper airway obstruction produced by laryngeal edema.

PATHOPHYSIOLOGY

The clinical manifestations of allergy are the result of an antigen-antibody reaction. Such reactions form a part of the body's defense mechanisms (i.e., immune system), which are described in the following material to provide a better understanding of the processes involved in allergy.

In order for acute, immediate allergy or for anaphylaxis to occur, three conditions must be met[10]:

1. An antigen-induced stimulation of the immune system with specific IgE antibody formation
2. A latent period after the initial antigenic exposure for sensitization of mast cells and basophils
3. Subsequent reexposure to that specific antigen

Anaphylactoid reactions are similar to anaphylaxis, but do not require an immunologic mechanism. Anaphylactoid reactions may occur following a single, first-time exposure to certain substances.

Antigens, Haptens, and Allergens

An antigen is any substance capable of inducing the formation of an antibody. Antigens are foreign to the species into which they are injected or ingested and may be harmful or harmless. Most antigens are proteins with a molecular weight between 5,000 and 40,000. Materials under a molecular weight of 5,000 are usually not allergenic or antigenic. Virtually all proteins, whether of animal, plant, or microbial origin, possess antigenic potential.

Drugs, however, are not proteins and commonly possess a very low molecular weight (500 to 1000), which makes them unlikely antigens. The hapten theory of drug allergy explains the mechanism through which drugs may act as antigens. A *hapten* is a specific, protein-free substance that can combine to form a hapten-protein complex with a carrier protein: circulating albumin. The hapten itself is not antigenic; however, when coupled with the carrier protein, it may provoke an immune response. The hapten may combine with the carrier protein outside the body and then be injected into the individual, or the hapten may combine with tissue proteins of the host after administration into the body. The latter mechanism is the one by which

most drugs become antigens and thus become capable of inducing antibody formation and causing an allergic reaction.[10] Penicillin, aspirin, and barbiturates are examples of haptens. Haptens are also called incomplete antigens. An allergen is an antigen that is capable of eliciting allergic symptoms. It is obvious that not every antigen is an allergen. An antigen or allergen may stimulate the production of several classes of immunoglobulins, each of which possesses different functions.

NOTE. **All drugs must be viewed as potential antigens and should be administered only when clinically indicated.**[49]

Antibodies (Immunoglobulins)

An antibody is a substance found in the blood or tissues that responds to the administration of an antigen or that reacts with it. The molecular weights of antibodies range from 150,000 (IgG = immunoglobulin G) to 900,000 (IgM). The basic structure of an antibody molecule consists of two heavy and two light polypeptide chains linked in a Y configuration by covalent disulfide bonds. The base of the heavy chain (called Fc for crystallizable unit) binds the antibody to the surface of a cell, while the arms of the antibody bind with receptor sites on the antigen. Immunoglobulins are produced by B lymphocytes, which constitute 10% to 15% of the circulating lymphocyte population, and are classified as IgA, IgD, IgE, IgG, and IgM according to structural differences in the heavy chains. Each immunoglobulin differs in its biologic functions and in the type of allergic response it may produce (Tables 24-1 and 24-7).[50]

IgA is found principally in the serum and in external secretions such as saliva and sputum. It represents 10% to 15% of all immunoglobulins. It plays a role in the defense mechanisms of the external surfaces of the body, including the mucous membranes. The fetus begins to produce IgA during the last 6 months in utero, and adult levels are reached by 5 years of age.

IgD is found in serum only in small amounts, representing only 0.2% of immunoglobulins. It is probably important as an antigen receptor on B lymphocytes.

IgE, the antibody responsible for immediate hypersensitivity, is synthesized by plasma cells in the nasal mucosa, respiratory tract, gastrointestinal tract, and lymphoid tissues. It is only found in the serum in trace amounts. It binds to tissue mast cells and basophils. When mast cell-bound IgE combines with an antigen, the mast cell releases histamine and other vasoactive substances. The half-life of IgE is approximately 2 days, serum levels normally

Table 24-7. Properties of human immunoglobulins

	IgA	IgD	IgE	IgG	IgM
Molecular weight	180,000	150,000	200,000	150,000	900,000
Normal serum concentration (mg/100 mL)	275	5	0.03	1200	120
Primary function	Local or mucosal reactions and infections	Antigen receptor on B lymphocytes	Type I hypersensitivity	Infection, type III hypersensitivity	Possible role in particular antigens

being quite low—0.03 mg/100 mL.

IgG represents approximately 75% to 80% of antibodies in normal serum, and its chief biologic functions are the binding to and enhancement of the phagocytosis of bacteria and neutralization of bacterial toxins. IgG also crosses the placenta and imparts immune protection to the fetus, which continues for the first 6 months after birth. Shortly after birth the infant begins to synthesize IgG, and by the age of 4 to 5 years, IgG levels approach adult levels.

IgM, the heaviest of the antibodies, is active in both agglutinating and in cytolytic reactions and accounts for 5% to 10% of all immunoglobulins. The fetus begins production of IgM during the final 6 months of fetal life, and adult levels are reached by 1 year of age.

Antibodies possess the ability to bind with the specific antigen that induces their production. This immunologic specificity is based on similarities in the structures of the antigen and antibody. Antibodies possess at least two specific antigen-binding sites per molecule (the Fab fragments). IgM possesses five, and IgA probably has more than two. Antibodies are not entirely specific, and cross-sensitivity is possible between chemically similar substances.

Defense Mechanisms of the Body

When a person is exposed to a foreign substance, the body attempts to protect itself through a number of mechanisms. These include anatomic barriers, which attempt to exclude entry of the antigen into the body. Examples of barriers include the epithelium of the gastrointestinal tract, the sneeze and cough mechanisms, and the mucociliary blanket of the tracheobronchial tree. Once the foreign substance is inside the body, two other nonspecific defense mechanisms are brought into play. These include mobilization of phagocytic blood cells such as leukocytes, histiocytes, and macrophages, and the production of nonspecific chemical substances such as lysozymes and proteolytic enzymes, which assist in removal of the foreign substance. A more specific defense mechanism is also employed. IgA antibody is produced by plasma cells in response to the antigen, and IgA then acts to aid in the removal or the detoxification of the antigen from the host.

Through these processes of anatomic localization, phagocytosis, and destruction, the antigen is usually eliminated, resulting in little or no damage to the host. If, however, the antigen remains because of genetic defects in the patient such as atopy or because of the nature of the antigen itself, additional defense mechanisms may be called into play that may ultimately prove harmful to the host. These include reactions that result in formation of antibodies that, on subsequent exposure to the antigen, may result in the formation of precipitates of antigen-antibody complexes within cells or blood vessels (type III response), or may result in the subsequent release of the chemical mediators of the type I allergic response.

There are at least three possible results of an antigen-antibody reaction:

1. The production of antibodies that combine with the antigen to neutralize it or change it so that it becomes innocuous
2. The antigen-antibody combination occurs within blood vessels in a magnitude sufficient to produce actual precipitates within small blood vessels, resulting in vascular occlusions with subsequent ischemic necrosis (e.g., the Arthus reaction—type III)
3. The antigen-antibody union, activating proteolytic enzymes that release certain chemicals from cells, which in turn act to produce the anaphylactic response

---

DEFENSE MECHANISMS OF THE BODY

Anatomic barriers
Mobilization of phagocytic blood cells
Production of enzymes
IgA antibody production

The first response is of benefit to the host, leading to elimination of the foreign material; the second and third reactions are capable of producing injury and death.

Type I Allergic Reaction—Anaphylaxis

The type I (anaphylactic or immediate) allergic reaction is of great concern to the doctor. For any true allergic reaction to occur, the patient must have previously been exposed to the antigen. This is called the sensitizing dose, and the subsequent exposure to the antigen is called the challenge dose.

Sensitizing Dose

During the sensitization phase the patient receives the initial exposure to the antigen. In response to the antigen, β lymphocytes are stimulated to develop into mature plasma cells that produce increasing amounts of immunoglobins specific for that antigen. When a susceptible (atopic) individual is exposed, antigen-specific immunoglobulin E (IgE) antibodies are formed, which interact only with that particular antigen (or with very closely related antigens, that is, cross-sensitivity). IgE antibodies are cytophilic and selectively attach themselves to the cell membranes of circulating basophils and tissue mast cells.

Sensitization occurs when the complement-fixing (F_c) portion of the IgE antibody affixes to receptor sites on the cell membranes of mast cells in the interstitial space and circulating basophils in the vascular space.[51,52] A latent period of variable duration (several days to possibly years) ensues, during which time IgE antibody continues to be produced (attaching to basophils and mast cells) while the level of antigen progressively decreases. Following this latent period, antigen is no longer present, but high levels of IgE-sensitized basophils and mast cells remain. The patient is then sensitized to the specific antigen.

Challenge (Allergic) Dose

Reexposure to the antigen results in an antigen-antibody interaction thought to be initiated by the antigen bridging the antibody fixing (Fab) arms of two adjacent IgE antibodies on the surface of sensitized mast cells or basophils.[53] In the presence of calcium, this bridging initiates a complex series of intramembrane and intracellular events that culminates in structural and functional membrane changes, granule solubilization, exocytosis, and the release of preformed chemical mediators of allergy into the circulation.[54] The primary preformed mediators of allergy are histamine, eosinophilic chemotactic factor of anaphylaxis (ECF-A), high mo-

lecular weight-neutrophil chemotactic factor (HMW-NCF), and the kallikreins.[55] Other preformed chemical mediators are enzymatic proteases (e.g., tryptase), acid hydrolases, and proteoglycans. These preformed mediators in turn may directly produce local and systemic pharmacologic effects, cause the release of other spontaneously generated mediators, or activate reflexes that ultimately produce the clinical picture of anaphylaxis. Spontaneously generated mediators include the leukokreines, prostaglandins, and platelet aggregating factor (PAF).[56]

Chemical Mediators of Anaphylaxis

The endogenous chemicals released from tissue mast cells and circulating basophils act on the primary target tissues, including the vascular, bronchial, and gastrointestinal smooth muscle, vascular endothelium, and exocrine glands, and are ultimately responsible for the clinical manifestations of allergy. These chemicals explain the similarity in allergic reactions regardless of the antigen that induces the response (e.g., penicillin, aspirin, procaine, shellfish, strawberries). The level of intensity of an allergic reaction may vary greatly (e.g., anaphylaxis, mild urticaria) from patient to patient. Factors involved in determining the variability of magnitude of an allergic response include (1) the amount of antigen or antibody present, (2) the affinity of the antibody for the antigen, (3) the concentration of chemical mediators, (4) the concentration of receptors for mediators, and (5) the affinity of the mediators for receptors. All of these factors, except for the antigen, are endogenous, which explains the wide variation in individual susceptibility. The major chemical mediators of allergy are briefly described with their primary biologic functions.

Histamine. Histamine is a widely distributed normal constituent of many tissues of the body, including the skin, lungs, nervous system, and gastrointestinal tract. In many tissues it is stored in preformed granules within the mast cell (a fixed-tissue cell) or in the circulating blood in basophils.[57] It is stored in these sites in a physiologically inactive form and is electrostatically bound to heparin in granule form. When an IgE-induced antigen-antibody reaction occurs, these granules undergo a process in which they are activated and released from the basophils and mast cells without damage to the cell. The actions of histamine within the body (which is described in the following paragraphs) are mediated by two different tissue histamine receptors called H_1 and H_2.[58,59] The clinical manifestations of histamine are influenced by the ratio of H_1 and H_2 activation.[56]

Particularly important pharmacologic actions of histamine include those on the cardiovascular system, smooth muscle, and glands. Cardiovascular actions of histamine include capillary dilation and increased capillary permeability. The action of capillary dilation, an H_1 and H_2 effect, is probably the most important action effected by histamine. All capillaries are involved following histamine administration. The effect is most obvious in the skin of the face and upper chest, the so-called blushing area, which becomes hot and flushed. Increased capillary permeability also leads to an outward passage of plasma protein and fluid into extracellular spaces, resulting in the formation of edema.

Other cardiovascular responses to histamine include the triple response. When administered subcutaneously or released in the skin, histamine produces (1) a localized red spot extending a few millimeters around the site of injection, (2) a brighter red flush or flare that is irregular in outline and extends for about 1 cm beyond the original red spot, and (3) localized edema fluid, which forms a wheal that is noted in about 1.5 minutes and occupies the same area as the original red spot. Histamine is also the chemical mediator of pain and itch.

Because of the cardiovascular actions of histamine, there is a decrease in venous return and a significant reduction in the systemic blood pressure and cardiac output. The resulting hypotension is normally of short duration because of the rapid inactivation of histamine and because of other compensatory reflexes that are activated in response to histamine release, such as increased catecholamine release from the adrenal medulla.

Histamine relaxes vascular smooth muscle in humans; however, most nonvascular smooth muscle is contracted (H_1). Smooth muscle constriction is most prominent in the uterus and bronchi. Bronchiolar smooth muscle constriction leads to the clinical syndrome of asthma (e.g., bronchospasm). Smooth muscle of the gastrointestinal tract is moderately constricted, whereas that of the urinary bladder and gallbladder is only slightly constricted.

Actions of histamine on exocrine glands involve the stimulation of secretions. Stimulated glands include the gastric, salivary, lacrimal, pancreatic, and intestinal glands. Increased secretion from mucous glands leads to the clinical syndrome of rhinitis, which is prominent in many allergic reactions.

Histamine is considered to be the major chemical mediator of anaphylaxis. Many of the physiologic responses to histamine may be moderated or blocked by the administration of pharmacologic doses of antihistamines before the release of histamine has occurred.

Slow-reacting substance of anaphylaxis. Slow-reacting substance of anaphylaxis (SRS-A) is a spontaneously generated mediator thought to be produced from the interaction of the antigen-IgE-mast cell and the subsequent transformation of cell membrane lipids to arachidonic acid. Arachidonic acid is then metabolized to either the prostaglandins, thromboxanes, and prostacyclins, or to the leukotrienes. SRS-A was recently identified as a mixture of leukotrienes (LTC_4, LTD_4, LTE_4).[60] The leukotrienes produce a marked and prolonged bronchial smooth muscle contraction. This effect is 6000 times as potent as that of histamine.[61] This bronchoconstrictive action is slower in onset, thus its original name: SRS-A, and longer lasting than that of histamine. Leukotrienes also increase vascular permeability and potentiate the effects of histamine.[62] The actions of leukotrienes are not diminished or reversed by antihistaminic drugs.

Eosinophylic chemotactic factor of anaphylaxis (ECF-A). ECF-A is a preformed mediator that has the ability to attract eosinophils to the target organ involved in the allergic reaction.[63] Eosinophils, through their release of secondary enzymatic mediators, are major regulatory leukocytes of anaphylaxis.

Another preformed mediator, **high molecular weight-neutrophil chemotactic factor** (HMW-NCF), is released rapidly into the circulation, has a half-life of several hours, and has a second peak level that correlates with the late phase asthmatic response.[64]

Basophil kallikreins, preformed mediators, are responsible for the generation of kinins. **Bradykinins** have been implicated as the mediators responsible for cardiovascular collapse in clinical situations in which no other manifestations of anaphylaxis are present.[65] Pharmacologic actions of the bradykinins include vasodilation, increased permeability of blood vessels, and the production of pain. Blood levels of bradykinin are significantly increased during anaphylaxis.

Prostaglandins (PG) are spontaneously generated mediators that are metabolites of arachidonic acid. Almost all cells are capable of producing these potent mediators. PGD_2 causes smooth muscle contraction and increased vascular permeability; PGE_1 and PGE_2 produce bronchodilation, whereas PGF_2 is a potent bronchoconstrictor.[66]

Platelet activating factor (PAF), has recently been described in humans,[67] and is the most potent compound known to cause the aggregation of human platelets.[68] PAF produces many important clinical findings in anaphylaxis, including cardiovascular collapse, pulmonary edema, and a prolonged increase in total pulmonary resistance.[69]

The chemical mediators described here act on the primary target organs to produce the clinical signs and symptoms of allergy and anaphylaxis.

Respiratory signs and symptoms: Vasodilation and increased vascular permeability result in transudation of plasma and proteins into interstitial spaces, which, along with increases in the secretion of mucus, laryngeal edema, and angioedema, may result in asphyxia from upper respiratory tract obstruction.[70] Bronchospasm resulting from bronchial smooth muscle constriction, respiratory mucosal edema, and increased mucus production can produce coughing, chest tightness, dyspnea, and wheezing.[10]

Cardiovascular signs and symptoms: Decreased vasomotor tone and increases in venous capacitance secondary to vasodilation can produce cardiovascular collapse. Circulatory collapse may develop suddenly and without prior respiratory or dermatologic manifestations.[71] Lightheadedness and syncope, tachycardia, dysrrhythmia, orthostatic hypotension, and shock are all results of these cardiovascular responses.

Gastrointestinal signs and symptoms: Cramping, abdominal pain, nausea and vomiting, diarrhea and tenesmus are produced by gastrointestinal mucosal edema and smooth muscle contraction.[72]

Urticaria, rhinitis, and conjunctivitis: These are end points of increased vascular permeability and vasodilation.[10]

In cases of fatal anaphylaxis the most prominent clinical pathological features are observed in the respiratory and cardiovascular systems, and include laryngeal edema, pulmonary hyperinflation, peribronchial vascular congestion, intraalveolar hemorrhage, pulmonary edema, increased tracheobronchial secretions, eosinophilic infiltration of the bronchial walls, and varying degrees of myocardial damage.[73]

MANAGEMENT

The clinical expression of allergy may be quite varied. Of concern to the doctor are the signs and symptoms of immediate allergy, which range from mild skin lesions to angioedema to generalized anaphylaxis. The speed with which symptoms of allergy appear and the rate at which they progress have a determining effect on the mode of management of the reaction.

Skin Reactions

Skin lesions may range from localized angioedema to diffuse erythema, urticaria, and pruritis. Management of these reactions is based on the speed at which they appear following antigenic challenge (e.g., drug administration).

Delayed Reactions

Skin reactions that appear after a considerable lapse of time following antigenic exposure (60 minutes or more) and do not progress may be considered non-life threatening. These include a mild skin reaction or a localized mucous membrane reaction following application of topical anesthetics.

Diagnostic clues to the presence of an allergic skin reaction include[74]:
- Hives, itching
- Edema
- Flushed skin

Step 1: Terminate the dental procedure. Stop treatment immediately upon recognition of clinical manifestations of an allergic skin reaction.

Step 2: Position the patient. As this patient is not in distress except for that produced by any itching that might be present, positioning is based upon comfort.

Step 3: Basic life support, as indicated. Assess airway, breathing, and circulation and implement basic life support as needed. At this juncture, airway, breathing, and circulation will be adequate.

Step 4: Definitive management. Immediate management of a mild, delayed-onset skin reaction will be to consider the administration of an antihistamine.

In the presence of a very localized response, such as with a small area of the lower lip appearing slightly swollen, erthematous, and itching following topical anesthetic application, observation might be considered the initial mode of treatment. The patient, or his or her parent or guardian, should be advised that if the reaction appears to increase, to call the dental office immediately so that a suitable drug (antihistamine) may be prescribed. An alternative, in this case of a very mild, localized reaction, is to give the patient a prescription for an oral antihistamine and either advise not to take the drug unless the reaction becomes bothersome, or to begin taking the drug immediately. When taken orally, the antihistamine should be administered as recommended for 2 to 3 days.

The oral dose of diphenhydramine is 25 mg to 50 mg (for adults) three to four times a day and 12.5 mg to 25 mg for children over 20 lbs. Chlorpheniramine 2 to 4 mg for adults, three or four times a day; for children, 2 mg every 4 to 6 hours may be administered in its place.

There is rarely an indication for summoning outside medical assistance for this type of response.

When a more generalized slow-onset skin reaction develops, recommended management will be somewhat more aggressive. This situation is most likely to develop in a patient who has received oral antibiotic prophylaxis about 1 hour prior to the

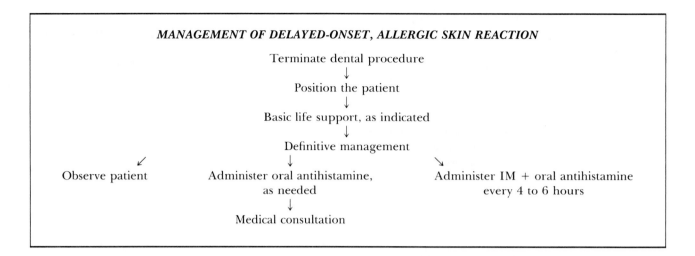

MANAGEMENT OF DELAYED-ONSET, ALLERGIC SKIN REACTION

Terminate dental procedure
↓
Position the patient
↓
Basic life support, as indicated
↓
Definitive management
↓

Observe patient   Administer oral antihistamine,   Administer IM + oral antihistamine
                              as needed   every 4 to 6 hours
                                   ↓
                         Medical consultation

onset of symptoms and has developed a more generalized allergic skin reaction. Examination of the patient demonstrates no involvement as yet of other systems. Management of this patient should involve the intravenous or intramuscular administration of an antihistamine such as diphenhydramine (50 mg for adults; 25 mg for children); or chlorpheniramine (10 mg for adults; 5 mg for children). Onset of action of an intravenously administered antihistamine will be within a few minutes, whereas 10 to 30 minutes might be required for the relief of symptoms following intramuscular administration. The patient is then given a prescription for either diphenhydramine or chlorpheniramine to be taken orally every 4 to 6 hours for 2 to 3 days.

Do not permit this patient to leave the dental office until the clinical signs and symptoms have resolved. In addition, the patient who has received a parenteral antihistamine should not be permitted to leave the dental office alone, nor should he or she be permitted to operate a motor vehicle. Varying degrees of central nervous system (CNS) depression (e.g., drowsiness, fatigue, sedation) are noted following antihistamine administration by any route, but is much more likely to be noted when administered parenterally.

Step 5: Medical consultation: A consultation with the patient's physician or an allergist should follow, and a thorough evaluation of the allergic reaction should be completed before continuing with any future dental treatment. A complete list of all drugs and chemicals administered to the patient should be compiled for use by the allergist.

If the skin reaction does not develop until the patient has left the dental office, the patient should be requested to return to the office where one of the therapies just described will be employed.*

Should the reaction occur at a time when the patient is unable to return to the dental office, the patient should be advised to see his or her physician or to report to the emergency room of a hospital.

Antihistamines reverse the actions of histamine by occupying H_1 receptor sites on the effector cell (competitive antagonism). Antihistamines thereby prevent the agonist molecules (histamine) from occupying these sites without initiating a response themselves. The protective responses of antihistamine include the control of edema formation and pruritis. Other allergic responses such as hypotension and bronchoconstriction are influenced little, if at all, by antihistamines. It can be seen therefore that antihistamines are of value only in mild allergic responses in which small quantities of histamine have been released or in the prevention of allergic reactions in allergic individuals. The accompanying box outlines the steps to follow to manage delayed-onset, allergic skin reactions.

Drugs used in management: Antihistamine, oral or parenteral

Medical assistance: No

Immediate Skin Reactions

Allergic skin reactions that arise in less than 60 minutes should be managed more aggressively. Other allergic symptoms of a relatively minor nature included in this section are conjunctivitis, rhinitis, urticaria, pruritus, and erythema.

Diagnostic clues to the presence of an allergic skin reaction include[74]:

---

*Though most delayed-onset, localized skin reactions do not progress to systemic involvement and anaphylaxis, extreme caution must be observed with all allergic reactions. It is impossible to effectively evaluate a patient by telephone.

- Same as delayed skin reaction
- Conjunctivitis
- Rhinitis

Step 1: Terminate the dental procedure. Stop treatment immediately upon recognition of clinical manifestations of an allergy.

Step 2: Position the patient. As this patient is not in acute distress, positioning is based upon comfort.

Step 3: Basic life support, as indicated. Assess airway, breathing, and circulation and implement basic life support as needed. At this juncture, airway, breathing, and circulation will be adequate.

Step 4: Monitor vital signs. Vital signs—heart rate and rhythm, blood pressure, and respirations—should be monitored and recorded.

Step 5: Provide definitive management. Management of the more rapid-onset allergic reaction will be predicated upon the presence or absence of signs of respiratory and/or cardiovascular involvement. Allergy that appears shortly following antigenic exposure is more likely to progress rapidly and to be more intense than the delayed-onset reaction. Treatment will necessarily be more aggressive the more rapid the onset.

Step 5a: Administer antihistamine. In the *absence of signs of cardiovascular and respiratory involvement* (absence of tachycardia, hypotension, dizziness, lightheadedness, dyspnea, wheezing), definitive management involves the administration of a parenteral antihistamine. Either diphenhydramine or chlorpheniramine may be administered intravenously or intramuscularly as described in the previous section. When the clinical signs and symptoms resolve, oral antihistamine should be prescribed for 2 to 3 days. The patient should not be permitted to leave the office alone or to operate a motor vehicle. Medical evaluation should be completed prior to any further dental treatment.

Step 5b: Reposition patient. In the *presence of signs of either cardiovascular or respiratory involvement* (tachycardia, hypotension, dizziness, lightheadedness, dyspnea, wheezing), additional steps are necessary. If hypotension is evident, reposition the patient in the supine position with legs elevated. Should respiratory distress be present in the absence of cardiovascular involvement, position is determined by patient comfort.

Step 6b: Oxygen and venipuncture, if available. Oxygen should be administered via nasal cannula, nasal hood, or face mask, as soon as it becomes available. In addition, if equipment and trained personnel are available, an intravenous line should be established.

Step 7b: Administer epinephrine: Recommended management of this mild anaphylactic reaction involves the immediate intramuscular or subcutaneous administration of 0.3 to 0.5 mL (0.3 to 0.5 mg) of a 1:1000 epinephrine solution (adult), 0.25 mg (child), or 0.125 mg (infant). Epinephrine may be administered every 5 to 20 minutes as needed, to a total of three doses. If the intravenous route is available, 1 mL of 1:10,000 (0.1 mg) should be administered by slow intravenous push over 3 to 5 minutes. Observe the patient for either the desired therapeutic effect or the development of complications. Additional 0.1 mL doses may be administered over a 15-to 30-minute period to a maximum dose of 5 mL.

Step 8b: Summon medical assistance. It is the author's firm conviction that any allergic reaction requiring the administration of epinephrine also requires additional medical assistance.

Step 9b: Administer antihistamine. Following the resolution of the cardiovascular and/or respiratory signs and symptoms of the allergic reaction, an antihistamine (diphenhydramine, 50 mg, or chlorpheniramine, 10 mg) should be administered intramuscularly. The pediatric dose of diphenhydramine is 25 mg, and chlorpheniramine is 5 mg. Antihistamines are administered intramuscularly to provide a more prolonged duration of clinical activity.

Step 10b: Monitor patient. Continue to monitor and record the cardiovascular and respiratory responses of the patient throughout the episode. The need for additional drug therapy (e.g., epinephrine) will be based upon these findings.

Step 11b: Recovery and discharge. With the arrival of emergency medical personnel, an intravenous infusion will be started, if not previously done, and appropriate drug therapy administerd. The patient who has had a mild anaphylactic reaction (e.g., urticaira, rhinitis, conjunctivitis, with respiratory and/or cardiovascular involvement) will be stabilized and then transported to the emergency department of a hospital for observation and possible additional treatment. The accompanying box outlines the steps to take to manage rapid-onset skin reactions.

Drugs used in management: Oxygen, antihistamine (IM), epinephrine (SC, IM, IV)

Medical assistance: No, if skin only; yes, if respiratory and/or cardiovascular involvement

Respiratory Reactions
Bronchial Constriction (Bronchospasm)

The most likely situations in dentistry in which an allergic reaction will manifest itself as a respiratory problem (bronchospasm) are in the asthmatic patient who is allergic to bisulfites and comes

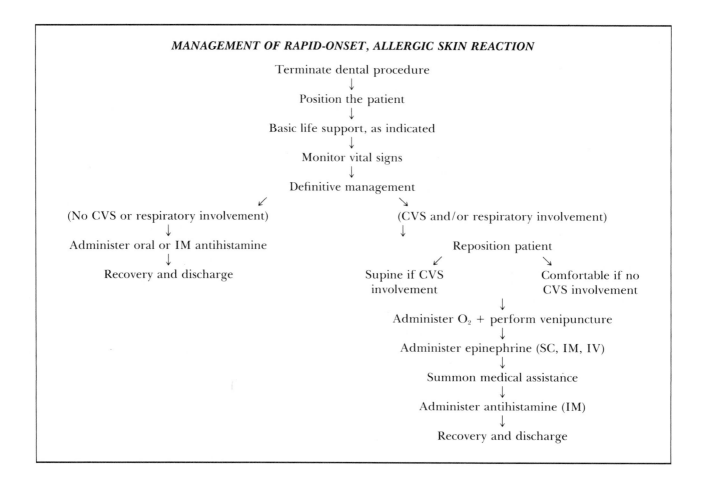

MANAGEMENT OF RAPID-ONSET, ALLERGIC SKIN REACTION

Terminate dental procedure
↓
Position the patient
↓
Basic life support, as indicated
↓
Monitor vital signs
↓
Definitive management
↙ ↘
(No CVS or respiratory involvement)　(CVS and/or respiratory involvement)
↓ ↓
Administer oral or IM antihistamine　Reposition patient
↓ ↙ ↘
Recovery and discharge　Supine if CVS　Comfortable if no
involvement　CVS involvement
↓
Administer O₂ + perform venipuncture
↓
Administer epinephrine (SC, IM, IV)
↓
Summon medical assistance
↓
Administer antihistamine (IM)
↓
Recovery and discharge

into contact with them during dental care, and in the patient who is allergic to aspirin.

Diagnostic clues to the presence of an allergy involving bronchospasm include:

• Wheezing
• Use of accessory muscles of respiration

Bronchial smooth muscle constriction results in asthmatic-like reactions. Management of the acute asthmatic episode is described in depth in Chapter 13 and includes the following:

Step 1: Terminate the dental treatment.

Step 2: Position the patient comfortably. An upright or semierect position is usually preferred by the patient.

Step 3: Remove materials from the patient's mouth.

Step 4: Calm the patient. The conscious patient who is experiencing respiratory distress may be quite fearful. Try to allay any apprehensions.

Step 5: Basic life support, as indicated. Assessment of airway and circulation will initially prove adequate. Breathing may show varying degrees of inadequacy, ranging from mild bronchospasm to almost complete obstruction and cyanosis.

Step 6: Summon medical assistance. With clinically evident respiratory distress associated with wheez-

ing and cyanosis, immediate summoning of emergency medical aid is warranted.

Step 7: Administer bronchodilator. Epinephrine may be administered by means of an aerosol inhaler (Medi-haler Epi) (Fig. 24-2) or by intramuscular or subcutaneous injection (0.3 mL of a 1:1000 dilution for adults) or intravenously, 0.1 mL of 1:10,000 every 15 to 30 minutes. The potent bronchodilating actions of epinephrine usually terminate bronchospasm within a few minutes of administration. Epinephrine is the drug of choice as a bronchodilator because it effectively reverses the actions of one of the major causes of bronchospasm—histamine; but like the antihistamines, epinephrine does not relieve bronchospam produced by the leukotrienes.[75] Other inhaled bronchodilators, such as metaproterenol, may be used in the management of bronchospasm.

Step 8: Monitor the patient. The patient should remain in the dental office for observation, because a recurrence of bronchospasm is possible as the epinephrine undergoes rapid biotransformation. Should symptoms reappear, epinephrine is readministered intramuscularly, subcutaneously, or by inhalation (aerosol).

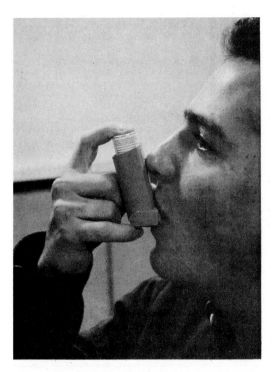

Fig. 24-2. Aerosol spray of bronchodilator for management of bronchial spasms.

MANAGEMENT OF RESPIRATORY ALLERGIC REACTION

Terminate dental treatment
↓
Position the patient (comfortably)
↓
Remove materials from the patient's mouth
↓
Calm patient
↓
Basic life support, as indicated
↓
Summon medical assistance
↓
Administer bronchodilator, epinephrine (inhalation, SC, IM, IV)
↓
Monitor vital signs
↓
Administer antihistamine (IM)
↓
Recovery and discharge

Step 9: Administer antihistamine. The intramuscular administration of an antihistamine minimizes the risk of recurrence of bronchospasm because the antihistamine occupies the histamine receptor site, preventing a relapse. Diphenhydramine, 50 mg intramuscular for adults, or 2 mg/kg intramuscularly or intravenously for children, is recommended.

Step 10: Recovery and discharge. With arrival of emergency medical personnel the victim will be stabilized, and definitive treatment will be started, if necessary. Additional treatment may involve the administration of one or more of the following: intravenous aminophylline; atropine, steroids (methylprednisolone), and intubation and ventilation if bronchospasm is persistent and severe. In most cases the patient exhibiting an allergic reaction consisting primarily of respiratory signs and symptoms will require hospitalization. The accompanying box outlines the steps to take to manage respiratory allergic reaction.

Drugs used in management: Oxygen, bronchodilators: epinephrine (inhalation, IV, IM, SC), antihistamine (IM)

Medical assistance required: Yes, if significant respiratory distress

Laryngeal Edema

The second and probably more life-threatening respiratory allergic manifestation is the development of laryngeal edema. It may be diagnosed when little or no air movement can be heard or felt through the mouth and nose despite exaggerated spontaneous respiratory movements by the patient, or when a patent airway cannot be obtained. A partially obstructed larynx in the presence of spontaneous respiratory movements produces a characteristically high-pitched crowing sound, in contrast to the wheezing of bronchospasm, whereas total obstruction is accompanied by silence in the presence of chest movement. The patient soon loses consciousness from lack of oxygen (e.g., hypoxia or anoxia). Laryngeal edema is not common, fortunately, but may arise in any acute allergic reaction that involves the airway.

Diagnostic clues to the presence of laryngeal edema include:
- Respiratory distress
- Exaggerated chest movements
- High-pitched crowing sound (partial obstruction), no sound (total obstruction)
- Cyanosis
- Loss of consciousness

Step 1: Terminate the dental treatment.

Step 2: Position the patient. If the degree of edema is severe, the patient's level of consciousness will be significantly altered and the supine position with feet elevated is most appropriate. Should the patient be unwilling or unable to tolerate the supine position, then position based on comfort is recommended.

Step 3: Summon medical assistance.

Step 4: Basic life support, as indicated. Airway will be the most critical factor in management of laryngeal edema. Initial management should include extension of the neck via head tilt–chin lift, or jaw thrust–chin lift, followed by the insertion of either a nasopharyngeal tube or oropharyngeal airway. The conscious patient will be able to tolerate the nasopharyngeal airway, whereas the orpharyngeal airway is likely to produce a gag reflex.

Step 5: Administer epinephrine. The immediate administration of 0.3 to 0.5 mL of 1:1000 epinephrine intramuscularly (0.125 to 0.25 mL for infant or child) or 0.1 mL of 1:10,000 epinephrine intravenously over 5 minutes, repeated every 3 to 5 minutes as necessary, is recommended. A maximum dose of 5.0 mL every 15 to 30 minutes should not be exceeded.

Step 6: Maintain airway. In the presence of a partially obstructed airway, epinephrine administration may halt or even reverse the progress of laryngeal edema.

Step 7: Administer oxygen. Oxygen should be administered as soon as it becomes available.

Step 8: Additional drug management. An antihistamine (diphenhydramine, 50 mg for adults; 25 mg for children) and corticosteroid (hydrocortisone, 100 mg) should be administered intramuscularly or intravenously following clinical recovery, as noted by airway improvement: normal, or at least improved, breath sounds; absence of cyanosis; and less exaggerated chest excursions. Corticosteroids inhibit edema and capillary dilation by stabilizing basement membranes. They are of little immediate value because of their slow onset of action, even when administered intravenously. Corticosteroids have an onset of action approximately 6 hours following their administration.[76] Corticosteroids function to prevent a relapse, whereas the function of epinephrine, a more rapidly acting drug employed during the acute phase, is to halt or reverse the deleterious actions of histamine and other mediators of allergy.

These procedures (steps 1 through 8) are normally adequate to maintain the patient. With the arrival of medical assistance, the patient will be stabilized and transferred to a hospital for further observation and treatment.

MANAGEMENT OF LARYNGEAL EDEMA

Terminate dental treatment
↓
Position the patient
↓
Summon medical assistance
↓
Basic life support, as indicated
↓
Administer epinephrine (SC, IM, IV)
↓
Maintain airway
(head tilt–chin lift; jaw thrust; use oro- or nasopharyngeal airways)
↓
Administer oxygen
↓
Additional drugs:
antihistamine, corticosteroid
↓
Cricothyrotomy, if needed

Step 9: Cricothyrotomy. A totally obstructed airway may not be reopened at all, or in adequate time by the administration of epinephrine and other drugs. In this case it will become necessary to create an emergency airway in order to maintain the life of the patient. Time is of the essence, and it is not possible to delay action until medical assistance arrives. A cricothyrotomy is the procedure of choice for the establishment of an airway in this situation. (The technique is described in Chapter 11.) Once an airway is obtained, oxygen must be administered, artificial ventilation employed if needed, and vital signs monitored.

Prior to the arrival of medical assistance, the drugs previously administered may halt the progress of the laryngeal edema and might even reverse it to a degree. The patient will require hospitalization following transfer from the dental office by the paramedics. The accompanying box outlines the steps to take to manage laryngeal edema.

Drugs used in management: Oxygen, epinephrine (IV, IM), antihistamine (IM), corticosteroid (IV,IM)

Medical assistance required: Yes

Epinephrine and Allergy

Epinephrine is the most important drug in the initial management of all immediate allergic reactions. Its actions effectively counteract the effects of histamine and the other chemical mediators of allergy. Although antihistamines reverse several allergic symptoms, especially edema and itch, they are of little value with other symptoms such as bronchospasm and hypotension. Epinephrine possesses properties to reverse all of these actions and has a more rapid onset of action than do antihistamines.

The actions of epinephrine are classified as β-adrenergic and α-adrenergic agonist effects. The β-adrenergic effects of epinephrine mimic those produced by efferent sympathetic (adrenergic) nerve activity on the heart (β₁) and lungs (β₂), whereas α-adrenergic properties mimic those of the sympathetic nerves on the peripheral vasculature. Useful β-adrenergic actions of epinephrine include bronchodilation, increased myocardial contractility, increased heart rate, and constriction of arterioles with a redistribution of blood to the systemic circulation. Useful α-adrenergic actions include cutaneous, mucosal, and splanchnic vasoconstriction, with a total increase in systemic vascular resistance. This action, in addition to the β₁-adrenergic actions (e.g., increased heart rate and myocardial contractility), leads to an increased cardiac output. Increased cardiac output, in addition to the increased systemic vascular resistance, produces an increased systemic blood pressure. Through as yet unknown mechanisms, epinephrine also reverses rhinitis and urticaria.

Although epinephrine is rapid acting, it is also a relatively short-acting drug, owing to its rapid biotransformation. Therefore, whenever epinephrine is used in an emergency situation, the patient should be observed for a long enough period of time to ensure that symptoms of allergy do not recur. In addition, care must be taken when considering the reinjection of epinephrine. Administration of epinephrine produces dramatic increases in heart rate and blood pressure (epinephrine injection has produced cerebrovascular hemorrhage) and increases the risk of the development of dysrhythmias. Before reinjection of epinephrine (0.3 mL of 1:1000 in adults, 0.125 to 0.25 mL in infants and children), the cardiovascular status of the patient must be evaluated and the risk of reinjection carefully weighed against the benefits. Epinephrine is relatively contraindicated in elderly patients and in those with known coronary artery disease and hypertension, and it must be avoided in those patients with life-threatening tachydysrhythmias.[10] In these situations it may be prudent to delay the (re)administration of epinephrine and to administer an antihistamine and/or corticosteroid (whichever is/are appropriate) in its place. However, in the presence of continued deterioration of the patient, epinephrine must be readministered.

The route of epinephrine administration is dependent upon the severity of the clinical situation. Epinephrine may be given subcutaneously when the reaction is mild and the patient is normotensive. However, when generalized urticaria or hypotension exist, subcutaneous absorption may be variable and slow and intramuscular administration is indicated.[10] When possible, the intravenous route should be used in more acute and life-threatening allergic reactions.

Generalized Anaphylaxis

In generalized anaphylaxis a wide range of clinical manifestations may occur; however, the cardiovascular system is involved in virtually all reactions. In a rapidly progressing anaphylactic reaction, cardiovascular collapse may occur within minutes of the onset of symptoms. Immediate and aggressive management of the situation is imperative if the patient is to survive.

In the dental office this reaction is most likely to occur during or immediately following administration of penicillin or aspirin to a previously sensitized patient. A much more remote possibility might be the injection of an ester local anesthetic. Two other life-threatening situations may also develop during this latter situation that may occasionally mimic anaphylaxis: vasodepressor syncope and a local anesthetic overdose. In the immediate management of this situation, there must be an attempt to diagnose the actual cause.

Signs of Allergy Present

Should any clinical signs, such as urticaria, erythema, pruritus, or wheezing be noted before the patient's collapse, the diagnosis of the problem is obvious: allergy, and management proceeds accordingly.

Step 1: Position the patient. The unconscious patient is placed into the supine position with the legs elevated slightly.

Step 2: Basic life support, as indicated. The airway is opened via head tilt and steps of basic life support are carried out as needed.

Step 3: Summon medical assistance. As soon as a severe allergic reaction is considered a possibility, emergency medical care should be summoned.

Step 4: Administer epinephrine. The doctor should have previously called for the office emergency team. Epinephrine from the emergency kit (0.3 mL of 1:1000 for adults, 0.15 mL for children, and 0.075 mL for infants) is administered intramuscularly as quickly as possible, or intravenously. Because of the immediate need for epinephrine in this situation, a preloaded syringe of epinephrine is recommended for the emergency kit. Epinephrine is the only injectable agent that need by kept in a preloaded form to prevent confusion when looking for the drug in this near-panic situation.

The site for intramuscular injection should be based upon muscle perfusion in the presence of what is likely to be profound hypotension. With decreased perfusion, the absorption of epinephrine from muscle will be delayed. It is recommended that consideration be given to the administration of epinephrine in this situation into the body of the tongue (intralingual) or the floor of the mouth (sublingual) (Fig. 24-3). The needle may enter from either an extraoral or intraoral puncture site. The vascularity of the oral cavity, even in the presence of hypotension, will provide a more rapid onset of activity than seen in the more traditional intramuscular sites.

Epinephrine, in one or more doses, usually produces clinical improvement in the patient. The respiratory and cardiovascular signs and symptoms should decrease in severity: breath sounds improve as bronchospasm decreases, and blood pressure increases.

Should the clinical picture fail to improve or continue to deteriorate (i.e., increased severity of symptoms) within 5 minutes of the initial epinephrine dose, a second dose is administered. Subsequent doses may be administered as needed every 5 to 10 minutes, if the potential risk of epinephrine administration (e.g., excessive cardiovascular stimulation) is kept in mind and the patient is adequately monitored.

Step 5: Administer oxygen.

Step 6: Monitor vital signs. The patient's cardiovascular and respiratory status must be monitored continuously. Blood pressure and heart rate (at the carotid artery) should be recorded at least every 5 minutes, and closed chest compression should be started if cardiac arrest occurs.

During this acute, life-threatening phase of what is obviously an anaphylactic reaction, management consists of basic life support; the administration of oxygen and epinephrine; with continual monitoring of vital signs. Until an improvement in the patient's status is noted, no additional therapy is indicated.

Step 7: Additional drug therapy. Once clinical improvement is noted (e.g., increased blood pressure, decreased bronchospasm), additional drug therapy may be started. This includes the administration of an antihistamine and a corticosteroid (both drugs intramusculary or intravenously, if possible). Their function is to prevent a possible recurrence of symptoms and to obviate the need for the continued administration of epinephrine. They are not administered during the acute phase of the reaction because they are too slow in onset and they do not do enough immediate good to justify their use at this time. Epinephrine and oxygen are the only drugs to administer during the acute phase of the anaphylactic reaction.

Throughout this text it has been stressed that definitive treatment of emergencies with drugs is of secondary importance to the ABCs of basic life support. Drugs need not be administered in all emergency situations. The anaphylactic reaction is the exception. Once a diagnosis of an acute, generalized anaphylactic reaction has been made, it is

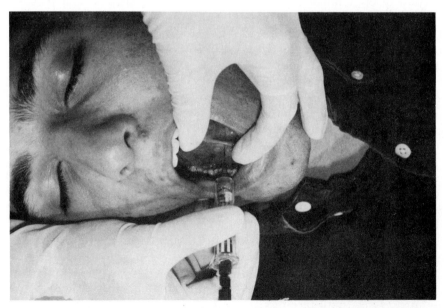

Fig. 24-3. Sublingual epinephrine injection.

```
┌─────────────────────────────────────────┐
│        MANAGEMENT OF GENERALIZED          │
│               ANAPHYLAXIS                 │
│                                           │
│   (Signs and symptoms of allergy present) │
│        Terminate dental treatment         │
│                    ↓                      │
│            Position the patient           │
│         (supine with legs elevated)       │
│                    ↓                      │
│        Basic life support, as indicated   │
│                    ↓                      │
│         Summon medical assistance         │
│                    ↓                      │
│     Administer epinephrine (SC, IM, IV)   │
│                    ↓                      │
│           Administer oxygen               │
│                    ↓                      │
│           Monitor vital signs             │
│                    ↓                      │
│ Additional drugs: antihistamine, corticosteroid │
└─────────────────────────────────────────┘
```

imperative that drug therapy (i.e., epinephrine) be initiated as soon as possible following the start of basic life support. Review of clinical reports demonstrates the effectiveness of immediate drug therapy in anaphylaxis. Recovery from anaphylaxis is related to the rapidity with which effective treatment is instituted. Delay in treatment increases the mortality rate. Eighty-seven percent of those experiencing anaphylaxis provoked by bee stings survived if treated within the first hour, but only 67% of dying patients were treated in this first hour.[77] The accompanying box outlines the steps to take to manage generalized anaphylaxis.

Drugs used in management: Oxygen, epinephrine (IV,IM), antihistamine (IM), corticosteroid (IV,IM)

Medical assistance required: Yes

No Clinical Signs of Allergy Present

A second clinical picture of anaphylaxis might well be one in which the patient receiving a potential allergen loses consciousness without any obvious signs of allergy being observed.[71,78]

Step 1: Terminate dental treatment.

Step 2: Position the patient. Management of this situation, which might prove to result from any of a number of causes, will require immediate positioning of the patient in the supine position with the legs elevated slightly.

Step 3: Basic life support, as indicated. Victims of vasodepressor syncope or postural hypotension rapidly recover consciousness once they are properly positioned with an ensured airway. Patients who do not recover at this point should continue to have the elements of basic life support applied (breathing, circulation).

Step 4: Summon medical assistance. If consciousness does not return rapidly following the institution of the steps of basic life support, emergency medical assistance should be sought immediately.

Step 5: Administer oxygen.

Step 6: Monitor vital signs. Blood pressure, heart rate and rhythm, and respirations should be monitored at least every 5 minutes, and the elements of basic life support should be started at any time they are required.

Step 7: Definitive management. On arrival, the emergency medical personnel will seek to make a diagnosis of the cause of the loss of consciousness. If this is possible, appropriate drug therapy will be instituted, the patient will be stabilized, and then transferred to a local hospital emergency department.

In the absence of any definitive signs and symptoms of allergy such as edema, urticaria, or bronchospasm, epinephrine and other drug therapy are not indicated. Any of a number of other situations may be the cause of the unconsciousness: for example, drug overdose, hypoglycemia, cerebrovascular accident, acute adrenal insufficiency, or cardiopulmonary arrest may be causative factors. Continuation of the steps of basic life support until medical assistance arrives is the most rational mode of management in this situation. The accompanying box outlines the steps to take to manage generalized anaphylaxis.

Drugs used in management: Oxygen

Medical assistance required: Yes

```
┌─────────────────────────────────────────┐
│        MANAGEMENT OF GENERALIZED          │
│               ANAPHYLAXIS                 │
│                                           │
│     (No signs or symptoms of allergy)     │
│        Terminate dental treatment         │
│                    ↓                      │
│            Position the patient           │
│         (supine with legs elevated)       │
│                    ↓                      │
│        Basic life support, as indicated   │
│                    ↓                      │
│         Summon medical assistance         │
│                    ↓                      │
│           Administer oxygen               │
│                    ↓                      │
│           Monitor vital signs             │
│                    ↓                      │
│          Definitive management            │
└─────────────────────────────────────────┘
```

Laryngeal Edema

Laryngeal edema is yet another possible development during the generalized anaphylactic reaction. Should the airway become difficult to maintain in spite of adequate head-tilt and a clear pharynx (obtained by suctioning), it may become necessary to perform a cricothyrotomy to obtain a patent airway. Laryngeal edema is a serious manifestation of allergy. Once airway patency has been ensured by cricothyrotomy, epinephrine may be administered (0.125 to 0.3 mL of 1:1000 solution), followed by administration of an antihistamine and corticosteroid, as described eariler. Once stabilized, the patient should be transferred to a hospital for definitive management and observation.

REFERENCES

1. *Mosby's medical & nursing dictionary*, St Louis, 1983, Mosby–Year Book.
2. Gell PGH, Coombs RRA: *Clinical aspects of immunology*, ed 3, Oxford and London, 1973, Blackwell Scientfic.
3. Chen MD, Greenspoon JS, Long TL: Latex anaphylaxis in an obstetrics and gynecology physician, *Amer J Obstetr Gynecol* 166(2):968-969, 1992.
4. Leynadier F, Dry J: Allergy to latex, *Clin Rev Allergy* 9(3-4):371-377, 1991.
5. Portier P, Richet C: De l'action anaphylactique des certain venins, *CR Soc Biol (Paris)* 54:170, 1902.
6. Caranasos GJ: Drug reactions. In Schwartz GR, Safar P, Stone JH, and others, editors: *Principles and practice of emergency medicine*, Philadelphia, 1978, WB Saunders.
7. Buisseret PD: Allergy, *Sci Am* 247:86, 1982.
8. Pascoe DJ: Anaphylaxis. In Pascoe DJ, Grossman J, editors: *Quick reference to pediatric emergencies*, ed 3, Philadelphia, 1984, JB Lippincott.
9. Patterson R, Anderson J: Allergic reactions to drugs and biologic agents, *JAMA* 248:2637, 1982.
10. Lindzon RD, Silvers WS: Anaphylaxis. In Rosen P, Baker FJ, Barkin RM, and others, editors: *Emergency medicine*, ed 2, St Louis, 1988, Mosby–Year Book,
11. Idsoe O, and others: Nature and extent of penicillin side-reactions, with particular reference to fatalities from anaphylactic shock, *Bull WHO* 38:159, 1968.
12. Barnard JH: Studies of 400 Hymenoptera sting deaths in the United States, *J Allergy Clin Immunol* 52:259, 1973.
13. Lieberman P, Siegle RL, Taylor WW Jr: Anaphylactoid reactions to iodinated contrast material, *J Allergy Clin Immunol* 62:174, 1978.
14. Settipane GA: Adverse reactions to aspirin and related drugs, *Arch Intern Med* 141:328, 1981.
15. Smith VT: Anaphylactic shock, acute renal failure, and disseminated intravascular coagulation: suspected complications of zomepirac, *JAMA* 247:1172, 1982.
16. Waldbott GL: Anaphylactic death from penicillin, *JAMA* 139:526, 1949.
17. Sogn DD: Penicillin allergy, *J Allergy Clin Immunol* 74:589, 1984.
18. Erffmeyer JE: Adverse reactions to penicillin: a review, *Ann Allergy* 47:288, 1981.
19. Spark RP: Fatal anaphylaxis to oral penicillin, *Am J Clin Pathol* 56:407, 1971.
20. Levine BB: Antigenicity and cross-reactivity of penicillins and cephalosporins, *J Infect Dis* 128:8364, 1974.
21. Samter M, Beers RF Jr: Intolerance to aspirin: clinical studies and consideration of its pathogenesis, *Ann Intern Med* 68:975, 1968.
22. Yurchak AM, Wicher K, Arbesman CE: Immunologic studies on aspirin: clinical studies with aspiryl-protein conjugates, *J Allergy* 46:245, 1970.
23. Spector SL, Farr RA: *Aspirin idiosyncrasy: asthma and urticaria.* In Middleton E Jr, Reed CE, Ellis FF, editors: *Allergy: principles and practice*, ed 2, St Louis, 1983, Mosby–Year Book.
24. Lowell FC: "Asthma," "rhinitis," and "atopy," reconsidered (editorial), *N Engl J Med* 300:669, 1979.
25. Speer F: Aspirin allergy: a clinical study, *South Med J* 68:314, 1975.
26. Moore ME, Goldsmith DP: Nonsteroidal anti-inflammatory intolerance: an anaphylactic reaction to tolmetin, *Arch Intern Med* 140:1105, 1980.
27. Wasserman SI: Anaphylaxis. In Middleton E, Ellis FF, Reed CE, editors: *Allergy: principles and practice*, ed 2, St Louis, 1983, Mosby–Year Book.
28. Aldrete JA, Johnson DA: Allergy to local anesthetics, *JAMA* 207:356, 1969.
29. deShazo RD, Nelson HS: An approach to the patient with a history of local anesthetic hypersensitivity: experience with 90 patients, *J Allergy Clin Immunol* 63:387, 1979.
30. Swanson JG: Assessment of allergy to local anesthetic, *Ann Emerg Med* 12:316, 1983.
31. Aldrete JA, Johnson DA: Evaluation of intracutaneous testing for investigation of allergy to local anesthetic agents, *Anesth Analg* 49:173, 1970.
32. Malamed SF: Evaluation of 188 patients with presumed "allergy to local anesthesia," unpublished data, 1991.
33. Prenner BM, Stevens JJ: Anaphylaxis after ingestion of sodium bisulfite, *Ann Allergy* 37:180, 1976.
34. Stevenson DD, Simon RA: Sensitivity to ingested metabisulfites in asthmatic subjects, *J Allergy Clin Immunol* 68:26, 1981.
35. Sher TH, Schwartz HJ: Bisulfite sensitivity manifesting as an allergic reaction to aerosol therapy, *Ann Allergy* 54:224, 1985.
36. Clayton DE, Busse W: Anaphylaxis to wine, *Clin Allergy* 10:341, 1980.
37. Twarog FJ, Leung DYM: Anaphylaxis to a component of isoetharine (sodium bisulfite), *JAMA* 248:2030, 1982.
38. Slavin RG: Skin tests in the diagnosis of allergies of the immediate type, *Med Clin N Am* 58:65, 1974.
39. Kamada MM, Twarog F, Leung DY: Multiple antibiotic sensitivity in a pediatric population, *Allergy Proceed* 12(5):347-350, 1991.
40. Dajani AS, Bisno AL, Chung KJ, and others: Prevention of bacterial endocarditis, *JAMA* 264(22):2919, 1990.
41. Glauda NM, Henerfer EO, Super S: Nonfatal anaphylaxis caused by oral penicillin: report of a case, *J Am Dent Assoc* 90:159, 1975.
42. Malamed SF: The use of diphenhydramine HCl as a local anesthetic in dentistry, *Anesth Prog* 20:76, 1973.
43. Benadryl package insert, Parke-Davis, Morris Plains, NJ, 1990.
44. Kelly JK, Patterson R: Anaphylaxis: course, mechanisms and treatment, *JAMA* 227:1431, 1974.
45. Siegel SC, Heimlich EM: Anaphylaxis, *Pediatr Clin N Am* 9:29, 1962.
46. Frank MM, Gelfand JA, Atkinson JP: Hereditary angioedema: the clinical syndrome and its management, *Ann Intern Med* 84:580, 1976.

47. Hopkinson RB, Sutcliffe AJ: Hereditary angioneurotic oedema, *Anaesthesaia* 34:183, 1979.

48. James LP Jr, Austen KF: Fatal systemic anaphylaxis in man, *N Engl J Med* 270:597, 1964.

49. Van Arsdel PP Jr: Drug allergy, an update, *Med Clin N Amer* 65:1089, 1981.

50. Katz WA, Kaye D: Immunologic principles. In Rose LF, Kaye D, editors: *Internal medicine for dentistry*, ed 2, St Louis, 1983 Mosby–Year Book.

51. Ishizaka K, Tomioka H, Ishizaka T: Mechanisms of passive sensitization. I. Presence of IgE and IgG molecules on human leukocytes, *J Immunol* 105:1459, 1970.

52. Isizaka T, Soto CS, Ishizaka K: Mechanisms of passive sensitization. III. Number of IgE molecules and their receptor sites on human basophil granulocytes, *J Immunol* 111:500, 1973.

53. Sullivan TJ, Kulcyzcki A Jr: Immediate hypersensitivity responses. In Parker CW, editor: *Clinical immunology*, vol 1, Philadelphia, 1980, WB Saunders.

54. Ishizaka T, Ishizaka K, Tomioka H: Release of histamine and slow reacting substance of anaphylaxis (SRS-A) by IgE-anti-IgE reactions on monkey mast cells, *J Immunol* 108:513, 1972.

55. Kaliner M, Austen KF: A sequence of biochemical events in the antigen-induced release of chemical mediator from sensitized human lung tissue, *J Exp Med* 138:1077, 1973.

56. Wasserman SI: Mediators of immediate hypersensitivity, *J Allergy Clin Immunol* 72:101, 1983.

57. Piper PJ: Mediators of anaphylactic hypersensitivity. In Brent L, Holborow J, editors: *Progress in immunology II*, vol 4, London, 1974, North-Holland.

58. Black JW, and others: Definition and antagonism of histamine H_2-receptors, *Nature* 236:385, 1972.

59. Beaven MA: Histamine, the classic antihistamines (H_1 inhibitors), *N Engl J Med* 294:320, 1976.

60. Sammuelson B: Leukotrienes: mediators of allergic reactions and inflammation, *Int Arch Allergy Appl Immunol* 66(suppl 1):98, 1981.

61. Israel E, Drazen JM: Leukotrienes and asthma: a basic review, *Curr Concepts Aller Clin Immunol* 14:11, 1983.

62. Levi R, Burke JA: Cardiac anaphylaxis: SRS-A potentiates and extends the effects of released histamine, *Eur J Pharmacol* 62:41, 1980.

63. Wasserman SI, Goetzl EJ, Austen KF: Preformed eosinophiltactic tetrapeptides of human lung tissue; identification of eosinophilic chemotactic factor of anaphylaxis (ECF-A), *Proc Nat Acad Sci USA* 72:4123, 1975.

64. Nagy L, Lee TH, Kay AB: Neutrophil chemotactic activity in antigen-induced late asthmatic reactions, *N Engl J Med* 306:497, 1982.

65. Newball HH, and others: Anaphylactic release of a basophil kallikrein-like activity. I. Purification and characterization, *J Clin Invest* 64:457, 1979.

66. Schulman ES, and others: Anaphylactic release of thromboxane A_2 prostaglandin D_2, and prostacyclin from human lung parenchyma, *Am Rev Respir Dis* 124:402, 1981.

67. Wanderer AA, and others: Detection and management of cold urticaria patients at high risk for cold-induced systemic reactions (abstract), *J Allergy Clin Immunol* 75:114, 1985.

68. Hanahan DJ, and others: Identification of platelet activating factor isolated from rabbit basophils as acetyl glyceryl ether phosphorylcholine, *J Biol Chem* 255:5514, 1980.

69. Pinkard RN, and others: Intravascular aggregation and pulmonary sequestration of platelets during IgE-induced systemic anaphylaxis in the rabbit: abrogation of lethal anaphylactic shock by platelet depletion, *J Immunol* 119:2185, 1977.

70. Orange RP, Donsky GJ: Anaphylaxis. In Middleton E, Ellis FF, Reed CE, editors: *Allergy: principles and practice*, ed 2, St Louis, 1983, Mosby–Year Book.

71. Lockey RF, Bukantz SC: Allergic emergencies, *Med Clin N Amer* 58:147, 1974.

72. Austen KF: Systemic anaphylaxis in the human being, *N Engl J Med* 291:661, 1974.

73. Delage C, Irey NS: Anaphylactic deaths: a clinicopathologic study of 43 cases, *F Forensic Sci* 17:525, 1972.

74. Pollakoff J, Pollakoff K: *EMT's guide to signs and symtoms*, 1991.

75. Brocklehurst WE: Slow reacting substance and related compounds, *Prog Allergy* 6:539, 1962.

76. Morris HG: Pharmacology of corticosteroids in asthma. In Middleton E, Ellis FF, Reed CE, editors: *Allergy: principles and practice*, ed 2, St Louis, 1983, Mosby–Year Book.

77. Peters GA, Karnes WE, Bastron JA: Near fatal and fatal reactions to insect sting, *Ann Allergy* 41:268, 1978.

78. Hanashiro PK, Weil MH: Anaphylactic shock in man: report of two cases with detailed hemodynamic and metabolic studies, *Arch Intern Med* 119:129, 1967.

25 Drug-Related Emergencies: Differential Diagnosis

The use of drugs is never undertaken without risk. In this section several adverse drug reactions (ADRs) were described that are potentially life threatening. These reactions are compared here so that the doctor called on to manage them may be better able to rapidly diagnose the precise cause of the reaction and initiate appropriate therapy. Included in the differential diagnosis is vasodepressor syncope, because it is a common drug-related reaction.

PAST MEDICAL HISTORY

Past medical history is of great importance in the prevention of ADRs. Careful evaluation of a patient's prior response to drugs is a major factor in prevention of these reactions. Allergy must be documented; however, the drug or drugs producing the reaction must be avoided until the patient undergoes more definitive evaluation. When a documented allergy does exist, alternative drugs may be used.

Drug overdose reactions are more difficult to evaluate from the medical history. Patients commonly record all adverse drug reactions as "allergy." Only a thorough dialogue history and knowledge of the pharmacology of the drug in question can lead to a diagnosis of prior overdose reaction.

Vasodepressor syncope is commonly associated with parenteral drug administration, particularly the administration of local anesthetics. A history of "blacking out" whenever an injection is administered should lead the doctor to suspect vasodepressor syncope and take measures to prevent its recurrence.

AGE OF PATIENT

Allergy and overdose may occur at any age. Children appear to have a greater potential to develop allergy than do adults; however, many children outgrow their childhood allergies, especially food allergies. Interestingly, over 90% of fatalities from anaphylaxis occur in patients over 19 years of age.[1]

Drug overdose reactions may also develop in any patient, but patients on either end of the age spectrum, children and the elderly, represent a greater risk, especially with central nervous system (CNS)-depressant drugs such as sedative-hypnotics, narcotic agonist analgesics, and local anesthetics. Adult dosages of these agents should not be administered to children.

Vasodepressor syncope, on the other hand, is only rarely observed in younger patients or in patients over the age of 40 years. The age span from late teens to late thirties, primarily in males, represents the high risk category for vasodepressor syncope.

SEX OF PATIENT

Drug overdose and allergic reactions are not found more often in one sex than the other. However, vasodepressor syncope is much more common in males. The most likely candidate for vasodepressor syncope is the male under the age of 35 years.

POSITION OF PATIENT

The patient's position when clinical signs and symptoms appear is relevant primarily during the administration of local anesthetics. Position has no bearing on the development of allergy or overdose.

376

Both may develop with the patient in an upright or supine position. Vasodepressor syncope, however, is rarely observed if local anesthetics are administered with the patient in the supine position. Injection of local anesthetics into a patient seated upright is much more likely to lead to vasodepressor syncope.

Positioning of the patient once clinical symptoms develop also aids in diagnosing the cause of the reaction if unconsciousness is a clinical sign. Placing the unconscious patient into a supine position leads to rapid improvement in the case of vasodepressor syncope (assuming patent airway), but produces no significant improvement in the patient suffering from drug overdose or allergy.

ONSET OF SYMPTOMS

Vasodepressor syncope, drug overdose, and allergy may develop immediately following drug administration, or they may develop more slowly. Vasodepressor syncope most often occurs immediately before the actual administration of a drug, but may also develop during or after its administration. Syncope occurring just before drug administration is caused by neither allergy nor drug overdose and is most often related to fear. Clinical symptoms developing during drug administration may be related to any of these reactions; however, in this situation the dose of drug injected is of great importance (see text that follows).

Signs and symptoms that appear following the administration of a drug most probably represent drug overdose or allergy. Vasodepressor syncope may also occur at this time, but in this situation the acute precipitating factor is most probably related to a different stimulus, such as the sight of blood or of dental instruments.

PRIOR EXPOSURE TO DRUG

Prior exposure to a specific drug or to a closely related drug is essential for an allergic response to occur. Vasodepressor syncope is not truly a drug-related situation except in the sense that the psychologic aspect of receiving a drug may precipitate the reaction. (The injection of sterile water might just as readily precipitate vasodepressor syncope. The main factor in the reaction is the injection.)

Prior exposure to a drug is not relevant in drug overdose. It may occur with the first exposure to the agent or with any subsequent exposure.

DOSE OF DRUG ADMINISTERED

Vasodepressor syncope is unrelated to the dose of drug administered, whereas drug overdose re-

actions are, in most instances, related to the quantity of the drug administered. Overdose represents an extension of the normal pharmacologic actions of a drug beyond its desired therapeutic effect and is related to elevated blood levels of that drug. Relative overdose may develop in patients for whom a normal therapeutic dose produces adverse effects, illustrating the phenomenon of biologic variability as represented by the normal distribution curve.

Allergy is not normally related to the absolute dosage of drug administered. Allergy testing using 0.1 mL of an agent may produce fatal systemic anaphylaxis in a previously sensitized patient.

OVERALL INCIDENCE OF OCCURRENCE

Vasodepressor syncope is the most commonly occurring adverse reaction. Of true adverse drug reactions, minor side effects (nonlethal, undesirable drug actions that develop at therapeutic levels, e.g., nausea or sedation) are encountered most frequently. Drug overdose represents the most common of the life-threatening situations that occur, whereas only 15% of ADRs are truly allergic in nature.[2]

SIGNS AND SYMPTOMS
Duration of Reaction

Overdose reactions to local anesthetics are normally self-limiting. Inadvertent intravascular injection of one cartridge of local anesthetic may lead to acute clinical symptoms (e.g., seizures) for 1 to 2 minutes before the blood level falls below overdose levels. Overdose reaction to epinephrine is of extremely short duration because of the rapid biotransformation of the agent into inactive forms.

Vasodepressor syncope is commonly self-limiting, with the patient regaining consciousness once he or she is placed into the supine position. Allergy, on the other hand, may persist for extended periods. As long as any antigen exists within the patient's body, the allergic response may continue. It is not uncommon for allergic reactions to persist for hours or days in spite of vigorous treatment.

Changes in Appearance of Skin

Allergy occurs frequently as a skin reaction. Flushing (i.e., erythema) may occur with other emergency situations, as well as with allergy; however, when flushing is accompanied by urticaria, pruritus (itching), or both, the clinical diagnosis of allergy is appropriate.

Epinephrine overdose may also produce erythema, yet other clinical signs allow for the ready differentiation of this reaction from allergy. The signs of epinephrine overdose include intense headache, tremor, increased anxiety, tachycardia, and greatly elevated blood pressure.

Pallor and cold, clammy skin are observed in vasodepressor syncope and possibly in local anesthetic overdose as hypotension develops. Pallor may also be noted in the epinephrine overdose reaction. Edema is noted only in allergic reactions.

Appearance of Nervousness

An increase in outward nervousness, described as fear, apprehension, or agitation, after completion of the injection may be observed in the local anesthetic overdose and in epinephrine overdose. The patient with vasodepressor syncope is nervous before and during the administration of the drug, but does not normally become progressively more nervous during the postinjection period. This patient's major complaint is one of "feeling bad" or "feeling faint." Allergic patients do not develop marked nervousness; most of these patients simply complain of "feeling terrible."

Loss of Consciousness

Local anesthetic overdose, acute systemic anaphylaxis, and vasodepressor syncope may all lead to the loss of consciousness. All may also produce milder reactions that do not evolve to this degree. Epinephrine overdose seldom produces unconsciousness unless serious cardiovascular complications develop.

Presence of Seizures

Local anesthetic overdose is most likely to produce generalized seizures of a tonic-clonic variety, whereas milder convulsive movement (e.g., individual muscles such as a finger or facial muscle twitching) may occur in vasodepressor syncope. Mild tremor of the extremities is normally observed in epinephrine overdose. Seizures do not usually occur with allergy unless hypoxia is present.

Respiratory Symptoms

Dyspnea, or difficulty in breathing, may be present with any of these situations. Respiratory symptoms are most marked in the allergic reaction. Wheezing produced by bronchial smooth muscle constriction leads to a definitive diagnosis of asthma or allergy. Because management of both of these clinical entities is identical, precise diagnosis is not immediately required.

A high-pitched crowing sound should lead the doctor to consider laryngeal obstruction. This may be produced by a foreign object in the posterior pharynx or by laryngeal edema resulting from an allergic reaction. In the absence of other signs of allergy, such as a skin reaction, the airway should be suctioned in order to remove any foreign material before further management.

Total airway obstruction is most probably produced by the tongue in an unconscious patient. If, following airway maneuvers and suctioning, the obstruction persists, lower airway obstruction should be considered. Regardless of the cause (e.g., edema or foreign object), an airway must be established rapidly through manual thrust or cricothyrotomy techniques.

Cardiovascular Symptoms
Heart Rate

The heart rate increases during the presyncopal phase of vasodepressor syncope, but it decreases dramatically to approximately 40 beats per minute once consciousness is lost and remains low during the postsyncopal period.

Local anesthetic overdose and allergic reactions are also associated with increases in heart rate, but the rate does not decrease to lower levels if consciousness is lost. A shock reaction develops that is characterized by rapid heart rate (tachycardia) and low blood pressure (hypotension), producing a weak, thready pulse.

Epinephrine overdose, on the other hand, produces a dramatic increase in heart rate and blood pressure, leading to a full and bounding pulse. In addition, the heart rate may become irregular during the epinephrine reaction, owing to the effects of the drug on the myocardium.

Blood Pressure

Blood pressure remains at or near the baseline level during the presyncopal phase of vasodepressor syncope. With the loss of consciousness, however, blood pressure drops significantly.

In acute allergic reactions the blood pressure may fall precipitously because of the massive vasodilation that occurs. Indeed, this reaction (acute systemic anaphylaxis) is one of the most likely of all the ADRs to lead to cardiovascular collapse (cardiac arrest).

During the early phase of a local anesthetic overdose, blood pressure is usually slightly elevated. As the reaction progresses, the blood pressure returns to baseline or falls below this level. Blood pressure during an epinephrine overdose reaction is dramatically increased. Pressures greatly in excess of 200 mmHg systolic and 120 mmHg diastolic may be observed during this reaction.

Table 25-1. Comparison of drug-related emergencies (by common factors)

Related (common) factors	Vasodepressor syncope	Overdose: local anesthetic or epinephrine	Drug allergy
Age of patient	18-40 years most common	Any age; more likely in children than in adults	Any age
Sex of patient	More common in males	No sexual difference in occurrence	No sexual difference in occurrence
Position of patient	Unlikely in supine position	Not related to position	Not related to position
Onset of symptoms	Before, during, or immediately following administration	During or following administration	During or following administration
Prior exposure to drug	Not related	May occur with any drug, any administration	Prior exposure; "sensitizing dose" required
Dose of drug administered	Not related	Dose-related	Not dose-related
Overall incidence of occurrence	Most common drug-related emergency	Overdose is the most common *true* drug-related emergency (85% of all ADRs)	Rare; represents 15% of all ADRs

Table 25-2. Comparison of drug-related emergencies (by signs and symptoms)

Signs and symptoms	Vasodepressor syndope	Overdose		Drug allergy
		Local anesthetic	Epinephrine	
Duration of acute symptoms	Brief, following positioning	Self-limiting (2-30 minutes)	Extremely brief (usually seconds)	Long; hours to days
Appearance of skin	Pale, cold, and moist	Not relevant	Erythematous	Erythematous, presence of urticaria, itching, edema
Appearance of nervousness	No drastic increase	Increased anxiety, agitation	Fear, anxiety present	Not present
Loss of consciousness	Yes—vasodepressor syncope is most common cause of loss of consciousness	Yes—in severe reaction	No—rarely, if ever	Yes—in severe reaction
Presence of seizures	Rare—limited to mild, localized	Yes; tonic-clonic seizure	Mild tremor	No—unless hypoxia present
Respiratory symptoms	Not diagnostic	Not diagnostic	Not diagnostic	Wheezing, laryngeal edema
Cardiovascular symptoms				
Heart rate (pulse)	Initial elevation (presyncope), then depression (syncope)	Increased Weak and thready	Dramatic increase in palpitations Full and bounding	Increased Weak and thready
Blood pressure	Initially normal (presyncope); then depression	Initial increase, then depression	Dramatic increase	Significant depression
Most significant diagnostic criteria	Presyncopal manifestations; rapid recovery following positioning	CNS "stimulation" following drug administration	Palpitations; intense headache; brief duration	Erythema, urticaria, and pruritis; bronchospasm

SUMMARY

Each of these clinical syndromes is presented with several outstanding features. Vasodepressor syncope has a presyncopal phase of relatively long duration. The patient feels faint and lightheaded, the skin loses color, and perspiration is evident. Consciousness is regained rapidly following placement of the patient in the supine position. This reaction commonly results from fear and is the most frequent drug-related emergency.

Local anesthetic overdose is related to high blood levels of local anesthetic. It is commonly produced by rapid intravascular injection or the administration of too large a dose. Signs and symptoms of stimulation (e.g., agitation, increased heart rate and blood pressure, and possibly seizures) are followed by depression (e.g., lethargy, cardiovascular depression, respiratory depression, and loss of consciousness).

Epinephrine overdose is most frequently produced by the use of excessive concentrations of epinephrine in gingival retraction cord and much less commonly by local anesthetics. The most prominent clinical signs include greatly increased nervousness; mild tremor; an intense, throbbing headache; and greatly increased blood pressure and heart rate. Epinephrine reactions are usually brief. The patient seldom loses consciousness.

Allergy may manifest itself in a variety of ways. However, obvious clinical signs of allergy include the skin reactions of flushing, urticaria, and itching. Edema may also occur. The presence of wheezing with respiratory efforts also signifies allergy. Allergy is the least common of these three ADRs, but is usually the most dangerous of these reactions. Tables 25-1 and 25-2 compare the different types of adverse drug reactions.

REFERENCES

1. Parrish HM: Analysis of 460 fatalities from venomous animals in the United States, *Am J Med Sci* 245:129, 1963.
2. Caranasos GJ: Drug reactions. In Schwartz GR, Safar P, Stone JH, and others, editors: *Principles and practice of emergency medicine*, ed 2, Philadelphia, 1986, WB Saunders.

26 *Chest Pain: General Considerations*

There are a great many specific causes for the clinical symptom of chest pain that are entirely non-cardiac in origin. Yet the sudden onset of chest pain is invariably a frightening experience because it immediately invokes thoughts of heart attack in the mind of the victim. Because cardiovascular disease is the major cause of death in the United States today, this concern is not entirely unfounded. The almost universal presence of signs of cardiovascular disease in adults means that we all are potential victims of one or more of the clinical manifestations of cardiovascular disease. If we add to this the stress involved in dental therapy, it becomes evident that many medically compromised dental patients represent an increased risk during treatment. Recognition of these potentially high-risk patients and the use of specific treatment modifications will go far to diminish the chances of life-threatening situations developing.

Although chest pain is a major clue to the possible presence of ischemic heart disease (IHD), the underlying disease process has normally been present for a considerable time before the appearance of clinical symptoms. Indeed, chest pain need not be the presenting symptom of IHD. Previous chapters have discussed two other clinical expressions of cardiovascular disease: heart failure, presented as respiratory distress (Chapter 14), and cerebrovascular ischemia and infarction (Chapter 19), presented as altered consciousness. In this section three additional clinical manifestations of heart disease are discussed. Two of these, angina pectoris (Chapter 27) and myocardial infarction (Chapter 28), most commonly present as chest pain. Another clinical syndrome of cardiovascular disease, cardiac arrest, is discussed in Chapter 30. Cardiac arrest is a possible acute complication of all forms of cardiovascular disease, or it may be the initial indication of the presence of cardiovascular disease.[1]

The more common causes of acute chest pain that may be encountered in dental situations include angina pectoris, hyperventilation, and myocardial infarction (Table 26-1). There are numerous other causes, both cardiac and noncardiac, which present as chest pain and must be differentiated from true cardiac pain. These include hiatal hernia, esophageal spasm, peptic ulcer, cholecystitis, musculoskeletal pain associated with the chest wall syndrome, pulmonary embolism, pneumothorax, mitral valve prolapse, pericarditis, and acute dissecting aortic aneurysm.[2-6] A differential diagnosis of chest pain, both cardiac and noncardiac, is presented in Chapter 29.

A major etiologic factor underlying virtually all forms of cardiovascular disease is atherosclerosis. Atherosclerosis represents a special type of thickening and hardening of medium- and large-sized

Table 26-1. Causes of chest pain

Cause	Frequency	Where discussed
Angina pectoris	Most common	Chest pain (Section VII)
Hyperventilation	Common	Respiratory difficulty (Section III)
Acute myocardial infarction	Less common	Chest pain (Section VII)

Table 26-2. Estimated leading causes of death in the United States, 1984-1985

Cause	Number	% of CVD
Deaths		
Diseases of the heart and blood vessels	991,332	
Heart attack (myocardial infarction)	540,400	54.8
Stroke (CVA)	155,000	15.7
High blood pressure	30,000	3.1
Rheumatic heart disease	6,900	0.7
Other CVD	253,500	25.7
Cancer	457,670	
Accidents	92,070	
Chronic obstructive pulmonary disease (COPD)	74,420	
Pneumonia and influenza	66,630	
All other causes	401,878	

Source: National Center for Health Statistics, US Public Health Service, DHHS, 1988.

arteries that accounts for a very large proportion of acute myocardial infarcts (AMI or heart attack) and cases of ischemic heart disease. It also accounts for many strokes (those caused by cerebral ischemia and infarction[7]), numerous instances of peripheral vascular disease, and most aneurysms of the lower abdominal aorta, which can rupture and cause sudden fatal hemorrhage.[8] Atherosclerosis is present in approximately 90% of patients with significant noncongenital heart disease.[9] When present in arteries that supply blood to the myocardium, the disease state is called coronary artery disease (CAD). Other common names for CAD are: coronary heart disease (CHD), ischemic heart disease (IHD), and atherosclerotic heart disease. Coronary artery disease may be defined as a narrowing or an occlusion of the coronary arteries, usually by atherosclerosis, which results in an imbalance between the requirement for and the supply of oxygen to the myocardium, leading to myocardial ischemia. An understanding of CAD and atherosclerosis leads to a greater knowledge of their clinical expressions. The remainder of this chapter discusses the important factors of cardiovascular disease, a disease responsible for approximately 50% of all deaths in the United States.[10]

The following are definitions of terms to be used in this section:

Hypoxia. Reduced oxygen supply to tissue despite adequate perfusion

Anoxia. Absence of oxygen supply to tissue despite adequate perfusion

Ischemia. Oxygen deprivation accompanied by inadequate removal of metabolites consequent to inadequate perfusion

Infarction. Area of coagulation necrosis in a tissue caused by local ischemia, resulting from obstruction of circulation to the area

PREDISPOSING FACTORS

In 1985 diseases of the heart and blood vessels were responsible for an estimated 991,332 deaths in the United States.[11] Of this figure, 540,400 (54.8%) died from myocardial infarction and the remainder succumbed to cerebrovascular accident, high blood pressure, rheumatic heart disease, and other causes such as aneurysms and pulmonary emboli (Table 26-2).[11]

The death rate due to cardiovascular disease increased in each decade in the United States until the 1970s. Since that time there has been a dramatic decline in the death rates from myocardial ischemia and its complications (Fig. 26-1).[12] A decline of 20.7% in the death rate was noted between 1968 and 1976.[12] This decline occurred each year and was noted in both sexes, all age groups, and in the three major ethnic groups. This decline continues at the present time with a 37% decline in cardiovascular deaths reported in the past 20 years.[13] The reasons for the decline in IHD mortality are not well understood, but are thought to be due to factors including[14-16]:

- Improved detection and treatment of high blood pressure
- Decreased cigarette use by middle-aged men
- A change toward a more prudent diet
- Improvements in the medical and surgical care for cardiovascular disease

These modifications in cardiovascular disease risk factors are thought to account for only one half of the decline in mortality for men and one third of the decline in mortality for younger women.[12] In addition the impact of emergency medical services and coronary artery bypass surgery is believed not to account for this decline in cardiovascular mortality.[12]

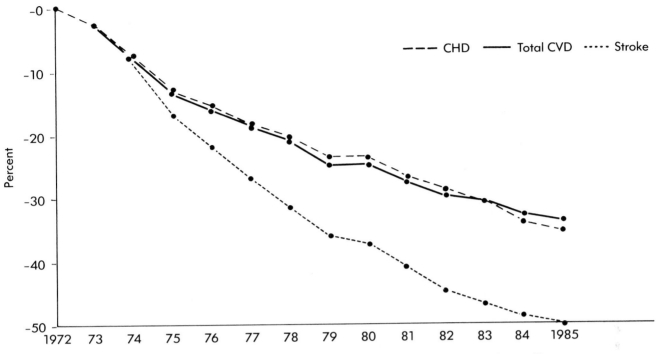

Fig. 26-1. Cumulative percent change in age-adjusted death rates for major cardiovascular diseases, 1972-1985.   — — — CHD   ——— CVD   — — — — Stroke   (From: *Textbook of advanced cardiac life support,* American Heart Assoc., 1987).

Despite these advances and the unexplained decline in cardiovascular mortality, death from cardiovascular disease is still a formidable problem. Cardiovascular disease is still the leading cause of death in the United States (see Table 26-2). Of an estimated 2,047,000 deaths that occurred in the United States in 1984, just under half (48%) were due to cardiovascular disease, two thirds of which were caused by underlying coronary and ischemic heart disease.[17]

An even more disturbing figure, however, is the overall incidence of cardiovascular disease in the United States. According to the American Heart Association,[10] more than 42 million persons have clinical evidence of one or more forms of cardiovascular disease. These persons represent a great potential risk to the dentist. Most of these persons are ambulatory, and a significant number may be asymptomatic, perhaps even unaware of their cardiovascular disease, when appearing in the dental office for routine dental care. As is evident, any procedure or incident that results in an increase in the workload of such an individual's cardiovascular system is potentially dangerous.

In 1987 it was estimated that 1.5 million persons in the United States suffered a myocardial infarction and that 540,000 (36%) died, 350,000 of those before they reach a hospital.[17] Thus, more than two thirds of deaths due to ischemic heart disease occur

outside of the hospital, the vast majority occurring within 2 hours of the onset of symptoms.[18] Though infrequent, it is entirely likely that such deaths will occur within the dental office setting.

Recent advances in emergency cardiac care have decreased mortality rates for patients with CAD suffering acute myocardial infarction who reach the hospital.[19,20] Additional decreases in mortality rates from acute ischemic heart disease have occurred from the increased use of thrombolytic therapy and/or percutaneous transluminal angioplasty.[21] Yet in those instances in which cardiopulmonary arrest occurs outside of the hospital, the survival rate for those victims who are not resuscitated prior to their arrival at the hospital is dismal.[22]

Coronary artery disease occurs more frequently in males, demonstrating an overall male to female incidence of 4:1. Of all deaths in men between the ages of 55 and 64, 40% are from coronary artery disease. In whites between the ages of 35 and 44 years, there is a 5.2:1 male to female ratio for CAD, which progressively falls until between the ages of 65 and 74, the male to female ratio for whites with CAD is 2.3:1. For nonwhites, these male to female ratios are 2.5:1 and 1.5:1, respectively. In general, the female rate lags behind the male rate by about 10 years in whites and by about 7 years in nonwhites.[10,23,24]

MAJOR RISK FACTORS OF HEART DISEASE

Factors that cannot be changed
Heredity
Sex
Race
Age

Factors that can be changed
Tobacco smoking
High blood pressure
High blood cholesterol levels
Diabetes

Data show that 2% of clinically significant CAD occurs before the age of 30 years. This incidence increases with age; 80% of CAD occurs between the sixth and eighth decades of life (ages 50 to 70 years), with the peak incidence in men occurring between 50 and 60 years of age and in women, between 60 and 70 years of age.[10,24]

The widespread occurrence and increasing incidence of coronary artery disease has prompted much research into its causes. In addition, possible methods are being researched to prevent CAD from progressing to the point of clinical morbidity and mortality. To date, a number of factors have been identified which, when present, can increase the probability of an individual exhibiting clinical manifestations of CAD.[25] Major risk factors for heart disease are listed in the accompanying box. Although the evidence relating these factors to a significant increase in morbidity and mortality from CAD is obvious, uncertainty remains about the degree of benefit to be obtained by removing or managing these factors.[1,14,15]

Major Modifiable Risk Factors

The following are major risk factors of heart disease that can be modified with a resulting decrease in risk.

Tobacco Smoking

Tobacco smoking is a major risk factor for acute myocardial infarction and death from CAD. Results of several studies demonstrate that total mortality (all causes), total cardiovascular morbidity and mortality, and the incidence of CAD are about 1.6 times higher in male smokers than in male nonsmokers. There is also a direct relationship between these events and the number of cigarettes smoked daily.[26,27]

Fortunately, the excessive risk factor for CAD declines in ex-smokers within a year or two after they discontinue smoking, but it does remain slightly greater than the risk associated with nonsmokers.[28]

Several reasons for the increased risk caused by smoking have been postulated, including the effects of nicotine and carbon monoxide on the heart, coronary arteries, and blood. Nicotine increases the myocardial demand for oxygen, increases the adhesiveness of platelets, and lowers the threshold for ventricular fibrillation.[29] Carbon monoxide prevents oxygen from forming oxyhemoglobin, thereby decreasing oxygen availability to tissues. Blood carbon monoxide levels in smokers range from 1% to 20%, compared with normal levels of 0.5% to 1.0% (blood levels from 20% to 80% occur in carbon monoxide poisoning).[30] When a person stops smoking, carbon monoxide blood levels fall and the increased risk of CAD falls to approximately that of the nonsmoker. This factor also explains the increased incidence of cardiovascular abnormalities noted in automobile passengers on crowded Los Angeles freeways.[31] These subjects were exposed to a significantly higher level of gasoline engine exhausts, of which carbon monoxide is a major part. Carbon monoxide levels in their blood reached 1.4% to 3.0%.

Blood Lipids

Among the recognized risk factors for the development of atherosclerosis, one of the most well documented is the relationship between blood lipid levels and CAD.[32] The evidence associating increased serum cholesterol levels with increased incidence of CAD is extensive and unequivocal.[33] Stated quite simply, persons with the highest cholesterol levels are at greatest risk to develop CAD, but even those with lower serum cholesterol levels are not completely risk free.

Several types of lipoproteins have been identified. Low-density lipoprotein (LDL) is known to be atherogenic and is the lipoprotein most directly associated with coronary artery disease.[34] High-density lipoprotein (HDL) demonstrates an inverse association with risk of CAD (higher HDL levels equate with lower risk of development of CAD).[35] There is, however, no cutoff point in serum cholesterol levels below which there is no risk.[25] Persons with blood cholesterol levels in excess of 300 mg% have a risk of devoping CAD four times greater than do those with blood cholesterol levels less than 200 mg%. Mean levels for total plasma cholesterol (mg/dL) in white men are 200 between the ages of 35 and 39, 213 between the ages of 45 and 49, and 221 between the ages of 65 and 69, whereas plasma LDL cholesterol levels in these same groups are 133, 143, and 150, respectively.[24]

Blood Pressure

The risk of morbidity and mortality from CAD, as well as the risk of other diseases produced or exacerbated by atherosclerosis, show a smooth, direct relationship to blood pressure levels over the entire range of values. As with blood lipids, there is no cutoff point at which risk suddenly changes from low to high.[36]

Management of high blood pressure through the administration of antihypertensive medications can decrease the risk to the patient.[37] Damage that has developed within arteries over the years from high blood pressure cannot be undone (see section on pathophysiology); however, the atherosclerotic process will be slowed if the patient's blood pressure is lowered.

Abnormal Glucose Tolerance

Hyperglycemia and glucose intolerance are associated with an increased risk of developing CAD. Overt diabetes mellitus has long been recognized as a precursor of vascular disease.[38] Males with glucose intolerance have a 50% greater chance of developing CAD than do those with normal values, whereas in females the risk is doubled.[39] In non–insulin-dependent diabetes the major cause of mortality is CAD. Both non–insulin-dependent and insulin-dependent adult-onset diabetics are at increased risk for developing CAD.[38] Mortality in juvenile-onset insulin-dependent diabetes is primarily associated with renal disease.[40]

Major Unmodifiable Risk Factors

Several other major risk factors of heart disease are unable to be modified at this time. These include heredity, sex, race, and age.

Heredity

Persons with either parents or siblings who are affected by CAD before the age of 50 years have a significantly greater risk of developing the disease themselves at a younger age than those who do not have such a history. This risk may be as great as 5:1.

Sex

As was previously discussed, CAD remains predominantly a male disease. The premenopausal female is relatively unaffected by CAD. Following menopause, the incidence of CAD in females increases, but it never reaches that of males.[24]

Race

Nonwhite men and women have higher rates of CAD up to the age of 65 years. Among specific ethnic groups in the United States, Japanese men in Hawaii and California, and Hispanic men in Puerto Rico have been found to have about half the amount of CAD as Caucasians.[41]

Age

The incidence of CAD increases with age. By 55 to 64 years, 40% of deaths in males are due to CAD.

Minor Risk Factors

Other factors related to an increased risk of significant CAD that are not as well supported by clinical evidence include gout,[42] menopause and oral contraceptives,[43,44] obesity,[45] physical activity,[46] and type of personality and behavior.[47,48] In addition, it is known that individuals with certain noncardiac diseases demonstrate a higher incidence of significant CAD. Hypercholesterolemia, high blood pressure, and diabetes mellitus have been mentioned previously. Another disease with significant CAD rates includes uncontrolled hypothyroidism. Fig. 26-2 illustrates the increased risk of death that is presented by some of these factors.

PREVENTION

Unfortunately, primary prevention (i.e., prevention of initial development) of atherosclerosis and coronary artery disease has not yet been effectively demonstrated. Research into the known risk factors may ultimately demonstrate the feasibility of prevention of clinical CAD. To date, however, secondary prevention (i.e., prevention of death following the onset of clinical symptoms) is the norm, but in too many cases this effort proves to be too late to prevent death or the occurrence of significant morbidity.

Emphasis is currently being placed on the elimination of any known risk factors that may be present. Smoking is discouraged, optimal weight and physical fitness are encouraged, and special diets and medications are recommended for those with elevated cholesterol levels in the blood. Uncontrolled hyperthyroidism or diabetes mellitus is brought under control, and elevations in blood pressure are corrected. However, conflicting evidence has been gathered concerning the effectiveness of many of these therapies in preventing morbidity and mortality.

Management of elevated blood pressure has been effectively demonstrated to produce a significant decrease in the morbidity and mortality rate from CAD. The Veterans Administration studies

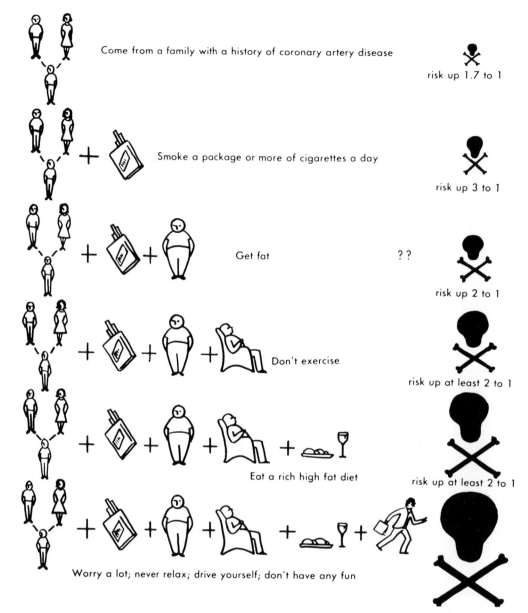

Fig. 26-2. How to die from coronary heart disease. The total increase in risk of death from coronary disease from all factors is at least 10 to 1, and may be more like 30 to 1. (From Phibbs B: *The human heart: a guide to heart disease,* ed 5, St Louis, 1982, Mosby–Year Book.)

(Tables 26-3 and 26-4) proved conclusively that reduction of elevated blood pressure leads to a highly significant decrease in the incidence of fatal and nonfatal cardiovascular events.[49] The Hypertension Detection and Follow-up Program Cooperative Group[50] has demonstrated that vigorous drug management of even mild elevations in blood pressure (diastolic blood pressure 90 to 104 mmHg) leads to significant reductions (a decline of 20.3%) of cardiovascular morbidity and mortality (Table 26-5).

It stands to reason therefore that monitoring and recording blood pressure of all dental patients before dental treatment commences might well prove to be a life-saving procedure. A suggested protocol for the management of dental patients with elevated blood pressure is presented in Chapter 2.

Another significant factor that may be applied to the dental office setting is the reduction of stress related to the planned dental care through treatment modification. Physical and psychologic stress increases the work of the myocardium and there-

Table 26-3. Death and major nonfatal events in untreated and treated hypertensive patients

| | Initial diastolic blood pressure | | | |
| | 115-129 torr* | | 90-114 torr* | |
	70 Untreated men†	73 Actively treated men	194 Untreated men	186 Actively treated men
Cardiovascular deaths	4	0	19	8
Major nonfatal events‡	23	2	57	14

From Veterans Administration Cooperative Study Group on Antihypertensive Agents (1970). II. Results in patients with diastolic blood pressure averaging 90-114 mm Hg, *JAMA* 213:1143, 1970.
*Average period of observation for men with diastolic blood pressure of 115-129 was 18 months; for men with diastolic blood pressure of 90-114, it was 40 months.
†Includes 20 patients whose diastolic blood pressure exceeded 124 torr at three separate clinic visits.
‡Includes congestive heart failure, cerebrovascular thrombosis, cerebral hemorrhage, myocardial infarction, grade 3 or 4 retinopathy, and azotemia.

Table 26-4. Effectiveness of antihypertensive treatment in reducing death and major nonfatal events

| | Percentage of patients with events | | Effectiveness of treatment (%)* |
Initial diastolic blood pressure	Control	Treated	
90-114 torr	33.3	11.8	70
115-129 torr	33.6	2.7	93

From Veterans Administration Cooperative Study Group on Antihypertensive Agents (1970). II. Results in patients with diastolic blood pressure averaging 90-114 mm Hg, *JAMA* 213:1143, 1970.
*Effectiveness of treatment is the difference between percentages of incidence of events in control and treated groups, divided by percentage of incidence in control group.

Table 26-5. Mortality from all causes for stepped care (SC) and referred care (RC) participants* during 5-year followup, by diastolic blood pressure (DBP) at entry

| DBP at entry (torr) | Sample size | | Deaths | | Life table death rate per 100 (SE)† | | 95% confidence limits for difference in RC and SC rates | Percentage of reduction in mortality for SC group‡ |
	SC	RC	SC	RC	SC	RC		
TOTAL	5485	5455	349	419	6.4 (0.3)	7.7 (0.4)§	0.37-2.29	16.9
90-104	3903	3922	231	291	5.9 (0.4)	7.4 (0.4)§	0.40-2.62	20.3
105-114	1048	1004	70	77	6.7 (0.8)	7.7 (0.8)	−1.25-3.21	13.0
115+	534	529	48	51	9.0 (1.2)	9.7 (1.3)	−2.84-4.18	7.2

From Hypertension Detection and Follow-up Program Cooperative Group. Five-year findings of the hypertension detection and follow-up program. I. Reduction in mortality of persons with high blood pressure, including mild hypertension, *JAMA* 242:2562, 1979.
*Stepped care (SC) patients received rigorous antihypertensive drug therapy from time of diagnosis of their elevated blood pressure; referred care (RC) patients were managed in a manner consistent with usually accepted techniques, which might not include immediate use of antihypertensive drugs.
†SE indicates standard error.
‡(RC rate − SC rate)/(RC rate) × 100.
§P < 0.1.

fore its oxygen requirement. In a patient with impaired coronary blood flow, this additional requirement for oxygen may not be met and may lead to an acute exacerbation of some form of heart disease. The Stress Reduction Protocol (see Chapter 2) is invaluable in the management of most patients with CAD. Of particular importance will be the administration of supplemental oxygen through a nasal cannula or nasal hood to higher risk patients during dental treatment.

CLINICAL MANIFESTATIONS

Atherosclerosis does not produce clinical manifestations of disease. It is only when the degree of atherosclerosis becomes great enough to produce a deficit in blood supply and ischemia to an area of the body that symptoms become apparent. The nature of the subsequent clinical syndrome depends on these factors:

1. The size and location of the tissue inadequately supplied with blood
2. The severity of the deficiency
3. The rate of development of the deficiency
4. The duration of the deficiency

For example, cerebrovascular ischemia is a manifestation of atherosclerosis occurring in the brain. If the oxygen deficiency is mild and of short duration, transient ischemic attacks (TIA) may be the sole clinical manifestation, whereas a CVA develops with infarction of neuronal tissues if the ischemia is of greater duration and more complete. A TIA is normally of short duration, usually resolving itself without residual neuronal deficiency; CVA produces permanent neuronal damage. The clinical manifestations of atherosclerosis in coronary blood vessels (e.g., angina pectoris, myocardial infarction, heart failure, cardiac dysrhythmias, and sudden death) are summarized in Table 26-6.

Angina pectoris (see Chapter 27) is a transient, localized ischemia of the myocardium (similar to the TIA), whereas a myocardial infarction (see Chapter 28) results from a prolonged arterial occlusion (similar to CVA). Heart failure and cardiac dysrhythmias quite frequently develop following myocardial infarction as chronic complications, but they may also occur through a process of gradual fibrosis of the myocardium and the conduction system of the heart in the absence of myocardial infarction. Sudden death (e.g., cardiopulmonary arrest) may develop following any of the aforementioned mechanisms or through the occurrence of ventricular fibrillation (see Chapter 30).

PATHOPHYSIOLOGY
Atherosclerosis

Atherosclerosis is an ongoing process that starts in utero as soon as blood begins to flow in rudimentary blood vessels. It is found in all individuals at certain sites of predilection. Atherosclerosis may therefore be considered a reactive biologic response of arteries to the forces being generated by the flow of blood. Texon[51] has described athero-

Table 26-6. Clinical manifestations of atherosclerosis

	Manifestation	Mechanism
Noncardiac		
Diabetes mellitus	Diabetic retinopathy and blindness	Atherosclerosis of retinal vessels
	Increased infection and poor healing of lower limb, with possible amputation of toes or feet	Atherosclerosis of arteries to legs
Cerebral arteries	Transient ischemic attack	Transient occlusion of vessels
	Cerebrovascular infarction	Prolonged occlusion of vessels
Cardiac		
Coronary artery disease	Angina pectoris	Transient, localized myocardial ischemia
	Unstable angina	Prolonged myocardial ischemia, with or without myocardial necrosis
	Myocardial infarction	Prolonged arterial occlusion
	Heart failure	Gradual fibrosis of myocardium; occurs commonly following MI
	Dysrhythmias	Gradual fibrosis of myocardium; occurs commonly following MI
	Sudden death (cardiopulmonary arrest)	Any of the above and/or ventricular dysrhythmias

sclerosis as "the price we pay for blood flow as a requirement of life."

The basic factor in the development of an atherosclerotic lesion (called an atheroma) is a multiplication of the smooth muscle cells of the intimal layer of the blood vessel in response to pressure changes within the vessel (Fig. 26-3). In a normal blood vessel, there is constant movement of lipids into and out of the intimal layer. However, when proliferative changes occur within the intimal smooth muscle cells, the ability of these cells to maintain a steady level of lipids is altered, and the influx of lipids into the intima becomes predominant. This influx is initially made up of cholesterol, triglycerides, and phospholipids and appears as a yellowish streak or plaque that is visible within the lumen of the artery (Fig. 26-4). As the lesion progresses, cholesterol becomes the predominant lipid. Fibrous tissue next grows into and around the atheroma, and finally, calcium is deposited into the lesion. The atheroma, which began as a soft fatty lesion, becomes a larger, harder lesion.[52] With the increase in size, the lesion may cause obstruction of blood flow through the vessel at the point of the lesion, leading to chronic ischemia (e.g., heart failure, dysrhythmias), acute ischemia (e.g., angina pectoris, TIA), or infarction (e.g., myocardial or cerebrovascular infarction). If the endothelial layer of the blood vessel breaks down, the atheromatous material is exposed to circulating blood platelets, which then clump and initiate thrombus formation with subsequent acute clinical manifestations (e.g., myocardial infarction, CVA, or cardiac arrest).

Location

Atherosclerosis of the coronary vessels occurs predominantly in the proximal segments of medium-sized coronary arteries, especially at branching points. Interestingly, only those vessels that run over the surface of the myocardium are susceptible to the development of atheromatous lesions.[53] Vessels that enter the myocardium (the penetrating or muscular branches) do not demonstrate atheromata. The explanation for this is not yet known. The most common site in which clinically significant atherosclerosis develops in the heart, leading to major morbidity and mortality, is the anterior descending branch of the left coronary artery. Occlusion of this vessel leads to infarction of the anterior portion of the left ventricle. The blood supply to the myocardium is shown in Fig. 26-5.

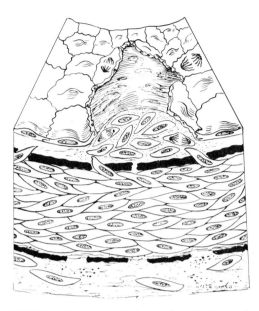

Fig. 26-3. Development of atherosclerosis. Smooth muscle cells migrate from media into the intimal layer through fenestrae in internal elastic lamina. (From Ross R, Glomset JA: The pathogenesis of atherosclerosis, *N Engl J Med* 295:369, 1976.)

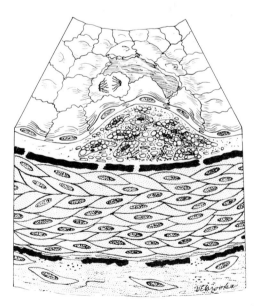

Fig. 26-4. Development of atherosclerosis. Lipid deposition within intimal cells and their surrounding connective tissue matrix. Lumen of vessel progressively narrows. (From Ross R, Glomset JA: The pathogenesis of atherosclerosis, *N Engl J Med* 295:369, 1976.)

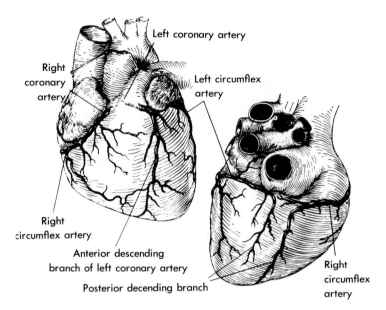

Fig. 26-5. Myocardial blood supply. *Left,* anterior portion of heart. *Right,* posterior portion of heart. (From Goldman MJ: *Principles of clinical electrocardiography,* ed 9, Los Altos, Calif., 1976, Lange Medical.)

Chest Pain

The basic mechanism of cardiac pain is a decrease or cessation of blood flow to the myocardium. Episodes of cardiac pain occur when critical myocardial ischemia is produced by an absolute decrease of the coronary blood flow or by oxygen demand of the myocardium that exceeds that which is available from the blood supply.

The precise mechanism of cardiac pain production is unknown. Theories suggest that cardiac pain results from an accumulation of metabolites within the ischemic portion of the myocardium. The rapid accumulation of metabolites within heart muscle, occurring with transient ischemia (e.g., angina pectoris) or prolonged ischemia (e.g., myocardial infarction), is responsible for triggering pain impulses.[54] Other theories on the genesis of cardiac pain include those suggesting that vasomotor reflexes or vasospasms produce paroxysms of cardiac pain (the pain arising from the coronary vessels themselves), or that cardiac pain is provoked by distention of the walls of coronary vessels proximal to the site of an occlusion.[55] Sudden obstruction of a major coronary vessel, primarily by thrombosis, and the occurrence of myocardial infarction are often associated with violent pain, yet if the vessel occlusion develops gradually, there may be no clinically evident signs. This is primarily because of the gradual development of an effective collateral circulation between the left and right coronary arteries.[56] In the presence of an adequate collateral circulation, an occlusion of the right coronary artery may not lead to infarction of that part of the tissue that is also supplied by the left coronary artery (see Fig. 26-5). Unfortunately, in the normal heart there is usually a minimally developed collateral circulation, which in part explains the greater incidence of acute episodes of cardiac disease.[57]

MANAGEMENT

Management of the acute clinical manifestations of ischemic heart disease is directed toward the specific clinical entity that develops. In the patient with congestive heart failure, primary management of the acute episode is directed at alleviation of respiratory distress, which is the major immediate symptom. Angina and acute myocardial infarction produce acute paroxysms of chest pain of varying intensity and duration. Immediate management of these clinical entities is directed at the alleviation of this pain. In all instances of clinical IHD, the goals of management include (1) decreasing the workload of the myocardium, thereby decreasing the myocardial oxygen requirement, and (2) providing the victim with an increased supply of oxygen. When sudden death is imminent, as in cardiopulmonary arrest, the goal of immediate therapy is of course the prevention of biologic death. The principles of basic life support must be applied as rapidly and as effectively as possible. Cardiac arrest is a possible complication of all forms of coronary artery disease.

REFERENCES

1. Gordon GS, Silverstein S: Ischemic heart disease. In Rosen P, Baker FJ, Barkin RM, and others, editors: *Emergency medicine*, ed 2, St Louis, 1988, Mosby–Year Book.
2. Braunwald E: Valvular heart disease. In Petersdorf RG, Adams RD, Braunwald E, and others, editors: *Harrison's principles of internal medicine*, New York, 1983, McGraw-Hill.
3. Fisch S: On the origin of cardiac pain: a new hypothesis, *Arch Intern Med* 140:754, 1980.
4. Minami H, McCallum RW: Chest pain: differentiating esophageal disease from angina pectoris, *Comp Ther* 8:50, 1982.
5. Benjamin SB, Castrell DO: Chest pain of esophageal origin: where are we and where should we go? *Arch Intern Med* 143:772, 1983.
6. Epstein SE, Gerber LH, Borer JS: Chest wall syndrome: a common cause of unexplained cardiac pain, *JAMA* 241:2793, 1979.
7. Khaw KT, Barrett-Conner E, Suaret L, and others: Prediction of stroke-associated mortality in the elderly, *Stroke* 15:244, 1984.
8. Hsu Y, Guzman L: Abdominal aortic aneurysm: diagnosis and treatment, *Milit Med* 145:807, 1980.
9. Kannel WB, Castell WP, Gordon T: Cholesterol in the prediction of atherosclerotic disease: new perspectives based on the Framingham study, *Ann Intern Med* 90:85, 1979.
10. American Heart Association: *Heart facts 1992*, Dallas, 1992, The American Heart Association.
11. National Center for Health Statistics, U.S. Public Health Service, DHHS, 1988.
12. Stern MP: The recent decline in ischemic heart disease mortality, *Ann Intern Med* 91:630, 1979.
13. Kannel WB, Thom TJ: Incidence, prevalence and mortality of cardiovascular disease. In Hurst JW, editor: *The heart*, ed 6, New York, 1986, McGraw-Hill.
14. Kannel WB, Thom TJ: Implication of the recent decline in cardiovascular mortality, *Cardiovasc Med* 4:983, 1979.
15. Goldman L, Cook EF: The decline in ischemic heart disease mortality rates: an analysis of the comparative effects of medical interventions and changes in lifestyle, *Ann Intern Med* 101:825, 1984.
16. TIMI Study Group: The thrombolysis in myocardial infarction (TIMI) trial: phase I findings, *N Engl J Med* 312:983, 1985.
17. American Heart Association: *Textbook of advanced cardiac life support*, Dallas, 1987, The American Heart Association.
18. Kuller LH: Sudden death—definition and epidemiologic considerations, *Prog Cardiovasc Dis* 23:1, 1980.
19. Koster RW, Dunning AJ: Intramuscular lidocaine for prevention of lethal arrhythmias in the prehospitalization phase of acute myocardial infarction, *N Engl J Med* 313:1105, 1985.
20. Gruppo Ittalino per lo studio della streptochinasi nell'infarto miocardico (GISSI): Effectiveness of intravenous thrombolytic treatment in acute myocardial infarction, *Lancet* 1:297, 1986.
21. O'Neill W, Timmis GC, Bourdelln PD, and others: A prospective randomized clinical trial of intracoronary streptokinase vs coronary angioplasty for acute myocardial infarction, *N Engl J Med* 314:812, 1986.
22. Gray WA, Capone RJ, Most AS: Unsuccessful emergency medical resuscitation—are continued efforts in the emergency department justified? *N Engl J Med* 325:1393, 1991.
23. Keys A: Coronary heart disease—the global picture, *Atherosclerosis* 22:149, 1975.
24. Levy RI, Feinleib M: Risk factors for coronary artery disease and their management. In Braunwald E, editor: *Heart disease*. ed 3, Philadelphia, 1986, WB Saunders.
25. Stamler J: Lifestyles, major risk factors, proof, and public policy, *Circulation* 58:3, 1978.
26. Feinleib M, Williams RR: Relative risks of myocardial infarction, cardiovascular disease, and peripheral vascular disease by type of smoking, *Proc Third World Conf Smoking and Health* I:243, 1976.
27. Ball K, Turner R: Smoking and the heart: the basis for action, *Lancet* 2:822, 1974.
28. Oslo Study Group: Effect of diet and smoking intervention on the incidence of coronary heart disease: report from the Oslo Study Group of a randomised trial in healthy man, *Lancet* 2:1301, 1981.
29. Bellet S, DeGuzmas NT, Kostis JB: The effect of inhalation of cigarette smoke on ventricular fibrillation threshold in normal dogs and dogs with acute myocardial infarction, *Am Heart J* 83:67, 1972.
30. Astrup P, Kjeldsen K: Carbon monoxide, smoking, and atherosclerosis, *Med Clin N Am* 58:323, 1973.
31. Aronow WS: Smoking, carbon monoxide and coronary heart disease, *Circulation* 48:1169, 1973.
32. Inter-society Commission for Heart Disease Resources: Primary prevention of the atherosclerotic diseases, *Circulation* 42:A55, 1970.
33. Kannel WB, Castelli WP, Gordon T: Cholesterol in the prediction of athersclerotic disease: new perspectives based on the Framingham study, *Ann Intern Med* 90:85, 1979.
34. Stone NJ, Levy RI, Fredrickson DS, and others: Coronary artery disease in 116 kindred with a familial type II hyperlipoproteinemia, *Circulation* 49:476, 1974.
35. Castelli WP, Doyle JT, Gordon T, and others: HDL cholesterol and other lipids in coronary heart disease: the cooperative lipoprotein phenotyping study, *Circulation* 55:767, 1977.
36. Kannel WB: Role of blood pressure in cardiovascular disease: the Framingham study, *Angiology* 26:1, 1975.
37. Wassertheil-Smoller S, Oberman A, Blaufox MD, and others: The trial of antihypertensive interventions and management (TAIM) study: final results with regard to blood pressure, cardiovascular risk, and quality of life, *Am J Hypertension* 5(1):37-44, 1992.
38. Garcia MJ, McNamara PM, Gordon T, and others: Morbidity and mortality of diabetes in the Framingham population. Sixteen-year follow-up study, *Diabetes* 23:105, 1976.
39. Shurtleff D: *Some characteristics related to the incidence of cardiovascular disease and death: the Framingham study, 18-year follow-up*, DHEW Publ. No. (NIH) 74-599, Section No. 30, Washington D.C., 1974.
40. Knowles HC Jr: *Magnitude of the renal failure problem in diabetic patients*. In *Kidney international*, vol 6, no. 4, suppl 1, New York, 1974, Springer-Verlag.
41. Gordon T, Garcia-Palmieri MR, Kagan A, and others: Differences in coronary heart disease in Framingham, Honolulu and Puerto Rico, *J Chronic Dis* 27:329, 1974.

42. Persky VW, Dyer AR, Idris-Soven E, and others: Uric acid: a risk factor for coronary heart disease? *Circulation* 59:969, 1979.

43. Kannel WB, Hjortland MC, McNamara PM, and others: Menopause and risk of cardiovascular disease: The Framingham study, *Ann Intern Med* 85:447, 1976.

44. Jick H, Dinan B, Rothman KJ: Oral contraceptives and nonfatal myocardial infarction, *JAMA* 239:1403, 1978.

45. Gordon T, Kannel WB: Obesity and cardiovascular disease: the Framingham study, *Clin Endocrinol Metab* 5:367, 1976.

46. Wyndham CH: The role of physical activity in the prevention of ischemic heart disease, *S Afr Med J* 36:7, 1979.

47. Rosenman RH, Brand RJ, Sholtz RI, and others: Multivariate prediction of coronary heart disease during 8.5 year follow-up in the western collaborative group study, *Am J Cardiol* 37:903, 1976.

48. Friedman H, Rosenman RH: *Type A behavior and your heart*, New York, 1974, Alfred A. Knopf.

49. Veterans Administration Cooperative Study Group on Antihypertensive Agents (1970): II. Results in patients with diastolic blood pressure averaging 90-114 mm Hg, *JAMA* 215:1143, 1970.

50. Hypertension Detection and Follow-up Program Cooperative Group: Five-year findings of the hypertension detection and follow-up program. I. Reduction in mortality of persons with high blood pressure, including mild hypertension, *JAMA* 242:2562, 1979.

51. Texon M: Atherosclerosis, its hemodynamic basis and implications, *Med Clin N Am* 58:257, 1974.

52. Ross R, Glamset JA: The pathogenesis of atherosclerosis, *N Engl J Med* 295:369, 1976.

53. Mitchell JRA, Schwartz CJ: *Arterial disease*, Oxford, 1965, Blackwell Scientific.

54. Sampson JJ, Cheitlin MD: Pathophysiology and differential diagnosis of chest pain, *Prog Cardiovasc Dis* 13:507, 1971.

55. Prinzmetal M, Kennamer R, Merliss R, and others: Angina pectoris. I. A variant form of angina pectoris, *Am J Med* 27:375, 1959.

56. Gorlin R: Coronary collaterals. In *Coronary artery disease*, Philadelphia, 1976, WB Saunders.

57. Baroldi G, Scomazzoni G: *Coronary circulation in the normal and pathologic heart*, Washington, D.C., 1965, Armed Forces Institute of Pathology, Office of the Surgeon General, Department of the Army.

27 *Angina Pectoris*

Angina is a Latin word describing a spasmodic, cramplike, choking feeling or suffocating pain; *pectoris* is the Latin word for chest.[1] These words aptly describe the basic clinical manifestations of angina pectoris, commonly known as angina, the classic expression of ischemic heart disease (IHD). The term *angina pectoris* was first used in 1768 in a lecture by Dr. William Heberden to distinguish the "strangling" sensation of angina from the word *dolor,* which means pain.[2] A working definition of angina is that of a characteristic thoracic pain, usually substernal; precipitated chiefly by exercise, emotion, or a heavy meal; relieved by vasodilator drugs and a few minutes' rest; and a result of a moderate inadequacy of the coronary circulation.[1] The major clinical characteristic of angina is chest pain. However, the pain is seldom described as such by the victim. Much more commonly, the sensation is described as a dull, aching discomfort, "suffocating," "heavy," or "squeezing."

Angina is clinically important to dentistry because it is usually a sign indicating the presence of a significant degree of coronary artery disease (CAD). However, anginal pain is not specific for CAD; it may also be found with aortic stenosis, hypertensive heart disease, or even in the absence of demonstrable heart disease.[3] The onset of anginal pain indicates that the victim's coronary arteries are not providing the myocardium with an adequate oxygen supply and that myocardial ischemia has developed. If this inadequacy is prolonged excessively, actual infarction of the myocardium may occur. The patient with a history of angina will represent an increased risk during dental care. Any factor that might produce an increase in the myocardial oxygen requirement can precipitate an acute episode of chest pain, which, though usually readily managed with vasodilator drug therapy, can ultimately lead to myocardial infarction, acute dysrhythmias, or cardiac arrest. The prevention of acute episodes of chest pain proves ultimately more satisfactory than management of the episode after it develops.

PREDISPOSING FACTORS

The factors that lead to the initial development of angina are discussed in Chapter 26 (see box on p. 384). In most patients acute episodes of angina pectoris are usually precipitated by factors that produce a relative inability of the coronary arteries to supply adequate volumes of oxygenated blood to the myocardium. Commonly observed precipitating factors are listed in the accompanying box.

The type of angina described here is called stable angina. Synonyms for stable angina are chronic, classic, or exertional angina. Stable angina is usually caused by coronary artery disease.[4] The prevalence of coronary artery disease in groups of patients with stable angina, atypical angina, and nonanginal chest pain was 90%, 50%, and 16% respectively,[5] whereas the incidence of CAD in asymptomatic adults was estimated at 3% to 4%. Stable angina is triggered by strenuous activity, emotional stress, or cold weather. The pain of stable angina normally lasts from 1 to 15 minutes, builds gradually and reaches maximum intensity quickly. The pain of stable angina is usually relieved by rest or nitro-

---

PRECIPITATING FACTORS IN ANGINA PECTORIS

Physical activity
Hot, humid environment
Cold weather
Large meals
Emotional stress (argument, anxiety, or sexual excitement)
Caffeine ingestion
Fever, anemia, or thyrotoxicosis
Cigarette smoking
Smog
High altitudes
Smoke from *another* person's cigarettes

---

glycerin. Two other forms of angina are described: variant angina and unstable angina.

Variant angina is also termed Prinzmetal's angina, atypical angina, or vasoplastic angina. It is more likely to occur with the patient at rest rather than during physical exertion or emotional stress; it may develop at odd times during the day or night (even awakening patients from sleep); and is often associated with dysrhythmias or conduction defects. Coronary artery spasm is the cause of variant angina. Spasm of a coronary artery produces a sudden brief occlusion of an epicardial or large septal coronary artery. Normal and diseased coronary arteries may become constricted. Variant angina may recur at the same time each day in an individual. It is thought that diurnal fluctuations in circulating endogenous catecholamine levels, highest during the early AM hours, are partially responsible for nocturnal angina. Variant angina is more common in women under the age of 50 years, whereas stable angina is uncommon in women in this age group in the absence of severe hypercholesterolemia, high blood pressure, or diabetes mellitus. Signs and symptoms of variant angina include syncope, dyspnea, and palpitation. Nitroglycerin usually provides prompt relief of pain.

Another syndrome, called unstable angina, is described. Other names for this syndrome are preinfarction angina, crescendo angina, intermediate coronary syndrome, premature or impending myocardial infarction, and coronary insufficiency. Unstable angina is a syndrome that lies intermediate between stable angina and acute myocardial infarction. It is very significant because of the adverse prognosis and of the unpredictability of sudden onset of acute myocardial infarction in some of the patients with unstable angina. Unstable angina is the result of the progression of atherosclerosis. The percentage of patients with unstable angina who progress to acute myocardial infarction is high.[6] Episodes of pain associated with unstable angina may persist for up to 30 minutes and may be precipitated by any of the factors mentioned for the other forms of angina, or for no apparent reason. Three characteristics are used to define unstable angina:

1. Angina of recent onset, caused by minimal exertion
2. Increasingly severe, prolonged, or frequent angina in a patient with relatively stable, exertion-related angina
3. Angina both at rest and with minimal exertion

A recent classification of unstable angina based on pain symptoms describes three subsets:[7]

Group I: Angina upon effort of recent origin (within 4 weeks)

Group II: Angina upon exertion with a changing pattern (more severe, more frequent, radiation to new sites, incomplete relief with use of nitroglycerin)

Group III: Angina at rest lasting 15 minutes or longer

The degree of risk increases from group I to group III.

In an early study, which did not include angina of recent onset, of 167 patients with unstable angina, 16% developed an acute myocardial infarction (AMI) and 2% died within 3 months.[8] Gazes and others[9] reported on 140 patients diagnosed prior to 1961 and followed for 10 years. All met the three aforementioned criteria. At 3 months the incidence of AMI was 21% with a 10% mortality rate; at 1 year mortality was 18%, at 5 years 39%, and 10 years 52%.

Most patients with unstable angina have severe obstructive CAD. As it is a complicated syndrome that may be a prodrome of myocardial infarction, patients with unstable angina should be managed in the dental office as if they had recently had an acute myocardial infarction. This syndrome will be discussed in depth in this chapter. Table 27-1 compares the three anginal syndromes.

PREVENTION

As has been stressed previously, the prevention of life-threatening situations is much preferred to their management after they occur. In no other category is this more true than that of chest pain, because the outcome frequently is the death of the patient. With the multitude of stresses placed on both the doctor and the dental patient, it is probable that most persons (doctor as well as patient) experience an increase in their cardiac workload during dental treatment. Identification of the patient at increased risk permits modifications of dental care that will, in most instances, prevent the development of chest pain. Because both emotional and physical stress are major elements known to precipitate chest pain, the elimination of stress is our chief preventive measure.

Medical History Questionnaire

QUESTION 9. Circle any of the following that you have had or have at present:

• Heart disease
• Angina pectoris
• Heart surgery

COMMENT. An affirmative answer to any part of this question should be followed with the dialogue history to determine the nature of the cardiac prob-

Table 27-1. Comparison of anginal syndromes

Anginal syndrome	Synonyms	Precipitating factors	Duration	Response to nitroglycerin
Stable	Chronic, classic, exertional	Emotional stress, physical exertion, cold weather	1-15 minutes	Good
Variant	Prinzmetal's, atypical, vasoplastic	Coronary artery spasm	Variable	Good
Unstable	Preinfarction, crescendo, acute coronary insufficiency, intermediate coronary syndrome, impending MI	Any factor or no factor	Up to 30 minutes	Questionable

lem and its severity. Percutaneous transluminal coronary angioplasty (PTCA) and/or coronary artery bypass graft (CABG) surgery are frequently indicated for patients with severe angina pectoris as a means of providing myocardial revascularization in the presence of significant CAD.[10,11] Atherectomy[12] and laser angioplasty[13] are newer approaches to myocardial revascularization.

QUESTION 10. When you walk up stairs or take a walk, do you ever have to stop because of pain in your chest or shortness of breath, or because you are very tired?

COMMENT. Pain occurring in the chest during exertion, such as walking or climbing a flight of stairs, that is relieved by rest or nitroglycerin is a symptom of angina pectoris.

QUESTION 6. Have you taken any medicine or drugs during the past 2 years?

COMMENT. Patients with angina pectoris normally have with them a supply of sublingual nitroglycerin tablets or spray that is used to terminate an acute episode of anginal pain. Since its introduction in January of 1986, increasing numbers of anginal patients use the more stable oral spray form of nitroglycerin in place of the sublingual tablets. Many patients with angina also receive other medications, such as the long-acting nitrates, β-adrenergic blockers,[14] and calcium channel blockers, in an effort to prevent the occurrence of acute anginal episodes. Although the frequency of anginal episodes may be decreased with the long-acting nitrates,[15] there is no convincing evidence that these agents prolong life. Calcium channel blockers are especially useful when coronary artery spasm is present, although they may relieve anginal pain in the absence of spasm because they also produce vasodilation.[16] Additionally, nitroglycerin ointment and transdermal nitroglycerin have recently been added to the treatment armamentarium. Nitroglycerin ointment provides relief for 4 to 6 hours,

whereas transdermal nitroglycerin provides slow, continuous release of the drug over a 24-hour period. Table 27-2 lists those drugs used in the prevention or management of anginal episodes.

Dialogue History

For patients with a history of angina, the dialogue history should be used to determine the following information concerning their anginal pains.

QUESTION. **Describe a typical anginal episode.**

COMMENT. The quality of chest discomfort of anginal episodes should be determined by asking patients to describe, in their own words, the nature of the episode and the radiation pattern associated with it. In place of the word *pain,* many patients describe their anginal attacks as "an unpleasant sensation," "squeezing," "pressing," "strangling," "constricting," "bursting," and "burning." If the patient describes the episodes with terms such as: "shooting," "knifelike," "sharp," "stabbing," "fleeting," or "tingling," the pain is probably not anginal.[4]

Observe patients as they describe their pain. Clenching of the fist in front of the chest while describing the sensation (Fig. 27-1) is a very strong indication of an ischemic origin for the pain.[17]

QUESTION. **Where does the "pain" hurt or radiate?**

COMMENT. Determine the location of the pain. Anginal pain is usually substernal, across both sides of the chest. Pain may radiate to various regions. Common sites of radiation of ischemic chest pain include: the neck and jaw; the upper epigastric region (stomach); intrascapular (between the shoulder blades); substernal radiating to the neck and jaw (mandible); substernal radiating to the left arm; epigastric radiating to the neck, jaw, and both arms; and the left shoulder and the inner aspect of both arms (Fig. 27-2).[4]

If the pain or discomfort can be localized (i.e., the patient can point to a spot where it hurts), the

Table 27-2. Drugs used to prevent anginal episodes

Generic name	Proprietary name	Route of administration	Side effects
Long-acting nitrates			
Isosorbide dinitrate	Isordil	Sublingual	Headache
	Sorbitrate	Oral	Flushing
			Tachycardia
			Dizziness
Pentaerythritol tetranitrate	Peritrate	Oral	Postural hypotension
Erythrityl tetranitrate	Cardilate	Sublingual and oral	Tachyphylaxis to nitroglycerin with prolonged use
Beta-blockers			
Propranolol	Inderal	Oral	For all beta blockers: develop-
Metoprolol	Lopressor	Oral	ment of asthma, severe brady-
Nadolol	Corgard	Oral	cardia, atrioventricular con-
Atenolol	Tenormin	Oral	duction defects, left ventricu-
Pindolol	Visken	Oral	lar failure
Timolol	Blocadren	Oral	
Calcium channel blockers			
Verapamil	Calan, Isoptin	Oral	For all calcium channel blockers:
Diltiazem	Cardizem	Oral	peripheral edema, hypoten-
Nifedipine	Procardia, Adalat	Oral	sion, dizziness, lightheaded-
			ness, headache, weakness,
			nausea, constipation
Nitroglycerin			
	Nitrostat	Sublingual	For all forms of nitroglycerin:
	Nitrolingual spray	Sublingual spray	headache, postural hypoten-
	Nitrobid	Ointment	sion
	Nitrol	Ointment	
	Nitrong	Ointment	
	Nitrostat	Ointment	
	Nitrodisc	Transdermal patch	
	Nitro-dur	Transdermal patch	
	Transderm-Nitro	Transdermal patch	

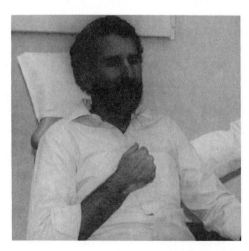

Fig. 27-1. The Levine sign, an indicator of angina pectoris.

origin is usually not ischemic, but from the skin or the chest wall. Ischemic pain, arising from deeper structures (e.g., the heart) tends to be more generalized in location, hurting over a larger area, as opposed to a more well-defined spot.[17]

QUESTION. **How long do your anginal episodes last?**

COMMENT. Determine the duration of the typical episode. Angina is by definition of short duration. If the episode is precipitated by exertion and the patient stops and rests, the discomfort normally ceases within 2 to 10 minutes. Chest pain lasting less than 30 seconds is usually not anginal. This brief duration commonly points to a problem of noncardiac origin, such as musculoskeletal pain, hiatal hernia, or functional pain. Chest pain lasting for hours suggests acute myocardial infarction,

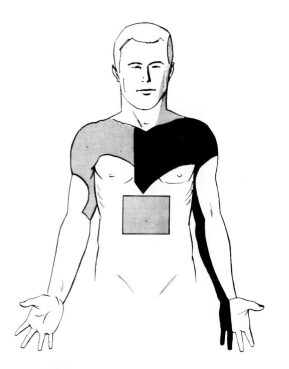

Substernal pain projected to left shoulder and arm (ulanar nerve distribution)

Less frequent referred sites including right shoulder and arm, left jaw, neck, and epigastrium

Fig. 27-2. Radiation patterns of chest pain. (From Jastak, JT and Cowan EF, Jr.,: *Dent Clin North Am* 17:363, 1973).

pericarditis, dissecting aortic aneurysm, musculoskeletal disease, herpes zoster, or anxiety. Anginal episodes developing after a large meal or emotional stress tend to be longer lasting and more difficult to treat. The longer the duration of ischemia, the greater the risk of irreversible myocardial damage.

QUESTION. What precipitates your anginal episode?

COMMENT. Determine the precipitating factors of the anginal episode. Most commonly, anginal pain occurs during exertion. The amount of exertion required to precipitate angina varies from patient to patient, but is usually relatively constant for each patient. Can the patient walk two level city blocks or climb one flight of stairs without developing chest pain? This is a question that will provide helpful information. Of particular importance for the doctor is the relationship of emotional factors to anginal episodes and the patient's attitude toward dentistry.

QUESTION. How frequently do you suffer anginal attacks?

COMMENT. The frequency of anginal episodes varies from patient to patient. Attacks may occur infrequently, perhaps once a week or once a month, or the patient may experience acute episodes several times a day. On average the patient with stable angina experiences one or two episodes per week. The risk of an episode being precipitated in the dental office is obviously increased in a patient with a greater frequency of episodes under other conditions.

QUESTION. How does nitroglycerin affect the anginal episode?

COMMENT. Determine what the patient does for the relief of pain. Nitroglycerin and rest characteristically relieve the discomfort of angina in approximately 2 to 4 minutes. Nitroglycerin in tablet, spray, or ointment form greatly shortens the duration of the anginal episode. Clinical management of chest pain in the dental patient is initiated by the administration of nitroglycerin, and any subsequent treatment will be based on the patient's response or lack of response to this antianginal drug. Chest pain lasting 10 minutes or more may prove to be acute myocardial infarction or unstable angina. Pain of esophageal spasm or esophagitis may also be relieved by nitroglycerin; however, pain of esophagitis and peptic ulcer is also relieved by ingestion of food and antacids, whereas anginal pain is not. Chest pain relieved by leaning forward is secondary to acute pericarditis, whereas chest pain relieved by holding the breath in deep expiration is commonly due to pleurisy.[17]

QUESTION. Describe any symptoms, other than chest pain, that are associated with your anginal attacks.

COMMENT. The presence of other accompanying signs and symptoms may help the doctor to determine the cause of the patient's chest pain. For example, severe chest pain that is accompanied by nausea and vomiting is often due to myocardial infarction. Chest pain associated with palpitation may be produced by ischemia that is secondary to a tachydysrhythmia in a patient with underlying CAD. Chest pain accompanied by hemoptysis (coughing up of blood from the respiratory tract) may be produced by a pulmonary embolis or a lung tumor. Pain associated with fever is noted in pneumonia and pericarditis.[17] Medical consultation is suggested if any accompanying symptoms appear disturbing.

The diagnosis of angina pectoris depends almost entirely on the dialogue history, and it is quite important to permit the patient sufficient time to describe the symptoms without interruption. Patients frequently use gestures to describe the location and quality of the symptom, such as placing a closed fist against the sternum—the "Levine sign" (Fig. 27-1).

Physical Examination

Physical examination of a patient with a history of angina will yield essentially normal findings during the period between episodes. Physical findings during the acute episode are described on p. 402.

Unstable Angina

Unstable angina is extremely significant to dentistry because of the increased risk of acute myocardial infarction (MI), as well as the unpredictability of the occurrence of MI. Patients developing unstable angina should be managed in the dental office as would patients having recently (within the past 6 months) suffered a myocardial infarction. They represent an ASA IV risk and should not be considered for elective dental care.

Unstable angina will be recognized from the dialogue history obtained from the anginal patient. As mentioned previously, the characteristics of the acute anginal episode for a given patient have a fair degree of consistency from episode to episode. In unstable angina the pain differs in character, duration, radiation, and severity—in which the pain, over a period of hours or days, demonstrates a crescendo or increasing quality, or occurs at rest or during the night.

Not all patients with unstable angina will develop signs of myocardial infarction. However, they are considered to be in a precarious balance between myocardial oxygen supply and demand, and prudence dictates that they be treated as if they had a minor myocardial infarction.

Medical management of unstable angina includes bed rest; the administration of nitrates (including intravenous nitroglycerin), beta-blockers, and calcium channel blockers; and psychologic rest and reassurance. Nitroglycerin ointment or transdermal nitroglycerin are frequently employed.

When medical treatment has not improved or eliminated the patient's symptoms, or if they become worse, surgical intervention may be indicated. Surgical options include percutaneous transluminal coronary angioplasty, coronary artery bypass graft surgery, atherectomy, and laser angioplasty.

Evidence shows that patients who are admitted to a coronary care unit because of unstable angina

Table 27-3. Dental therapy considerations in angina pectoris

Frequency of angina	Patient's abilities	ASA physical status	Considerations
0-1 per month	Patient can walk two level city blocks or climb one flight of stairs	II	Usual ASA II considerations and supplemental oxygen
2-4 per month	Patient can walk two level city blocks or climb one flight of stairs	II	Usual ASA II considerations to include possible premedication with nitroglycerin 5 minutes before therapy and supplemental oxygen
2-3 per week	Pain develops before patient walks two level city blocks or climbs one flight of stairs	III	Usual ASA III considerations to include possible premedication with nitroglycerin 5 minutes before therapy and supplemental oxygen
Daily episodes *or* recent (within past 2-3 weeks) changes in character of episode: Increased frequency, duration, or severity Radiation to new site Precipitated by less activity Decreased pain relief with usual nitroglycerin dose	Patient unable to walk two level city blocks or climb one flight of stairs	IV	Usual ASA IV considerations

suggestive of myocardial infarction, but in whom infarction is never demonstrated, have a higher death rate over the next 1 to 2 years than ordinary anginal patients.[18,19] Only emergency dental care should be considered for patients with unstable angina, and then only after consultation with their physician and preferably within a hospital environment.

DENTAL THERAPY CONSIDERATIONS

Prevention of acute episodes of angina during dental treatment is predicated on minimizing stress so that the amount of oxygen delivered through the coronary arteries is adequate to meet the requirements of the myocardium. The stress reduction protocol is particularly important to the anginal patient. Specific consideration must be given to the intraoperative aspects of the protocol, in particular, the length of the appointment, pain control during therapy, and the use of psychosedation. The average patient with angina pectoris is an ASA physical status III (Table 27-3). Patients with unstable or daily anginal episodes should be considered ASA IV risks, with dental treatment limited to emergency care and then only following consultation with the patients' physician.

Length of Appointment

An important factor in preventing the occurrence of anginal episodes during dental treatment is to avoid overstressing the patient. No absolute time limit for treatment can be given, because patient tolerance to stress varies considerably. However, treatment should cease when the anginal patient demonstrates signs or symptoms of fatigue, such as sweating, fidgety movements, or increased anxiety. Permit the patient to rest before permitting discharge.

Supplemental Oxygen

Anginal patients are excellent candidates to receive supplemental oxygen through a nasal cannula or nasal hood during dental treatment. A flow of 3 to 5 L per minute via cannula or 5 to 7 L per

Table 27-4. Catecholamine blood levels

	Epinephrine (μg/min)	Norepinephrine (μg/min)
Resting adrenal medullary secretion	7.0	1.5
Stress	280.0	56.0
Local anesthesia (1:50,000 epinephrine in 1.8 mL)	<1.0	—

minute via nasal hood will minimize the possibility of inadequate oxygenation of the myocardium.

Pain Control During Therapy

Pain is quite stressful; therefore, its control in the anginal patient is extremely important. The prevention of pain during dental therapy can best be ensured by the appropriate use of local anesthesia. The question that arises all too frequently concerns the advisability of using a vasoconstrictor in conjunction with the local anesthetic in the cardiac-risk patient.

A wealth of clinical evidence has accumulated that supports the statement that, for most cardiac patients, local anesthetics containing a vasoconstrictor (e.g., epinephrine or levonordefrin) are indicated for pain control during dental treatment.[20-26] The American Dental Association, in conjunction with the American Heart Association, published the findings of a joint committee that researched this potential problem.[21]

To summarize the available clinical data concerning this question, it may be stated that, if pain control proves inadequate, cardiac patients are potentially at greater risk from the effects of endogenously released catecholamines (e.g., epinephrine and norepinephrine) than they are from a properly administered (aspiration negative, slowly injected) local anesthetic containing epinephrine. Under the stress of pain or anxiety, the adrenal medulla releases extremely high levels of epinephrine (approximately 280 μg per minute) and norepinephrine (approximately 56 μg per minute) into the circulation, whereas with proper injection technique of a local anesthetic containing 1:50,000 epinephrine, less than 1 μg per minute of epinephrine is added to the circulatory system.[24] Table 27-4 summarizes these clinical findings.

Adequate depth of anesthesia to permit tooth manipulation (e.g., extraction, cavity preparation) without the patient experiencing pain is the major factor determining the ultimate blood level of catecholamines. Local anesthetics that contain no vasoconstrictor (e.g., plain lidocaine, prilocaine, and mepivacaine) are less likely to provide pulpal anesthesia of sufficient duration to permit the completion of the planned dental care before the patient experiences pain. The addition of minimal concentrations of epinephrine (1:200,000 and 1:100,000) to the local anesthetic prolongs the duration of pulpal anesthesia in most cases well beyond the time required for treatment, so that the anginal patient does not experience any pain and the release of endogenous catecholamines is minimized.

The maximal dose of epinephrine recommended for administration to the cardiac risk patient (ASA II or III) at one appointment is 0.04 mg.[27,28] To put this figure in terms of commonly used epinephrine concentrations, this is equivalent to one cartridge (1.8 mL) of a local anesthetic containing a 1:50,000 concentration of epinephrine (0.02 mg/mL), two cartridges with 1:100,000 epinephrine (0.01 mg/mL), or four cartridges with 1:200,000 epinephrine (0.005 mg/mL). Patients with poorly controlled IHD (ASA IV) should not be administered local anesthetics with vasoconstrictors.[26-28]

If the doctor is confronted with a patient who states that he or she cannot receive epinephrine, consultation with the patient's physician should be completed before initiating dental treatment. If considerable doubt persists concerning a particular patient following the medical consultation about the proper use of epinephrine in local anesthetics, it is recommended that a second opinion be obtained, or that a local anesthetic with a different vasoconstrictor, or an agent that provides sufficient duration of pulpal anesthesia without a vasoconstrictor be employed. Examples of these are mepivacaine with levonordefrin, and prilocaine without vasoconstrictor (when used for block anesthesia only). A textbook on local anesthesia and the drug package insert should be consulted before selecting the local anesthetic. One absolute contraindication to the use of vasoconstrictors in local anesthetics is the presence of cardiac dysrhythmias that persist in spite of antidysrhythmic therapy.

Patients who are receiving β-adrenergic blockers (e.g., propranolol) for the management of their angina or other cardiovascular disorders are at potential risk when receiving vasoconstrictors. Acute hypertensive episodes have been reported following the administration of local anesthetics containing vasoconstrictors.[29,30] A rapid-acting, short-duration vasodilator should be available for administration in the event such a reaction develops.

One additional factor must be mentioned regarding the use of epinephrine in the cardiac risk patient: 8% racemic epinephrine, a combination of the dextrorotatory and levorotatory forms commonly used in gingival retraction cord before taking impressions, contains approximately 4% (40 mg/mL) of the pharmacologically active levo form of epinephrine, which is 40 times the epinephrine concentration used in acute emergency situations (e.g., 1 mg/mL in anaphylaxis).[22,31-36] Absorption of epinephrine through unabraded mucous membranes into the cardiovascular system is normally rapid and is even more rapid with the gingival abrasion and active bleeding such as occur following subgingival tooth preparation. Blood levels of epinephrine rise rapidly in this situation, leading to manifestations (primarily cardiovascular) of epinephrine overdose (see Chapter 23).[32,34] Tachycardia, palpitation, sweating, tremor, and headache are the usual clinical symptoms.[36] In the patient with preexisting, clinically evident, or subclinical cardiovascular disease, this increase in cardiovascular activity may prove to be life threatening. The American Dental Association[22] recommends that racemic epinephrine cord not be used for any patient with a history of or suspicion of cardiovascular disease. Indeed, there are very few indications for the use of racemic epinephrine in any dental procedure in any patient.

Psychosedation

The use of psychosedation during the dental appointment may be indicated for the patient who experiences acute anginal episodes once a week or more often, or in any anginal patient who is fearful of dentistry. Of the various techniques currently in use, inhalation sedation with nitrous oxide and oxygen is the author's preferred technique for all cardiac risk patients.[37] Reasons for preferring this technique include (1) the increased percentage of oxygen that the patient is always receiving along with the nitrous oxide (most sedation units available in the United States do not deliver less than 27% to 30% oxygen), (2) the anxiolytic properties of nitrous oxide, which successfully reduce the stress of dental therapy, thereby minimizing endogenous catecholamine release, and (3) the minor but potentially highly significant analgesic properties of nitrous oxide. As discussed in Chapter 28, nitrous oxide and oxygen are commonly employed in the emergency management of acute myocardial infarction in many countries, including the United States.

Additional Considerations

Vital signs. Patients with a history of angina should have their vital signs monitored and recorded before the start of treatment at each visit to the dental office. Minimally, these recordings should include the blood pressure, heart rate and rhythm, and respiratory rate. It is suggested that measurements also be taken upon completion of the treatment.

Nitroglycerin. It has been suggested by some authorities that nitroglycerin be administered on a routine basis (prophylactically) to all anginal patients 5 minutes prior to the start of dental treatment.[38,39] Nitroglycerin exerts a clinical action within 2 to 4 minutes, with a duration of action of approximately 30 minutes. Being somewhat concervative in the administration of drugs, the author suggests that prophylactic premedication with nitroglycerin should be reserved for the anginal patient who experiences episodes of anginal pain more than once a week and who exhibits fear of dentistry (ASA III). However, the author does feel that before beginning dental treatment on the higher risk anginal patient, the doctor should request that the patient's nitroglycerin spray or tablets be placed where they will be accessible for immediate use if needed. Although nitroglycerin is present in the dental office emergency kit, the patient's own nitroglycerin should be used preferentially.

CLINICAL MANIFESTATIONS

The primary clinical manifestation of angina is chest pain. The doctor managing the anginal patient usually has been forewarned about this medical situation through the medical history questionnaire and is prepared to manage it. Although most instances of anginal pain are easily terminated, it is always possible that a supposed anginal attack is actually a more severe manifestation of ischemic heart disease—unstable angina or acute myocardial infarction. The initial clinical manifestations of all of these cardiovascular problems are quite similar; therefore, the immediate management of chest pain is based on the response of the patient to certain initial steps in treatment.

Signs and Symptoms
Pain

The patient becomes acutely aware of the sudden onset of chest pain and stops any activities. In the dental chair the patient will normally sit upright and press a fist against the chest. If questioned about the pain, the patient commonly describes it as a sensation of squeezing, burning, pressing, choking, aching, bursting, tightness, or "gas." In fact, on many occasions episodes of cardiac pain are mistaken for indigestion—not infrequently with a fatal outcome (see Chapter 28). The patient may state that it feels as if there is a heavy weight on the chest. In describing this sensation, many anginal victims hold a clenched fist to their chest as they describe their attacks (the Levine sign). Sharp pains are not typical of angina pectoris. In addition, respiratory movements (inspiration) do not exaggerate the discomfort. The sensation is more of a dull, aching, heavy pain than a searing hot or knifelike pain. The pain is located substernally, most commonly in the middle of the sternum, but it may appear just to the left of the sternum.

Finally, pain of cardiac origin tends to be more generalized than noncardiac pain, which can often be localized to one specific site (see discussion of radiation of pain that follows).

Radiation of Pain

Chest pain normally spreads or radiates to other locations in the body that are distant from the chest. Fig. 27-2 shows the more common pathways of radiation. Typically, the sensation radiates to the left shoulder and distally down the medial surface of the arm, occasionally as far as the hand and fingers, following the distribution of the ulnar nerve. The sensation felt is that of an ache, numbness, or tingling discomfort. Less commonly, the pain may radiate to the right shoulder only or to both shoulders. Other sites of radiation include the left side of the neck (usually described as a constricting sensation), with continuation up into the left side of the face and mandible. Mandibular pain, for which the victim may have sought dental care, has been reported as the sole clinical manifestation of chest pain in one case of angina.[40] Another possible yet relatively uncommon area of radiation is the upper epigastrium (Table 27-5).

Patient reaction to anginal pain varies. In some individuals the discomfort of angina subsides without their having to stop activities. Other individuals experience moderate pain that persists but does not become more intense. The victim is able to tolerate this level of discomfort and is not forced to stop activities. In most anginal patients, however, the clinical progression is of a different nature. In these persons the pain becomes progressively more intense, eventually forcing them to seek relief by terminating activities, taking medication, or both.

Table 27-5. Common causes of abdominal pain in the emergency department for all age groups

Cause	Percentage
Abdominal pain of unknown cause	41.3%
Gastroenteritis	6.9%
Pelvic inflammatory disease	6.7%
Urinary tract infection	5.2%
Ureteral stone	4.3%
Appendicitis	4.3%
Acute cholecystitis	2.5%
Intestinal obstruction	2.5%
Constipation	2.3%
Duodenal ulcer	2.0%
Other causes	22.0%

From Brewer RJ, and others: *Am J Surg* 131:219, 1976.

It must always be kept in mind that the clinical characteristics of acute anginal episodes are reasonably consistent for each patient from episode to episode. The intensity, frequency, radiation, and duration of the episodes demonstrate little variation. Recent changes in the usual pattern of the disease, with an increase in frequency, duration, or intensity, are signs of unstable angina and should be reported immediately to the patient's physician. It is commonly associated with recent obstructive disease of the coronary arteries and frequently precedes acute myocardial infarction or sudden death.

Physical Examination

During acute anginal episodes, the following signs and symptoms may be noted: The patient is apprehensive, is usually sweating, may press a fist to the sternum, and appears anxious to take nitroglycerin. The heart rate is markedly elevated, as is the blood pressure, with blood pressures of 200 mmHg/150 mmHg having been recorded in normotensive patients during acute anginal episodes. Respiratory difficulty (dyspnea) and a feeling of faintness may also be noted during the episode.

Complications

Although most anginal episodes resolve without residual complication, it is possible for more acute situations to develop. Acute cardiac dysrhythmias occurring during the episode are most common. Although these are normally not life threatening, ventricular dysrhythmias may occur with a possibility of ventricular fibrillation and sudden death. A second potential complication of angina is acute myocardial infarction.

Prognosis

The prognosis for the anginal patient depends largely on the severity of the underlying disorder (e.g., IHD, CAD) and the presence or absence of additional risk factors.[41-43] In men with angina the annual mortality rate is 1.4% if they have no history of myocardial infarction, a normal ECG, and normal blood pressure. This rate increases to 7.4% annually if they have elevated blood pressure, to 8.4% if they have an abnormal electrocardiogram (ECG), and to 12% annually if both the blood pressure is elevated and the ECG is abnormal. Other factors, such as the presence of diabetes mellitus, heart failure, cardiac dysrhythmias, and cardiac hypertrophy, tend to decrease life expectancy even further. Fifty percent of all anginal patients die suddenly (cardiac arrest). Thirty-three percent die following myocardial infarction, and most of the remainder succumb to heart failure.[43]

PATHOPHYSIOLOGY

Angina is caused by the temporary inability of the coronary arteries to provide adequate oxygenated blood to the myocardium. The patient with ischemic heart disease or coronary artery disease may be asymptomatic at rest or during moderate exertion because the coronary arteries may be able to deliver an adequate supply of oxygen to the myocardium under these circumstances. Any additional increase in the oxygen requirement of the myocardium above this critical level, which varies from patient to patient, results in a degree of oxygen deficiency and the development of myocardial ischemia, with the subsequent appearance of clinical manifestations of anginal pains (or of other IHD syndromes, e.g., AMI, dysrhythmias).

The pain of angina may be related to the metabolic changes produced in the ischemic myocardium. Agents such as adenosine, bradykinin, histamine, and serotonin are released from ischemic cells. These chemicals act on intracardiac sympathetic nerves that go to the cardiac plexus and to sympathetic ganglia at the C7 to T4 level. Impulses are then transmitted through the spinal cord to the thalamus and the cerebral cortex.[44]

Further evidence for this theory comes from patients with spontaneous angina (i.e., onset of anginal pain while the patient is at rest). The increases in blood pressure and heart rate seen during acute anginal episodes are consistently observed before the onset of pain. Changes in the electrocardiogram also occur from 1 to 3 minutes before the pain. These factors indicate that a buildup of the metabolic products of ischemia occurs before the stimulation of pain fibers.

Some of the most dangerous occurrences observed during the anginal episode include continuing elevation in blood pressure and tachycardia. Both of these produce a potentially dangerous feedback system. Myocardial oxygen requirements continue to increase as the workload of the heart continues to rise (with increasing blood pressure and rapid heart rate). If the coronary arteries are unable to deliver the oxygen required, the degree of myocardial ischemia increases, which in turn increases the chances of acute, possibly lethal, ventricular dysrhythmias and myocardial infarction. Rapid management of the anginal episode therefore becomes quite important.

Coronary artery spasm (Prinzmetal's variant angina) has been demonstrated to occur either spontaneously or upon exposure to cold, by exposure to ergot-derivative drugs used to treat migraine headaches, or by mechanical irritation from a cardiac catheter.[44-47] Spasm has been observed in the large coronary arteries, whether healthy or atherosclerotic, resulting in decreased coronary blood flow.[47] Prolonged spasm of the coronary arteries in angina may result in documented episodes of myocardial infarction—even in the absence of visible coronary artery disease.

MANAGEMENT

The primary goal in the management of the acute anginal episode is to decrease the myocardial oxygen requirement. Diagnostic clues to the presence of angina include:[48]

- Onset with exercise, activity, stress
- Symptoms that include pressure, tightness, a heavy weight
- Substernal, epigastric, or jaw pain
- Mild to moderate discomfort

Patient with a History of Angina Pectoris

Step 1: Terminate the dental procedure. When the patient experiences chest pain, all dental procedures should be stopped immediately. In many instances the precipitating factor may be a part of the dental treatment, such as the sight of a local anesthetic syringe, scalpel, or hand piece, and simply by terminating the procedure the acute episode of chest pain ends.

Step 2: Position the patient. The anginal patient is conscious and usually apprehensive. Position the patient in the most comfortable manner. Most commonly this will be sitting or standing upright.[49] The supine position is rarely preferred by the patient and in fact commonly makes the pain appear subjectively to be more intense.

Step 3: Basic life support, as indicated. The anginal patient is conscious, breathing spontaneously, and

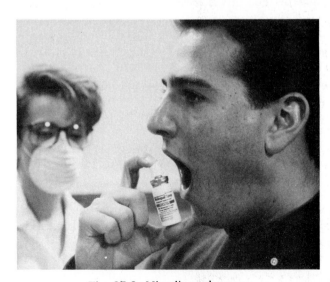

Fig. 27-3. Nitrolingual spray.

has a palpable pulse in the wrist, antecubital fossa, and carotid artery.

Step 4: Administer vasodilator. A member of the emergency team should immediately get the emergency kit and oxygen. Oxygen may be administered at any time to the anginal patient. A nasal cannula or nasal hood are preferred. As soon as possible (even before oxygen is available), nitroglycerin should be administered transmucosally (e.g., nitrolingual spray) or sublingually (e.g., tablet). The patient's own nitroglycerin supply is preferred because the dosage will be correct for the patient. The number of sprays or tablets administered is determined by the patient's usual requirement (0.3 to 0.6 mg is the usual dosage). One or two metered sprays are recommended initially with no more than three metered doses within a 15 minute period,[50] whereas sublingual nitroglycerin tablets are recommended at 1 tablet every 5 minutes as needed, with no more than 3 tablets every 15 minutes.[51] The use of nitrolingual spray is preferred to the sublingual tablets because of the relative instability of the tablets.[52] (See Fig. 27-3.)

Effects and side effects of nitroglycerin: Nitroglycerin normally reduces or eliminates anginal discomfort dramatically within 2 to 4 minutes. Commonly observed side effects of nitroglycerin administration include a fullness or pounding in the head, flushing, tachycardia, and possible hypotension (if the patient is sitting upright).

Action of nitroglycerin: Nitroglycerin is the single most effective agent available for the management of acute anginal episodes. In normal individuals the administration of nitroglycerin decreases coronary artery resistance and increases coronary blood flow. This mechanism is probably of little consequence in patients with significant CAD, however. The probable mechanism of action of nitroglycerin in anginal patients is its ability to produce a decrease in the systemic vascular resistance through arterial and venous dilation. This leads to a decrease in return of venous blood to the heart and a decrease in cardiac output, which results in a lessened cardiac workload. A decrease in cardiac work produces a lesser oxygen requirement of the myocardium and a reversal of the oxygen insufficiency that existed during the episode.[53,54]

Step 5: Administer additional vasodilators, if necessary: If the patient's nitroglycerin tablets are ineffective in terminating anginal pain within 5 minutes, a second dose should be administered either from the patient's drug supply or from the emergency kit supply, which will be fresher than the patient's. Nitroglycerin tablets lose potency unless they are stored in tightly sealed glass containers.

This is one possible explanation for the failure of the patient's nitroglycerin to relieve anginal pains. Nitroglycerin spray is considerably more stable than sublingual tablets and is preferred in this situation. A test for nitroglycerin potency is to place a tablet on the tongue; the drug is still potent if a tingling sensation is felt as the tablet dissolves, with a feeling of coolness throughout the mouth similar to that associated with mint candy but without the taste. A second possible explanation for the failure of nitroglycerin to provide relief is that the episode is not due to angina, but is an acute myocardial infarction. Administration of nitroglycerin and the patient's subsequent response to it is a major factor in the differential diagnosis of these two important cardiovascular syndromes.

The American Heart Association recommends that in a patient with known angina pectoris, emergency medical care be sought if chest pain is not relieved by three nitroglycerin tablets or spray doses over a 10-minute period. In a person with previously unrecognized coronary disease, the persistence of chest pain for 2 minutes or longer is an indication for emergency medical assistance.[55]

Step 6: Summon medical assistance, if necessary: If an episode of chest pain in a known anginal patient has not been terminated following the administration of oxygen and the suggested three doses of nitroglycerin, medical assistance should be sought immediately. This step should usually be unnecessary for patients with angina pectoris. The management of continued or increasing chest pain will be discussed in Chapter 28.

If nitroglycerin is unavailable or proves ineffective in terminating an episode of chest pain, the use of amyl nitrate or a calcium channel blocker should be considered. Amyl nitrate is available in 0.3-mL ampules, which are crushed and then inhaled. The patient should be in the recumbent position when amyl nitrate is administered. Amyl nitrate is not recommended for use unless the anginal episode is severe and unrelieved by nitroglycerin and unless the patient has high blood pressure with a markedly elevated diastolic pressure. Medical assistance should be sought in this situation.

Effects and side effects of amyl nitrate: Once inhaled, amyl nitrate normally produces relief of anginal discomfort within 10 seconds. Because of its extreme potency, there are uncomfortable side effects that invariably occur with its use. These include flushing of the face, pounding of the pulse, dizziness, and a pounding headache. (The person administering amyl nitrate may also experience the clinical effects of the drug if vapors are inadvertently inhaled.)

Action of amyl nitrate: Amyl nitrate causes profound peripheral arterial vasodilation. With the administration of one ampule, the blood pressure falls precipitously. Amyl nitrate has a negligible effect on the veins; therefore, little venous pooling occurs. Amyl nitrate markedly decreases cardiac output.[56]

Effects and side effects of calcium slow-channel blockers: Patients known to have coronary artery spasm as a component of their anginal episodes will usually respond well to the administration of nifedipine (10 to 20 mg) sublingually. Nifedipine, verapamil, and diltiazem are calcium entry-blocking agents.

Verapamil has been the most extensively studied agent in this relatively new group of drugs for emergency cardiac care. Its actions are representative of the other agents in the group. The therapeutic usefulness of verapamil is based on its slow channel-blocking properties, particularly the inward flow of calcium ions in cardiac and vascular smooth muscle. By blocking calcium influx and supply to the myocardial contractile mechanism, verapamil exerts a direct depressant effect on the inotropic state and therefore on the myocardial oxygen requirement. Verapamil also reduces contractile tone in vascular smooth muscle, which results in coronary and peripheral vasodilation, which in turn reduces systemic vascular resistance. Additionally, the calcium slow-channel blockers exhibit antidysrhythmic effects, specifically by slowing conduction and prolonging refractoriness in the AV (atrioventricular) node. The current primary use of verapamil and other calcium slow-channel blockers is as an antidysrhythmic agent. (It is highly effective in the management of PSVT [paroxysmal supraventricular tachycardia]). Its hemodynamic properties account for its beneficial actions in managing angina induced by coronary artery spasm.[57,58]

Pain-relieving narcotics such as morphine and meperidine (Demerol) should not be used because they do not treat the cause of pain (i.e., inadequate oxygen supply). The only indication for narcotic administration is acute myocardial infarction (see Chapter 28).

Step 7: Modify further dental therapy: Following termination of the anginal episode, it should be determined what factors might have caused it to occur. Modification of future dental treatment should be considered in order to prevent chest pain from recurring.

Dental treatment may resume at any time (immediately if necessary) following the cessation of the acute anginal episode. The patient should be

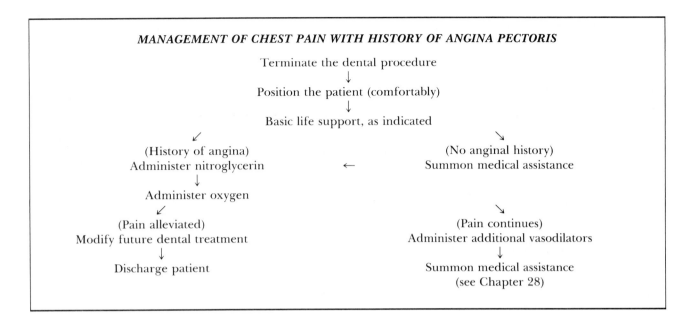

MANAGEMENT OF CHEST PAIN WITH HISTORY OF ANGINA PECTORIS

Terminate the dental procedure
↓
Position the patient (comfortably)
↓
Basic life support, as indicated

(History of angina)   ←   (No anginal history)
Administer nitroglycerin   Summon medical assistance
↓
Administer oxygen

(Pain alleviated)   (Pain continues)
Modify future dental treatment   Administer additional vasodilators
↓   ↓
Discharge patient   Summon medical assistance
(see Chapter 28)

permitted to rest until he or she is comfortable, again prior to resuming dental care or discharge. Vital signs should be monitored and recorded prior to discharge of the patient. The patient may be permitted to leave the office unescorted and to operate a motor vehicle if, in the opinion of the dentist, he or she is able to do so. In the unlikely situation that doubt persists about the degree of recovery, medical assistance or a medical consultation should be sought, or a friend or relative of the patient should be brought to the office to act as an escort.

Patients with No Prior History of Chest Pain

When no prior history of chest pain is present, but the patient experiences chest pain during dental treatment, the steps of angina management, discussed earlier, are appropriate, with the exception that medical assistance be sought immediately— even before the administration of nitroglycerin and oxygen.

Even when this initial episode of chest pain is alleviated by nitroglycerin and oxygen, a thorough evaluation of this very frightened patient is in order, thus the recommendation for seeking medical assistance immediately. The accompanying box outlines the steps to follow to manage chest pain in a patient with a history of angina pectoris.

Drugs used in management: Nitroglycerin, oxygen

Medical assistance: No if history of angina and relief of pain; yes if initial episode of chest pain or no relief of pain with three doses of nitroglycerin

REFERENCES

1. *Mosby's medical & nursing dictionary,* St Louis, 1983, Mosby–Year Book.
2. Heberden W: Some account of a disorder of the breast, *Med Trans Coll Physicians (London)* 2:59, 1872.
3. Cohn PF, Braunwald E: Chronic coronary artery disease. In Braunwald E, editor: *Heart disease,* ed 3, Philadelphia, 1986, WB Saunders.
4. Angst DM, Bensinger DA: Angina. In *Cardiopulmonary emergencies,* Springhouse, Pa, 1991, Springhouse.
5. Diamond GA, Forrester JS: Analysis of probability as an aid in the clinical diagnosis of coronary heart disease, *N Engl J Med* 300:1350, 1979.
6. Waters D, Lam J, Theroux P: Newer concepts in the treatment of unstable angina pectoris, *Am J Cardiol* 68(12):34C-41C.
7. Gazes PC, Mobley EM Jr., Faris HM Jr., Duncan RC, Humphries GB: Preinfarction (unstable) angina: a prospective study: ten year follow-up, *Circulation* 48:331, 1973.
8. Welch CC, Proudfit WL, Sones FM Jr, and others: Cinecoronary arteriography in young men, *Circulation* 42:647, 1970.
9. Gazes PC, Mobley EM Jr, Faris HM Jr, and others: Preinfarctional (stable) angina—a prospective study; ten-year follow-up. Prognostic significance of electrocardiographic changes, *Circulation* 48:331, 1973.
10. Hartzler GO, Rutherford BD, McConahay DR: Percutaneous transluminal coronary angioplasty: application for acute myocardial infarction, *Am J Cardiol* 53:117c, 1984.
11. Phillips SJ, Kongtahworm C, Zeff RH: Emergency coronary artery revascularization: a possible therapy for acute myocardial infarction, *Circulation* 60:241, 1979.
12. Ricci DR, Moscovich MD, Kinahan PJ: Preliminary experience at a Canadian centre with directional coronary atherectomy for complex lesions, *Can J Cardiol* 7(9):399-406, 1991.

13. Korsch KR, Haase KK, Voelker W, and others: Percutaneous coronary excimer laser angioplasty in patients with stable and unstable angina pectoris: acute results and incidence of restenosis during 6-month follow-up, *Circulation* 81(6):1849-1859, 1990.

14. Warren SG, Bremer DL, Orgain ES: Long-term propranolol therapy for angina pectoris, *Am J Cardiol* 37:420, 1976.

15. Markis JE, Gorlin R, Mills RM, and others: Sustained effect of orally administered isosorbide dinitrate on exercise performance of patients with angina pectoris, *Am J Cardiol* 43:265, 1979.

16. Maseri A: Aspects of the medical therapy of angina pectoris, *Drugs* 42(suppl 1):28-30, 1991.

17. Braunwald E: The history. In Braunwald E, editor: *Heart disease*, ed 3, Philadelphia, 1986, WB Saunders.

18. Guthrie RB, and others: Pathology of stable and unstable angina pectoris, *Circulation* 51:1059, 1975.

19. Conti CR, and others: Unstable angina pectoris: morbidity and mortality in 57 consecutive patients evaluated angiographically, *Am J Cardiol* 32:745, 1973.

20. New York Heart Association: Report of the special committee of the New York Heart Association, Inc., on the use of epinephrine in connection with procaine in dental procedures, *J Am Dent Assoc* 50:108, 1955.

21. American Dental Association Council on Dental Therapeutics: American Dental Association and American Heart Association joint report: management of dental problems in patients with cardiovascular disease, *J Am Dent Assoc* 68:533, 1964.

22. American Dental Association Council on Dental Therapeutics: *Accepted dental therapeutics*, Chicago, 1985, The American Dental Association.

23. Boakes AJ, and others: Adverse reactions to local anaesthetic/vasoconstrictor preparations, *Br Dent J* 133:137, 1972.

24. Glover J: Vasoconstrictors in dental anaesthetics contraindication—fact or fallacy, *Aust Dent J* 13:65, 1968.

25. Holroyd SV, Watts DT, Welch JT, Jr: The use of epinephrine in local anesthetics for dental patients with cardiovascular disease: a review of the literature, *J Oral Surg* 18:492, 1960.

26. Jastak JT, Yagiela JA: Vasoconstrictors and local anesthesia: a review and rationale for use, *J Am Dent Assoc* 107:623, 1983.

27. Bennett CR: *Monheim's local anesthesia and pain control in dental practice*, ed 7, St Louis, 1984, Mosby–Year Book.

28. Malamed SF: *Handbook of local anesthesia*, ed 3, St Louis, 1991, Mosby–Year Book.

29. Brummett RE: Warning to otolaryngologists using local anesthetics containing epinephrine: potential serious reaction occurring in patients treated with beta-adrenergic receptor blockers, *Arch Otolaryngol* 110(9):561, 1984.

30. Yagiela JA: *Deadfalls in drug interactions. 6th Annual review course in dental anesthesiology*, 1990, American Dental Society of Anesthesiology.

31. Harrison JD: Effect of retraction materials on gingival sulcus epithelium, *J Prosthet Dent* 11:514, 1961.

32. Houston JB, and others: Effect of r-epinephrine impregnated retraction cord on the cardiovascular system, *J Prosthet Dent* 24:373, 1970.

33. Munoz RJ: The cardiovascular effects of anxiety and epinephrine retraction cord in routine fixed prosthodontic procedures, *J Calif Dent Assoc* 46:10, 1970.

34. Pague WL, Harrison JD: Absorption of epinephrine during tissue retraction, *J Prosthet Dent* 18:242, 1967.

35. Timberlake DL: Epinephrine in tissue retraction, *Ariz Dent J* 17:14, 1971.

36. Phatak NM, Lang RL: Systemic hemodynamic effects of r-epinephrine gingival retraction cord in clinic patients, *J Oral Ther Pharmacol* 2:393, 1966.

37. Malamed SF: *Sedation: a guide to patient management*, ed 2, St Louis, 1989, Mosby–Year Book.

38. McCarthy FM: *Essentials of safe dentistry for the medically compromised patient*. Philadelphia, 1989, WB Saunders.

39. Winsor T, Berger HJ: Oral nitroglycerin as a prophylactic antianginal drug; clinical, physiologic, and statistical evidence of efficacy based on a three-phase experimental design, *Am Heart J* 90:611, 1975.

40. Godefroy JN, Batisse JP: Dental pain and cardiac pain, *Revue Francaise d'Endodontie* 9(1):17-21, 1991.

41. Kannel WB, Feinleib M: Natural history of angina pectoris in the Framingham study: prognosis and survival, *Am J Cardiol* 29:154, 1972.

42. Kent RI: Prognosis of symptomatic or mildly symptomatic patients with coronary artery disease, *Am J Cardiol* 49:1823, 1982.

43. Frank CW, Weinblatt F, Shapiro S: Angina pectoris in men: prognostic significance of selected medical factors, *Circulation* 47:509, 1973.

44. Cannon RO III: Microvascular angina: cardiovascular investigations regarding pathophysiology and management, *Med Clin N Amer* 75(5):1097–1108, 1991.

45. Carleton RA, Johnson AD: Coronary arterial spasm: a clinical entity, *Mod Concepts Cardiovasc Dis* 43:87, 1974.

46. Hillis LD, Braunwald E: Coronary artery spasm, *N Engl J Med* 299:695, 1978.

47. Maseri A, Chierchia S: Coronary artery spasm: demonstration, definition, diagnosis, and consequences, *Prog Cardiovasc Dis* 25:169, 1982.

48. Pollakoff J, Pollakoff K: *EMT's guide to signs and symptoms*, 1991.

49. Pollakoff J, Pollakoff K: *EMT's guide to treatment*, Los Angeles, 1991, Jeff Gould.

50. Nitrolingual spray: Drug package insert, Rhone-Poulenc Rorer Pharmaceuticals, 1990.

51. Nitrostat sublingual tablets: Drug package insert, Parke-Davis, 1990.

52. Mayer GA: Instability of nitroglycerin tablets, *Can Med Assoc J* 110:788, 1974.

53. DiCarlo FJ: Nitroglycerin revisited: chemistry, biochemistry, interactions, *Drug Metab Rev* 4:1, 1975.

54. Judge TE: Vasodilators, *Practitioner* 212:2, 1974.

55. American Heart Association: *Heart Attack: signals and actions for survival*, Dallas, 1976, The American Heart Association.

56. Skidmore-Roth L: *Mosby's 1990 Nursing Drug Reference*, St Louis 1990, Mosby–Year Book.

57. Gerstenblith G, and others: Nifedipine in unstable angina: a double-blind, randomized trial, *N Engl J Med* 306:885, 1982.

58. Singh BN: The pharmacology of slow channel blocking drugs, *Cardiovasc Rev Rep* 4:179, 1983.

28 *Acute Myocardial Infarction*

Myocardial infarction may be defined as a clinical syndome resulting from a deficient coronary arterial blood supply to a region of myocardium that results in cellular death and necrosis. The syndrome is usually characterized by severe and prolonged substernal pain similar to, but more intense and of longer duration, than that of angina pectoris. Common complications of myocardial infarction include shock, heart failure, and cardiac arrest. Synonyms for myocardial infarction include coronary occlusion, and heart attack.

Each year more than 1.5 million Americans experience acute myocardial infarction (AMI).[1] It is the single leading cause of death in the United States and is responsible for 35% of deaths occurring in men between the ages of 35 and 50 years. A male living in North America has a 20% chance of suffering a myocardial infarction or sudden death before the age of 65 years; for women this risk is 10%.[2] Although a relatively common clinical occurrence, myocardial infarction unfortunately still has a high mortality rate; approximately 36% of acute myocardial infarction victims (540,000) will die, 350,000 of those before reaching a hospital.[1] In 1987 1,500,000 persons in the United States sustained a myocardial infarction. Over 60% of deaths from acute myocardial infarction occur within 2 hours of the onset of signs and symptoms.[3] Most of these result from development of lethal dysrhythmias, usually ventricular fibrillation.[3]

For the victim of an acute myocardial infarction to have a greater chance of survival, the dentist must be aware of ways to prevent its occurrence, how to recognize its signs and symptoms, and how to manage it effectively. Killip[4] has stated that, once admitted to a hospital, the patient has already survived a significant risk. Indeed, recent advances in resuscitation and in management of acute myocardial infarction have lead to a substantially reduced mortality rate amongst AMI victims who reach the hospital.[5,6]

In addition to management of the acute myocardial infarction, dentists are asked to manage the needs of those patients who have survived a myocardial infarction. The American Heart Association[7] estimates that there are 4,600,000 victims of myocardial infarction still living in the United States. Most patients who survive a myocardial infarction are returned by their physician to their normal activities within 6 to 8 weeks.[1] As with the status post-CVA patient and patients with angina, there is always a greater risk of reinfarction when status postmyocardial infarction patients are treated. Patients discharged from the hospital following myocardial infarction have a 6% to 10% mortality rate in the first year, with most of the deaths occurring within the first 3 months.[7,8] Major risk factors associated with these deaths include the severity of the left ventricular damage,[9] continued myocardial ischemia,[10] and the predisposition to ventricular dysrhythmias.[11] Of the survivors of AMI, 30% will develop significant angina pectoris.[8] As a group, compared to the population at large, survivors of AMI face a tenfold risk of heart failure and a fourfold risk of sudden death.[8]

In myocardial infarction a portion of myocardium dies. Depending on the extent of myocardial damage and the presence or absence of acute complications such as dysrhythmias, heart failure, and cardiac arrest, the victim either survives or succumbs during the acute phase of the disease. After the acute phase further complications such as continued myocardial ischemia or heart failure may develop. The latter decreases the ability of the heart to carry out its primary function—that of a pump—because of the size of the infarcted area of myocardium. Varying degrees of heart failure are common following myocardial infarction. Knowledge of the presence of a compromised myocardium will enable the dentist to modify dental treatment to decrease the potential risk presented by the patient.

PREDISPOSING FACTORS

The primary cause of acute myocardial infarction is coronary artery disease (atherosclerosis; CAD). Coronary artery disease is a factor in more than 90% of all episodes of AMI.[12] Other risk factors in myocardial infarction include obesity, being a male (especially during the fifth to seventh decades of life), and undue stress (see also Chapter 26). Friedman[13,14] has described the cardiac risk patient as a "coronary prone" individual. This person is further characterized as having a type A behavior pattern, described as follows[15]:

Foremost is a frightening and often obsessive sense of time urgency. He is determined to accomplish too much in too little time. He struggles both with his environment and with himself, but mainly with the latter. He is alert, very intense, and usually hostile. He is very competitive and ambitious; he wants recognition and seeks advancement. He tends to speed up his ordinary activities by looking at his watch often, by being on time, by hating to wait in line at the bank, movie, or restaurant. He is usually in occupations subject to deadlines. These patients themselves have labeled the type-A behavior pattern as the "hurry-up" disease.

In addition, a strong family history of cardiovascular disease, an abnormal electrocardiogram, elevated blood pressure, enlarged heart size, and/ or an elevated blood cholesterol level add to the risk of a person suffering acute myocardial infarction.

Immediate predisposing factors in myocardial infarction include a significant decrease in blood flow through the coronary arteries, as in coronary thrombosis, or an increase in the level of cardiac work without a corresponding increase in the supply of oxygen to the myocardium, as seen in stress. This situation of decreased perfusion is called myocardial ischemia. Factors other than severe CAD that are implicated in the pathogenesis of myocardial infarction include the rupture (fissuring or hemorrhage) of atherosclerotic plaque,[16] and arterial spasm.[17] On very rare occasion, AMI can occur in the absence of coronary artery narrowing if there is a marked disparity between myocardial oxygen supply and demand. The abuse of cocaine has been implicated as a cause of such a disparity.[18]

Location and Extent of Infarction

As described in Chapter 26, the anterior descending branch of the left coronary artery is the most common site of clinically significant atherosclerosis within the heart. Not surprisingly, this vessel is the most common site of thrombosis, leading to myocardial infarction. With occlusion of this vessel, the anterior portion of the left ventricle becomes ischemic, and in the absence of adequate collateral circulation, infarction occurs with subsequent myocardial necrosis throughout the distribution of the occluded artery. Occlusion of the left circumflex artery produces anterolateral infarction. Thrombosis of the right coronary artery leads to infarction of the posteroinferior portion of the left ventricle and might also involve the right ventricular myocardium.[19] The extent of infarction is therefore related to several factors, including the anatomic distribution of the occluded vessel, the adequacy of collateral circulation, the extent of existing coronary artery disease throughout the myocardium (one vessel versus multivessel involvement), and whether or not previous infarctions have occurred.[20]

PREVENTION

Prevention of a first myocardial infarction in a high-risk patient (see CAD risk factors, p. 384), although a seemingly impossible task, may be attempted by the dentist through strict adherence to the stress reduction protocol. This protocol minimizes the potentially adverse effects of undue stress on the workload and oxygen requirement of the myocardium, thereby reducing the risk from one of the immediate predisposing factors of acute myocardial infarction (i.e., increased cardiac workload). The other immediate predisposing factors—thrombosis, occlusion, or spasm of a coronary blood vessel—obviously cannot be prevented by the doctor.

The dental patient with a history of prior myocardial infarction must be identified, and the doctor must attempt to obtain as much information concerning the current physical status of this patient as is possible so that an accurate determination of risk may be established before the start of dental treatment. This necessitates the use of the medical history questionnaire, physical examination of the patient, and the dialogue history.

Medical History Questionnaire

QUESTION 9. Circle any of the following that you have had or have at present:
- Heart disease
- Heart attack

COMMENT. An affirmative reply must be followed by a detailed dialogue history to determine the degree of risk represented by this patient.

QUESTION 6. **Have you taken any medicine or drugs during the past 2 years?**

COMMENT. Survivors of myocardial infarction (called status postmyocardial infarction) will be receiving medications according to the degree of residual myocardial damage and the presence of post-MI complications.

Postmyocardial infarction patients frequently receive one or more of the following drug groups: diuretics—for management of heart failure and high blood pressure; digitalis or dopamine—for heart failure; antidysrhythmics—if significant cardiac dysrhythmias are present; nitrates (e.g., nitroglycerin)—if anginal pains are present in the post-MI period; and possibly antiplatelet agents, such as sulfinpyrazone (Anturane) and aspirin. Beta-adrenergic blockers such as propranolol are also frequently prescribed as studies have demonstrated reduced mortality during the first several years following myocardial infarction.[21,22] Table 28-1 summarizes the drugs used in the post-MI period. Anticoagulants such as coumarin, heparin, and Dicumarol are only infrequently employed today in the management of the status post-myocardial infarction patient.

QUESTION 10. **When you walk up stairs or take a walk, do you ever have to stop because of pain in your chest or shortness of breath, or because you are very tired?**

COMMENT. The presence of one or more of these symptoms of poor cardiopulmonary reserve indicates a greater risk during management of this patient.

Dialogue History

In the presence of a positive history of cardiovascular disease (e.g., angina, myocardial infarction), the doctor should continue with the following dialogue history:

QUESTION. **Has there been any alteration in the pattern of your episodes of angina in the last month?**

COMMENT. As discussed in Chapter 27, anginal episodes are usually fairly constant for each patient. Any increase in the rate of frequency, duration, or severity, or a decrease in the level of precipitating factors may well be an indication of unstable angina. Immediate consultation with the patient's physician is desirable in this instance.

QUESTION. **When did you have your last myo-**

Table 28-1. Medications employed for patients with status postmyocardial infarction

Drug category	*Example(s)*	*Rationale*
Diuretics	Hydrochlorothiazide	High blood pressure, heart failure
Inotropic agents	Digitalis	Heart failure
	Dopamine	
	Dobutamine	
	Amrinone	
Antidysrhythmics	Digitalis	Atrial fibrillation with rapid ventricular rate
	Lidocaine/tocainide	Ventricular dysrhythmias
	Procainamide	
	Quinidine sulfate	
	Disopyramide (Norpace)	
Nitrates	Nitroglycerin—ointment, transdermal, or sublingual tablet or spray forms	Anginal pains
	Long-acting nitrates (see Table 27-2)	
Antiplatelet agents	Sulfinpyrazone (Anturane)	Shown in two studies to reduce incidence of sudden death and recurrent myocardial infarction (for up to 7 months post-MI)
	Aspirin	Still prescribed, although a large, multicenter study found no reduction in deaths from recurrent myocardial infarction
B-adrenergic agents	Propranolol	Several studies have shown beta-blockers to decrease likelihood of sudden death and reinfarction in months following acute myocardial infarction
	Timolol	
	Alprenolol	
	Metoprolol	

cardial infarction?

COMMENT. Length of time elapsed since the last myocardial infarction is significant in relation to the risk involved in dental treatment. Following myocardial infarction, there is an increased risk of reinfarction. The patient represents an increased risk during dental therapy regardless of the amount of time elapsed since the initial episode.[8] However, in the immediate postinfarction period there is a significantly higher risk of reinfarction. In a survey by Weinblatt and others,[23] the reinfarction rate (noted during surgery or in the immediate postoperative period [24 hours]) was 37% if the surgical procedure occurred within 3 months of the initial episode. If performed within 4 to 6 months of the episode, the reinfarction rate dropped to 16%; whereas if surgery was postponed for longer than 6 months following the episode, the reinfarction rate fell to 5%. These figures compare to an infarction rate of 0.1% in persons with no prior history of infarction. During the recovery period collateral circulation to the infarcted area improves, thereby allowing the heart to heal and minimizing the size of the residual infarct.[24,25] This process of healing normally requires approximately 6 months.[26] The increased risk represented by the status postmyocardial infarction patient is illustrated by an overall mortality rate of 30% within the first month after the infarction.[7,8] The majority of these deaths are related to the presence of significant dysrhythmias. Although this high mortality rate does decrease with time, after 10 years the postinfarction mortality rate is still ten times that of a normal group.[8]

Physical Examination

Vital signs should be recorded before and immediately following all dental appointments for the status postmyocardial infarction patient. (See Table 2-1 for suggested management of patients according to their blood pressures.)

Additional examination of the patient may not provide any reliable indication of previous myocardial infarction. Many survivors of a mild myocardial infarction appear to be in extremely fine physical and mental condition. Research has looked into the role of physical exercise in the rehabilitation of myocardial tissues following infarction. Findings have led to comprehensive physical training programs for many of these persons.[27-29] Patients are permitted to resume normal activities, such as walking and sexual activity, in a graded manner during convalescence. Such programs result in both subjective and objective improvement, recorded as decreases in heart rate and blood pressure, as well as a return to a normal or near-normal life style and improved morale. Unfortunately, there is much less evidence for improvement in ventricular function and little convincing evidence that these programs, with exercise, decrease the recurrence of myocardial infarction or the mortality rate.[30] It must always be remembered, therefore, that regardless of the apparent state of physical fitness of postmyocardial infarction patients, they must still be considered a high risk during all dental procedures.

Status postmyocardial infarction patients who have a significant degree of ventricular damage may also have clinical signs and symptoms of congestive heart failure (CHF). (See Chapter 14 for a discussion of this clinical entity.) Visual examination of these patients may reveal a degree of peripheral cyanosis (e.g., seen in nailbeds, mucous membranes), coolness of the extremities, peripheral edema (in ankles), and possible orthopnea (difficulty in breathing that is relieved by sitting upright). These patients represent a considerable risk during dental treatment.

DENTAL THERAPY CONSIDERATIONS

Dental therapy considerations for the status postmyocardial infarction patient include reduction in stress that is related to dental therapy and possible alteration in drug therapy, dental therapy, or both.

The status postmyocardial infarction patient represents an ASA III or IV risk depending upon the time elapsed since the previous infarction, the number of prior infarcts, and the presence of continued signs or symptoms of cardiovascular disease (e.g., dyspnea, chest pain, dysrhythmias). Table 28-2 presents the ASA classification of the status postmyocardial infarction patient.

Stress Reduction

The status postmyocardial infarction patient is relatively stress-intolerant; therefore, implementation of appropriate steps in the stress reduction protocol should receive serious consideration. Of special importance in this patient are intraoperative stress reduction and adequate pain control.

Supplemental oxygen: The administration of supplemental oxygen to the status postmyocardial infarction patient will minimize the risk of development of hypoxia and myocardial ischemia. A flow of 3 to 5 L per minute of oxygen through a nasal cannula (humidified) or nasal hood (5 to 7 L per minute) is recommended.

Sedation: Oxygen may also be delivered in conjuction with nitrous oxide. Nitrous oxide-oxygen inhalation sedation is the most highly recom-

Table 28-2. Dental therapy considerations for status postmyocardial infarction patients

Number of episodes	ASA physical status	Considerations
One documented myocardial infarction at least 6 months previously; no residual cardiovascular complications	III	Usual ASA III considerations to include follow-up after therapy by telephone; supplemental oxygen during treatment
One documented episode at least 6 months previously; angina, CHF, or dysrhythmia present	III or IV	Use of dialogue history to determine level of risk; usual ASA III considerations include possible premedication with nitroglycerin 5 minutes preop (if angina); oxygen through nasal cannula or nasal hood; and follow-up after therapy by telephone
More than one documented episode, most recent one at least 6 months previously; no further cardiovascular complications	III	Usual ASA III considerations to include supplemental oxygen during treatment and follow-up after therapy by telephone
Documented episode less than 6 months previously, or severe post-MI complications	IV	Usual ASA IV considerations

mended sedation technique for the cardiac risk patient. Its value in the management of acute episodes of myocardial infarction is discussed later in this chapter. Other sedation techniques may be used if deemed necessary by the doctor. In all sedation techniques hypoxia should be avoided. The use of supplemental oxygen will minimize this risk.

Pain control: Adequate pain control during the dental procedure is a critical factor in increasing safety during dental treatment of the cardiac risk patient. As discussed in Chapter 27, endogenous catecholamine release is potentially more dangerous to the cardiac risk patient than is the 0.01 mg/mL of exogenous epinephrine introduced into the tissues with a properly administered local anesthetic containing epinephrine in a 1:100,000 concentration. However, vasoconstrictors are contraindicated in patients with intractable cardiac dysrhythmias or any ASA IV cardiovascular risk patient (as in *any* elective dental care in this patient). The use of vasoconstrictor-containing local anesthetics is relatively contraindicated in patients receiving beta-blocking agents, such as propranolol.[31]

Duration of treatment: The duration of an appointment for the status postmyocardial infarction patient is variable but should never exceed a patient's level of tolerance. Signs of discomfort such as dyspnea, diaphoresis, and increased anxiety should lead to questioning of the patient and possible termination of treatment.

Six months post-MI: It is strongly recommended that no elective dental care, even procedures as seemingly inocuous as a prophylaxis, be considered for a status postmyocardial infarction patient for at least 6 months following the infarction.[32,33] Emergency care, such as that for infection and pain,

should not be managed within the dental office setting during this 6-month period. The acute clinical problem may initially be managed pharmacologically, through the administration of oral drugs (e.g., antibiotics and/or analgesics) alone, with any necessary invasive treatment, such as extraction or pulpal extirpation, being carried out in a more controlled environment, such as a hospital dental clinic.

It must be stressed that only emergency procedures should be considered on the status postmyocardial infarction patient within 6 months of the acute cardiac event, and then, only after medications have been ineffective in resolving the problem, immediate invasive care is warranted, and a hospital setting is available for the comtemplated treatment.

Medical consultation: Medical consultation should be considered before the dental management of a status myocardial infarction patient if any doubt remains in the doctor's mind after a full dental, medical, and psychological evaluation of the patient. If the doctor is contemplating emergency dental treatment for this patient within the 6-month waiting period, medical consultation is strongly suggested before commencing with treatment.

Anticoagulant or Antiplatelet Therapy

Medical consultation is also indicated before any treatment that involves a degree of hemorrhage (e.g., periodontal surgery, oral surgery) if the patient is currently receiving anticoagulant or antiplatelet therapy. The post-MI use of anticoagulants is much less common today than it was in the recent past.

Dental surgery is frequently performed in patients whose prothrombin time is 20% to 30% of normal without the development of bleeding problems.[32] In most instances, therefore, the proposed dental procedure does not have to be postponed, and the patient's anticoagulant medication does not need to be altered. The doctor, however, should take precautions to prevent postoperative hemorrhage from occurring. Possible steps include a hemostatic dressing placed within the socket, multiple sutures in the surgical area, intraoral pressure packs, ice packs (extraoral), the avoidance of mouth rinses, and a soft diet for 48 hours following the procedure.

CLINICAL MANIFESTATIONS
Pain

The chief clinical manifestation of acute myocardial infarction is the sudden onset of severe pain of the anginal type. Pain is experienced in 80% of patients with AMI. Acute myocardial infarction may occur without an obvious precipitating cause, often arising during a period of rest or sleep, or it may occur during or immediately following a period of unusually strong exercise (Table 28-3).[34] There is considerable evidence that emotional stress is a precipitating factor.[35,36] The pain builds rapidly to maximal intensity, lasting for prolonged periods of time (30 minutes to several hours) if unmanaged.[12]

The pain is usually described as a pressing or crushing sensation, like a deep ache within the chest. The patient may state that "it feels like there is a heavy rock or someone sitting on my chest." Rarely is the pain described as sharp or stabbing. It is located over the middle to upper third of the sternum and, much less commonly, over the lower third of the epigastrium.[1] Unfortunately, when the pain of AMI occurs in the epigastrium and is as-sociated with nausea and vomiting (see text that follows), the clinical picture may easily be confused with that of acute gastritis, cholecystitis, or peptic ulcer.[12]

Rest does not reduce the pain, nor does the use of nitroglycerin. The pain of myocardial infarction is most effectively relieved through the administration of narcotics such as morphine. Radiation of pain occurs throughout the same pattern as that of angina (see Fig. 27-2).

In 20% to 25% of cases pain is either absent or minor, and is overshadowed by immediate complications such as acute pulmonary edema, CHF, profound weakness, shock, syncope, or cerebral thrombosis. This type of infarction is called a painless infarction.[37]

Other Clinical Signs and Symptoms

The patient with acute myocardial infarction may appear to be in acute distress. A cold sweat is usually present, and the patient feels quite weak. The patient appears apprehensive and expresses an intense fear of impending doom. Although "intense fear of impending doom" may appear to the reader to be an overly dramatic and silly statement, rest assured that many victims of AMI do indeed verbally report this feeling. In contrast to anginal patients who lie, sit, or stand still, realizing that any activity will increase the discomfort of angina, patients with acute myocardial infarction will often be restless, moving about in a futile attempt to find a comfortable position for themselves. They may clutch at the chest with a fist—the Levine sign (a sign of ischemic pain popularized by Dr. Samuel A Levine).

Dyspnea is usually present, with the patient complaining that the crushing pressure on the chest prevents normal breathing. Respiratory movements do not intensify the painful sensation. Nausea and vomiting frequently occur, especially if the pain is severe.

Other clinical signs and symptoms associated with AMI may include a feeling of lightheadedness or faintness, coughing, wheezing, and abdominal bloating. This last symptom may lead victims to think that they are suffering from a upset stomach or indigestion, thereby delaying the initiation of proper treatment and increasing the chance of death.

The doctor should suspect an acute myocardial infarction in the following three situations:

1. New onset of chest pain suggestive of myocardial ischemia either at rest or with ordinary activity; chest pain appearing for the first time in a patient during dental treatment will usually be indicative of occlusion of a coronary

Table 28-3. Patient activity at onset of myocardial infarction

Activity	Percentage of patients
At rest	51
Modest or usual exertion	18
Physical exertion	13
Sleep	8
During surgical procedure	6
Other	4

Data from Phipps C: Contributory causes of coronary thrombosis, *JAMA* 106:761, 1936.

artery—it is unlikely to be simple angina of effort

2. A change in a previously stable pattern of anginal pain—either an increased frequency or severity, or the occurrence of rest angina for the first time.

3. Chest pain suggestive of myocardial ischemia in a patient with known coronary artery disease if unrelieved by rest and/or nitroglycerin

Physical Findings

The patient appears restless and apprehensive and is possibly in severe pain. Color may be poor, the face an ashen gray color, and the nailbeds and other mucous membranes cyanotic. The skin is cool, pale, and moist. The heart rate (pulse) may be weak, thready, and rapid, although a slow rate (bradycardia) may occasionally be present. Significant dysrhythmias are often present: premature ventricular contractions (PVCs) are seen in 93% of patients with acute myocardial infarction within the first 4 hours after acute myocardial infarction.[38] Blood pressure may be normal but much more commonly is low, decreasing dramatically over the first few hours and possibly falling to shock levels. Respirations appear rapid and shallow. If the left ventricle is the major site of the infarction, left ventricular failure may become clinically evident with labored breathing, a frothy sputum, and other signs of congestive heart failure (dependent edema), or pulmonary edema may gradually develop (Table 28-4).

Acute Complications

The greatest risk of death from myocardial infarction is during the first 4 to 6 hours after the onset of signs and symptoms. Complications such as acute dysrhythmias and cardiac arrest can occur abruptly during this time. More than 60% of the deaths associated with AMI occur within an hour of the event and are associated with acute lethal dysrhythmias, such as ventricular tachycardia and ventricular fibrillation.[39] Premature ventricular contractions are very common (93%). Their presence indicates increased irritability of the damaged myocardium and may presage the development of ventricular tachycardia or ventricular fibrillation. Ventricular fibrillation is 15 times more likely to occur in the first hour after the onset of signs and symptoms than in the following 12 hours.[40,41] Ventricular fibrillation develops in the first hour in approximately 36% of persons with acute myocardial infarction.[42] The significant mortality rate from myocardial infarction is in part based on the average delay between the onset of signs and symp-

Table 28-4. Clinical manifestations of acute myocardial infarction

Symptoms	*Signs*
Pain	Restlessness
Severe to intolerable	In acute distress
Prolonged, >30 min	Skin—cool, pale, moist
Crushing, choking, knifelike	Heart rate—bradycardia to tachycardia; PVCs common
Retrosternal	
Radiates: left arm, hand, epigastrium, shoulders, neck, jaw	
Nausea and vomiting	
Weakness	
Dizziness	
Palpitations	
Cold perspiration	
Sense of impending doom	

toms of myocardial infarction and entering the emergency medical system, which is 3 hours.[43]

The doctor must prepare for acute complications. Survival of the patient through the prehospitalization period is indeed a good omen, because once the patient is hospitalized in the emergency department and then in a specialized cardiac care unit (CCU), the chances for ultimate survival increase significantly. The most dangerous period is that time spent waiting for medical assistance to arrive.[40-43] Adequate preparation by the dental office staff can improve the chances of a successful outcome of this situation.

PATHOPHYSIOLOGY

Acute myocardial infarction is usually the direct result of a sudden occlusion of a major coronary vessel. The obstruction may result from acute thrombosis, subintimal hemorrhage, or the rupture of an atheromatous plaque, which then initiates the formation of a clot. The artery most often involved in coronary occlusion is the anterior descending branch of the left coronary artery, which supplies the anterior left ventricle. There are two major types of myocardial infarction; the transmural infarct and the nontransmural infarct. In the transmural infarct the myocardial necrosis involves the full thickness of the ventricular wall. Necrosis in the nontransmural infarct involves subendocardium, the intramural myocardium, or both, without extension all the way through the ventricular wall to the epicardium.[12]

An occlusion may occur rapidly, or it may develop over a prolonged period. In either case it is possible that even total occlusion of a coronary vessel may not lead to ischemia and infarction. In the presence of an adequate collateral circulation, the myocardial tissue supplied by the occluded vessel still receives an adequate blood supply through collateral vessels. Collateral circulation in the normal heart is usually poorly developed; however, it has been demonstrated that, immediately following occlusion of a coronary artery, collateral blood flow doubles.[44] The significance of this increase in collateral circulation is debatable.[24] The enlargement of these vessels over the next 3 to 4 weeks is a major element in the finding that the size of the area of myocardial necrosis is usually smaller than would be expected.[45]

Myocardial infarction may occur even though the vessel is not totally occluded. In an area dependent for its blood supply on collateral circulation (e.g., a previously infarcted area with adequate collateral circulation), a minimal change in blood supply through the vessel may lead to infarction. This may come about through a partial occlusion of the vessel or from a change in vascular resistance in the vessel (e.g., spasm).

Infarction of the myocardium produces alterations in the contractility of the heart due to a loss of functioning myocardial segments. The degree of depression of cardiac function in myocardial infarction is directly related to the extent of left ventricular damage.[46] Because the left ventricle is most commonly involved in AMI, the blood supply to the periphery may become inadequate. This leads to many of the clinical signs and symptoms observed in myocardial infarction, such as cool, moist skin, peripheral cyanosis, and tachycardia. The larger the infarct, the greater the degree of circulatory inadequacy that is noted (e.g., signs and symptoms of heart failure). Left ventricular filling pressures increase significantly even in the presence of a small infarct. If the infarction is larger, there is a greater increase in the left ventricular filling pressure and clinical evidence of left ventricular failure. Infarction of 35% or more of left ventricular mass leads to clinical evidence of hypotension, decreased cardiac output, and cardiogenic shock.[47]

Cardiogenic shock occurs in approximately 10% to 15% of patients with AMI who survive long enough to reach the hospital.[48,49] Its presence is ominous because it is associated with a higher mortality rate. It normally develops approximately 10 hours following the onset of the infarction and may be produced by cardiac dysrhythmias, the continued presence of severe pain, the onset of acute pulmonary edema, or pulmonary embolism. Clinical evidence of cardiogenic shock includes hypo-

tension (systolic blood pressure below 80 mmHg) and signs of an inadequate peripheral circulation (e.g., mental confusion, cool skin, peripheral cyanosis, tachycardia, and a decreased urinary output).[49]

Probably the most threatening feature of the early postinfarction period (1 to 2 hours) is the presence of cardiac dysrhythmias. Most patients (95%) exhibit abnormalities in heart rhythm. They are significant in that they may produce alterations in the normal sequence of atrial and ventricular contraction, thereby leading to inadequate cardiac output, and/or they may produce an aberrant focus of electrical depolarization in the myocardium. They also may adversely affect the ventricular rate, producing bradycardia (slow heart rate), ventricular tachycardia (an extremely rapid contraction rate with insufficient time for ventricular filling), ventricular fibrillation (irregular, uncoordinated, ineffective contraction of individual muscle bundles), or asystole (complete absence of contractions). Commonly observed dysrhythmias are shown in Fig. 30-1. Death occurring in the early postinfarction period, although it may be produced by the infarction of a large mass of myocardium, is normally the result of an acute dysrhythmia.[41,42]

Survival following myocardial infarction depends of many factors. Most important of these are the state of left ventricular function and the severity of obstructive lesions in the coronary vascular bed. Complete clinical recovery (i.e., no chronic complications) and a normal ECG are compatible with a 10- to 20-year period of survival. However, patients who exhibit residual congestive heart failure usually die within 1 to 5 years.[50,51]

MANAGEMENT

Clinical management of acute myocardial infarction is based on its recognition and the application of the steps of basic life support. It may be difficult to differentiate immediately between the pain of angina and that of acute myocardial infarction. Although there are slight differences initially, the doctor may find it difficult to determine which of these clinical entities is present at the onset of the episode of acute chest pain.

Diagnostic clues to the presence of acute myocardial infarction include[52]:

- Symptoms of pressure, tightness, a heavy weight
- Substernal, epigastric pain that may radiate to jaw
- Moderate to severe discomfort
- Longer duration (>30 minutes) than anginal pain

- Nausea and vomiting
- Diaphoresis
- Dyspnea
- Irregular pulse
- Generalized weakness

Step 1: Terminate the dental procedure. With the onset of chest pain, immediately stop the dental treatment.

Step 2: Diagnosis. The suspicion of AMI must be based on the patient's clinical appearance. If the history (record of clinical signs and symptoms) is consistent with a diagnosis of acute myocardial infarction, the patient must be treated accordingly. Although the ECG, if available, may confirm acute myocardial infarction, the ECG may also appear to be entirely normal.[42] For this reason a single, normal ECG tracing cannot reliably exclude the diagnosis of past acute myocardial infarction.

Three possible clinical situations follow:

1. Anginal patient/angina: A patient with a history of angina will usually be able to tell if the episode is indeed anginal. If angina is thought to be the problem, management follows the steps presented in Chapter 27. The patient, who is accustomed to treating his or her angina, will usually be more calm about the situation than will the doctor, who is unaccustomed to patients experiencing acute chest pain during treatment.

2. Anginal patient/not angina: An anginal patient in whom the chest pain is more intense than usual will become frightened, convinced that "the big one" is happening. Recommended management follows the steps outlined below for acute myocardial infarction.

3. No cardiac history: Chest pain developing in a patient with no prior history of acute chest pain normally frightens the patient, who is also convinced that a heart attack is occurring. Management of this situation is presented below.

It is suggested that management of chest pain be approached as if it were angina pectoris (situation 1) unless it is obviously not of anginal origin, as it is in situations 2 and 3.

Step 3: Position patient.

Step 4: Administer nitroglycerin.

Step 5: Administer oxygen.

The initial steps in management of these patients include termination of dental treatment (step 1) and allowing the patient to find a comfortable position (step 3). If the patient has a history of angina, the nitroglycerin, which should always be available, is used at this time (step 4). (See Fig. 28-1.) Nitroglycerin from the emergency kit is used only if the patient does not have his or her own supply or if the patient's supply fails to alleviate the pain. The

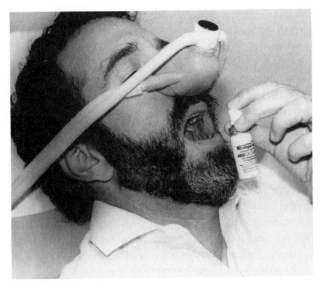

Fig. 28-1. Administration of 100% oxygen and nitroglycerin.

patient's vital signs should be recorded either before administering the nitroglycerin or shortly thereafter. Nitroglycerin should not be administered if the systolic blood pressure is below 100 mmHg, because it can decrease the mean arterial pressure. Nitroglycerin normally acts within 2 to 4 minutes to dramatically reduce or terminate the discomfort of angina. Oxygen is administered as soon as it becomes available (step 5).

Angina: If angina is present the pain will subside and the acute problem is terminated. Dental care may resume if desired and/or the patient can be dismissed from the office. There is no need to seek outside medical assistance or hospitalization with stable angina. This protocol is presented in depth in Chapter 27.

Myocardial infarction: Should the pain continue or increase in severity in spite of the administration of nitroglycerin and oxygen, or if nitroglycerin alleviates the pain, but the pain returns in but a few minutes, we must consider the very real possibility of an acute myocardial infarction.

NOTE: Chest pain that is alleviated by nitroglycerin but returns should be managed as though it were acute myocardial infarction

Step 6: Basic life support, as indicated. At this point in the AMI, the patient will be experiencing more extreme discomfort and may be showing clinical signs of decreased cardiac output (i.e., diaphoresis; cool, moist extremities; ashen-gray pallor, cyanosis of mucous membranes and nailbeds). The airway, breathing, and circulation are assessed and deemed adequate. Permit the patient to remain in a comfortable position.

Continue to administer oxygen to the patient. There is evidence suggesting that increased arterial oxygen tension (PaO_2) may decrease the size of the infarct.[53] Oxygen should be delivered through a nasal cannula or nasal hood at a flow rate of 4 to 6 L per minute.

Step 7: Summon medical assistance. With the failure of nitroglycerin to ease the patient's discomfort, medical assistance should immediately be sought. It must always be remembered that mortality from myocardial infarction is greatest during the first few hours, with the majority of deaths occurring before the patient is admitted to the hospital. Over 60% of all deaths from myocardial infarction occur within the first few hours after the onset of symptoms. Three quarters of all deaths occur within the first 24 hours. Most deaths occurring before hospitalization are the result of life-threatening dysrhythmias that frequently occur in the immediate postinfarction period, as well as the misinterpretation or denial of signs and symptoms by the patient or medical personnel. Early entry into the emergency medical services (EMS) system is often vital for patient survival. The average time from onset of symptoms of IHD to entry into the EMS is more than 3 hours.

The availability of trained paramedical personnel in mobile coronary care units has led to a significant decrease in the mortality rate from myocardial infarction.[54] Definitive therapy (e.g., advanced cardiac life support) can be started at the scene or while en route to the hospital. In the city of Seattle, Washington, which has a model EMS system, basic life support was provided for victims of out-of-hospital cardiac arrest within 2.9 minutes and advanced cardiac life support within an average of 4 minutes from dispatch to arrival of EMS. By 1978, 60% of 290 patients with cardiac arrest were resuscitated in the field and 30% (88 patients) were eventually discharged home.[54]

Step 8: Monitor vital signs. Vital signs (e.g., blood pressure, heart rate and rhythm, and respirations) should be monitored on a regular basis (every 5 minutes) and recorded.

Step 9: Relieve pain. Prolonged pain during AMI is potentially life threatening. It will lead to increased patient anxiety, and it contributes to excessive activity of the autonomic nervous system, producing an increase in cardiovascular workload and oxygen requirement. In addition, prolonged, intense pain is one of the causative factors of cardiogenic shock, which has a high mortality rate.

Nitroglycerin has previously been administered,

to no effect. Nitroglycerin will usually be inadequate to alleviate the pain associated with AMI.[55]

Parenteral analgesics: The use of narcotic analgesics is recommended for relief of the pain of myocardial infarction. Intravenous administration of 2 to 5 mg of morphine sulfate repeated every 5 to 15 minutes provides adequate pain relief and allays apprehension.[1] Additionally, morphine increases venous capacitance and systemic vascular resistance, relieving pulmonary congestion, thereby decreasing myocardial oxygen requirements.[56] Morphine sulfate may be administered subcutaneously in a dose of 5 to 15 mg. Morphine should not be readministered if the respiratory rate is less than 12 respirations per minute. Meperidine (50 to 100 mg intramuscularly) may be administered in place of morphine. Intramuscular injection of these analgesic drugs provides adequate pain relief of long duration. Intravenous administration may also be considered, but the drugs require readministration in a shorter period to time. Naloxone, a narcotic antagonist, should always be available when narcotics are administered.

Other analgesics: Another useful analgesic medication for administration in AMI may already be present in the dental office. A mixture of nitrous oxide and oxygen, more commonly employed as an inhalation sedation technique in dental practice, has been employed in Great Britain and several other countries since 1967 in premixed cylinders containing 50% nitrous oxide (N_2O) and 50% oxygen (O_2) (Entonox).[57] (See Fig. 28-2.) Premixed cylinders of nitrous oxide (35%) and oxygen (65%) (Dolonox) have also been used in the United States in the treatment of myocardial infarction.[58] In Britain, the nitrous oxide-oxygen mixture is employed on emergency ambulances and serves as the primary agent for pain relief in acute cardiovascular emergency situations. The primary advantage of this agent is that it provides the patient with a gaseous analgesic agent that by itself has little effect on blood pressure. This contrasts with the use of parenteral analgesics, which are more likely to reduce blood pressure and produce adverse side effects (e.g., excessive CNS depression, respiratory depression, nausea, and vomiting). The use of this mixture also provides the patient with a source of enriched oxygen (50% to 65% versus 21% in atmospheric air).[57-62]

Although premixed nitrous oxide and oxygen is available through medical suppliers in the United States, any available source of these gases may be employed in this situation. A 35% concentration of nitrous oxide is administered through the nasal hood or by means of a full face mask. When the

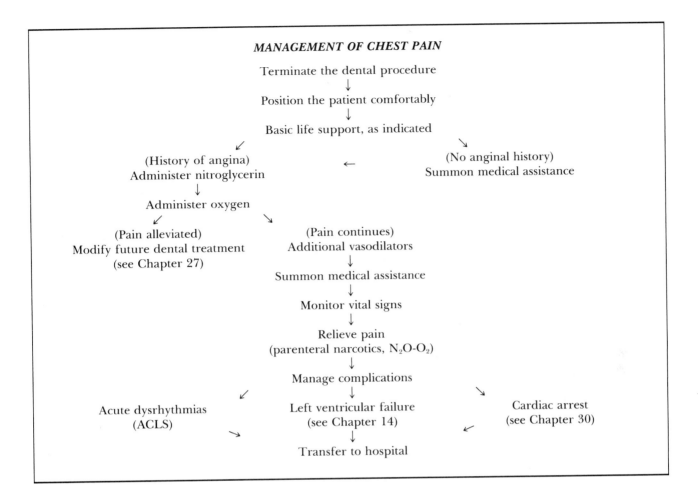

MANAGEMENT OF CHEST PAIN

Terminate the dental procedure
↓
Position the patient comfortably
↓
Basic life support, as indicated

(History of angina)
Administer nitroglycerin
↓
Administer oxygen

(No anginal history)
Summon medical assistance

(Pain alleviated)
Modify future dental treatment
(see Chapter 27)

(Pain continues)
Additional vasodilators
↓
Summon medical assistance
↓
Monitor vital signs
↓
Relieve pain
(parenteral narcotics, N_2O-O_2)
↓
Manage complications
↓
Left ventricular failure
(see Chapter 14)
↓
Transfer to hospital

Acute dysrhythmias
(ACLS)

Cardiac arrest
(see Chapter 30)

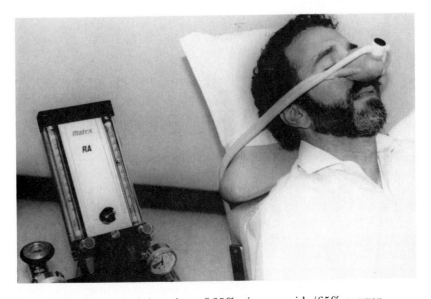

Fig. 28-2. Administration of 35% nitrous oxide/65% oxygen.

patient is ready to be transported from the dental office to the hospital, the medical or paramedical personnel will administer a parenteral analgesic to provide continuing pain relief during the journey should portable sources of N_2O-O_2 be unavailable.

Step 10: Manage complications. The major complications of acute myocardial infarction likely to develop while awaiting the arrival of emergency medical assistance are acute dysrhythmias, congestive heart failure, and cardiac arrest.

The management of acute dysrhythmias requires intravenous administration of various drugs. In addition, the presence of an electrocardioscope and the training to interpret the ECG are essential. Agents that may be employed to manage dysrhythmias include lidocaine and atropine.[1] It must be emphasized that without an electrocardiographic monitor, no antidysrhythmic drugs should be administered to a patient with dysrhythmias. Oxygen must continue to be administered to this patient.

Left ventricular failure may develop if a significant portion of the myocardium has been infarcted. Respiratory symptoms are most prominent, with dyspnea and acute pulmonary edema occurring. (Management of this complication is discussed fully in Chapter 14.) Essentials of management include positioning the patient and reducing the circulating blood volume through the use of a bloodless phlebotomy. In addition, oxygen should continue to be administered to this patient.

Cardiac arrest, indicative of acute cardiorespiratory collapse, needs immediate effective management. Chapter 30 covers this important subject in depth.

Step 11: Transport patient to hospital. Once the patient's condition has been stabilized (i.e., relief of pain and stabilization of heart rhythm and blood pressure), he or she will be transported to a primary care facility (e.g., emergency department of a hospital). It is desirable for the doctor to accompany the patient in the ambulance or by car from the dental office to the hospital and to remain with the patient until a physician is in attendance. The box on page 417 outlines the steps to follow to manage chest pain.

Drugs used in management: Nitroglycerin; oxygen; morphine or meperidine, N_2O-O_2

Medical assistance: Yes

REFERENCES

1. American Heart Association: *Textbook of advanced cardiac life support*, Dallas, 1987, American Heart Association.
2. Stamler J: The primary prevention of coronary heart disease. In Braunwald E, editor: *The myocardium: failure and infarction*, New York, 1974, HP Publishing.
3. Kuller LH: Sudden death—definition and epidemiologic considerations, *Prog Cardiovasc Dis* 23:1, 1980.
4. Killip T: Arrhythmias in myocardial infarction, *Med Clin N Am* 60:233, 1975.
5. Simoons ML, Serruys PW, vd Brand M, and others: Improved survival after early thrombolysis in acute myocardial infarction: A randomized trial conducted by the Inter-University Cardiology Institute in the Netherlands, *Lancet* 1:578, 1985.
6. O'Neill W, Timmis GC, Bourdellon PD, and others: A prospective, randomized clinical trial of intracoronary streptokinase vs coronary angioplasty for acute myocardial infarction, *N Engl J Med* 314:812, 1986.
7. American Heart Association: *Heart facts*, Dallas, 1984, The American Heart Association.
8. Kannel WB: Some lessons in cardiovascular epidemiology from Framingham, *Am J Cardiol* 37:269, 1976.
9. Norris RM, Barnaby PF, Brandt PWT, and others: Prognosis after recovery from first acute myocardial infarction: determinants of reinfarction and sudden death, *Am J Cardiol* 53:408, 1984.
10. DeFeyter PJ, Van Eenige MJ, Dighton DH, and others: Prognostic value of exercise testing, coronary angiography and left ventriculography 6-8 weeks after myocardial infarction, *Circulation* 66:527, 1982.
11. Schulze RA Jr, Strauss HW, Pitt B: Sudden death in the year following myocardial infarction: relation to ventricular premature contractions in the late hospital phase and left ventriculat ejection fraction, *Am J Med* 62:192, 1977.
12. Alpert JS, Braunwald E: Pathological and clinical manifestations of acute myocardial infarction. In Braunwald E, editor: *Heart disease*, ed 3, Philadelphia, 1986, WB Saunders.
13. Friedman EH: Type A or B behavior, *JAMA* 228:1369, 1974.
14. Friedman M, Rosenman RH: *Type A behavior and your heart*, New York, 1974, Alfred A. Knopf.
15. Elek SR: Psychological management of patients with coronary-prone type-A behavior pattern, *JAMA* 229:1805, 1974.
16. Wilson RF, Holida MD, White CW: Quantitative angiographic morphology of coronary stenosis leading to myocardial infarction or unstable angina, *Circulation* 73:286, 1986.
17. Maseri A, L'Abbate A, Baroldi G, and others: Coronary vasospasm as a possible cause of myocardial infarction: a conclusion derived from the study of "preinfarction" angina, *N Engl J Med* 299:1271, 1978.
18. Howard RE, Hueter DC, Davis GJ: Acute myocardial infarction following cocaine abuse in a young woman with normal coronary arteries, *JAMA* 254:95, 1985.
19. Dolter K: Myocardial infarction. In *Cardiopulmonary emergencies*, Springhouse, Pa., 1991.
20. Little WC, Downes TR, Applegate RJ: The underlying coronary lesion in myocardial infarction: implications for coronary angiography, *Clin Cardiol* 14(11):868-874, 1991.
21. B-Blocker Heart Attack Trial Research Group: A randomized trial of propranolol in patients with acute myocardial infarction. I. Mortality results, *JAMA* 247:1707, 1982.
22. Pedersen TR: Six-year follow-up of the Norwegian Multicenter Study in Timolol after acute myocardial infarction, *N Engl J Med* 313:1055, 1985.
23. Weinblatt E, and others: Prognosis of men after first myocardial infarction: mortality and first recurrence in relation to selected parameters, *Am J Public Health* 58:1329, 1968.
24. Gorlin R: Coronary collaterals. In *Coronary artery disease*, Philadelphia, 1976, WB Saunders.
25. Bolooki H, and others: Myocardial revascularization after acute infarction, *Am J Cardiol* 36:395, 1975.

26. Fishbein MC, Maclean D, Maroko PR: The histopathological evolution of myocardial infarction, *Chest* 73:843, 1978.

27. Cohen BS: A program of rehabilitation after acute myocardial infarction, *South Med J* 68:145, 1975.

28. Horgan JH: Rehabilitation after myocardial infarction, *J Irish Med Assoc* 66:661, 1973.

29. Kavanagh T, Shephard RH, Pandit V: Marathon running after myocardial infarction, *JAMA* 229:1602, 1974.

30. Neill WA, Oxendine JM: Exercise can promote coronary collateral development without improving perfusion of ischemic myocardium, *Circulation* 60:1513, 1979.

31. Yagiela JA: Deadfalls in drug interactions. 6th Annual review course in dental anesthesiology, 1990, American Dental Society of Anesthesiology.

32. McCarthy FM: *Essentials of safe dentistry for the medically compromised patient*, Philadelphia, 1989, WB Saunders.

33. Little JW, Falace DA: *Dental management of the medically compromised patient*, ed 3, St Louis 1988, Mosby–Year Book.

34. Phipps C: Contributory causes of coronary thrombosis, *JAMA* 106:761, 1936.

35. Jenkins CD: Recent evidence supporting psychologic and social risk factors for coronary disease, *N Engl J Med* 294:1033, 1976.

36. Rahe RH, Romo M, Bennett L, and others: Recent life changes, myocardial infarction, and abrupt coronary death. Studies in Helsinki, *Arch Intern Med* 133:221, 1974.

37. Margolis JR, Kannel WB, Feibleib M, and others: Clinical features of unrecognized myocardial infarction—silent and symptomatic. Eighteen year follow-up: The Framingham study, *Am J Cardiol* 32:1, 1973.

38. Adgey AAJ, and others: Acute phase of myocardial infarction: prehospital management of the coronary patient, *Minnesota Med* 59:347, 1976.

39. Schaffer WA, Cobb LA: Recurrent ventricular fibrillation and modes of death in survivors of out-of-hospital ventricular fibrillation, *N Engl J Med* 293:259, 1975.

40. Pantridge JE, Geddes JS: A mobile intensive care unit in the management of myocardial infarction, *Lancet* 2:271, 1967.

41. Pantridge JF, Webb SW, Adgey AAJ: Arrhythmias in the first hours of acute myocardial infarction, *Prog Cardiovasc Dis* 23:265, 1981.

42. Rose RM, and others: Occurrence of arrhythmias during the first hour in acute myocardial infarction, *Circulation* 50 (suppl 3):111, 1974.

43. Moss AJ, Goldstein S: The prehospital phase of acute myocardial infarction, *Circulation* 41:737, 1970.

44. Gensini GG: Coronary arteriography. In Braunwald E, editor: *Heart disease.* ed 3, Philadelphia, 1986, WB Saunders.

45. Levin DC: Pathways and functional significance of the coronary collateral circulation, *Circulation* 50:831, 1974.

46. Pfeiffer MA, Pfeiffer JM, Fisgbein MC, and others: Myocardial infarct size and ventricular function in rats, *Circ Res* 44:503, 1979.

47. Page DL, Caulfield JB, Kastor JA, and others: Myocardial changes associated with cardiogenic shock, *N Engl J Med* 285:133, 1971.

48. Loeb HS, Johnson SA, Gunnar AM: Cardiogenic shock, *Triangle* 13:121, 1974.

49. Rackley CE, Russell RO Jr., Mantle JA, and others: Cardiogenic shock: recognition and management, *Cardiovasc Clin* 7:251, 1975.

50. Wolk MJ, Scheidt S, Killip T: Heart failure complicating acute myocardial infarction, *Circulation* 45:1125, 1972.

51. Lassers BW, and others: Left ventricular failure and acute myocardial infarction, *Am J Cardiol* 25:511, 1970.

52. Pollakoff J, Pollakoff K: *EMT's guide to signs and symptoms*, 1991.

53. Marokso PR, Radyany P, Braunwald E, and others: Reduction of infarct size by oxygen inhalation following acute coronary occluson, *Circulation* 52:360, 1975.

54. Cobb LA, Werner JA, Trobaugh GB: Sudden cardiac death, *Mod Concepts Cardiovasc Dis* 49:31, 1980.

55. Jaffe AS, Geltman EM, Tiefenbrunn AJ, and others: Reduction of infarct size in patients with inferior infarction with intravenous glyceryl trinitrate, *Br Heart J* 49:452, 1973.

56. Todres D: The role of morphine in acute myocardial infarction, *Am Heart J* 81:566, 1971.

57. Nancekievill D: Apparatus for the administration of Entonox (50% N$_2$O: 50% O$_2$ mixture) by intermittent positive pressure, *Anaesthesia* 29:736, 1974.

58. Thompson PL, Lown B: Nitrous oxide as an analgesic in acute myocardial infarction, *JAMA* 235:924, 1976.

59. Eisele JH, and others: Myocardial performance and N$_2$O analgesia in coronary artery disease, *Anesthesiology* 44:16, 1976.

60. Kerr F, and others: A double blind trial of patient-controlled nitrous oxide/oxygen analgesia in myocardial infarction, *Lancet* 1:397, 1975.

61. Stern MS, and others: Nitrous oxide and oxygen in acute myocardial infarction, *Circulation* 58(suppl II):171, 1978.

62. Wynne J, and others: Beneficial effects of nitrous oxide in patients with ischemic heart disease, *Circulation* 55(suppl. III):18, 1977.

29 Chest Pain: Differential Diagnosis

The two major clinical syndromes that exhibit chest pain and confront the dentist are angina pectoris and acute myocardial infarction (AMI). Yet there are occasions when the dental patient or the doctor may have other forms of chest pain. Indeed, everybody experiences various forms of chest pain at times. Fortunately, most of these pains are unrelated to cardiac disease and for the most part are innocuous. However, most of those experiencing chest pain have stopped and thought, "This pain I am feeling now is the real thing." With this in mind, we will first discuss the major differences between noncardiac chest pain and the chest pain associated with cardiovascular disease. Following this discussion is a differential diagnosis of the two major forms of chest pain. Table 29-1 lists several of the possible causes of chest pain.

NONCARDIAC CHEST PAIN

Noncardiac chest pain can usually be differentiated from the pain of angina and myocardial infarction because a sharp, knifelike chest pain that increases in intensity with inspiration and diminishes with exhalation is usually not related to cardiac syndromes.

Chest pain that is aggravated by movement (e.g., twisting, turning, or stretching of the sore area) is most often related to muscle or nerve injuries, not to cardiac disease. It must be noted that the author has used the word *usually* when describing typical chest pains. Instances occur in which patients are aware of a sharp, knifelike pain that may in fact be related to cardiac disease. Variations from the typical are expected, and the dental health professional is well advised to take note of this.

Probably the most common cause of noncardiac chest pain is musculoskeletal, from muscle strain that occurs after exercise or physical exertion.[1] This form of pain is normally localized (the patient can point to a specific site of discomfort), does not radiate, and is made worse by breathing and movement. A heating pad or mild analgesic medication may give relief.

Pericarditis is an inflammation of the outer membrane covering the heart and is most commonly caused by viral infection. The pain of pericarditis is similar to that of angina or myocardial infarction, occurs in the midsternum, and is described as "oppressive." Clues to its differential diagnosis include aggravation of the pain of pericarditis when breathing and swallowing, characteristic relief of the pain when the patient bends forward from the waist, and very often the presence of a fever before the onset of pain.[2]

Table 29-1. Causes of chest pain

Cardiac related	Noncardiac related
Angina pectoris	Muscle strain
Myocardial infarction	Pericarditis
	Esophagitis
	Hiatal hernia
	Pulmonary embolism
	Dissecting aortic aneurysm
	Acute indigestion
	Intestinal "gas"

Esophagitis with or without hiatal hernia produces a substernal or epigastric burning pain that is precipitated by eating or lying down after a meal. The pain is relieved by antacids. There often is an acid reflux into the mouth.[3]

Pulmonary embolism usually indicates the sudden occlusion of a blood vessel within the lungs by an embolus that has been "thrown" (broken loose) from the legs. The patient experiences a sudden severe chest pain that is commonly associated with the coughing up of blood-tinged sputum.[4]

A less common cause of acute chest pain is the dissecting aortic aneurysm. The patient experiences sudden, acute, severe chest pain that is often greatest at onset. Typically, it spreads up and down the chest and back over a period of hours. The dissecting aortic aneurysm may rapidly lead to death.[5]

Two other very common causes of chest pain often make it difficult to differentiate between cardiac and noncardiac pain. These are the pains of acute indigestion and "gas." It has been mentioned previously that one of the major factors leading to the high initial mortality rate associated with AMI is the misinterpretation or denial of clinical symptoms by the patient or the attending physician. The symptoms are commonly written off as indigestion or gas pains and are later discovered to have been produced by AMI. The pain of gas is normally sharp and knifelike and increases in intensity upon breathing. This fact should assist in differentiating gas pain from the pain of ischemic heart disease (IHD). Acute indigestion is similar to the pain of angina or myocardial infarction, and therefore all patients with this symptom should receive careful evaluation. Epigastric discomfort may be a manifestation of myocardial ischemia or infarction and should not be dismissed lightly. Unusual or prolonged indigestion should rouse suspicion, particularly in a high-risk individual. The American Heart Association recommends that a patient with previously unrecognized coronary disease seek medical assistance if a suspicious chest pain persists for 2 minutes or longer.[6]

CARDIAC CHEST PAIN

Angina and AMI are the two most common causes of IHD-related chest pain in the dental office. Differential diagnosis is essential because these two syndromes represent quite different risks to the patient and are ultimately managed differently. The following discussion is offered to assist in making this differential diagnosis.

Prior Medical History

The patient with angina is usually aware of its existence and is receiving medications to manage acute anginal episodes as they occur. It is possible, though highly unlikely, that a patient without a history of heart problems will suffer a first episode of angina within the dental office setting. Most first episodes of chest pain for patients in the dental environment will prove to be either myocardial infarction or unstable angina. A medical history of a prior myocardial infarction may also be available. Many patients who survive myocardial infarction later develop episodes of angina and have medication for it.

Age of Patient

Coronary artery disease (CAD) is present in all age groups. Clinical evidence may develop in young individuals, or it may never develop at all. There is no clinical difference between the age of patients developing either of these two coronary syndromes. Clinical evidence of CAD is most commonly noted in men between the ages of 50 and 60 years, whereas in women its greatest incidence is found between the ages of 60 and 70 years.

Sex of Patient

Coronary artery disease remains primarily a disease of males. The overall male-to-female ratio is 4:1. Before the age of 40 years, the ratio rises to 8:1.

Circumstances Associated with Onset of Symptoms

The clinical symptomatology of angina is usually associated with exertion, whether physical or mental. Myocardial infarction, on the other hand, may occur during or immediately following a period of exertion, but it also commonly occurs during periods of rest. Angina rarely occurs during rest, although coronary artery spasm may provoke anginal pain at any time. Unstable angina, by definition, may occur at rest.

Clinical Symptoms and Signs
Location of Chest Pain

Location of chest pain is not a reliable indicator of the nature of the pain. Both anginal pain and the pain of AMI occur substernally or just to the left of the midsternal region.

Description of Chest Pain

Chest pain associated with either of these two syndromes is usually not described as pain by the patient. More commonly the sensation is described as "squeezing," "pressing," or "crushing." The pain associated with myocardial infarction is more intense than that of angina and is more commonly described as painful or intolerable.

Radiation of Chest Pain

Differentiation between the two syndromes is difficult to make using radiation of pain as a criterion. Radiation of chest pain commonly occurs to the left shoulder and medial side of the left arm, following the distribution of the ulnar nerve. Less frequently the pain may radiate to the right shoulder, the mandibular region, or the epigastrium. Both syndromes have similar radiation patterns.

Duration of Chest Pain

The pain associated with AMI is normally of long duration and lasts from 30 minutes to several hours if untreated. As mentioned in Chapter 28, untreated cardiac pain may produce cardiogenic shock. Pain associated with angina is almost always brief. Merely terminating the activity that induced the episode brings relief within 3 to 5 minutes. Anginal episodes that have been precipitated by eating a large meal or feeling angry are of a longer duration, perhaps lasting 30 minutes or more.

Response to Medication

Probably the most reliable diagnostic tool is the patient's response to the administration of medications. A vasodilator, preferably nitroglycerin but possibly amyl nitrate or nifedipine, is administered. The pain of angina will be relieved approximately 2 to 4 minutes following administration of nitroglycerin and within 1 minute following amyl nitrate administration. These agents may temporarily diminish the pain of myocardial infarction, but more commonly they will have no effect. The pain of myocardial infarction is commonly managed through administration of narcotic analgesics, such as morphine, or nitrous oxide and oxygen.

Administration of a vasodilator to the patient with presumed cardiac-related chest pain offers one of the most reliable methods of differentiating between the pain of angina and that of AMI. For this reason, the administration of nitroglycerin represents the first step in the clinical drug management of chest pain in the dental office.

Physical Examination
Heart Rate

The heart rate noted during episodes of angina is quite rapid and may feel full or bounding. A rapid heart rate may also be present during AMI; however, because the blood pressure is usually decreased, the pulse may feel weak or thready. The heart rate during AMI may also be slow.

Blood Pressure

Episodes of angina are normally accompanied by marked elevations in blood pressure, whereas blood pressure in AMI may be normal, but more commonly is decreased.

Respiration

Patients with either coronary syndrome may exhibit respiratory distress during the acute episode. The respiratory rate is more rapid, and the depth of each respiration may be more shallow than usual. During myocardial infarction the left ventricle may fail, producing clinical evidence of left ventricular failure.

Other Signs and Symptoms

Overall appearance. Most patients with AMI and some patients with angina will appear quite apprehensive and may be bathed in a cold sweat. Anginal patients can compare current episodes with previous episodes, which may give a clue to the seriousness of a present episode. Anginal episodes tend to be quite similar in an individual patient. Any change in severity, duration, or frequency may indicate the occurrence of unstable angina or myocardial infarction. Patients with AMI often have a great fear of impending doom.

Skin. During myocardial infarction facial skin may appear ashen gray. The nailbeds and other mucous membranes of the victim may demonstrate varying degrees of cyanosis. These changes rarely occur during anginal episodes.

Nausea and vomiting. Nausea and vomiting are common during AMI, especially in the presence of severe pain. Nausea and vomiting are uncommon with anginal pain.

SUMMARY

As is evident, the clinical diagnosis of chest pain is difficult to make. However, the management of cardiac-related chest pain invariably leads to an accurate diagnosis. This depends primarily on the response of the patient to the administration of nitroglycerin.

One other important factor that bears repetition at this time is that anginal episodes for a given patient are usually similar from episode to episode. Any change in the acute attacks that produces a more severe episode may indicate the occurrence of AMI.

Noncardiac chest pain is usually easily differentiated from cardiac-related chest pain because of the nature of the pain. However, two common forms of discomfort, acute indigestion and gas, are quite difficult to differentiate from cardiac-related chest pain. These symptoms must not be ignored. Careful evaluation is required, and medical consultation should be considered if doubt remains in the dental practitioner's mind.

REFERENCES

1. Dronen SC: Chest pain. In Rosen P, Baker FJ, Barkin RM, and others, editors: *Emergency medicine*, ed 2, St Louis, 1988, Mosby–Year Book.
2. Burchell HB: Pericarditis: some current concepts, *Cardiovasc Med* 11:287, 1977.
3. Henderson RD, Maryatt G: Characteristics of esophageal pain, *Acta Med Scand* 644:49, 1980.
4. Zimmerman D, Parker BM: The pain of pulmonary hypertension: fact or fancy? *JAMA* 246:2345, 1981.
5. Wheat MW: Acute dissecting aneurysms of the aorta: diagnosis and treatment—1979, *Am Heart J* 99:373, 1980.
6. *Heart attack: signals and actions for survival*, Dallas, 1986, American Heart Association.

30 *Cardiac Arrest and Cardiopulmonary Resuscitation*

Angina pectoris, myocardial infarction, and heart failure are three clinical manifestations of ischemic heart disease (IHD). Associated with each of these clinical situations is the possible occurrence of acute complications. Among these are cardiac dysrhythmias and cardiopulmonary collapse, the latter also called cardiac arrest or sudden death. It should be noted that cardiac arrest can also occur as an acute clinical entity in the absence of other cardiovascular manifestations. Of the victims of cardiac arrest, 25% do not exhibit clinical signs or symptoms before the onset of sudden death.[1] Stated another way, the first clinical indication of the presence of IHD may be the death of the patient.

Sudden death is defined by the World Health Organization as clinical death that occurs within 24 hours after the onset of symptoms.[2] Clinical death that occurs within 30 seconds of the onset of symptoms is termed instantaneous death.[2] For the purpose of our discussion in this section, the term *sudden death* is defined as death occurring within 1 hour of the onset of signs and symptoms.[3]

Death, as referred to in these definitions, is clinical death as opposed to biologic death. Clinical death occurs at the moment of cardiopulmonary arrest but may, on occasion, be reversed if promptly recognized and effectively managed, thereby preventing biological death. Biologic death follows when permanent cellular damage has occurred, primarily from a lack of oxygen. Biologic or cellular death of neuronal (brain) tissue takes place when delivery of oxygen is inadequate for approximately 4 to 6 minutes.[4]

The magnitude of the problem of sudden death becomes apparent when it is noted that of the more than 944,688 deaths occurring in 1988[5] from cardiovascular disease, of which 497,850 were due to coronary artery disease (including 350,000 cardiac arrests[6]), at least two thirds of the deaths take place outside of the hospital setting—usually within 1 hour after the onset of symptoms.[1] Sudden, unexpected death from myocardial infarction is therefore—in terms of absolute loss of life—the greatest single acute medical problem today.[7]

With the introduction of closed chest cardiac massage by Kouwenhoven, Jude, and Knickerbocker in 1960,[8] a new era in cardiac resuscitation began. Sudden death, previously an irreversible situation, became reversible in many instances with the effective application of these new procedures.

Today this is no longer the case. Death is not a surety. The overall outcome for victims of out-of-hospital cardiac arrest has improved. Though the rates of successful resuscitation from out-of-hospital cardiac arrest have shown but modest gains in the years since the 1960s, it must be remembered that before emergency medical services (EMS) became available, cardiac arrest was almost universally fatal, and that given the circumstances necessary for resuscitation to be successful, it is remarkable that anyone survives.[9]

The rationale for cardiac resuscitation outside the hospital is based on the fact that in most cases cardiac arrest is unexpected and cannot be predicted accurately in individual patients, thus effective preventive measures are lacking. Immediate efforts at resuscitation offer the only realistic hope for most victims.[9]

In some communities, such as Seattle, Washington, where advanced EMS systems exist, the rate of successful resuscitation and ultimate discharge home has more than doubled during the past decade.[10] Response time from dispatch until the arrival of a basic life support team averages less than 3 minutes in Seattle, with a paramedic unit capable of administering advanced cardiac life support (ACLS) arriving 4 minutes later. A result of this expeditious response is that up to 60% of cases of ventricular fibrillation are successfully resuscitated at the scene, with 25% surviving to leave the hospital.[10] In addition to Seattle's advanced EMS system, more than 33% of the population now know cardiopulmonary resuscitation (CPR).

Unfortunately, the results of Seattle's experience with out-of-hospital cardiac arrest have not been duplicated in many cities, although in cities with equivalent programs similar survival rates occur. Gray and others[11] found that in several New England communities, rates of resuscitation from out-of-hospital cardiac arrest average 20%, with even fewer patients surviving until hospital discharge. Other studies have reported discharge rates of 2% to 33% after cardiac arrests outside the hospital.[12] The low likelihood of survival after resuscitation efforts from out-of-hospital cardiac arrest are the result of several factors, some of which are related to fate (witnessed or unwitnessed arrest and the cardiac rhythm) and others related to the emergency response itself (length of time from collapse to the initiation of resuscitation efforts and defibrillation.[13,14] The absence of any single favorable condition in this "chain of survival" will result in an unsuccessful resuscitation.[15]

Eisenberg developed the "A-C-L-S" score to help estimate the likelihood of survival from out-of-hospital cardiac arrest.[3] These are the four factors comprising the more recent chain of survival.[15]

A—was the *A*rrest witnessed?

C—What was the original *C*ardiac rhythm documented by the paramedics upon arrival?

L—Was *L*ay bystander CPR performed?

S—How long did it take for help to arrive (i.e., *S*peed of paramedic response?)

Witnessed versus unwitnessed: During a 3-year period (1976 to 1979), 28% of 380 patients whose cardiac arrests were witnessed were ultimately discharged from the hospital, whereas only 3% of 231 victims of unwitnessed arrest survived.[3]

Initial rhythm: When the initial rhythm was either ventricular tachycardia (VT) (Fig. 30-1, *A*) or ventricular fibrillation (VF) (Fig. 30-1, *B*), survival rates are higher,[3,16] 28% of 389 patients survived, compared to a dismal 3% of 222 patients in asystole.[3] Survival is unusual (<5% of patients) when either electromechanical dissociation (EMD) (Fig. 30-1, *C*) or asystole (Fig. 30-1, *D*) is initially recorded.[9] In a series of nearly 1100 attempted resuscitations of patients found to have asystole, only 13 survived (0.012%).[17]

It is unlikely that EMD or asystole are the initial rhythms that precipitate the cardiac arrest. In patients sustaining cardiac arrest while undergoing continuous cardiac monitoring (Holter monitoring), ventricular tachycardia of varying duration is frequently noted as the precipitating mechanism of arrest.[18,19] Asystole and EMD probably represent secondary dysrhythmias succeeding VT and VF as the time from patient collapse to EMT arrival elapsed.

Bystander CPR: When bystander CPR was initiated, a 32% survival rate was noted, whereas the survival rate fell to 14% when basic life support (BLS) was delayed until the arrival of EMTs (emergency medical technicians).[9]

Response time: In situations in which paramedics were able to initiate ACLS within 4 minutes, 56% of the patients survived.[9] In other cities with response times as short as 3 to 5 minutes, survival rates of 25% to 33% are reported.[20,21] This rate fell to 35% when response time was between 4 and 8 minutes, and to 17% if response time exceeded 8 minutes.[9]

One factor that unites all four links of the chain of survival is time. The more quickly cardiac arrest is recognized, the more quickly resuscitation efforts are instituted by a bystander, and the more quickly advanced management is begun (ACLS), the greater the likelihood that the initial rhythm noted will be either VT or VF, and the greater the likelihood of an ultimately successful resuscitation.

Basic life support, by itself, is not a substitute for definitive treatment. Without the administration of adjunctive drugs, such as epinephrine, BLS will not result in adequate perfusion of vital organs such as the heart and the brain.[22] The performance of BLS simply buys a small quantity of time until definitive therapy can be provided.[23] Basic life support does not prevent VT or VF from deteriorating into EMD or asystole.[24]

The advent, in the 1960s, of emergency medical services systems involving mobile coronary care units staffed by trained paramedical personnel increased the likelihood of the chain of survival remaining intact. Early use of definitive therapy (defibrillation) led to a more than doubling of survival rates from out-of-hospital cardiac arrest.[12] Para-

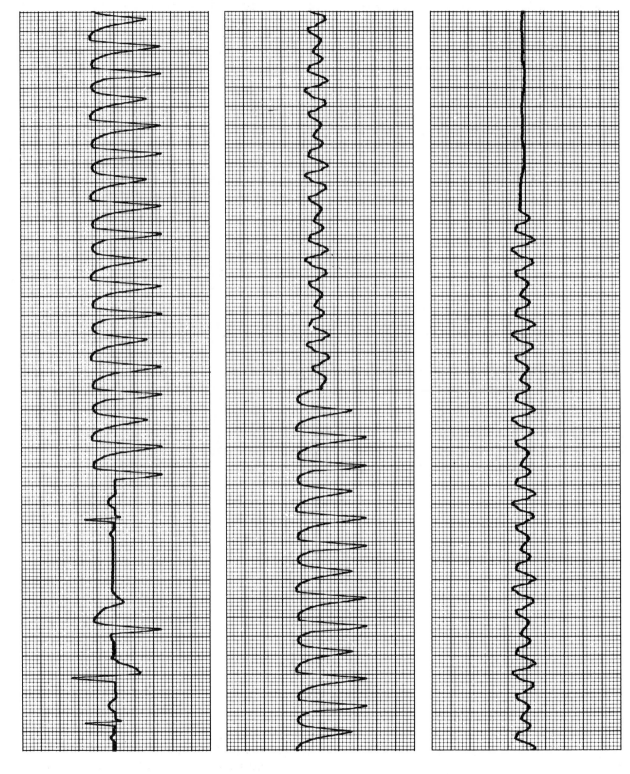

Fig. 30-1. Dysrhythmias leading to cardiac arrest. *Top,* premature ventricular contraction (PVC) leading to ventricular tachycardia (VT); *middle,* VT leading to ventricular fibrillation (VF); *bottom,* VF leading to asystole.

medical personnel have been taught to identify VF and to defibrillate effectively with as little as 10 hours of formal training.[12] Even when such persons were not permitted to administer drugs or to intubate, (i.e., defibrillation alone was permitted), lives were saved.[25]

The dental office: In the typical dental office situation it is highly unlikely that a cardiac arrest would go unwitnessed for more than a few seconds. Bystander CPR (BLS) would be initiated within a minute or so of the collapse of the victim, thereby providing that little extra time for the initiation of advanced resuscitative techniques.

As has been stressed throughout this text, the ability to effectively employ the steps of basic life support—airway, breathing, circulation—is absolutely critical in saving a life in an emergency situation. Up to this point, however, the emergencies presented have been situations in which one step (airway), or two steps (airway + breathing) of BLS were all that were required for effective patient management. The need for closed chest cardiac compression has been unnecessary. In the unlikely event that cardiopulmonary arrest does occur, rapid action by the entire dental office emergency team is required if the victim is to be successfully resuscitated.

Basic life support or cardiopulmonary resuscitation is readily carried out without the use of any adjunctive equipment or drug therapy. As described shortly, basic life support consists of airway maintenance, artificial ventilation, and external chest compression so that a continuous supply of oxygenated blood is delivered to the brain and heart, thereby preventing nonreversible (biologic) death and providing some additional time until advanced resuscitation procedures can be initiated.

CARDIOPULMONARY ARREST

Although disease of the cardiovascular system is the most common cause of sudden death (cardiopulmonary arrest), many other life-threatening situations may also terminate in this clinical entity (Table 30-1). Regardless of the precise nature of its cause, it is imperative that cardiac arrest be recognized and managed in as short a period of time as possible, minimizing the period of anoxia and increasing the likelihood of a successful outcome.

Cardiopulmonary arrest is comprised of two specific entities: pulmonary arrest and cardiac arrest. Pulmonary, or respiratory arrest occurs with cessation of effective respiratory movement, whereas cardiac arrest refers to the cessation of circulation or to circulation that is inadequate to sustain life.

Respiratory arrest may develop in the absence of cardiac arrest. However, if respiratory arrest is unmanaged or if managed ineffectively, cardiac function deteriorates, with cardiac arrest supervening in a short period of time, depending in part on the degree of oxygen deprivation and the underlying status of the patient's myocardium and coronary arteries. Cardiac arrest can occur in the absence of respiratory arrest (e.g., with electric shock); however, this is quite rare, especially within the dental environment, and in such circumstances respiratory arrest inevitably follows within a few seconds. In most instances, respiratory arrest precedes cardiac arrest.

Pulmonary (Respiratory) Arrest

Recognition and management of respiratory arrest have previously been described. The reader is referred to Chapter 5 for a complete discussion.

Cardiac Arrest

The term *cardiac arrest* must be defined to avoid possible confusion. At one time cardiac arrest was used to indicate that the heart had stopped beating, a situation referred to today as ventricular standstill or asystole. The meaning of the term cardiac arrest has been expanded to include other clinical situations in which the circulation of blood is absent or, if present, is inadequate to maintain life. Cardiac arrest as defined today may therefore result from

Table 30-1. Possible causes of cardiac arrest*

Cause	Frequency	Where discussed in text
Myocardial infarction	Most common	Chest pain (Section VII)
Sudden death (no other symptoms)	Most common	Cardiac arrest (Chapter 30)
Airway obstruction	Common	Respiratory difficulty (Section III)
Drug overdose reaction	Common	Drug-related emergencies (Section VI)
Anaphylaxis	Less common	Drug-related emergencies (Section VI)
Seizure disorders	Less common	Seizure disorders (Section V)
Acute adrenal insufficiency	Less common	Unconsciousness (Section II)

*All medical emergency situations may ultimately lead to cardiac arrest. In most instances prompt recognition and initiation of effective management of the specific situation prevents cardiac arrest from occurring.

any of the following: electromechanical dissociation (EMD), (pulseless) ventricular tachycardia (VT), ventricular fibrillation (VF), or ventricular standstill (asystole).

In electromechanical dissociation, the heart continues to beat but so weakly that effective circulation of blood throughout the cardiovascular system is not accomplished. This situaion may be caused by drugs, including local anesthetics, barbiturates, and narcotics, all of which are used in dentistry (see Chapter 23). Electromechanical dissociation more commonly results from severe hemorrhage and shock.

Ventricular fibrillation is a dysrhythmia in which the individual myocardial muscle bundles contract independently of each other as opposed to the normal, regular, coordinated, and synchronized contraction of myocardial fibers. Although myocardial elements are still contracting, little or no effective circulation is present. Ventricular fibrillation is a common occurrence in the period immediately following myocardial infarction (within the first 2 to 4 hours), and is the leading cause of death from ischemic heart disease. In humans, VF is 15 times more frequent during the first hour after the onset of signs and symptoms of acute myocardial infarction than during the following 12 hours.

Ventricular asystole or standstill refers to the absence of contractile movements of the myocardial fibers. Cardiac arrest in its strictest sense refers to ventricular standstill. A severe lack of oxygen to the myocardial muscle is the most common cause of this situation.

Although there are several forms of cardiac arrest (asystole, pulseless VT, VF, and electromechanical dissociation), in an emergency the precise nature of the arrest is not immediately known. The clinical picture of all three is the same: the victim loses consciousness, and respiration, blood pressure, and pulse are absent. Time is of the essence, because every second that passes without effective circulation adds to the degree of hypoxia or anoxia in the tissues of the body, to the development of respiratory and metabolic acidosis, and to rhythms such as asystole and EMD, from which effective resuscitation is unlikely.

The immediate clinical management of cardiopulmonary arrest is therefore based on the need to furnish the victim with a supply of well-oxygenated blood adequate to maintain life (prevent clinical death) until definitive management (ACLS) may be initiated.

CARDIOPULMONARY RESUSCITATION

The technique of cardiopulmonary resuscitation (CPR) has undergone intensive scrutiny by various segments of the medical community. Standardization of technique is being sought so that teaching the procedures will not lead to confusion among those called upon to use them.

In May 1973, the American Heart Association and the National Academy of Sciences National Research Council cosponsored a National Conference on Standards of Cardiopulmonary Resuscitation (CPR) and Emergency Cardiac Care (ECC), which for the first time presented standardized procedures for basic and advanced life support (American Heart Association, 1974). In the years since the first conference a significant body of research has added to our understanding of the phenomenon of cardiac arrest and cardiopulmonary resuscitation. In 1979 and 1985, a second and third conference, respectively, were called to update these standards. The technique of basic life support described in the following material and elsewhere in this text are those recommended by the 1985 conference.[7] In February 1992, a fourth conference was convened to reconsider and, if necessary, to update these guidelines. Though the recommendations of this conference have not yet been published (October, 1992), their suggestions have been included in the following discussion of technique, and it is expected that the formal guidelines for CPR will be published by early 1993.

Two broad areas of training in life support were established at these conferences. Basic life support and advanced cardiac life support represent differing degrees of training and responsibility in the management of the victim of cardiac arrest and implementation of cardiopulmonary resuscitation to maintain life until a victim recovers sufficiently to be transported to a hospital or until advanced cardiac life support becomes available. Basic life support includes the ABC steps of cardiopulmonary resuscitation (Fig. 30-2). Advanced cardiac life support consists of training in the following areas: basic life support; use of adjunctive equipment and techniques, such as endotracheal intubation and open chest internal cardiac compression; cardiac monitoring (electrocardiography) for recognition of dysrhythmias; defibrillation technique; establishment of an intravenous infusion; stabilization of the victim's condition; and the employment and use of definitive therapy, including the administration of drugs to correct acidosis and to assist in establishing and maintaining an effective cardiac rhythm and circulation.

The level of training in life support varies according to an individual's requirements. It is the author's recommendation that all dental office personnel receive certification in the basic life support

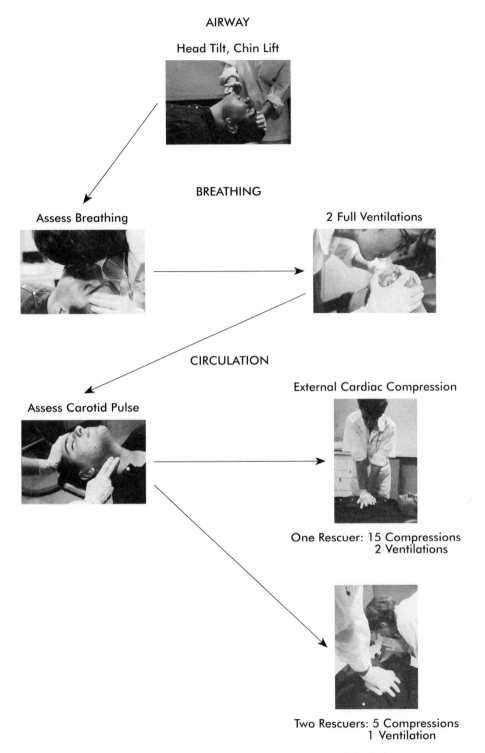

Fig. 30-2. Summary of basic life support for adult victim.

provider level C course, at the very minimum. More frequently today, dentists are receiving training and certification in advanced cardiac life support. Training at this level is invaluable because of the potential for complications arising that are associated with the administration of drugs, such as local anesthetics, antibiotics, analgesics, and sedatives. All other dental office personnel (dental hygienists, dental assistants, and nonchairside personnel) should be knowledgeable in and capable of proper application of the techniques of basic life support (BLS provider level C course).

Training in BLS should be repeated at least annually by all office personnel and more frequently if possible. Weaver and others[26] demonstrated that retention of skills by trainees who do not perform CPR regularly is quite limited. Only 11.7% of 61 trainees were capable of properly performing one-person CPR on mannequins, compared to 85% of the same group 6 months earlier.

Basic life support courses are sponsored by many organizations, including the American Heart Association, American Red Cross, dental societies, and fire departments. The BLS provider level C program involves training in four areas:

1. Single-rescuer CPR
2. Two-rescuer (team) CPR
3. Obstructed airway
4. Pediatric basic life support

Team Approach

In no other life-threatening situation is prompt recognition and management of greater importance than in cardiac arrest. Although it is possible for a single individual to effectively perform cardiopulmonary resuscitation, the procedure becomes even more efficient when a trained team of rescuers is available. The team approach to basic life support is described shortly (two-rescuer sequence). Dental office personnel should receive their training together so that they may interact effectively as a team when called on to do so.

Basic Life Support

As mentioned earlier, basic life support consists of the application, as needed, of the procedures of airway maintenance (A), breathing (B), and circulation by means of chest compression (C) to the victim of any medical emergency, including cardiac arrest, until recovery, or until the victim can be stabilized and transported to an emergency care facility or until advanced life support is available.

Two of the three components of cardiopulmonary resuscitation have previously been discussed. Airway maintenance and artificial ventilation in the

unconscious patient are outlined in Chapter 5; lower airway obstruction is discussed in Chapter 11. Together these comprise the A and B portions of cardiopulmonary resuscitation. Fig. 30-2 summarizes the important steps of basic life support.

Witnessed and Unwitnessed Cardiac Arrest

In the management of cardiac arrest, two separate clinical situations are considered (see accompanying box and on p. 432). In an unwitnessed cardiac arrest the victim is unconscious when discovered by the rescuer. The rescuer did not see the victim collapse and consequently has no knowledge about the length of time since the cessation of breathing and effective circulation. In such circumstances, it must be assumed that the collapse occurred more than 1 minute before the victim was discovered and the institution of basic life support procedures. In this situation the myocardium is considered to be hypoxic, with the sequencing of basic life support predicated on this fact. The witnessed cardiac arrest differs in that it develops in an ECG-monitored patient in the presence of the rescuer, and effective basic life support is administered within 1 minute of the collapse. The management sequence differs slightly in this situation because of the probability that the myocardium is still fairly well oxygenated at the time life support procedures are begun.

Cardiopulmonary arrest that occurs in a patient not monitored by ECG, even if the arrest is witnessed, is categorized and managed as an unwitnessed cardiac arrest.

MANAGEMENT OF WITNESSED, MONITORED CARDIAC ARREST

Recognize unconsciousness
↓
Call for help; position patient
↓
Deliver single precordial thump
↓
Open airway
↓
Check for breathing
↓
Ventilate four times
↓
Check carotid artery
↓
Begin external chest compression

The recommended sequence of steps in the management of each of these situations is presented shortly. Unless the rescuer is absolutely certain that the cardiopulmonary collapse occurred within 1 minute of discovery, it must be assumed that the heart is hypoxic, and the sequence for unwitnessed cardiac arrest is followed. Overall, most cardiac arrests are unwitnessed; however, within the dental office setting it is highly likely that office personnel will be available within 60 seconds of the collapse. In June 1979, the American Heart Association changed the criteria for the witnessed cardiac arrest to include only those situations in which the cardiac arrest occurs in an ECG-monitored patient,[27] the major emphasis of this section is on the unwitnessed cardiac arrest.

Cardiac Arrest in the Dental Office

Cardiac arrest, as well as any other life-threatening situation, may occur anywhere within the dental office. Medical emergencies have occurred in the waiting room, rest room, laboratory, and doctor's office, as well as in the treatment room.[28] In all situations the collapsed victim must be placed into the supine position so that BLS may be initiated. It is possible that the victim of cardiopulmonary arrest may be seated in the dental chair at the time of collapse. The question that must then be asked is: "Can effective cardiopulmonary resuscitation be performed with the victim remaining in the dental chair?" In past years before the advent of the contoured dental chair, the answer might have been yes. However, with the introduction of dental chairs designed for maximal comfort, it has become more difficult to adequately carry out chest compression if the victim is permitted to remain in the chair. The heart lies between two bony masses—the sternum, located anteriorly, and the spinal column, located posteriorly. With compression of the sternum toward the spinal column, intrathoracic pressure is raised, compressing the heart and blood vessels and thereby producing cardiac output. If the victim is lying on a soft surface (mattress or comfortable dental chair), the spinal column flexes and the force of the compression is partially absorbed by the soft surface, thereby lessening the effectiveness of the sternal compression. When properly performed against a hard surface, external chest compression can produce systolic blood pressure peaks of 100 torr, but the diastolic blood pressure is 0. The mean arterial blood pressure is rarely greater than 40 torr as measured in the carotid arteries. Blood flow through the carotid arteries to the cerebral circulation therefore is approximately only one quarter to one third of normal, at best. Basic life support performed on a soft backing is less effective and is contraindicated.

It is usually recommended that the victim of cardiac arrest be moved from the dental chair and placed onto the floor, if at all possible, so that BLS may be performed in a more effective manner. In most dental treatment rooms, however, there is little or no room available on the floor to place the victim and still permit one or two rescuers to perform BLS. In such a situation, or if it is difficult or impossible to move the victim to the floor, BLS should be initiated with the patient kept in the chair. If possible, a hard object such as a solid board (e.g., a removable cabinet top or a molded CPR backboard) should be placed under the victim to support the spinal cord (Fig. 30-3). Under no circumstances should basic life support be withheld or delayed because of the inability to move the victim to a more suitable location. "Bad CPR is better than no CPR."

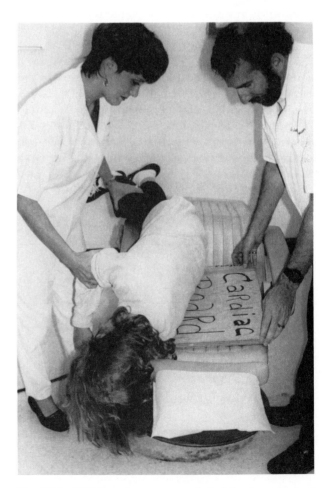

Fig. 30-3. CPR board to support victim's back and spinal cord during external chest compression.

In all of the following sequences, it is assumed that the patient (victim) has suffered a cardiac arrest—that is, the victim is unconscious and there is an absence of both respiration and circulation. It is critically important for the reader to fully understand that these basic steps (ABC) are equally important in the management of *all* emergency situations—not just cardiac arrest.

As has been demonstrated throughout this book, one of the initial steps in the management of every emergency situation is the implementation, as needed, of the steps of basic life support. This means that in every situation considered to be an emergency by the doctor or by any rescuer, the steps listed in the accompanying box must be followed.

Patient response to these steps will guide the rescuers in their management. In many instances in which the victim is conscious (e.g., with respiratory distress and/or altered consciousness), the rescuer need only to assess A, B, and C—a process requiring a few seconds. The patient will be effectively managing A, B, and C by himself or herself, permitting the rescuer to continue to step D—definitive management.

In another situation the rescuer may determine that the victim is unconscious (lack of response to sensory stimulation). Assessment of the airway and head tilt–chin lift are required; however, assessment of B and C may demonstrate the adequacy of spontaneous breathing and effective pulse. The rescuer need only maintain an airway while considering the definitive management of the situation.

These possibilities must be kept in mind as the following material is reviewed. Although A, B, and C are always assessed in every emergency situation, only those elements that are necessary for the victim's survival will be instituted clinically.

BASIC LIFE SUPPORT
Unwitnessed Cardiac Arrest

When cardiac arrest occurs in an unmonitored victim, the procedures described below for unwitnessed cardiac arrest must be instituted promptly. Following a description of these steps, we will review the basic sequences for the one-person rescue and the team rescue.

The following sequence of steps should be rapidly carried out by the rescuer in the unwitnessed cardiac arrest:

Step 1: Recognize unconsciousness. Stimulate the victim by gently shaking the shoulders and shouting. Lack of response to these sensory stimuli is a suitable criterion for establishing a diagnosis of unconsciousness (Fig. 30-4).

Many factors may be responsible for the loss of consciousness (see Table 5-1), most of which do not lead immediately to respiratory and cardiac arrest. However, prompt management of unconsciousness from any cause follows the identical format—basic life support. A differential diagnosis of uncon-

Assess level of consciousness
↓
Summon assistance
↓
Properly position the victim
↓
Assess and maintain airway (A), if necessary
↓
Assess spontaneous respirations (breathing, B) and perform artificial ventilation, if required
↓
Assess the adequacy of circulation (C); if absent, activate the emergency medical services system and perform external chest compressions

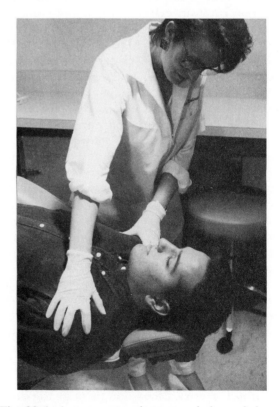

Fig. 30-4. Assess unconsciousness; shake and shout.

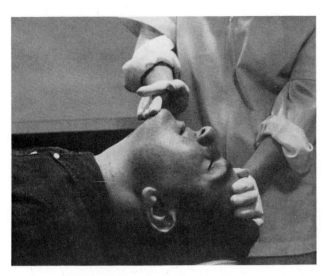

Fig. 30-5. Head tilt–chin lift.

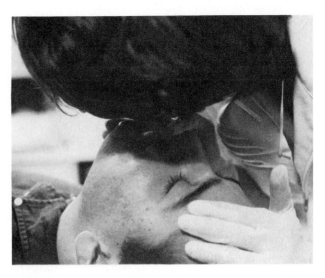

Fig. 30-6. Assess breathing: look, listen, and feel while maintaining head tilt–chin lift.

sciousness will be reached by assessing the response or lack of response of the victim to each of these steps.

Step 2: Summon assistance and position patient. The rescuer will not want to treat the victim alone, therefore assistance should be called for as soon as unconsciousness is recognized. Members of the office emergency team should report to the emergency area with the emergency drug kit and a supply of oxygen, and should be prepared to assist member one as required. This step does *not* involve activation of the emergency medical services system, just the dental office emergency team.

The patient should be placed into the supine position. The head and chest of the victim are placed parallel to the floor and the feet elevated slightly (10°) to facilitate return of blood from the periphery. At this time, before the determination of cardiovascular collapse, it is not yet necessary to place the victim on a hard surface. Once pulselessness is established, this procedure will be necessary.

Step 3: Assess and maintain airway. Head-tilt combined with chin-lift may be employed to obtain a patent airway. The rescuer places one hand on the victim's forehead, the other hand on the bony prominence of the chin (symphysis). The head is extended backward, stretching the tissues in the neck and lifting the tongue off of the posterior wall of the pharynx (Fig. 30-5). Head-tilt is the single most important procedure in airway maintenance. Should head-tilt be ineffective in establishing a patent airway, the jaw-thrust maneuver can be employed.

Step 4: Assess breathing and ventilate, if needed. While maintaining head-tilt, the rescuer places his or her ear approximately 1 inch from the victim's mouth and nose so that any exhaled air may be felt and heard. The rescuer looks toward the chest of the victim to see if spontaneous respiratory efforts are visible (Fig. 30-6). With cardiopulmonary arrest, respiratory efforts are absent or are so weak as to be essentially nonexistent.

Step 5: Artificial ventilation. In the absence of effective respiratory movement, artificial ventilation must immediately be started. Several techniques of artificial ventilation are discussed in Chapter 5; however, in this section only one—mouth-to-mouth (or mask) ventilation—is considered. Other techniques may also be used, but it must be remembered that no technique of artificial ventilation is effective unless a patent airway is maintained throughout the ventilatory process. Most other devices for artificial ventilation require advanced training (advanced cardiac life support) to adequately prepare the rescuer to use them.

To perform mouth-to-mouth ventilation, head-tilt must be maintained and the nose of the victim sealed (Fig. 30-7). The first ventilatory cycle is comprised of two full ventilations with adequate time (1 to 1½ seconds per breath) allowed to provide good chest expansion and to minimize the risk of gastric distention. Effective artificial ventilation is noted by expansion of the victim's chest. In the normal adult the minimal volume of air should be 800 mL per breath but need not exceed 1200 mL for adequate ventilation. The process of exhalation is passive, with the rescuer removing his or her

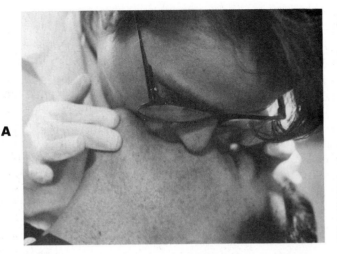
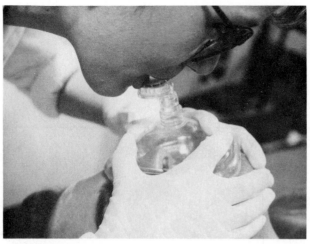

Fig. 30-7.. A, Mouth-to-mouth ventilation. **B,** Mouth to mask ventilation.

mouth from that of the victim, taking in a breath of fresh air, and watching the chest fall. Subsequent ventilations are performed at a rate of one every 5 seconds (12 per minute) for the adult victim. In the child, ventilations are carried out at a rate of one every 4 seconds (15 per minute), and in the infant, one every 3 seconds (20 per minute). Immediately following the first ventilatory cycle of two full breaths, the rescuer should determine the victim's cardiovascular status.

When using mouth-to-mask ventilation, the mask is held in position with one or two hands as needed, maintaining both an air-tight seal and a patent airway. The mouth of the rescuer is placed on the breathing port and air is forced into the victim until the chest is seen to rise. The rates of ventilation are the same as those already mentioned.

Step 6: Assess circulation. Having oxygenated the blood, the rescuer next determines the presence or absence of effective circulation. A large artery must be located and carefully palpated. The femoral artery in the groin and the carotid artery in the neck are two large, central arteries. Although either may be palpated, the carotid artery is preferred. It is located in the neck region and can be accessed easily without disrobing the victim. In addition, the carotid artery transports oxygenated blood to the victim's brain, the organ that must be adequately perfused if successful resuscitation is to occur.

The carotid artery is located in a groove between the trachea and the sternocleidomastoid muscle on the anterolateral aspect of the neck (Fig. 30-8). The fleshy portions of the first and second fingers of the rescuer should be used to feel for a pulse. Up

to 10 seconds should be allowed for this procedure because the pulse, if present, may be very slow or very weak and rapid. The thumb should never be used to monitor a pulse because the thumb contains a medium-sized artery and the heart rate recorded may be that of the rescuer instead of the victim's. Unless the carotid pulse is unquestionably present, external chest compression should be initiated immediately. At this point the victim should be placed on the floor, if this is practical (it often is not), or left in the dental chair with a stable support, such as a CPR board, placed under the victim's back.

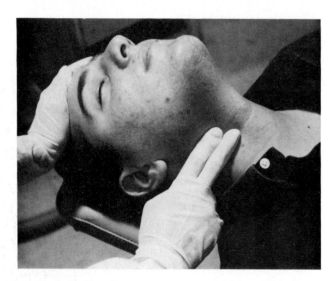

Fig. 30-8. Locate carotid artery in groove between trachea and sternocleidomastoid muscle. Head-tilt must be maintained.

Step 7: Activate emergency medical system (EMS). The EMS should be activated following the pulse check. Many communities employ the universal emergency number, 9-1-1; however, the appropriate telephone number for your locality should be called. Information given to the EMS dispatcher should include the following:

1. Location of the emergency (with names of cross streets, if possible)
2. Number of telephone from which the call is made
3. What happened (e.g., heart attack, seizure, accident)
4. How many persons need help
5. Condition of the victim(s)
6. What aid is being given to the victim(s)
7. Any other information requested

To ensure that EMS personnel have no more questions, the caller should hang up last. When more than one rescuer is available, one person is sent immediately to activate the EMS. Eisenberg and others[29] demonstrated that the shorter the time interval between collapse and the initiation of BLS and advanced cardiac life support, the greater the likelihood of survival for the victim of cardiac arrest (Table 30-2).

If only one rescuer is present, it is recommended that he or she continue BLS for 1 minute and then telephone for assistance as quickly as possible. Should the solo rescuer feel that there is a good chance of someone else arriving on the scene shortly, it may be decided to continue BLS until help arrives instead of making a telephone call. Should the rescuer be alone with no telephone available, the only option is to continue BLS.

Step 8: External chest compression. External chest compression consists of the rhythmic application of pressure over the lower half of the adult sternum. The heart lies under and just to the left of the

Table 30-2. Survival rate from cardiac arrest resulting from ventricular fibrillation, as related to promptness of initiation of CPR and ACLS*

Initiation of CPR (minutes)	Arrival of ACLS (minutes)	Survival rate (%)
0-4	0-8	43
0-4	16+	10
8-12	8-16	6
8-12	16+	0
12+	12+	0

From Eisenberg MS, Bergner L, Hallstrom A: Cardiac resuscitation in the community: importance of rapid provision and implications for program planning, *JAMA* 241:1905, 1979.
*Data from Project Restart, King County, Washington.

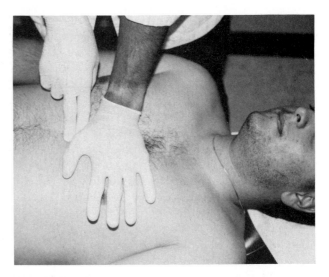

Fig. 30-9. Proper location for adult external chest compression.

midline under the lower half of the sternum and above the spinal column. When the sternum is compressed, intrathoracic pressure is increased; it is this increased pressure that produces the cardiac output by compressing the vessels within the chest cavity and forcing blood back to and through the heart. With release of this pressure, blood from the periphery flows back into the heart to refill its chambers.

Effective artificial ventilation and artificial circulation can provide sufficient oxygen to prevent cellular death. Two theories, the cardiac pump theory[30] and the thoracic pump theory,[31] seek to explain the mechanism of blood flow during external chest compression.

Location of pressure point. To perform effective external chest compression and to minimize injury to other organs (lungs, liver, heart), the rescuer's hands must be properly positioned. This area may be located by using the following maneuver (Fig. 30-9). The rescuer, located at the victim's shoulders, runs his or her middle finger in a superior direction along the lower border of the rib cage until the midline is reached. Directly below this midline notch, created by the convergence of the ribs, is the cartilaginous xiphoid process, which curves downward, and the liver. The rescuer's middle finger should be located in the notch, the index finger lying beside it on the lower border of the sternum. The rescuer then places the heel of the second hand over the midline of the sternum immediately next to the index finger. This is the proper location for external chest compression in an adult.

In the child (ages 1 through 8 years) the proper site for chest compression is located in a manner similar to that described for the adult:

1. The lower margin of the victim's rib cage is located with the rescuer's middle and index fingers.
2. The margin of the rib cage is followed with the middle finger to the notch in the midline where the right and left side ribs meet.
3. With the middle finger in this notch, the index finger is placed next to the middle finger.
4. The heel of the hand is placed next to the index finger with the long axis of the heel parallel to that of the sternum.
5. The chest is compressed with one hand to a depth of 1 to 1½ inches (2.5 to 3.8 cm) at a rate of 80 to 100 compressions per minute.

In the infant (under 1 year of age) the site of compression is somewhat different (Fig. 30-10). Recent evidence has shown that the heart of the infant is lower in relation to external chest landmarks than was previously thought.[32] Proper hand position for chest compression in the infant is located in the following manner:

1. An imaginary line is drawn between the nipples located over the sternum (intermammary line).
2. The index finger of the hand farthest from the infant's head is placed just under this intermammary line where it intersects the sternum. The area of compression is one finger's width below this intersection, at the location of the middle and ring fingers.

3. Using two or three fingers, the sternum is compressed to a depth of ½ to 1 inch (1.3 to 2.5 cm) at a rate of at least 100 compressions per minute.

Hand position. Having determined the proper location for chest compression, the rescuer must align the hands properly so that maximal effectiveness may be achieved. In the adult victim the heel of the first hand is already in position on the midsternum of the victim approximately 1.5 to 2 inches (4 to 5 cm) above the xiphoid process. It is essential that only the heel of this hand contact the chest wall. The heel of the second hand is next placed directly over the first hand, parallel to it (Fig. 30-11). The fingers of the two hands are then interlaced, with the fingers of the top hand pulling the fingers of the lower hand upward. In this manner only the heel of the lower hand remains in contact with the victim's chest. An alternative hand position, especially useful for persons with arthritis of the hand or wrist, is to grasp the wrist of the hand on the chest wall with the hand that had been locating the lower end of the sternum.

These procedures are important because if the fingers of the hand contact the chest wall, the pressures exerted in chest compression will be delivered over a larger area and will therefore be less effective in increasing intrathoracic pressure. In addition, this pressure will be extended to the ribs, not just the sternum, leading to an increased probability of costochondral separation or rib fracture, with possible contusion and laceration of the heart and lungs.

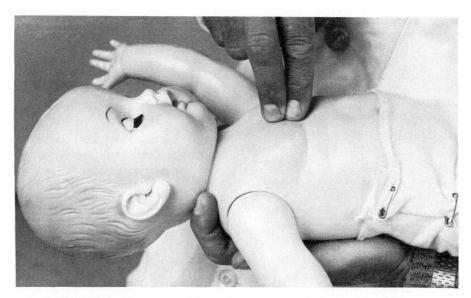

Fig. 30-10. Proper location for infant external chest compression.

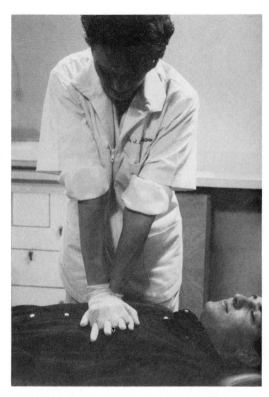

Fig. 30-11. Hand position for adult external chest compression.

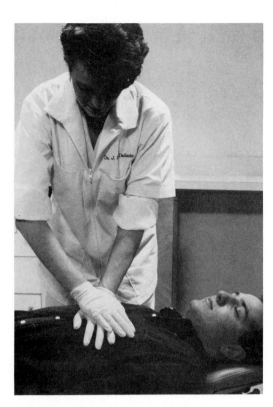

Fig. 30-12. Improper position: elbow of rescuer should be locked (straight), not bent.

Application of pressure. Having determined the location for chest compression and positioning the hands properly, the rescuer can begin chest compression. External chest compression (ECC) is strenuous. However, when ECC is performed properly, the trained rescuer does not become exhausted rapidly. Improperly performed, ECC is rapidly exhausting as well as ineffective. The following points facilitate the implementation of ECC with maximal effectiveness and minimal fatigue: The shoulders of the rescuer must be located directly over the sternum of the victim, and the rescuer's arms should be locked straight, not bent (Fig. 30-12). If the victim is lying on the floor, the rescuer must kneel beside the victim, close enough to the body so that the rescuer's shoulders are directly over the victim's sternum. If the victim is in the dental chair, the rescuer stands astride the victim, and the chair is lowered so that proper positioning may be achieved (Fig. 30-13, *A*).

Improper positioning of the shoulders at an angle to the sternum decreases the effectiveness of chest compression and increases the likelihood of complications related to costochondral separation from the stretching of ribs on one side, and fracture of ribs from the bending of ribs on the opposite side (Fig. 30-13, *B*). Bending the elbows greatly decreases the effectiveness of ECC and leads to rapid fatigue of the rescuer.

The rescuer then exerts pressure directly downward so that the sternum of the adult victim is depressed 1½ to 2 inches (3.8 to 5 cm). With proper shoulder and arm placement, the rescuer allows the weight of his or her body to compress the sternum of the victim. Movement of the rescuer occurs only at the hips; it should be a gentle back-and-forth rocking motion if the technique is properly executed. Compressions must be regular, smooth, and uninterrupted. Relaxation follows compressions immediately and is of equal duration. The heel of the rescuer's hand must not be removed from the chest during relaxation, but pressure on the sternum should be completely released so that the sternum returns to its normal position between compressions.

The infant's chest is compressed ½ to 1 inch (1.3 to 2.5 cm) just below the intermammary line using the tips of two or three fingers, while the chest of the child is compressed 1 to 1½ inches (2.5 to 2.8 cm) using the heel of one hand (Fig. 30-14). Basic life support techniques for the adult, infant, and child are summarized in Table 30-3.

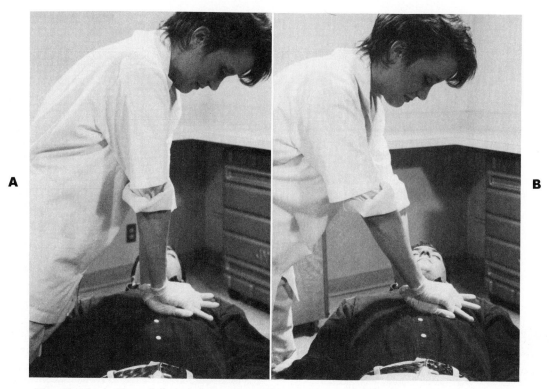

Fig. 30-13. A, Dental chair is lowered to allow rescuer to bring shoulders directly over sternum of victim. **B,** Improper positioning increases risk of injury to victim.

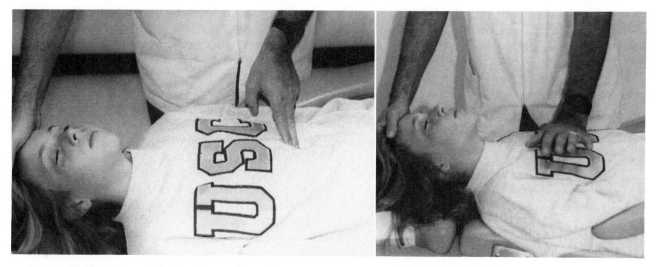

Fig. 30-14. Hand position for external chest compression in child.

Table 30-3. Summary of CPR techniques

Victim	Respirations per minute	Interval (seconds)	Ratio of compression to ventilation	Compressions				
				Rate/min	Depth (inches)	Depth (cm)	Hands	Site
Infant (<1 year of age)	20	3	5:1	100	½-1	1.3-2.5	2-3 fingers	One fingerwidth below intermammary line, midsternum
Child (1-8 years of age)	15	4	5:1	80-100	1-1½	2.5-3.8	1 heel	Midsternum
Adult (>8 years of age)	12	5	5:1	80-100	1½-2	3.8-5.0	2 hands	Lower half of sternum
One rescuer	8	—	15:2					
Two rescuers	12	—	5:1					

Rate of compression. A change in the rate of chest compression was recommended in the 1986 guidelines. The rate was increased to a minimum of 80 per minute, 100 per minute if possible. When BLS is being performed by a team of two persons, one rescuer is responsible for airway and breathing, whereas the second rescuer carries out chest compression. In this case chest compression is performed at a rate of 80 to 100 per minute with artificial ventilation interspersed after every fifth compression. In the two-rescuer sequence, the ratio of chest compression to artificial ventilation is 5:1 with a pause of 1 to 1.5 seconds for ventilation.

When only one rescuer is available, that person is responsible for both ventilation and chest compression. In the single-rescuer sequence the ratio of chest compression to artificial ventilation is 15:2. However, to compress the chest 60 times and to intersperse eight ventilations in 60 seconds, the rate of chest compressions must be faster than one per second. Fifteen chest compressions are followed by two full breaths, allowing 1 to 1.5 seconds per ventilation. Four complete cycles of 15 compressions and two ventilations should be completed in approximately 1 minute with a single rescuer. To do so effectively, it has been the author's experience that the 15 chest compressions should be completed in approximately 9 to 11 seconds. The remaining time permits the rescuer to move to the head, deliver two full breaths, relocate the site for chest compression, and prepare to restart chest compression.

In the infant and child, the compression to ventilation ratio is 5:1 in both single and team rescue situations. Compression rates are 100 per minute in infants and 80 to 100 per minute in the child. Fig. 30-2 summarizes the management of the unwitnessed cardiac arrest in the adult.

Single Rescue for Adults

Clinical application of the technique of basic life support for the single rescuer in a case of unwitnessed cardiac arrest is based on the techniques described earlier. When dealing with cardiac arrest and possible neurologic damage, the time element becomes critical. The chart on p. 440 presents performance criteria for one-rescuer CPR (American Heart Association).

The first steps in the sequence involve the recognition of unconsciousness, calling for assistance, and positioning the victim. The process of calling for help needs clarification. When the unconscious victim is found by a lone rescuer, calling for help simply means yelling loudly for assistance. It does not mean leaving the victim to seek assistance, nor does it mean taking time to place a telephone call. Every second that is not spent performing effective BLS decreases the chance of recovery for the victim.

The rescuer is positioned so that artificial ventilation and artificial circulation may be carried out with minimal movement. The most nearly ideal position for the rescuer is astride the shoulders of the victim so that both procedures may be performed merely by bending at the waist.

Airway patency is ensured through the head tilt–chin lift or the jaw-thrust maneuver, or both, and the rescuer checks for spontaneous respiratory movement (look, listen, feel). In the absence of such movement, the rescuer ventilates the victim with two full breaths at 1 to 1.5 seconds per ventilation. Chest deflation should be noted between breaths.

With the blood of the victim now oxygenated, the rescuer assesses circulatory status by palpating for the carotid pulse. This important step must not be hurried. Allow 5 to 10 seconds to determine pulselessness.

CPR and ECC Performance Sheet
One-Rescuer CPR: Adult
Name _____ Date: _____

Step	Activity	Critical performance	S	U
1. Airway	Assessment: Determine unresponsiveness	Tap or gently shake shoulder		
		Shout, "Are you OK?"		
	Call for help	Call out "Help!"		
	Position the victim	Turn on back as unit, if necessary, supporting head and neck (4-10 sec)		
	Open the airway	Use head tilt–chin lift maneuver		
2. Breathing	Assessment: Determine breathlessness	Maintain open airway		
		Ear over mouth, observe chest: look, listen, feel for breathing (3-5 sec)		
	Ventilate twice	Maintain open airway		
		Seal mouth and nose properly		
		Ventilate 2 times at 1-1.5 sec/inspiration		
		Observe chest rise (adequate ventilation volume)		
		Allow deflation between breaths		
3. Circulation	Assessment: Determine pulselessness	Feel for carotid pulse on near side of victim (5-10 sec)		
		Maintain head-tilt with other hand		
	Activate EMS system	If someone responded to call for help, send him/her to activate EMS system		
		Total time, Step 1—Activate EMS system: 15-35 sec		
	Begin chest compressions	Rescuer kneels by victim's shoulders		
		Landmark check prior to hand placement		
		Proper hand position throughout		
		Rescuer's shoulders over victim's sternum		
		Equal compression-relaxation		
		Compress 1½ to 2 inches		
		Keep hands on sternum during upstroke		
		Complete chest relaxation on upstroke		
		Say any helpful mnemonic		
		Compression rate: 80-100/min (15 per 9-11 sec)		
4. Compression/ventilation cycles	Do 4 cycles of 15 compressions and 2 ventilations	Proper compression/ventilation ratio: 15 compressions to 2 ventilations per cycle		
		Observe chest rise: 1-1.5 sec/inspiration; 4 cycles/52-73 sec		
5. Reassessment*	Determine pulselessness (If no pulse: step 6)†	Feel for carotid pulse (5 sec)		
6. Continue CPR	Ventilate twice	Ventilate twice		
		Observe chest rise; 1-1.5 sec/inspiration		
	Resume compression/ventilation cycles	Feel for carotid pulse every few minutes		

*Second rescuer arrives to replace first rescuer: (1) Second rescuer identifies self by saying "I know CPR. Can I help?" (2) Second rescuer then does pulse check in step 5 and continues with step 6. (During practice and testing only one rescuer actually ventilates the mannequin. The second rescuer simulates ventilation.) (3) First rescuer assesses the adequacy of second rescuer's CPR by observing chest rise during ventilations and by checking the pulse during chest compressions. †If pulse is present, open airway and check for spontaneous breathing: (1) If breathing is present, maintain open airway and monitor pulse and breathing. (2) If breathing is absent, perform rescue breathing at 12 times/min and monitor pulse.
Instructor _____ Check: Satisfactory _____ Unsatisfactory _____

CPR and ECC Performance Sheet
Two-Rescuer CPR: Adult*

Name _____ Date: _____

Step	Activity	Critical performance	S	U
1. Airway	One rescuer (ventilator): Assessment: Determine unresponsiveness	Tap or gently shake shoulder		
		Shout, "Are you OK?"		
	Positions the victim	Turn on back if necessary (4-10 sec)		
	Opens the airway	Use a proper technique to open airway		
2. Breathing	Assessment: Determine breathlessness	Look, listen, and feel (3-5 sec)		
	Ventilator ventilates twice	Observe chest rise: 1-1.5 sec/inspiration		
3. Circulation	Assessment: Determines pulselessness States assessment results	Palpate carotid pulse (5-10 sec)		
		Say, "No pulse"		
	Other rescuer (compressor): Gets into position for compressions	Hands, shoulders in correct position		
	Locates landmark notch	Landmark check		
4. Compression/ventilation cycles	Compressor begins chest compressions	Correct ratio compressions/ventilations: 5/1		
		Compression rate: 80-100/min (5 compressions/3-4 sec)		
		Say any helpful mnemonic		
		Stop compressing for each ventilation		
	Ventilator ventilates after every fifth compression and checks compression effectiveness	Ventilate 1 time (1-1.5 sec) Check pulse to assess compressions		
	(Minimum of 10 cycles)	Time for 10 cycles: 40-53 sec		
5. Call for switch	Compressor calls for switch when fatigued	Give clear signal to change		
		Compressor completes fifth compression		
		Ventilator completes ventilation after fifth compression		
6. Switch	Simultaneously switch:			
	Ventilator moves to chest	Move to chest		
		Become compressor		
		Get into position for compressions		
		Locate landmark notch		
	Compressor moves to head	Move to head		
		Become ventilator		
		Check carotid pulse (5 sec)		
		Say, "No pulse"		
		Ventilate once†		
7. Continue CPR	Resume compression/ventilation cycles	Resume step 4.		

*(1) If CPR is in progress with one rescuer (layperson), the entrance of the two rescuers occurs after the completion of one rescuer's cycle of 15 compressions and 2 ventilations. The EMS should be activated first. The two new rescuers start with step 6. (2) If CPR is in progress with one professional rescuer, the entrance of a second professional rescuer is at the end of a cycle after check for pulse by first rescuer. The new cycle starts with one ventilation by the first rescuer, and the second rescuer becomes the compressor. †During practice and testing only one rescuer actually ventilates the mannequin. The other rescuer simulates ventilation.

Instructor _____ Check: Satisfactory _____ Unsatisfactory _____

CPR and ECC Performance Sheet
One-Rescuer CPR: Infant
Name _____ Date: _____

Step	Activity	Critical performance	S	U
1. Airway	Assessment: Determine unresponsiveness	Tap or gently shake shoulder		
	Call for help	Call out "Help!"		
	Position the infant	Turn on back as unit, supporting head and neck		
		Place on firm, hard surface		
	Open the airway	Use head tilt–chin lift maneuver to sniffing or neutral position		
		Do not overextend the head		
2. Breathing	Assessment: Determine breathlessness	Maintain open airway		
		Ear over mouth, observe chest: look, listen, feel for breathing (3-5 sec)		
	Ventilate twice	Maintain open airway		
		Make tight seal on infant's mouth and nose with rescuer's mouth		
		Ventilate 2 times, 1-1.5 sec/inspiration		
		Observe chest rise		
		Allow deflation between breaths		
3. Circulation	Assessment: Determine pulselessness	Feel for brachial pulse (5-10 sec)		
		Maintain head-tilt with other hand		
	Activate EMS system	If someone responded to call for help, send him/her to activate EMS system		
		Total time, step 1—Activate EMS system: 15-35 sec		
	Begin chest compressions	Draw imaginary line between nipples		
		Place 2-3 fingers on sternum, 1 finger's width below imaginary line		
		Equal compression-relaxation		
		Compress vertically, ½ to 1 inches		
		Keep fingers on sternum during upstroke		
		Complete chest relaxation on upstroke		
		Say any helpful mnemonic		
		Compression rate: at least 100/min (5 in 3 sec or less)		
4. Compression/ventilation cycles	Do 10 cycles of 5 compressions and 1 ventilation	Proper compression/ventilation ratio: 5 compressions to 1 slow ventilation per cycle		
		Pause for ventilation		
		Observe chest rise: 1-1.5 sec/inspiration; 10 cycles/45 sec or less		
5. Reassessment	Determine pulselessness (If no pulse: step 6)*	Feel for brachial pulse (5 sec)		
6. Continue CPR	Ventilate once	Ventilate once		
		Observe chest rise; 1-1.5 sec/inspiration		
	Resume compression/ventilation cycles	Feel for brachial pulse every few minutes		

*If pulse is present, open airway and check for spontaneous breathing. (1) If breathing is present, maintain open airway and monitor breathing and pulse. (2) If breathing is absent, perform rescue breathing at 20 times/min and monitor pulse.
Instructor _____ Check: Satisfactory _____ Unsatisfactory _____

CPR and ECC Performance Sheet
One-Rescuer CPR: Child*
Name _____ Date: _____

Step	Activity	Critical performance	S	U
1. Airway	Assessment: Determine unresponsiveness	Tap or gently shake shoulder		
		Shout, "Are you OK?"		
	Call for help	Call out "Help!"		
	Position the victim	Turn on back as unit, if necessary, supporting head and neck (4-10 sec)		
	Open the airway	Use head tilt–chin lift maneuver		
2. Breathing	Assessment: Determine breathlessness	Maintain open airway		
		Ear over mouth, observe chest: look, listen, feel for breathing (3-5 sec)		
	Ventilate twice	Maintain open airway		
		Seal mouth and nose properly		
		Ventilate 2 times at 1-1.5 sec/inspiration		
		Observe chest rise		
		Allow deflation between breaths		
3. Circulation	Assessment: Determine pulselessness	Feel for carotid pulse on near side of victim (5-10 sec)		
		Maintain head-tilt with other hand		
	Activate EMS system	If someone responded to call for help, send him/her to activate EMS system		
		Total time, step 1—Activate EMS system: 15-35 sec		
	Begin chest compressions	Rescuer kneels by victim's shoulders		
		Landmark check prior to initial hand placement		
		Proper hand position throughout		
		Rescuer's shoulders over victim's sternum		
		Equal compression-relaxation		
		Compress 1 to 1½ inches		
		Keep hands on sternum during upstroke		
		Complete chest relaxation on upstroke		
		Say any helpful mnemonic		
		Compression rate: 80-100/min (5 per 3-4 sec)		
4. Compression/ventilation cycles	Do 10 cycles of 5 compressions and 1 ventilation	Proper compression/ventilation ratio: 5 compressions to 1 slow ventilation per cycle		
		Observe chest rise, 1-1.5 sec/inspiration (10 cycles/60-87 sec)		
5. Reassessment†	Determine pulselessness (if no pulse: step 6)‡	Feel for carotid pulse (5 sec)		
6. Continue CPR	Ventilate once	Ventilate once		
		Observe chest rise; 1-1.5 sec/inspiration		
	Resume compression/ventilation cycles	Palpate carotid pulse every few minutes		

*If child is above age of approximately 8 years, the method for adults should be used.
†Second rescuer arrives to replace first rescuer: (1) Second rescuer identifies self by saying, "I know CPR. Can I help?" (2) Second rescuer then does pulse check in step 5 and continues with step 6. (During practice and testing only one rescuer actually ventilates the mannequin. The second rescuer simulates ventilation.) (3) First rescuer assesses the adequacy of second rescuer's CPR by observing chest rise during ventilations and by checking the pulse during chest compressions. ‡If pulse is present, open airway and check for spontaneous breathing. (1) If breathing is present, maintain open airway and monitor breathing and pulse. (2) If breathing is absent, perform rescue breathing at 15 times/min and monitor pulse.
Instructor _____ Check: Satisfactory _____ Unsatisfactory _____

In the absence of effective circulation, the emergency medical services (EMS) system is activated, and external chest compression is immediately begun. The proper site for compression on the lower half of the adult sternum is located using the maneuver described earlier.

With elbows locked and shoulders directly over the sternum, the chest of the adult victim is depressed approximately 1½ to 2 inches (4 to 5 cm) at a rate of 80 to 100 compressions per minute. The rescuer should count silently or softly to himself or herself during this sequence and after 15 compressions immediately give two full lung inflations (1 to 1.5 seconds each), allowing complete lung deflation to occur between each breath.* One complete 15:2 sequence should take approximately 15 seconds. The rescuer then immediately relocates the pressure point on the sternum and repeats the cycle of 15 compressions and two ventilations so that four complete cycles may be performed in approximately 1 minute. After the first four cycles and periodically thereafter, the rescuer stops to reassess the pulse and breathing of the victim.

Two-Rescuer CPR for Adults (see chart on p. 441)

With two or more rescuers present to perform cardiopulmonary resuscitation, it is possible to carry out artificial ventilation and chest compressions without interruption. The 1986 guidelines present two scenarios for two rescuers, both of which follow.

One-rescuer CPR with entry of a second rescuer. This scenario is recommended for use by persons who are not health care professionals and may not be proficient in the two-person protocol.

When a second rescuer becomes available, he or she is sent immediately to activate the EMS system if this has not previously been done and to perform one-rescuer CPR in the event the first rescuer becomes fatigued. The following sequence is recommended:

1. Second rescuer identifies himself or herself as CPR certified and willing to help.
2. First rescuer stops CPR after the next two ventilations.
3. Second rescuer kneels down and checks for the carotid pulse for 15 seconds.

4. If pulse is absent, second rescuer gives two breaths.
5. Then second rescuer begins external chest compression at a 15:2 ratio at a rate of 80 to 100 compressions per minute.
6. Meanwhile, the first rescuer assesses the adequacy of the second rescuer's efforts.

CPR performed by two rescuers. This scenario is recommended for all health care professionals.

The use of mouth-to-mask ventilation is an acceptable alternative to mouth-to-mouth ventilation in this scenario because it is recommended that all health care professionals be adequately trained to use such devices.

One person performs external chest compression while the second rescuer remains at the victim's head, maintains a patent airway, monitors the carotid pulse for adequacy of external chest compressions, and provides rescue breathing. The compression rate for two-rescuer CPR is 80 to 100 per minute with a pause of 1 to 1.5 seconds per ventilation and a compression/ventilation ratio of 5:1. When the compressor becomes fatigued, the rescuers should change position as soon as possible.

The following sequence is used if one-rescuer CPR is in progress when the second rescuer arrives on the scene:

1. The most appropriate time for entry of the second rescuer is immediately following the completion of a cycle of 15 compressions and 2 ventilations.
   a. One rescuer moves to the head of the victim, opens the airway, and checks for a pulse.
   b. The second rescuer, positioned on the opposite side of the victim, locates the area for external chest compression and locates the proper hand position (Fig. 30-15).
2. If no pulse is present, the ventilator gives one breath and the compressor starts external chest compression at the rate of 80 to 100 per minute, counting "one-and, two-and, three-and, four-and, five."
3. After the fifth compression a pause of 1 to 1.5 seconds is allowed for ventilation.
4. The compression/ventilation ratio is 5:1.

In the event that no CPR is in progress and both professional rescuers arrive at the same time, the following sequence is followed: First, one rescuer ensures that the EMS system has been activated. If this person must leave the area, the second rescuer initiates one-rescuer CPR. However, if both persons are available for CPR:

---

*Studies have shown that rescuers counting silently or softly can perform CPR effectively for longer durations than those counting out loud. It requires more energy expenditure to count aloud; however, when a second rescuer appears to aid, counting aloud is essential.

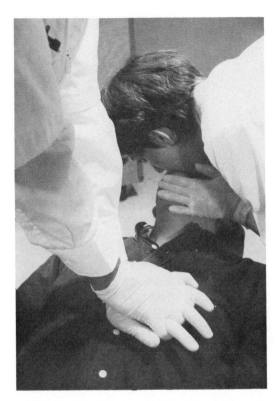

Fig. 30-15. Rescuer positions for two-person CPR.

1. One rescuer goes to the head of the victim and
   a. Determines unresponsiveness ("shake and shout")
   b. Positions the victim
   c. Opens the airway
   d. Assesses breathing
   e. If breathing is absent, says, "No breathing," and gives two ventilations
   f. Assesses circulation
   g. If pulse is absent, says, "No pulse"
2. The second rescuer simultaneously
   a. Finds the location for external chest compression
   b. Locates the proper hand position
   c. Initiates external chest compressions after the first rescuer states, "No pulse"

When one rescuer, usually the compressor, gets fatigued, the rescuers change position as rapidly as possible. The sequence for change in two-rescuer CPR was simplified in the 1986 guidelines. The compressor calls for a switch when fatigued and completes the fifth compression. The ventilator then gives one full ventilation. Both rescuers then switch positions. The original ventilator moves to the victim's chest, gets in position to administer external chest compressions, and locates the land-

---

BASIC LIFE SUPPORT

Recognize unconsciousness and call for help
↓
Position patient in supine position
↓
Open airway (head tilt–chin lift)
↓
Check for breathing and airway patency (look, listen, feel)
↓
Jaw-thrust maneuver, if necessary
↓
Recheck breathing and airway patency, if necessary
↓
Artificial ventilation, if necessary
↓
Check circulation
↓
Activate EMS system
↓
Perform external chest compression, if necessary

---

mark for compressions. The original compressor moves to the victim's head, checks the carotid pulse for 5 seconds, and if it is absent says, "No pulse," and ventilates once. The new chest compressor immediately begins chest compression at the rate of 5 compressions in approximately 3 to 4 seconds. A total of 10 cycles of 5:1 should be completed in approximately 40 to 53 seconds.

The two-rescuer sequence is a more effective method of carrying out cardiopulmonary resuscitation because it avoids interruptions in the cycle of chest compression that occur in the single-rescuer sequence. During two-rescuer CPR it is also possible for the rescuers to change position at any time, if desired. With the rescuers located on opposite sides of the victim, this may be readily accomplished with minimal interruption in the sequence of events. This allows the rescuers to perform BLS for longer periods of time by minimizing fatigue.

Practice, practice, and still more practice is absolutely essential if the team approach to BLS is to be effective. All members of the dental office staff should be capable of working with each other in either capacity (ventilation or chest compression).

Infant Resuscitation (see chart on p. 442)

For the purpose of BLS technique, the infant is a person under 1 year of age.

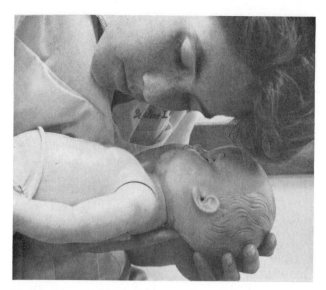

Fig. 30-16. Assess airway (look, listen, and feel) in infant victim.

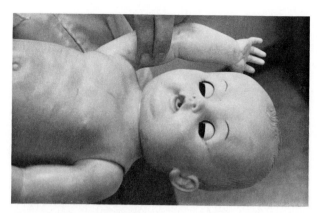

Fig. 30-17. Brachial artery in upper arm is assessed for pulse (5 to 10 seconds).

Lack of responsiveness is determined by the "shake and shout" technique, as with the adult or child victim. Once unresponsiveness is determined, the rescuer will immediately call for help and place the infant in the supine (horizontal) position.

The airway is opened and assessed for patency (look, listen, and feel) and the presence or absence of spontaneous ventilation (Fig. 30-16). Three to five seconds are allowed for assessment. Two ventilations are delivered (1 to 1.5 seconds per ventilation) forcefully enough to produce chest inflation and permit complete deflation between breaths. Overinflation is dangerous because it produces gastric distention, which reduces the effectiveness of subsequent ventilation and increases the risk of regurgitation. The adult rescuer's mouth or mask can usually cover both the mouth and nose of the infant victim. If this is not possible, mouth-to-mouth or mouth-to-nose ventilation is recommended.

The pulse is next assessed. The brachial artery in the upper portion of the arm is palpated for 5 to 10 seconds (Fig. 30-17), and if absent the EMS system is activated and external chest compression is begun. The proper site for finger placement is midsternum, one finger's width below the intermammary line (see Fig. 30-10). The chest is compressed at a rate of 100 per minute (5 in 3 seconds or less) with one ventilation interspersed after every fifth compression (ratio of 5:1). The depth of compression of the infant's chest is ½ to 1 inch (1.3 to 2.5 cm), using the fleshy tips of two or three fingers held in the long axis of the sternum. After 10 cycles (approximately 45 seconds) and period-

ically thereafter, the patient is reevaluated for the return of pulse and/or respiration.

Child Resuscitation (see chart on p. 443)

For the purpose of basic life support technique, the child is a person between the ages of 1 and 8 years.

Basic procedures for resuscitation of the child are similar to those previously described for the adult and infant. The "shake and shout" maneuver is employed to determine lack of responsiveness, help is called, and the patient is placed in the supine position. The airway of the child is maintained by head tilt–chin lift and is then assessed for the presence of spontaneous respiratory efforts (look, listen, and feel). If absent, two full ventilations are provided.

The carotid pulse is assessed for 5 to 10 seconds, and if absent, the EMS system is activated and external chest compressions are begun. Proper hand position for the child is located by placing the middle finger into the lower border of the sternum, as in the adult, and placing the heel of one hand onto the sternum immediately superior to the index finger. The sternum is compressed 1 to 1½ inches (2.5 to 3.8 cm) at a ratio of 5 compressions to 1 ventilation, at a rate of 80 to 100 compressions per minute (5 every 3 to 4 seconds).

After 10 cycles (60 to 87 seconds) and periodically thereafter, the patient should be evaluated for the return of spontaneous pulse and/or respiration.

Monitored-Witnessed Cardiac Arrest

The monitored-witnessed cardiac arrest is one in which cardiopulmonary arrest develops in a patient who has been monitored by means of electrocardiograph and the rescuer or rescuers are able to reach the victim and begin basic life support procedures within 60 seconds of the collapse. In this sequence the myocardium is presumed to be fairly well oxygenated because of the short period of time elapsed since the collapse. Because of this, it is possible that a small electrical stimulus delivered to the myocardium may convert ventricular tachycardia, complete AV block, or ventricular fibrillation to a functional rhythm. This stimulus may be provided by the precordial thump. Though most instances of cardiac arrest in the dental setting will be witnessed, few patients are monitored, therefore the unwitnessed sequence for BLS should be used.

Precordial Thump

In the monitored-witnessed cardiac arrest, the sequence of steps in BLS is altered slightly to allow for delivery of a precordial thump. The precordial thump, applied to the midsternum immediately following collapse, creates a small electrical stimulus that may be effective in reestablishing effective circulation in situations such as ventricular asystole caused by heart block and in converting ventricular tachycardia or ventricular fibrillation of recent onset.

The precordial thump is used to provide a stimulus to a potentially reactive heart. The precordial thump is not a substitute for effective external chest compression. In addition, only one precordial thump should be employed. After carrying out the precordial thump, the sequence of BLS previously described is begun; if the pulse remains absent following delivery of the precordial thump, closed chest compression is started immediately.

The precordial thump is carried out as follows (Fig. 30-18): The rescuer holds a closed fist approximately 8 to 12 inches above the midpoint of the victim's sternum, with the fleshy portion of the fist facing the chest. A single, sharp, quick blow (thump) is then delivered to the sternum. If there is no immediate response (carotid pulse not present), external chest compression is started.

Evaluation of Effectiveness

It is important to evaluate the status of the victim during the administration of BLS. This evaluation determines the effectiveness of the efforts being applied and determines if the victim resumes spontaneous and effective respiratory movements and cardiac function. There are four indicators that may be observed: (1) Color of the skin and mucous membranes, (2) carotid pulse, (3) respiratory movements, and (4) pupils of the eye. Depending on the number of rescuers present, this monitoring may be continually or periodically carried out.

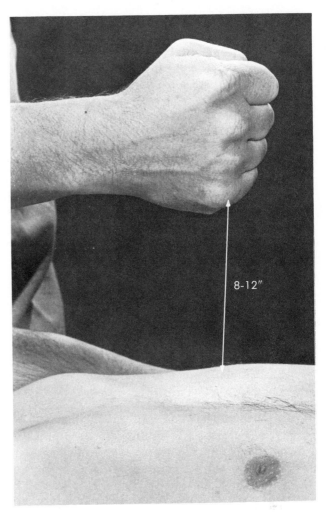

Fig. 30-18. Precordial thump used only in monitored-witnessed cardiac arrest.

With only one rescuer present, the color of the skin and mucous membranes is the only continually observable indicator of effectiveness. With effective BLS the skin and mucous membranes should lose any cyanotic or dusky gray coloration and return to a more normal color. When performing BLS alone, it is suggested that the rescuer pause after the first minute to check for a carotid pulse (maximum of 5 seconds) and observe for spontaneous respiratory movements. Subsequently, the rescuer should check these indicators every 4 to 5 minutes. Never pause for more than 5 seconds at a time, because during this time blood flow drops to zero.

With a second rescuer present it becomes possible to monitor these important indicators with minimal interruption. The ventilation rescuer is able to monitor these indicators, as well as determine the effectiveness of external chest compression. With a finger located on the carotid artery of the victim, a pulsation should be felt with each compression. After the first minute and every 4 to 5 minutes thereafter, the sequence may be stopped for no more than 5 seconds to determine the effectiveness of the BLS technique (color of skin and mucous membranes, presence or absence of spontaneous respiration, presence or absence of spontaneous cardiac rhythm, and pupillary reaction). The two-rescuer sequence described previously has a built-in delay that allows for monitoring of both respiratory and cardiac effectiveness.

Pupillary reaction to light is frequently employed as an indicator of the effectiveness of BLS. Pupils normally respond to light by constricting or narrowing. In the unconscious individual, pupils dilate. This is an indication that the brain is receiving a less than adequate supply of oxygen. If the pupils constrict when exposed to light, that is a sign that oxygenation and cerebral blood flow are adequate. Widely dilated pupils that do not react to light indicate that serious brain damage has occurred or is imminent. Pupils that are dilated but that react to light are a less ominous sign.

Pupillary response should not become the primary indicator of effectiveness of life support efforts. Many factors may produce variations in normal pupillary response, and for this reason it is recommended that other, more reliable factors such as skin color, respiratory movement, and cardiac activity be employed. In older persons it is not uncommon to have variations in pupillary reaction, and it is very common for alterations to occur in persons who are receiving medications (e.g., atropine and narcotic analgesics).

Beginning and Termination of BLS

Basic life support is most effective if begun immediately after cardiac arrest has occurred. If cardiac arrest has existed for 10 minutes or more, it is highly unlikely that the victim's central nervous system will be restored to its precardiac arrest status. In their study of unsuccessful resuscitation attempts, Gray and others[11] found an improved outcome with a total resuscitation time (collapse to recovery) of less than 15 minutes, confirming, according to researchers, the ineffectiveness of prolonged resuscitation. However, individual cases are reported in the literature of effective resuscitation with little or no residual central nervous system deficit after long periods of time (1 hour and longer), usually in situations of hypothermia (submergence in cold water).[33] The American Heart Association guidelines for basic life support continue to recommend that the steps of BLS be

started on all victims of cardiac arrest when any doubt exists about the duration of the arrest.[7] The victim should be given the benefit of the doubt when the decision must be made whether or not to start BLS.

Once cardiopulmonary resuscitation has been started, it should be continued until one of the following occurs: (1) the victim begins adequate spontaneous respiratory movement and/or adequate circulation is restored, (2) a second individual who is equally well trained in BLS is available to assist or take over the efforts of the first individual, (3) a physician arrives on the scene and assumes overall responsibility, (4) the victim is transferred to an emergency care facility that is able to continue with basic life support and/or advanced life support, or (5) the rescuer is exhausted and is physically unable to continue with resuscitation.[34]

MANAGEMENT OF CARDIAC ARREST

Unwitnessed cardiac arrest and witnessed, unmonitored cardiac arrest

↓

Recognize unconsciousness

↓

Position victim and call for assistance

↓

Open airway
(head tilt–chin lift)

↓

Check for breathing

↓

Perform jaw thrust maneuver, if needed;
reassess breathing, if needed

↓

Perform artificial ventilation
(Two full inflations, permitting deflation)

↓

Assess circulation
(palpate carotid pulse)

↓

Perform external chest compression

↓

Locate pressure point
(hand position: heel of hand on chest [adult])

↓

Apply pressure: compress sternum 1½ to 2
inches (adult)

↓

Compress at a rate of 80-100 compressions
per minute

↓

Single rescuer: 15 compressions, 2 ventilations
Team rescue: 5 compressions, 1 ventilation

Because of the dismal results in patients in whom resuscitation efforts in the field were unsuccessful, an impetus is underway by researchers to place greater emphasis on the treatment of cardiac arrest victims in the field.[11,35,36] Specifically, they recommend: (1) The establishment of protocol to allow termination of resuscitation efforts at the scene and the development of legislation in all states to support this practice; (2) efforts to increase the number of emergency medical units capable of providing rapid defibrillation; and (3) widespread CPR instruction for lay persons, Dr. Richard Kerber, the chairman of the AHA Committee on Emergency Cardiac Care, stated that "there is not much point in bringing a patient to the hospital who's had an adequate and full attempt at resuscitation in the field.[37]

The last factor listed for termination of resuscitation, fatigue of the rescuer, is not as unlikely as it might at first seem. Performing BLS is strenuous work. Cases have been reported in which the rescuer has suffered cardiac arrest or myocardial infarction while performing BLS, with one or both persons dying.[28] This factor should motivate the doctor to see to it that all members of the dental office staff are fully trained in all BLS procedures.

Transport of Victim

The victim of cardiac arrest is ultimately transferred from the scene of the incident (e.g., the dental office) to the emergency department of a hospital, where advanced resuscitation techniques are available (electrocardiography, defibrillation, and additional drugs to control acidosis and/or dysrhythmias), if not already started in the field. The doctor should accompany the victim in the ambulance to the hospital, assisting with BLS if necessary, or overseeing its administration by other individuals such as paramedics until the victim is under the care of a physician.

Availability of Training

Training in the procedures described in this section is essential if they are to be effectively applied in life-threatening situations. Training standards have been established, and many excellent programs in BLS and advanced cardiac life support are available. It is recommended that all members of the dental office staff receive certification at least annually so that a degree of proficiency may be maintained. For the location of these courses, interested individuals should contact their local dental society, dental school, American Heart Association, or American Red Cross. It is strongly suggested that training be received at basic life support provider level-C.

REFERENCES

1. Cobb LA, Werner JA, Trobaugh GB: Sudden cardiac arrest. I. A decade's experience with out-of-hospital resuscitation, *Mod Concepts Cardiovasc Dis* 49(6):31, 1980.
2. World Health Organization: *Manual of the international statistical classification of diseases, injuries, and causes of death: based on the recommendations of the Ninth Revision Congress, 1975,* and adopted by the Twenty-Ninth World Health Assembly, 1975 revision, Geneva, 1977, World Health Organization.
3. Eisenberg MS, Hallstrom A, Bergner L: The ACLS score—predicting survival from out-of hospital cardiac arrest, *JAMA* 246:50, 1981.
4. Rabkin SW, Mathewson FAL, Tate RB: Chronobiology of cardiac sudden death in men, *JAMA* 244:1357, 1980.
5. American Heart Association: *1992 Heart and stroke facts,* Dallas, 1991, American Heart Association.
6. McIntyre KM, Winslow EBJ, Parker MR: Sudden cardiac death. In *Textbook of advanced cardiac life support,* Dallas, 1983, American Heart Association.
7. American Heart Association and National Academy of Sciences, National Research Council: Standards for cardiopulmonary resuscitation (CPR) and emergency cardiac care (FCC), *JAMA* 255:2905, 1986.
8. Kouwenhoven WB, Jude JR, Knickerbocker GG: Closed chest cardiac massage, *JAMA* 173:1064, 1960.
9. Weaver WD: Resuscitation outside the hospital—what's lacking, *N Engl J Med* 325:1437, 1991 (editorial).
10. Cobb LA, Werner JA: Predictors and prevention of sudden cardiac death. In Hurst JW, editor: *The heart,* New York, 1982, McGraw-Hill.
11. Gray WA, Capone RJ, Most AS: Unsuccessful emergency medical resuscitation—are continued efforts in the emergency department justified? *N Engl J Med* 325:1393, 1991.
12. Eisenberg MS, Horwood BT, Cummins RO, and others: Cardiac arrest and resuscitation: a tale of 29 cities, *Ann Emerg Med* 19:179, 1990.
13. Roth R, Stewart RD, Rogers K, and others: Out-of-hospital cardiac arrest: factors associated with survival, *Ann Emerg Med* 13:237, 1984.
14. Weaver WD, Cobb LA, Hallstrom AP, and others: Factors influencing survival after out-of-hospital cardiac arrest, *J Am Coll Cardiol* 7:752, 1986.
15. Improving survival from sudden cardiac arrest: the "chain of survival" concept: a statement for health professionals from the Advanced Cardiac Life Support Subcommittee and the Emergency Cardiac Care Committee, American Heart Association, *Circulation* 83:1832, 1991.
16. Myerburg RJ, Kessler KM, Zaman L, and others: Survivors of prehospital cardiac arrest, *JAMA* 247:1485, 1982.
17. Weaver WD, Cobb LA, Hallstrom AP, and others: Considerations for improving survival from out-of-hospital cardiac arrest, *Ann Emerg Med* 15:1181, 1986.
18. Milner PG, Platia EY, Reid PR, and others: Ambulatory electrocardiographic recordings at the time of fatal cardiac arrest, *Am J Cardiol* 56:588, 1985.
19. Kempf FC, Josephson ME: Cardiac arrest recorded on ambulatory electrocardiogram, *Am J Cardiol* 53:1577, 1984.
20. Cummins RO, Eisenberg MS, Litwin PE, and others: Automatic external defibrillators used by emergency medical technicians: a controlled clinical trial, *JAMA* 257:1605, 1987.
21. Weaver WD, Hill D, Fahrenbruch CE, and others: Use of the automatic external defibrillator in the management of out-of-hospital cardiac arrest, *N Engl J Med* 319:661, 1988.
22. Saunders AB, Meislin HW, Ewy GA: The physiology of cardiopulmonary resuscitation: an update, *JAMA* 252:3283, 1984.

23. Stueven H, Troiano P, Thompson B, and others: Bystander/first responder CPR: ten years experience in a paramedic system, *Ann Emerg Med* 15:707, 1986.

24. Enns J, Tween WA, Donen N: Prehospital cardiac rhythm deterioration in a system providing only basic life support, *Ann Emerg Med* 12:478, 1983.

25. Eisenberg MS, Cummins RO, Hallstrom AP, and others: Defibrillation by emergency medical technicians, *Crit Care Med* 13:921, 1985.

26. Weaver EJ, Ramirez AG, Dorfman SB, and others: Trainees' retention of cardiopulmonary resuscitation, *JAMA* 241:901, 1979.

27. Standards and Guidelines for cardiopulmonary resuscitation (CPR) and emergency cardiac care (ECC), *JAMA* 244(suppl):453, 1980.

28. Brown D: Patient has heart attack, dies; dentist also stricken, *Los Angeles Times*, Feb 7, 1988.

29. Eisenberg MS, Bergner L, Hallstrom A: Cardiac resuscitation in the community: importance of rapid provision and implications for program planning, *JAMA* 241:1905, 1979.

30. Babbs CF: New versus old theories of blood flow during CPR, *Crit Care Med* 8:191, 1980.

31. Neimann JT, Garner D, Rosborough J: The mechanism of blood flow in closed chest cardiopulmonary resuscitation, *Circulation* 60(suppl 2):74, 1979.

32. Orlowski JP: Optimal position for external cardiac massage in infants and children, *Crit Care Med* 12:224, 1984.

33. Walpoth BH, Locher T, Leupi F, and others: Accidental deep hypothermia with cardiopulmonary arrest: extracorporeal blood rewarming in 11 patients, *Europ J Cardiothorac Surg* 4(7):390, 1990.

34. American Heart Association: *Instructors' manual for basic life support*, Dallas, 1985, American Heart Association.

35. Bonnin M, Swor R: Outcomes in unsuccessful field resuscitation attempts, *Ann Emerg Med* 18:507, 1989.

36. Kellermann A, Staves DR, Hackman BB: In-hospital resuscitation following unsuccessful prehospital advanced cardiac life support: 'heroic efforts' or an exercise in futility? *Ann Emerg Med* 17:689, 1988.

37. Kerber R: *New York Times*, February 23, 1992.

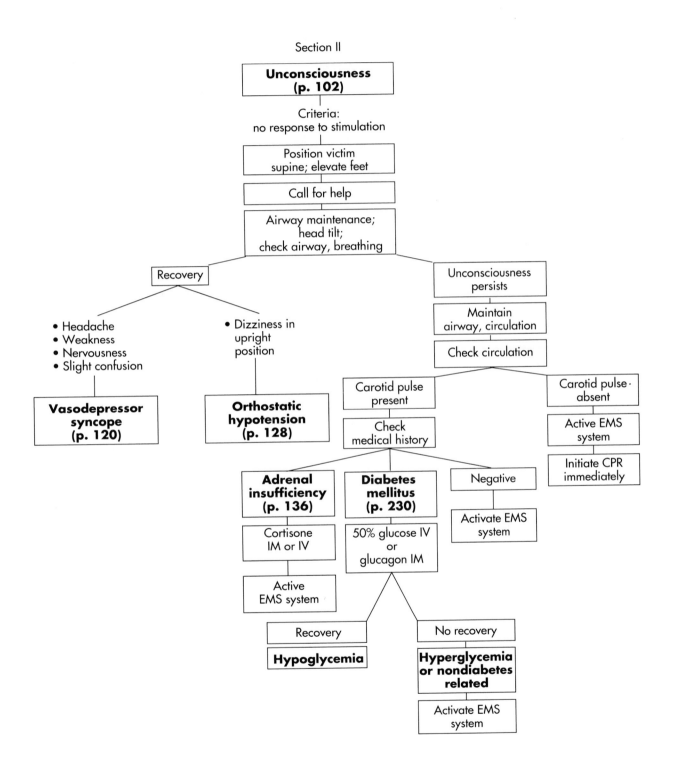

Section II

Unconsciousness (p. 102)

Criteria: no response to stimulation

Position victim supine; elevate feet

Call for help

Airway maintenance; head tilt; check airway, breathing

Recovery

- Headache
- Weakness
- Nervousness
- Slight confusion

Vasodepressor syncope (p. 120)

- Dizziness in upright position

Orthostatic hypotension (p. 128)

Unconsciousness persists

Maintain airway, circulation

Check circulation

Carotid pulse present

Check medical history

Carotid pulse absent

Active EMS system

Initiate CPR immediately

Adrenal insufficiency (p. 136)

Cortisone IM or IV

Active EMS system

Diabetes mellitus (p. 230)

50% glucose IV or glucagon IM

Negative

Activate EMS system

Recovery

Hypoglycemia

No recovery

Hyperglycemia or nondiabetes related

Activate EMS system

Section III

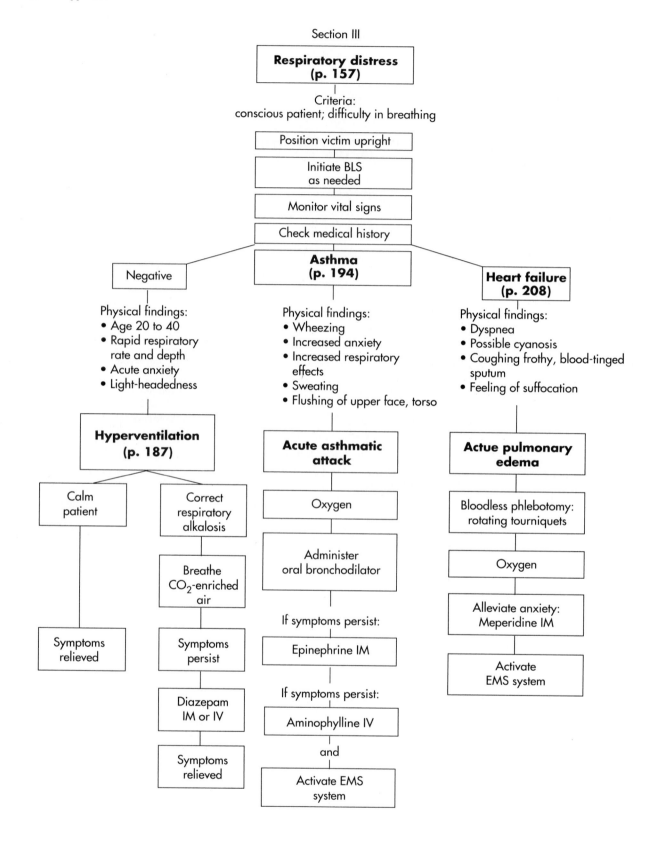

Section IV

**Altered consciousness
(p. 227)**

Criteria: conscious patient, unusual behavioral responses

Initiate BLS,
as needed

Check medical history

Negative

Physical findings:

- Alcohol breath odor
- Confused, "drunk"
  appearance

- Acute anxiety
- Mild tremor
- Profuse sweating
- Rapid speech
- Elevated blood pressure
- Rapid heart rate
- Flushed skin

- Slow speech
- Lethargy, sluggishness
- Dry skin
- Peripheral edema
- Puffy face, eyelids
- Carotenemic skin color
- Bradycardia

- Headache (intense)
- Weakness or paralysis
  of speech, extremities
- Dizziness, vertigo
- Nausea, vomiting

Alcohol overdose

Arrange patient
escort home

**Hyperthyroidism
(p. 251)**

**Hypothyroidism
(p. 251)**

Medical
consultation

**Cerebrovascular
accident (p. 262)**

Position victim
semierect

Manage
signs and symptoms

Monitor
vital signs

Activate
EMS system

Section IV

**Altered consciousness
(p. 227)**

Criteria: conscious patient, unusual behavioral responses

Check medical history

**Diabetes mellitus
(p. 230)**

Physical findings:

- Appears confused, "drunk"
- No alcohol breath odor
- Cool, moist skin
- Hunger present

- Acetone odor on breath
- Skin dry and flushed
- Intense thirst
- Abdominal pain
- Nausea, vomiting

Hypoglycemia

Administer
carbohydrate
orally

Hyperglycemia

Maintain patient

Activate
EMS system

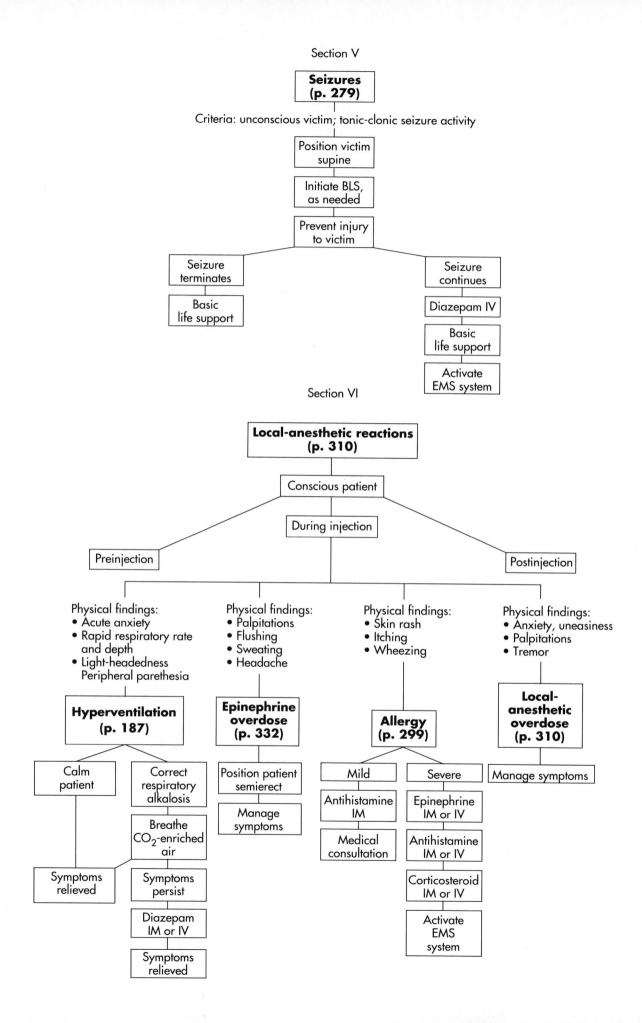

Section V

**Seizures
(p. 279)**

Criteria: unconscious victim; tonic-clonic seizure activity

Position victim
supine

Initiate BLS,
as needed

Prevent injury
to victim

Seizure
terminates

Basic
life support

Seizure
continues

Diazepam IV

Basic
life support

Activate
EMS system

Section VI

**Local-anesthetic reactions
(p. 310)**

Conscious patient

During injection

Preinjection

Postinjection

Physical findings:
• Acute anxiety
• Rapid respiratory rate
  and depth
• Light-headedness
  Peripheral parethesia

Physical findings:
• Palpitations
• Flushing
• Sweating
• Headache

Physical findings:
• Skin rash
• Itching
• Wheezing

Physical findings:
• Anxiety, uneasiness
• Palpitations
• Tremor

**Hyperventilation
(p. 187)**

**Epinephrine
overdose
(p. 332)**

**Allergy
(p. 299)**

**Local-
anesthetic
overdose
(p. 310)**

Calm
patient

Correct
respiratory
alkalosis

Position patient
semierect

Mild

Severe

Manage symptoms

Breathe
CO$_2$-enriched
air

Manage
symptoms

Antihistamine
IM

Epinephrine
IM or IV

Symptoms
relieved

Symptoms
persist

Medical
consultation

Antihistamine
IM or IV

Diazepam
IM or IV

Corticosteroid
IM or IV

Symptoms
relieved

Activate
EMS
system

Section VI

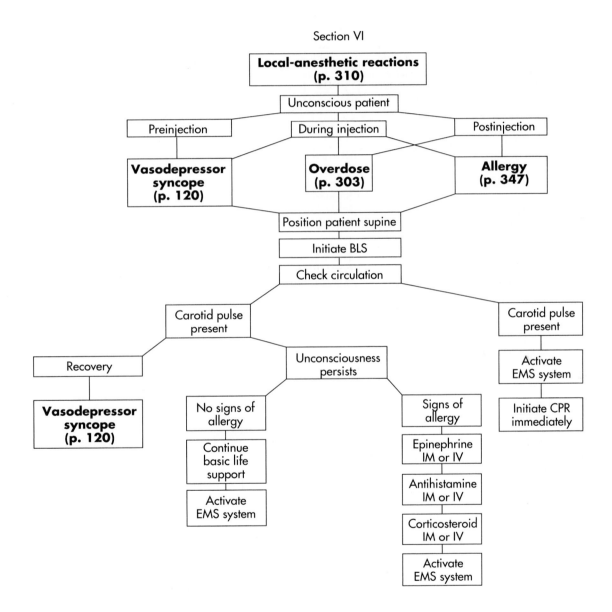

Section VII

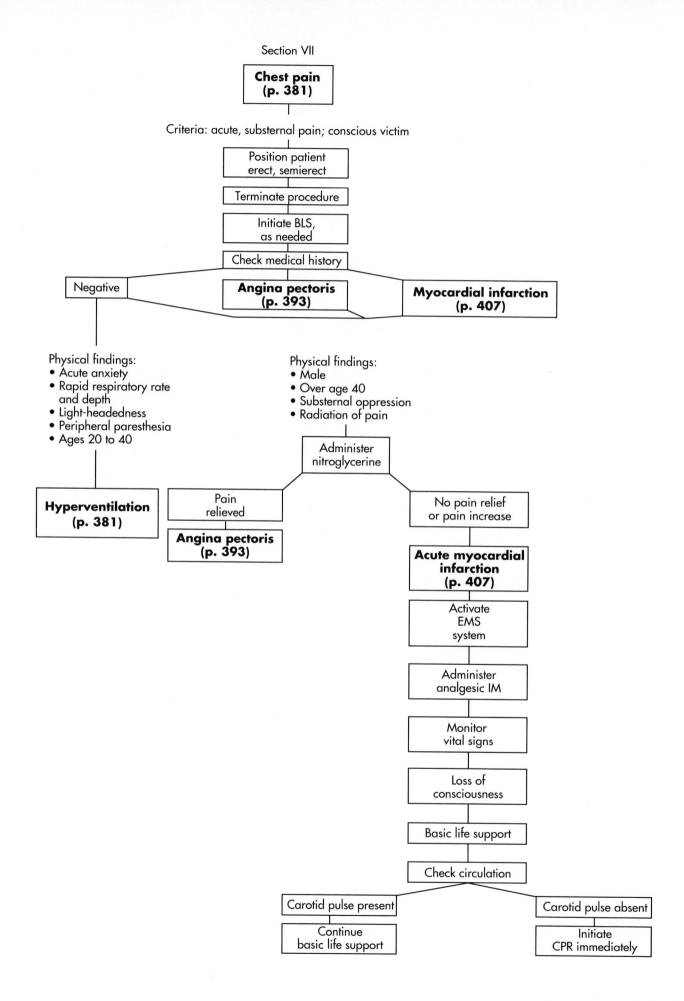

**Chest pain
(p. 381)**

Criteria: acute, substernal pain; conscious victim

Position patient
erect, semierect

Terminate procedure

Initiate BLS,
as needed

Check medical history

Negative | **Angina pectoris
(p. 393)** | **Myocardial infarction
(p. 407)**

Physical findings:
• Acute anxiety
• Rapid respiratory rate
  and depth
• Light-headedness
• Peripheral paresthesia
• Ages 20 to 40

Physical findings:
• Male
• Over age 40
• Substernal oppression
• Radiation of pain

Administer
nitroglycerine

**Hyperventilation
(p. 381)**

Pain
relieved

No pain relief
or pain increase

**Angina pectoris
(p. 393)**

**Acute myocardial
infarction
(p. 407)**

Activate
EMS
system

Administer
analgesic IM

Monitor
vital signs

Loss of
consciousness

Basic life support

Check circulation

Carotid pulse present

Carotid pulse absent

Continue
basic life support

Initiate
CPR immediately

Index

A

Abdominal thrust, 171, 173-174
Acetaminophen, 306
Acetone breath, 37, 155, 278
Acidosis, 243-244
ACLS; *see* Advanced cardiac life support (ACLS)
Acrylic resins, 351-352
Addison's disease, 136-137, 142-143
  postural hypotension and, 128, 130
Adrenal; *see* Epinephrine
Adrenal function, normal, 143-145
Adrenal insufficiency, acute, 136-151
  clinical indications for adrenocortical steroids in, 138
  clinical manifestations of, 136, 143
  death as result of, 137, 143
  emergency kit and, 76, 77
  pathophysiology of, 136, 145-148
  postural hypotension and, 128, 130
  prevention of, 139-141
  unconsciousness caused by, 156
Adrenergic agonist, 80, 81
ADRs; *see* Adverse drug reactions
Advanced cardiac life support (ACLS), 78, 425, 428
  training, 50, 51-52
Advanced trauma life support (ATLS) certification, 51
Adverse drug reactions (ADRs), 3, 15, 98, 378
  age of patient and, 311
  allergy vs. overdose, 348
  classification of, 302-304
  combinations of drugs and, 343-344
  dialogue history and, 301, 376
  frequency of, 299
Afterload, 218-219
Age of patient
  adverse drug reactions and, 311
  altered consciousness and, 276
  anxiety and, 187
  asthma and, 194
  chest pain and, 421
  coronary artery disease and, 385
  CVA and, 263
  drug-related emergencies and, 376

Age of patient—cont'd
  older, and life-threatening emergencies, 1, 4-6
  postural hypotension and, 128, 129
  respiratory difficulty and, 224
  seizures and, 283
  stress and, 4-5, 6
  unconsciousness and, 153-154
AIDS (acquired immunodeficiency syndrome), 23, 36
Airways; *see also* Ventilation
  acute adrenal insufficiency and, 150
  adjuncts to management of, 81-84
  artificial, 81-83, 114-117
  basic maneuvers for, 108-113, 170
  in cardiac arrest, 433-434
  in children, 111, 112
  emergency, establishment of, 170-171
  esophageal obturator, 83
  inflammation of, 200
  invasive procedures for, 179-185
  nasopharyngeal, 81-83
  noninvasive procedures for, 172-179
  obstructed, 108, 161-185
    completely, 168-169
    due to allergy, 358
    due to asthma, 21, 203
    from foreign object, 159, 161; *see also* Swallowed objects
    lower, 157, 159
    partial, 169
    recognition of, 168-169
    tongue as cause of, 157
    unconsciousness and, 106, 113, 118
  oropharyngeal, 81-83
  patent, determination of, 111, 125, 133, 433
  sensitivity of, in asthmatics, 200
  tonic-clonic movements and, 155
Albuterol, 80, 81
Alcohol, 139, 155, 227
  altered consciousness and, 277-278
Aldomet; *see* Methyldopa
Alkalosis, respiratory, 35
Allergens, 347
Allergies, 3, 22, 347-374; *see also* Anaphylaxis, generalized
  adrenal insufficiency and, 139

Allergies—cont'd
  to aspirin, 350
  asthma and, 194, 200-201
  blood pressure and, 378
  classification of, 347, 348
  clinical manifestations of, 357-361
  defined, 303
  drug-related emergencies and, 309, 376, 377, 380
  emergency kit and, 80
  emergency treatment for, 65-67, 80, 77
  hay fever, 21-22
  management of, 356-357, 365-374
  pathophysiology of, 361-365
  to penicillin, 349
  predisposing factors in, 348-352
  prevention of, 32
  questionnaire regarding, 15
  shock caused by, 378
  testing, 355
Alpha-blockade, 77-78
Alphaprodine, 335, 337
Altered consciousness, 227-229, 453
  differential diagnosis of, 276-278
Alveolar nerve blocks, 23
Ambulances, 54-55
American Dental Association (ADA), 3
  questionnaire forms of, 11, 14, 91-93
AMI; *see* Myocardial infarction, acute (AMI)
Aminophylline, 80
Ammonia, aromatic, 78, 79, 124, 126, 150
Amyl nitrite, 68, 404, 422
Analgesics, 306-307
  allergy to, 350
  asthma and, 198
  emergency kit and, 73, 75, 86
  narcotic, 340-342
  overdose, 335
  unconsciousness and, 103
Anaphylaxis, generalized, 22, 347, 358
  chemical mediators of, 363-365
  clinical symptoms of, 359-361
  diagnosis of cause of, 371-374
Anemia, 20, 24, 37